Surgical Management *of* Cerebrovascular Disease

Surgical Management *of* Cerebrovascular Disease

EDITOR

R. EUGENE ZIERLER, M.D.

Associate Professor of Surgery
Division of Vascular Surgery
University of Washington School of Medicine
Seattle, Washington

McGraw-Hill, Inc.
Health Professions Division

New York St. Louis San Francisco Auckland Bogotá Caracas Lisbon London
Madrid Mexico City Milan Montreal New Delhi
San Juan Singapore Sydney Tokyo Toronto

SURGICAL MANAGEMENT OF CEREBROVASCULAR DISEASE

1234567890 KGPKGP 987654

ISBN 0-07-072792-9

This book was set in Times Roman by Compset, Inc.
The editors were Michael J. Houston and Steven Melvin;
the production supervisor was Richard Ruzycka;
the cover designer was José Fonfrias;
the index was prepared by Mary Kidd.
Quebecor Printing/Kingsport, was printer and binder.
This book is printed on acid-free paper

LIBRARY OF CONGRESS CATALOGING-IN-PUBLICATION DATA

Surgical management of cerebrovascular disease / editor, R. Eugene Zierler.
p. cm.
Includes bibliographical references and index.
ISBN 0-07-072792-9 :
1. Cerebrovascular disease—Surgery. 2. Carotid artery—Surgery. 3. Cerebrovascular disease. I. Zierler, R. Eugene.
[DNLM: 1. Cerebrovascular Disorders—therapy. 2. Cerebrovascular Disorders—physiopathology. 3. Cerebrovascular Disorders—diagnosis. 4. Carotid Body—surgery. 5. Carotid Stenosis—surgery.
WL 355 S9599 1995]
RD594.2.S88 1995
617.4'81—dc20
DNLM/DLC
For Library of Congress 94-20311

To my wife, Brenda, who renewed my life,

and

to our children Keri, Erin, Jesse, and Andrew,

who remind me each day that it is what we leave behind

that truly matters.

Contents

Part Five
Surgical Management

Contributors

Dennis F. Bandyk, M.D. [20, 24]
Professor of Surgery
Division of Vascular Surgery
University of South Florida College of Medicine
Tampa, Florida

José Biller, M.D. [8]
Professor and Chairman
Department of Neurology
Indiana University School of Medicine
Indianapolis, Indiana

David L. Dawson, M.D. [21]
Assistant Professor of Surgery
F. Edward Hébert School of Medicine
Uniformed Services University of the Health Sciences
Bethesda, Maryland;
Staff Surgeon
Director, Vascular Laboratory
Wilford Hall USAF Medical Center
Lackland Air Force Base
San Antonio, Texas

Christopher DeMaioribus, M.D. [28]
Vascular Surgery Fellow
Department of Surgery
University of Kentucky
Lexington, Kentucky

Glenn E. Esses, M.D. [20]
Vascular Surgery Fellow
Division of Vascular Surgery
University of South Florida College of Medicine
Tampa, Florida

David Gordon, M.D. [3]
Professor of Pathology
University of Michigan Medical School
Ann Arbor, Michigan

John D. Harley, M.D. [14]
Professor of Radiology
University of Washington School of Medicine
Radiology Service
Seattle Veterans Affairs Medical Center
Seattle, Washington

Robert G. Hart, M.D. [15]
Associate Professor of Medicine
Department of Medicine
Division of Neurology
University of Texas Health Science Center
San Antonio, Texas

Thomas S. Hatsukami, M.D. [5]
Assistant Professor of Surgery
University of Washington School of Medicine
Vascular Surgery Section
Seattle Veterans Affairs Medical Center
Seattle, Washington

Numbers in brackets refer to chapters written or co-written by the contributors.

David R. Haynor, M.D., Ph.D. [14]
Assistant Professor of Radiology
University of Washington School of Medicine
Radiology Service
Seattle Veterans Affairs Medical Center
Seattle, Washington

Dean A. Healy, M.D. [25, 27]
Assistant Professor of Surgery
Department of Surgery
Vascular Surgery Section
Pennsylvania State University College of Medicine
Hershey, Pennsylvania

Robert W. Hobson, II, M.D. [17]
Professor of Surgery
Chief, Section of Vascular Surgery
UMDNJ-New Jersey Medical School
Newark, New Jersey

Kaj H. Johansen, M.D., Ph.D. [31]
Professor of Surgery
Division of Vascular Surgery
University of Washington School of Medicine
Seattle, Washington

Andris Kazmers, M.D. [28, 29]
Associate Professor of Surgery
Division of Vascular Surgery
Wayne State University
Detroit, Michigan

Richard R. Keen, M.D. [13]
Assistant Professor of Surgery
Rush Medical College
Attending Surgeon, Section of Vascular Surgery
Cook County Hospital
Chicago, Illinois

Ted R. Kohler, M.D. [3, 4]
Associate Professor of Surgery
University of Washington School of Medicine
Chief, Vascular Surgery Section
Seattle Veterans Affairs Medical Center
Seattle, Washington

Arthur M. Lam, M.D., F.R.C.P.C. [22]
Professor
Departments of Anesthesiology and Neurosurgery
University of Washington School of Medicine
Seattle, Washington

Basil F. Matta, M.B., F.R.C.A. [22]
Acting Assistant Professor
Departments of Anesthesiology and Neurosurgery
University of Washington School of Medicine
Seattle, Washington

Joseph L. Mills, M.D. [20]
Associate Professor of Surgery
Division of Vascular Surgery
University of South Florida College of Medicine
Tampa, Florida

David W. Newell, M.D. [12]
Associate Professor
Department of Neurological Surgery
University of Washington School of Medicine
Seattle, Washington

Stephen C. Nicholls, M.D. [19, 30]
Assistant Professor of Surgery
Division of Vascular Surgery
University of Washington School of Medicine
Seattle, Washington

Anthony J. Orencia, M.D., Ph.D. [8]
Assistant Professor
Department of Neurology
Northwestern University Medical School
Chicago, Illinois

William H. Pearce, M.D. [13]
Professor of Surgery
Northwestern University Medical School
Attending Surgeon
Northwestern Memorial Hospital
Chicago, Illinois

William J. Quiñones-Baldrich, M.D. [26]
Associate Professor of Surgery
Section of Vascular Surgery
UCLA School of Medicine
Los Angeles, California

Diane H. Solomon, M.D. [15]
Assistant Professor of Medicine
Department of Medicine
Division of Neurology
University of Texas Health Science Center
San Antonio, Texas

D. Eugene Strandness, Jr., M.D. [Foreword, 1, 16]
Professor and Chief
Division of Vascular Surgery
University of Washington School of Medicine
Seattle, Washington

Phillip D. Swanson, M.D. [6, 7, 9]
Professor of Medicine
Head, Division of Neurology
University of Washington School of Medicine
Seattle, Washington

Brian L. Thiele, M.D. [23]
Professor of Surgery and Chief
Section of Vascular Surgery
Department of Surgery
Pennsylvania State University College of Medicine
Milton S. Hershey Medical Center
Hershey, Pennsylvania

Henry Veldenz, M.D. [29]
Vascular Surgery Fellow
Department of Surgery
University of Kentucky
Lexington, Kentucky

Joseph A. Wasselle, M.D. [24]
Vascular Surgery Fellow
Division of Vascular Surgery
University of South Florida College of Medicine
Tampa, Florida

Mark Wengrovitz, M.D. [25, 27]
Vascular Surgery Fellow
Department of Surgery
Vascular Surgery Section
Pennsylvania State University College of Medicine
Hershey, Pennsylvania

R. Eugene Zierler, M.D. [2, 10, 11, 18, 32]
Associate Professor of Surgery
Division of Vascular Surgery
University of Washington School of Medicine
Seattle, Washington

Foreword

THERE ARE FEW AREAS in medicine that have been the source of such controversy as the surgical treatment of cerebrovascular disease. The debate initially concerned the efficacy of extracranial to intracranial bypass grafting and more recently focused on the role of carotid endarterectomy in the prevention of stroke. While extracranial to intracranial bypass grafting was largely discredited, carotid endarterectomy has been validated as an effective method of preventing stroke in selected patients with carotid bifurcation atherosclerosis. This latter fact makes the publication of this book timely and very important.

The extracranial and intracranial circulations form a complex anatomic configuration which is exemplified by the circle of Willis. From a theoretical standpoint, this arrangement is ideal for protecting the brain against the impact of extracranial arterial occlusive disease. However, as pointed out in the opening chapters, the circle of Willis is often not anatomically and functionally intact, and the clinical consequences of this observation are of critical importance. The chapters on atherosclerosis and the mechanisms of cerebral ischemia highlight the areas of agreement and disagreement regarding these critical issues. For reasons that are not completely understood, atherosclerosis preferentially involves some arterial segments while regularly sparing others. It appears that the potential for development of ischemic events depends largely on the degree of narrowing rather than on the mere presence of a plaque. Even though the emphasis of most published work in this field, including this book, is on atherosclerosis, it is also important to remember that other diseases affect the cerebrovascular circulation.

While the clinical manifestations of ischemic cerebrovascular disease are usually straightforward, the picture may not be clear-cut, and the assistance of a neurologist is frequently invaluable. This is particularly true for problems relating to the posterior circulation where it is often difficult to relate the presence of extracranial arterial lesions to the clinical presentation. In addition, not all strokes are due to extracranial arterial disease. It is important to keep these facts in mind, and the chapters on clinical manifestations will help us in this regard.

With the general availability of noninvasive testing methods, which are currently dominated by ultrasonic duplex scanning, we have the capability to study the extracranial circulation in considerable detail and monitor the changes that occur over time. This has provided us with some unique opportunities not only to detect and classify the degree of stenosis but to use these same tests to evaluate the results of therapy and study the natural history of the diseases we treat. With recently developed CT and MRI techniques, we can also study the impact of ischemic episodes on the brain. Contrast arteriography remains the standard diagnostic test prior to carotid surgery, but there is a rapidly growing body of evidence indicating that this may not be necessary except in carefully defined circumstances. All of these topics are covered in detail.

Medical therapy for atherosclerosis involving the cerebrovascular circulation has concentrated on control of those risk factors thought to be important in the pathogenesis of the disease. The greatest emphasis has been on the use of antiplatelet agents, particularly aspirin. However, as noted in the chapters on this subject, there are other strategies that can be used along with some new and emerging forms of antiplatelet therapy. It is clear that the medical therapy of cerebrovascular disease, both for limiting the progression of disease and altering its clinical impact once it is discovered, will continue to evolve.

The chapters on clinical trials and indications for operation will be of particular interest to the reader. It is here that discussions on the current status and clinical role of carotid endarterectomy can be found. As these chapters point out, some formerly controversial issues have been settled, especially for high-grade carotid stenoses. However, some areas of uncertainty remain that will require more time and work to resolve.

While the carotid bifurcation is the most common site for atherosclerosis of the extracranial arterial circulation, this process can also involve the vertebral arteries and the origins of the great vessels from the aortic arch. Effective and safe surgical management of these lesions requires both ingenuity and a clear understanding of the local anatomy. Chapters on these complex problems provide the necessary guidelines for all of us to use in our practice.

The perennial problem of combined carotid and coronary artery disease is covered in detail. It is often difficult to decide if and when these two problems should be treated at the same operation or with staged procedures. Clearly, this decision may have a major influence on the overall clinical outcome. While many questions remain, this is an issue that needs to be discussed whenever these two conditions occur together.

The critically important aspects of surgical and anesthetic management are covered in a series of chapters that forms the largest part of this book. As every surgeon performing carotid operations knows, these procedures often seem simple and straightforward. On the other hand, we all recognize that there is very little room for error. There is no place in the arterial circulation where a technically precise operation is more likely to produce a favorable outcome or, at the other extreme, where a technical problem can have more disastrous consequences. We certainly need to acknowledge how much advances in the field of anesthetic management have contributed to both the welfare of the patient and the comfort of the surgeon. While the issue of cerebral protection remains a source of debate, it is important to review this topic and to present the various approaches and discuss how they might affect clinical outcome.

The carotid artery is subject to direct and indirect injuries. Every metropolitan trauma center has become familiar with the difficult problems related to injuries of the extracranial vessels. Coverage of this topic brings us up to date on current practice. The treatment of carotid body tumors is another area that requires some special attention. While these lesions are rare, they require the combined attention and cooperation of both surgeon and radiologist. The important considerations in evaluating carotid body tumors and guidelines for management are covered in the last chapter.

For those interested in extracranial cerebrovascular disease, this book contains nearly all one needs to know from either a practical or scientific standpoint. It will not only provide the necessary background and current information to approach these problems intelligently, but will also serve as a valuable reference source. This book belongs on the shelf of vascular surgeons and other medical specialists who share an interest in this rapidly moving and complex field.

D. Eugene Strandness, Jr., M.D.

Preface

THE PREVENTION OF STROKE by treatment of cerebrovascular disease is a relatively new concept in the practice of medicine. Although the relationship between cerebrovascular disease and neurologic symptoms is now generally accepted, the current level of understanding has been reached by the gradual accumulation of knowledge and experience in a variety of fields. Consequently, the surgical management of cerebrovascular disease is based not only on advances in the specialty of surgery, but also on recent developments concerning the pathogenesis of carotid artery disease, diagnostic methods, and nonoperative treatment. The availability of this information has stimulated a growing interest in the problem of stroke and the critical issue of stroke prevention.

Recognizing the vast amount of data from the basic and clinical sciences that has been generated on cerebrovascular disease in recent years, there appeared to be a need for a complete but still concise work that could bring together information from a broad range of disciplines, including vascular biology, pathology, diagnostic imaging, epidemiology, clinical trials, and surgery. Thus, the goal of this book is to present information from these diverse fields in a logical way that facilitates the application of new developments to clinical practice. While the book is directed primarily to vascular surgeons and neurological surgeons, it will also be relevant to general surgeons with an interest in vascular problems, and neurologists or other nonsurgical specialists who treat patients with cerebrovascular disease.

The book is divided into five parts. Part I reviews the anatomy and pathophysiology of cerebrovascular disease, including aspects of atherosclerosis that are unique to the carotid system, mechanisms of cerebral ischemia, and nonatherosclerotic disorders. The clinical manifestations and epidemiology of cerebrovascular disease are covered in Part II. Discussions of both established and new approaches to the diagnostic evaluation of cerebrovascular lesions are contained in Part III. Therapeutic issues are addressed in Part IV, with emphasis on nonsurgical treatment, clinical trials, and indications for surgery. The various aspects of surgical management are covered in Part V, including anesthesia, operative techniques, cerebral protection, complications, recurrent stenosis, and trauma. Special or unusual problems in cerebrovascular disease, such as vertebral artery surgery, combined carotid and coronary artery disease, carotid surgery without angiography, reoperative carotid surgery, approaches to aortic arch branch lesions, and carotid body tumors, are also discussed in appropriate parts of the book.

Because the emphasis of this book is on the surgical aspects of cerebrovascular disease, the authors are predominantly vascular surgeons. However, the quality and scope of the book have been significantly enhanced by the expertise of specialists from other fields, including anesthesiology, pathology, neurology, neurological surgery, and vascular radiology.

The list of authors reflects the kind of multidisciplinary approach that is necessary for the optimal management of patients with cerebrovascular disease, and I am extremely grateful to all the authors for their comprehensive and up-to-date contributions.

The editing and final production of this book are the result of the efforts of a dedicated team. I especially want to thank Michael Houston, Senior Medical Editor at McGraw-Hill, for smoothly guiding this project from start to finish. His support, encouragement, and editorial judgment were invaluable. I also appreciate the help of Editing Supervisor, Steven Melvin, whose skill and attention to detail were critical during the final production phase of the book. The secretarial assistance of Kathy Pratt at the University of Washington was also vital to moving the project along.

Finally, I would like to give a special acknowledgment to my teacher, colleague, and friend, D. Eugene Strandness, Jr., M.D., who first introduced me to the study of cerebrovascular disease. The critical thinking and scientific rigor which mark his approach to clinical research are the foundation on which my career is based. Although research is often regarded as an entirely theoretical endeavor, it is only of value when the results can ultimately be used to benefit patients. The contributions Dr. Strandness has made to the diagnosis and treatment of cerebrovascular disease are an example of what can be achieved in academic surgery through time, hard work, and sacrifice.

1

Historical Perspectives in Cerebrovascular Disease

D. Eugene Strandness, Jr.

While the connection between disease of the carotid bifurcation and stroke seems so logical, given our knowledge about the localization, pathology, and outcome of atherosclerosis, this was one of the last areas in the arterial circulation where such a clinical-pathologic relationship became well known. Why did this take so long and what were the factors involved? As I will point out in this chapter, there were numerous clues along the historical path, but it was not until C. Miller Fisher published his observations in 1951 that the medical community began to focus more closely on this relationship.[1]

My own experiences and an observation given to me by a distinguished neurologist may shed some light on the lack of progress in this field. As a surgical resident in 1956, I spent six months on the autopsy service, and became familiar with most conditions that were common causes of death. The standard autopsy done at that time included examination of all major organ systems, including the brain. For the coronary arteries, great efforts were made not only to localize the areas of disease, but to do it literally millimeter by millimeter.

The same was true of the abdominal aorta and the iliac arteries. However, we never examined the vessels of the upper or lower limbs or the carotid arteries in the neck. Why was this the case? I was told such examinations caused problems for undertakers in embalming the body. In fact, undertakers were known to become quite angry if we sacrificed the carotid arteries for pathologic examination.

Our failure to examine the carotid arteries, even in cases of stroke, was never of much concern at that time; but this practice seriously limited our knowledge. Dr. Oscar Reinmuth, a distinguished neurologist and former editor of the journal *Stroke,* fully appreciated this failure when I asked him why it had taken so long for the medical community to understand that carotid bifurcation atherosclerosis could be a common cause of stroke.

How long did it take for this relationship to be discovered and widely known? When I reviewed my neurology textbook from medical school (1954) to see what it had to say about this problem, all I could find was a reference to "cerebral apoplexy." This also explained the practice of designating a stroke simply as a CVA (cerebrovascular accident), without attempting to define the etiology of the event further.

"CAROTID"

The potential of the carotid artery as a source of problems was clearly recognized by the Greeks. The etymology of the word "carotid" is from "karoo," which means "to stupefy." In fact, the carotid artery was often referred to as "the artery of sleep." This is evident in a statement by Ambroise Paré in 1634[2]:

> . . . two branches which they call carotides or soporales, the sleepy arteries, because they being obstructed or any way stopt we presently fall asleep.

Was this information generally appreciated? My own experience as a child is interesting. At age 13, I was talking to a close friend who was sitting on a log beside me. I told him that by simply pressing on his neck, I could make him pass out! He scoffed at the idea and challenged me to prove my point, which I did. Much to my surprise and horror, as I grasped my friend's neck, his eyes rolled back, he passed out, and fell off the log. What happened in the course of that experiment? It is most likely that massage of the carotid bifurcation may have induced a brief sinus arrest. On the other hand, since my grip was not calibrated or controlled in any way, it is conceivable that I showed how interruption of the blood supply to the brain can lead to a temporary condition of sleep. How did I originally come by this knowledge? Unfortunately, I do not remember, but perhaps this initial experiment was an indicator of my future interest in this fascinating area.

THOMAS WILLIS

One of the earliest recorded reports on carotid artery occlusion was by Willis in 1684. It was, of course, Willis who immortalized his name and observations by describing the Circle that now bears his name. In his work *Cerebri Anatome,* the function of the Circle was described in these terms[3]:

> But there is another reason far greater than this of these manifold ingraftings of the Vessels, to wit, that there may be a manifold way, and that more certain, for the blood about to go into divers Regions of the Brain, laid open for each; so that if by chance one or two should be stopt, there might easily be found another passage instead of them; as for example, if the Carotid of one side might provide either province. . . . Further, if both Carotids should be stopt, the offices of each might be supplied through the Vertebrals.

This classic description defines the potential role of the Circle, and is as relevant today as when Willis made his observations.

The relationship between atherosclerosis and the carotid artery did not surface until the observations of Ramsey Hunt in 1913.[4] More about this later. However, progress continued that proved essential for the growth of the field and our understanding of the potential for surgical correction of problems involving this artery. As might be expected, this progress developed along several lines, each of which was dependent on observations made by others.

JOHN HUNTER AND ASTLEY COOPER

The great English surgeon John Hunter, whose genius still shines today, can be given credit for many important observations, but the one most relevant to cerebrovascular disease is his description of the collateral circulation.[5] The simple experiment of ligating the artery to the stag antler and showing that it could continue to grow was proof that alternate arterial pathways were available and could be called on to provide perfusion to an organ or tissue deprived of its normal arterial blood supply. This observation and others led him to conclude that "vessels go where needed." He was not the first, but certainly the one who deserves the most credit for advocating ligation of a feeding artery in the treatment of aneurysmal disease. Even today, ligation of the femoral artery for the treatment of popliteal aneurysm is referred to as the "Hunterian operation."

Hunter had many distinguished pupils, but the one who had the most influence on the history of this field was Sir Astley Cooper.[6] Cooper was a striking and very handsome gentleman whose courage and foresight must have been derived in large part from his work with John Hunter. While Cooper made many contributions, his ligation of the common carotid artery and the impact of that procedure on one of his own pupils began a chain of events in surgery that is still evident.

In 1805, Cooper performed a ligation of the common carotid artery in a woman with an aneurysm of the vessel. She had no neurologic complications following the procedure, but apparently died of sepsis some 16 days later. The interesting thing about this approach, and also its relevance to the influence of John Hunter, was the fact that the surgery was to a large degree based on experimental data. Cooper had ligated both carotid and vertebral arteries in a dog, and the animal survived. In fact, he commented that the animal even became "a good house dog."

VALENTINE MOTT

As Cooper derived experience and perhaps inspiration from Hunter, it is very clear that Mott can trace his career and success to Cooper.[6,7] Mott spent six months with Cooper, returning to the United States in 1805. After his return, he continued to pursue many of the lessons learned from Cooper and to extend them to lengths that seem amazing even today. For example, he was involved in many ligations of arteries for the treatment of aneurysmal disease and trauma. These included one innominate artery, eight subclavian arteries, two common carotid arteries, and 51 external carotid arteries. Such ligations would not have been conceivable had it not been for the work of his predecessors. Mott is considered by some to be the father of vascular surgery in the United States.

The experiences reviewed above were instrumental in setting the stage for many surgical advances. However, as one might expect, knowledge of the pathophysiology of a disorder must precede any systematic attempts to identify and treat it by direct means.

RAMSEY HUNT

This distinguished physician was a neurologist whose suggestions would never be implemented during his lifetime. He made the following comments in an address to the American Neurological Association in 1913[4]:

> It would therefore seem proper in all cases with cerebral symptoms of vascular origin, to examine the pulsation of the carotids in the neck as possibly throwing some light on the source of the obstruction and rendering more exact our localization of the seat of the problem in this group of cases. For this purpose a section of the carotid artery is readily accessible to palpation, extending from the lower border of the thyroid cartilage to the angle of the jaw; the main trunk divides into the external and internal, the larger of the two vessels, is readily felt from this point to the angle of the jaw.

This observation is even more remarkable because Hunt appreciated the relationship between disease of the carotid artery and hemiplegia. Although Hunt was clearly on the right track, it is well known today that the physical examination of these arteries for pulsation is not only inaccurate but relatively useless in defining the status of the carotid circulation.

EGAS MONIZ

No matter how astute clinical observations might be, they cannot be verified or rejected until a proper diagnostic procedure is developed and tested. While there is little doubt that Hunt was right, the relationship between carotid artery disease and neurologic symptoms could be established with certainty only when a method to document the status of the carotid circulation became available. The development of arteriography by Moniz certainly fulfilled this requirement.[8] In 1927, he described the arteriographic method for visualization of the carotid arterial system. Finally, the observations of Hunt could be verified objectively. This landmark development permitted the field of vascular surgery to reach its current level of sophistication.

C. MILLER FISHER

As noted earlier, Fisher must be credited for bringing the carotid artery back to its position of importance as a cause of stroke.[1] After extensive autopsy experience, he was able to make several critically important observations. In his 373 postmortem examinations of the brains of patients who died of cerebrovascular causes, he reported that less than 20 percent died of cerebral hemorrhage, whereas the majority apparently died of embolic causes. He confirmed that disease of the carotid bifurcation was common and that emboli were the likely causative event. He also concluded that any evaluation of cerebrovascular disease would be incomplete without examination of the carotid bulb.

What is even more impressive is his prediction concerning the possible role of surgery for this problem:

> . . . it is even conceivable that some day vascular surgery will find a way to bypass the occluded portion of the artery during the period of ominous fleeting symptoms. Anastomosis of the external carotid artery, or one of its branches with the internal carotid artery above the narrowing should be feasible.

THE PRESENT ERA

The landmark observations of Fisher were rapidly followed by surgical attempts to address this important issue. The surgical procedure given the most credit for bringing this approach to our attention was the operation reported by Eastcott, Pickering, and Rob in 1954.[9] In this procedure, the carotid bifurcation was resected, with anastomosis of the common carotid artery to the internal carotid artery. This case report is the one most commonly cited, and is widely regarded as the first reconstructive surgical procedure to be performed on the carotid bifurcation. However, this is not true.

In 1951 in Argentina, Carrea and his colleagues resected a carotid bifurcation and anastomosed the external carotid to the internal carotid artery as Fisher had suggested.[10] This operation was referred to as a "carotid-carotideal anastomosis." These authors were apparently aware of Fisher's contributions and gave him much credit for the idea.

It appears that the first attempted carotid thromboendarterectomy was by Strully, Hurwitt, and Blankenberg in 1953.[11] In this case, the reconstruction was not followed by retrograde flow, presumably secondary to propagation of a thrombus into the distal internal carotid. This case was probably the first to show how difficult it is to restore flow in a carotid artery that has thrombosed. It is likely that the first successful carotid endarterectomy was performed in 1953 by DeBakey, who also confirmed patency of the internal carotid artery by an intraoperative arteriogram.[12]

These historic operations following the development of arteriography and the observations of Fisher set the stage for what has been a period of dramatic advances as well as confusion and controversy. As the number of surgical procedures for carotid artery disease increased, there was a need to evaluate the clinical role of carotid endarterectomy. In response to this need, surgeons and neurologists collaborated on the first randomized clinical trial of this procedure for the prevention of stroke.[13] It is unfortunate that both the operative techniques and anesthesia for carotid surgery were still evolving from many viewpoints during the time of this trial, and the results would be considered inadequate by present standards. For example, although it appeared that carotid endarterectomy was effective in the prevention of late stroke, when the perioperative morbidity and mortality were considered this benefit was lost.

The subsequent development of carotid endarterectomy and its clinical application will be covered later in this book. Fortunately, the early expectations of the pioneers have been accomplished, in spite of many periods of uncertainty.

REFERENCES

1. Fisher M: Occlusion of the internal carotid artery. *AMA Arch Neurol Psychiat* 65:346–377, 1951.
2. Paré A: *The works of that famous Chirurgeon Ambroise Paré*: Translated out of Latin and compared with the French, by Thomas Johnson. New York, Milford House, 1968, (originally published in 1634).
3. Friedman SG: Operation on the carotid artery, in *A History of Vascular Surgery*. Mt. Kisco, NY, Futura, pp 157–171, 1989.
4. Hunt JR: The role of the carotid arteries in the causation of vascular lesions of the brain, with remarks on certain special features of the symptomatology. *Am J Med Sci* 147:704, 1914.
5. Gloyne SR: John Hunter. Edinburgh, E. & S. Livingstone, 1950.
6. Brock RC: The life and work of Sir Astley Cooper. Edinburgh, E. & S. Livingstone, 1952.
7. Brock RC: Valentine Mott. Guys Hosp Rep, 94:75, 1945.
8. Moniz E: L'encephalographie arterielle: Son importance dans la localisation des tumeurs. Rev Neurol 2:72, 1927.
9. Eastcott HHG, Pickering GW, Rob CG: Reconstruction of internal carotid artery in a patient with intermittent attacks of hemiplegia. Lancet 2:994–996, 1954.
10. Carrea R, Molins M, Murphy G: Surgical treatment of spontaneous thrombosis of the internal carotid artery in the neck. Carotid-carotideal anastomosis. Report of a case. Acta Neurol Latinoamer 1:17, 1955.
11. Strully KJ, Hurwitt ES, Blankenberg HW:

Thrombo-endarterectomy for thrombosis of the internal carotid artery in the neck. J Neurosurg 10:474, 1953.

12. DeBakey ME: Successful carotid endarterectomy for cerebrovascular insufficiency. Nineteen year follow-up. JAMA 233:1083, 1975.
13. Fields WS, Maslenikov V, Meyer JS, et al: Joint study of extracranial arterial occlusion: V. Progress report of prognosis following surgery or nonsurgical treatment for transient cerebral ischemic attacks and cervical carotid lesions. JAMA 211:1993–2003, 1970.

Part One

Anatomy and Pathophysiology

2

The Cerebral Arteries and Collateral Circulation

R. Eugene Zierler

The blood supply to the brain is provided by the carotid arteries, often referred to as the anterior circulation, and the vertebral arteries, which constitute the posterior circulation. An understanding of the normal anatomy of the cerebral arteries, common anatomic variants, and collateral blood flow patterns is vital to the discussions of pathophysiology, diagnosis, and treatment in the chapters that follow. The purpose of this chapter is to review the embryologic development of the cerebral circulation, the normal anatomy of the anterior and posterior cerebral circulations, important anatomic variants, and the collateral circulation to the brain.

EMBRYOLOGY

The cardiovascular system is the first major organ system to function in the embryo. Blood begins to circulate by the end of the third week, at a time when the rapidly growing embryo is no longer able to satisfy its nutritional requirements by diffusion alone. Around the beginning of the third week, cells located in the visceral mesoderm of the wall of the yolk sac begin to differentiate into precursors of blood vessels and blood cells, called *angio-*

blasts. These cells form *angiogenic clusters,* which become canalized and coalesce to form small vessels. The cells in the lumen of these vessels give rise to primitive blood cells, while the cells lining the vessel walls flatten and become the vascular endothelium. By a process of continuous budding and fusion, the vessels within the embryo become continuous with the extraembryonic vessels, thus establishing the circulation of the embryo and placenta.

The angiogenic cell clusters initially are located along the lateral margins of the embryo, but they quickly move cephalad and unite to form a horseshoe-shaped network of small blood vessels (Fig. 2-1*A* and *B*).[1] This network, particularly the central cardiogenic area, will form the heart tube and give rise to all the cardiac structures (Fig. 2-1*C*). Other angiogenic cell clusters join to form a pair of longitudinal vessels, the *dorsal aortae,* running lateral to the midline of the embryo. These vessels eventually establish connections with the heart tube through the aortic arches (Fig. 2-2). As the six branchial or pharyngeal arches take shape during the fourth and fifth weeks of development, each is penetrated by an aortic arch derived from the aortic sac at the distal end of the heart tube (Fig. 2-2 and Fig. 2-3*A*). These six pairs of aortic arches terminate in the dorsal aortae (Fig. 2-3*A*). Although the paired dorsal aortae initially extend along the entire length of the embryo, they eventually fuse to form a single dorsal aorta just caudal to the branchial arches. Proximal to the aortic arches, the aortic sac forms right and left horns, which give rise to the brachiocephalic artery and the ascending aorta, respectively (Fig. 2-3*B* and *C*).

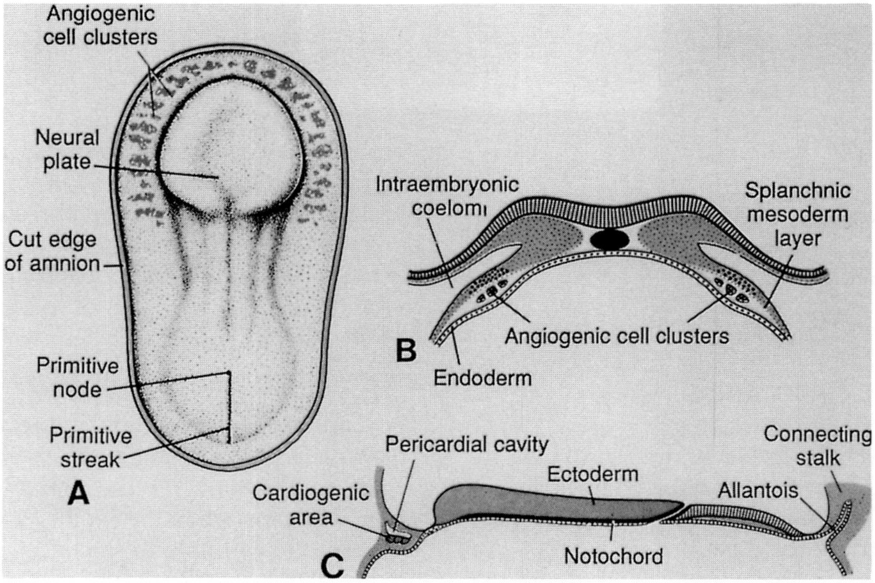

Figure 2-1. *A.* Dorsal view of a human embryo at about 18 days. The angiogenic cell clusters are located around the neural plate. *B.* Transverse section through the embryo shows the position of the angiogenic cell clusters in the splanchnic mesoderm layer. *C.* Midsagittal section through the embryo showing the cardiogenic area and pericardial cavity. (*From Sadler TW: Langman's Medical Embryology, 6th ed. Baltimore, Williams & Wilkins, 1990, p. 179. Used with permission.*)

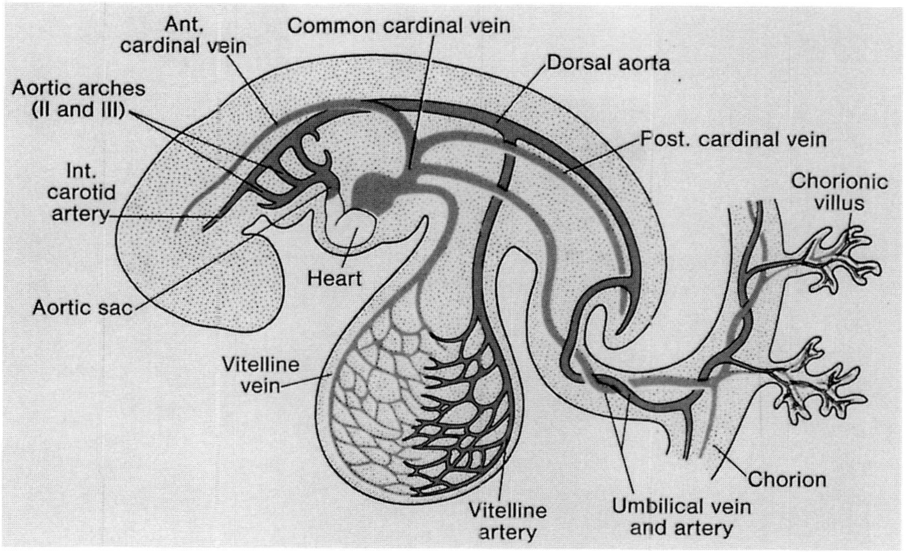

Figure 2-2. The main intra- and extraembryonic arteries and veins of an embryo at the end of the fourth week. Only vessels on one side of the embryo are shown. (*From Sadler TW: Langman's Medical Embryology, 6th ed. Baltimore, Williams & Wilkins, 1990, p. 208. Used with permission.*)

The original symmetric arrangement of aortic arches shown in Fig. 2-3*A* changes dramatically during subsequent development, as illustrated in Fig. 2-3*B* and *C*. Most of the first aortic arch disappears, although a small portion remains as the maxillary artery. The remnants of the second aortic arch form the hyoid and stapedial arteries.[2] The fifth aortic arch is small and disappears without giving rise to any important structures; however, the third, fourth, and sixth arches enlarge considerably. On each side, the third aortic arch forms the common carotid artery and the proximal segment of the internal carotid artery. The remaining portion of the internal carotid is derived from the cranial segment of the dorsal aorta. The external carotid arteries originate as branches of the third arches. The fourth aortic arch makes different contributions on the right and left sides. On the right, it forms the proximal portion of the right subclavian artery, while the distal portion of the right subclavian is derived from the right dorsal aorta and seventh intersegmental artery. The left fourth aortic arch becomes the arch of the aorta between the left common carotid and left subclavian arteries. The sixth aortic arch is the pulmonary arch and gives rise to the pulmonary arteries. On the right side, the connection between the sixth arch and the dorsal aorta disappears; on the left, the distal portion of the sixth arch persists during intrauterine life as the ductus arteriosus.

As the aortic arch system develops, the segments of the dorsal aortae between the third and fourth aortic arches disappear. On the right, the dorsal aorta between the seventh intersegmental artery and the junction with the left dorsal aorta also is obliterated (Fig. 2-3*B*). The heart descends into the thoracic cavity as the neck develops, resulting in considerable lengthening of the brachiocephalic and carotid arteries. Since the left subclavian artery is fixed distally in the left arm bud, its point of

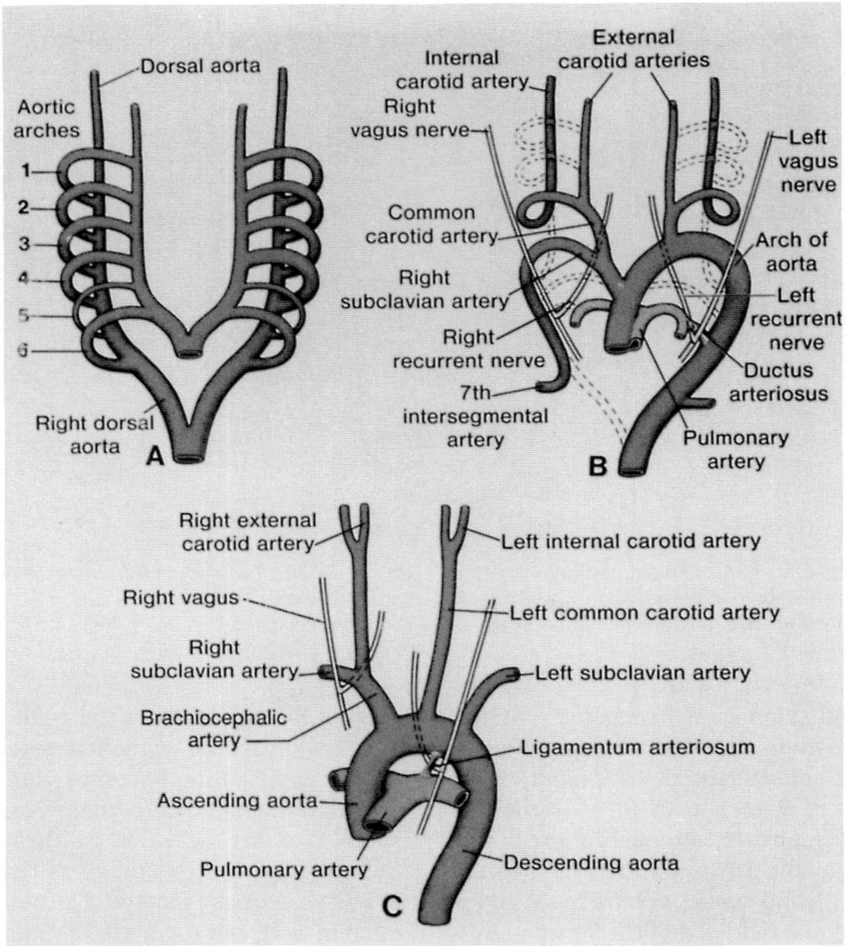

Figure 2-3. *A.* Diagram of the aortic arches and dorsal aortae before transformation into the definitive vascular pattern. *B.* Diagram of the aortic arches and dorsal aortae after the transformation. The obliterated components are indicated by dashed lines. *C.* The great arteries in the adult. Note the difference in the distance between the origins of the left common carotid and left subclavian arteries in *B* and *C*. (*From Sadler TW: Langman's Medical Embryology, 6th ed. Baltimore, Williams & Wilkins, 1990, p. 210. Used with permission.*)

origin gradually shifts from the aorta at the level of the left seventh intersegmental artery to a more proximal location near the origin of the left common carotid artery (Fig. 2-3*B* and *C*).[3] These asymmetric changes in the aortic arches account for the difference in the course of the recurrent laryngeal nerves on the right and left sides. The recurrent laryngeal branches of the vagus nerves initially supply the sixth branchial arches and follow a course around the sixth aortic arches (Fig. 2-3*B*). As the heart descends, the recurrent laryngeal nerves elongate and run upward to the larynx. When the distal portions of the right fifth and sixth aortic arches disappear, the recurrent laryngeal nerve on that side moves cephalad and hooks around the right subclavian artery. This does not occur on the left side, since the distal portion of the sixth aortic arch persists as the ductus arteriosus or ligamentum arteriosum (Fig. 2-3*C*).

Because of the complex changes involved in transforming the embryonic system of aortic arches into the adult arterial pattern, many variations occur. Most anomalies result from either the abnormal persistence of arterial segments or the disappearance of segments that normally should remain. For example, when the right dorsal aorta persists between the origin of the seventh intersegmental artery and its junction with the left dorsal aorta, two aortic arches arise from the ascending aorta. This creates a double aortic arch or vascular ring around the trachea and esophagus, which can compress these structures and cause difficulties with breathing or swallowing.[4] When this occurs, the right arch is usually larger and passes posterior to the trachea and esophagus. A right arch of the aorta is formed when the entire right dorsal aorta persists while the left fourth aortic arch and left dorsal aorta are obliterated.

If the right fourth aortic arch and adjacent segment of the right dorsal aorta disappear, the right subclavian artery is formed by the seventh intersegmental artery and the distal portion of the right dorsal aorta. As the segment of aorta between the left common carotid artery and left subclavian artery shortens, the origin of the right subclavian artery is carried proximally and is eventually located just distal to the origin of the left subclavian artery.[3] In this situation, the right recurrent laryngeal nerve does not hook around the right subclavian artery, but originates from the vagus near the carotid bifurcation and passes directly to the larynx. A non-recurrent laryngeal nerve lies deep to the common carotid artery and may be injured during carotid endarterectomy. Because it is derived from the right dorsal aorta, an anomalous right subclavian artery must cross the midline posterior to the trachea and esophagus to reach the right arm. Although this anatomic variant of the right subclavian artery is found in less than one percent of individuals, it typically does not constrict the trachea or esophagus enough to produce clinically apparent symptoms.[5,6] Rarely, this vessel compresses the esophagus against the posterior aspect of the trachea and causes swallowing difficulty, a condition known as *dysphagia lusoria*.[7] Aneurysmal changes have been reported in anomalous right subclavian arteries with symptoms related to esophageal and tracheal compression, as well as rupture.[6,8]

The most frequent developmental anomaly of the carotid arteries is a left common carotid artery which originates from the brachiocephalic artery.[9] This occurs in approximately 10 percent of individuals, but is of little clinical significance. The left vertebral artery originates directly from the aortic arch in about 5 percent of the population.[5] Kinks and coils typically involve the internal carotid artery and may represent either developmental anomalies or degenerative processes. Carotid coils seen in infants and young children probably are the result of a discrepancy between the growth rates of the vascular and skeletal systems. If the elongation of the spine does not keep pace with the descent of the heart and associated vessels into the thorax, a redundancy or coiling of the carotid artery can be produced in the neck. Thus, most children with this anomaly have it bilaterally and are likely to have other vascular anomalies such as aortic coarctation.[10] However, in most adults with kinks or coils of the internal carotid artery the underlying pathologic process appears to be atherosclerotic degeneration. The management of carotid kinks and coils is discussed in Chap. 5.

CAROTID ARTERIES

Common Carotid Artery

The paired common carotid arteries begin in the chest, with the right originating at the bifurcation of the brachiocephalic (innominate) artery along with the right subclavian, and the left arising directly from the aortic arch between the brachiocephalic and left subclavian arteries (Fig. 2-4). Each common carotid artery ascends in the neck medial to the internal jugular vein and anterior to the vagus nerve. The carotid sheath is a loose aggregation of connective tissue that surrounds the carotid artery, internal jugular vein, and vagus nerve from the base of the neck to the base of the skull. The cervical sympathetic chain is adherent to the posterior fibers of the carotid sheath, and the ansa cervicalis, which provides motor innervation to the strap muscles, is associated with the anterior fibers of the sheath.

The common carotid artery normally has no branches proximal to its bifurcation, although the superior thyroid or ascending pharyngeal arteries occasionally originate just before the internal and external carotid. In adults, the bifurcation of the common carotid artery usually is located at the level of the upper border of the thyroid cartilage or the C4 cervical vertebra. The bifurcation tends to be one or

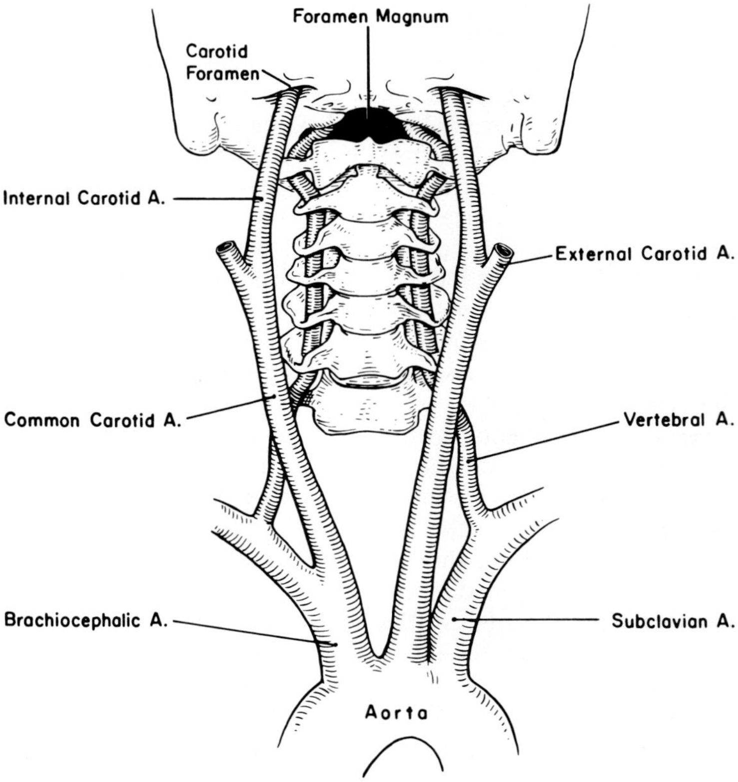

Figure 2-4. Normal origin and course of the extracranial cerebral vessels (anterior view).

two cervical levels higher in children. Variations in the level of the carotid bifurcation are frequent and are more often above the typical level than below. A small oval nodule of chemoreceptor tissue, the carotid body, is located on the medial side of the distal common or proximal internal carotid artery (see Chap. 32). The carotid bifurcation also contains the carotid sinus, a pressure receptor. Both the carotid body and carotid sinus are supplied by branches of the glossopharyngeal nerve.

External Carotid Artery

The external carotid artery is the smaller of the two terminal branches of the common carotid. It provides the main blood supply to the extracranial structures of the head and gives off branches that contribute to the blood supply of the dura of the basal and lateral brain surfaces. These latter branches communicate with the internal carotid and vertebral systems and are potential routes for collateral flow to the intracranial circulation (Fig. 2-5). Just beyond the common carotid bifurcation, the external carotid lies anteromedial to the internal carotid. The external carotid passes deep to the posterior belly of the digastric and the stylohyoid muscles. It then enters the substance of the parotid gland, where it is crossed by the facial nerve and divides into its terminal branches. There are characteristically eight branches of the external carotid artery: three anterior branches; two posterior branches; one medial branch; and two terminal branches. As illustrated in Fig. 2-5, the anterior branches are the superior thyroid, lingual, and facial (external maxillary); the posterior branches are the occipital and posterior auricular; the medial branch is the ascending pharyngeal; and the terminal branches are the superficial temporal and internal maxillary. The middle meningeal artery is the most important branch of the internal maxillary artery. It enters the cranial cavity through the foramen spinosum in the sphenoid bone and communicates with branches of the internal carotid artery.

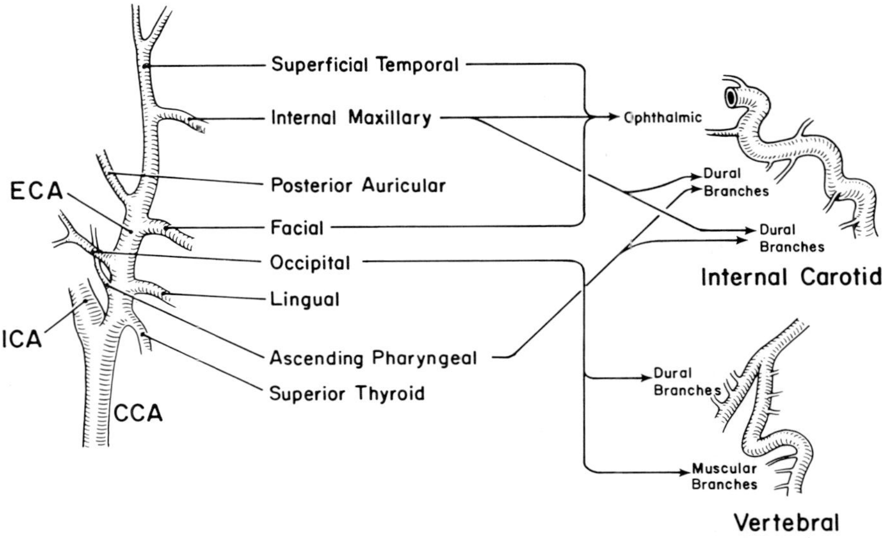

Figure 2-5. Branches of the external carotid artery (ECA). Arrows indicate potential anastomoses with intracranial branches of the internal carotid (ICA) and vertebral arteries. CCA = common carotid artery.

Internal Carotid Artery

The internal carotid artery proceeds posteromedially from the common carotid bifurcation and enters the carotid canal of the temporal bone without giving off any branches in the neck. It passes deep to the posterior belly of the digastric and the stylohyoid muscles and lies medial to the internal jugular vein. Each internal carotid normally supplies the ipsilateral eye and cerebral hemisphere.

The distal portion of the extracranial internal carotid artery is closely associated with the last four cranial nerves. The glossopharyngeal (IX), vagus (X), and spinal accessory (XI) nerves exit from the jugular foramen just posterior and lateral to the carotid canal. The hypoglossal (XII) nerve emerges from the hypoglossal canal medial to the jugular foramen. The glossopharyngeal nerve runs anteriorly, passing superficial to the internal carotid artery and along the stylopharyngeus muscle. A small branch of the glossopharyngeal, the carotid sinus nerve, descends to the carotid bifurcation. The vagus nerve usually lies posteriorly between the internal jugular vein and internal carotid artery; however, the vagus occasionally is in a more anterior position, particularly lower in the neck. The spinal accessory nerve runs posteriorly and penetrates the sternomastoid muscle on its way across the posterior triangle of the neck to the trapezius muscle. The hypoglossal nerve initially passes between the internal carotid artery and internal jugular vein before looping forward under the occipital branch of the external carotid. This nerve then passes over the lateral surfaces of the internal and external carotid arteries and deep to the stylohyoid and digastric muscles. The hypoglossal nerve is typically found crossing the carotid arteries 1 to 2 cm distal to the bifurcation, although its location is variable.

The internal carotid artery can be divided into four anatomic segments: cervical; petrous; cavernous; and supraclinoid (Fig. 2-6).

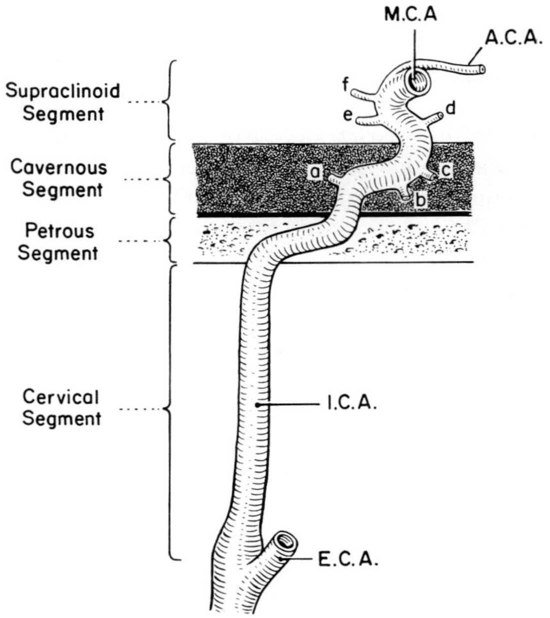

Figure 2-6. Segments and branches of the internal carotid artery (ICA). Branches include the (a) meningohypophyseal trunk (b) artery of the inferior cavernous sinus, (c) McConnell's capsular artery, (d) ophthalmic artery, (e) posterior communicating artery, and (f) anterior choroidal artery. The terminal branches are the anterior cerebral artery (ACA) and middle cerebral artery (MCA). ECA = external carotid artery.

The cervical segment, which has no named branches, begins at the origin of the internal carotid and ends where the artery enters the temporal bone at the base of the skull. A dilated area of extremely variable size, the carotid bulb, occupies the most proximal portion of this segment. While the cervical segment usually is straight, varying degrees of tortuosity occur, ranging from sharp angulation or kinking to elongation with coiling (Figs. 2-7 and 2-8).[11] The petrous segment includes the portion of the internal carotid artery that traverses the carotid canal in the petrous temporal bone. Initially, the carotid canal runs vertically, but it then curves anteriorly and medially to enter the middle cranial fossa.

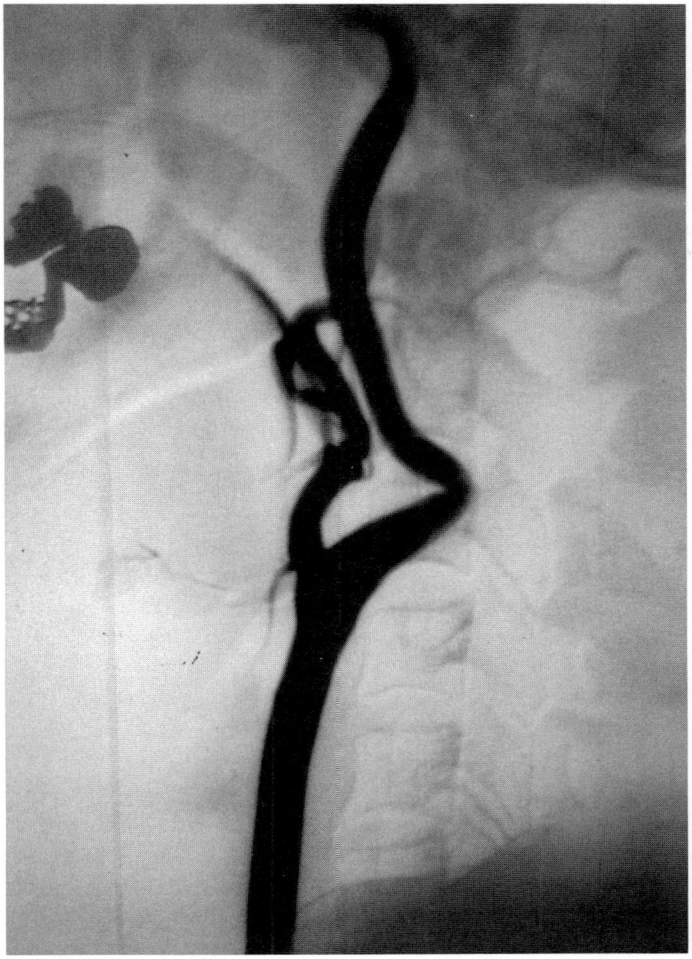

Figure 2-7. Arteriogram of an adult carotid bifurcation with a kink in the proximal internal carotid artery. Such kinks are often associated with atherosclerotic plaque and narrowing of the arterial lumen.

Along this course, the internal carotid is closely related to the middle ear. The only branches of the petrous segment are small caroticotympanic branches.

The cavernous segment of the internal carotid artery passes through the cavernous sinus and is covered by the endothelial lining and dural sheaths of the sinus. The artery runs in an anterior and superior direction, lateral to the wall of the sphenoid sinus. Branches arising from this segment include the meningohypophysial trunk, the artery of the inferior cavernous sinus, and McConnell's capsular artery (Fig. 2-6). These small branches supply the dura surrounding the pituitary gland. The cavernous segment terminates when the internal carotid ascends and pierces the dural roof of the cavernous sinus medial to the anterior clinoid process, entering the subarachnoid space. The last part of the internal carotid artery is the supraclinoid segment, also referred to as the subarachnoid or intracranial segment. After entering the subarachnoid space, the internal carotid continues upward and pos-

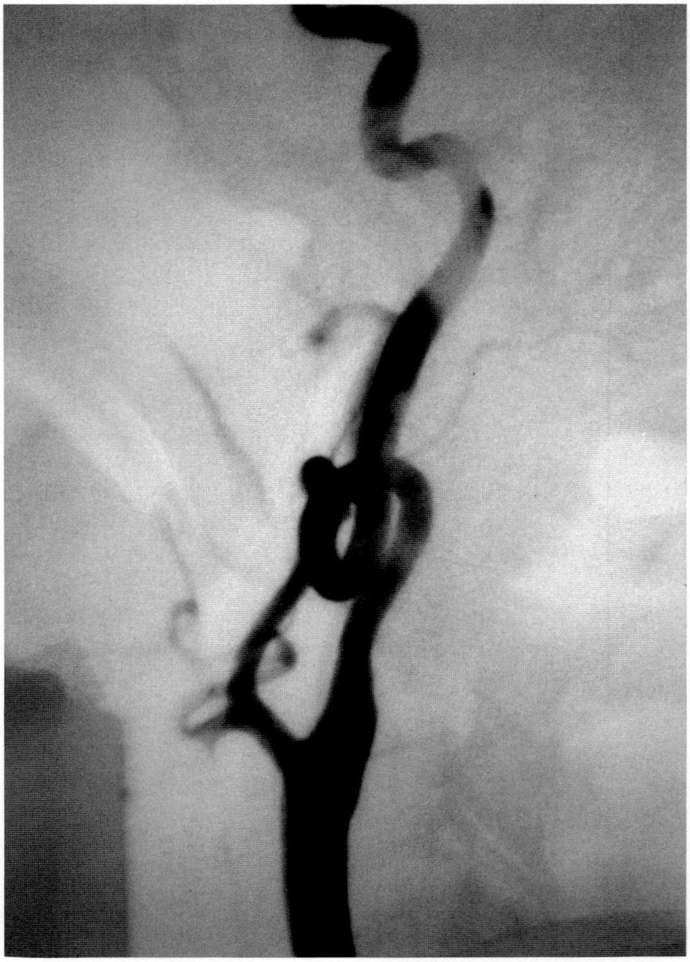

Figure 2-8. Arteriogram of an adult carotid bifurcation showing a coil in the internal carotid artery.

teriorly below the optic nerve and reaches the lateral aspect of the optic chiasm. The artery then turns anteriorly again and bifurcates into the middle and anterior cerebral arteries. Because of the S-shaped course of the cavernous and supraclinoid segments, this portion of the internal carotid artery is called the *carotid siphon*. The other branches of the supraclinoid segment include the ophthalmic artery, the posterior communicating artery, and the anterior choroidal artery (Fig. 2-6).

The ophthalmic artery is the first branch of the supraclinoid segment. It passes forward through the optic canal beneath the optic nerve, where it divides into the central retinal artery, which provides the major blood supply to the eye, and a variety of smaller branches. These include the lacrimal artery, which gives off a recurrent meningeal branch that ultimately connects with branches of the middle meningeal artery, the ciliary arteries, the ethmoidal arteries, and the supraorbital, supratrochlear, and lateral nasal arteries that supply the upper eyelid, forehead, and scalp. The latter three branches also form connections with branches of the external carotid artery.

The posterior communicating artery runs posteriorly from the internal carotid artery to join the posterior cerebral artery (Fig. 2-9). During embryologic development, both the posterior communicating artery and posterior cerebral artery originate from the internal carotid or anterior circulation. However, the posterior communicating artery usually does not persist, and the posterior cerebral artery becomes part of the vertebral or posterior circulation. In about 20 percent of individuals the posterior communicating artery remains widely patent, an arrangement referred to as a "fetal" posterior communicating artery.[12]

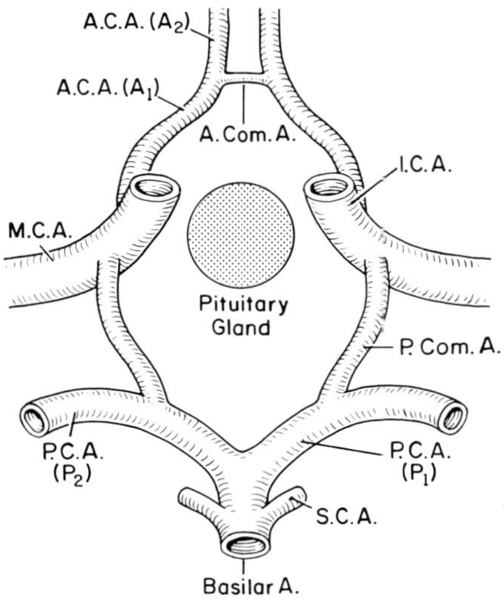

Figure 2-9. Normal circle of Willis. ICA = internal carotid artery; ACA = anterior cerebral artery (A_1 = precommunicating segment, A_2 = postcommunicating segment); MCA = middle cerebral artery; AComA = anterior communicating artery; PComA = posterior communicating artery; PCA = posterior cerebral artery (P_1 = precommunicating segment, P_2 = postcommunicating segment); SCA = superior cerebellar artery.

The anterior choroidal artery arises near the termination of the internal carotid artery. It passes posteriorly along the optic tract and enters the choroid fissure, giving off numerous small branches to the deep structures of the brain, including the choroid plexus and lateral ventricle.

The distribution of the major cerebral arteries is illustrated in Fig. 2-10. The anterior cerebral artery is the smaller of the two terminal branches of the internal carotid. It passes forward and medially above the optic chiasm and enters the longitudinal fissure of the brain (Fig. 2-11). At the point where the two anterior cerebral arteries approach the midline, they are joined by one or more anterior communicating arteries which form the anterior portion of the circle of Willis (Figs. 2-9 and 11*A*).[13] The initial portion of the anterior cerebral artery is called the A_1 segment and gives off numerous perforating branches to the hypothalamus and septal region. Distal to the anterior communicating artery, the A_2 segment of the anterior cerebral artery enters the longitudinal fissure and curves around the corpus callosum on the medial aspect of the cerebral hemisphere (Fig. 2-11*B*). The distal portion of the anterior cerebral artery is also referred to as the pericallosal artery and terminates as a posterior pericallosal branch. Throughout its course, the anterior cerebral artery gives off small perforating branches to the adjacent structures (Fig. 2-10).

The middle cerebral artery is the largest terminal branch of the internal carotid. It originates as the continuation of the internal carotid lateral to the optic chiasm (Fig. 2-11*A*). The initial portion of the middle cerebral artery (the M_1 segment) runs horizontally, giving off perforating branches; it divides into two major trunks (Fig. 2-12). These trunks continue to the cortical surface and supply the majority of the lateral aspect of the cerebral hemisphere, including portions of the frontal,

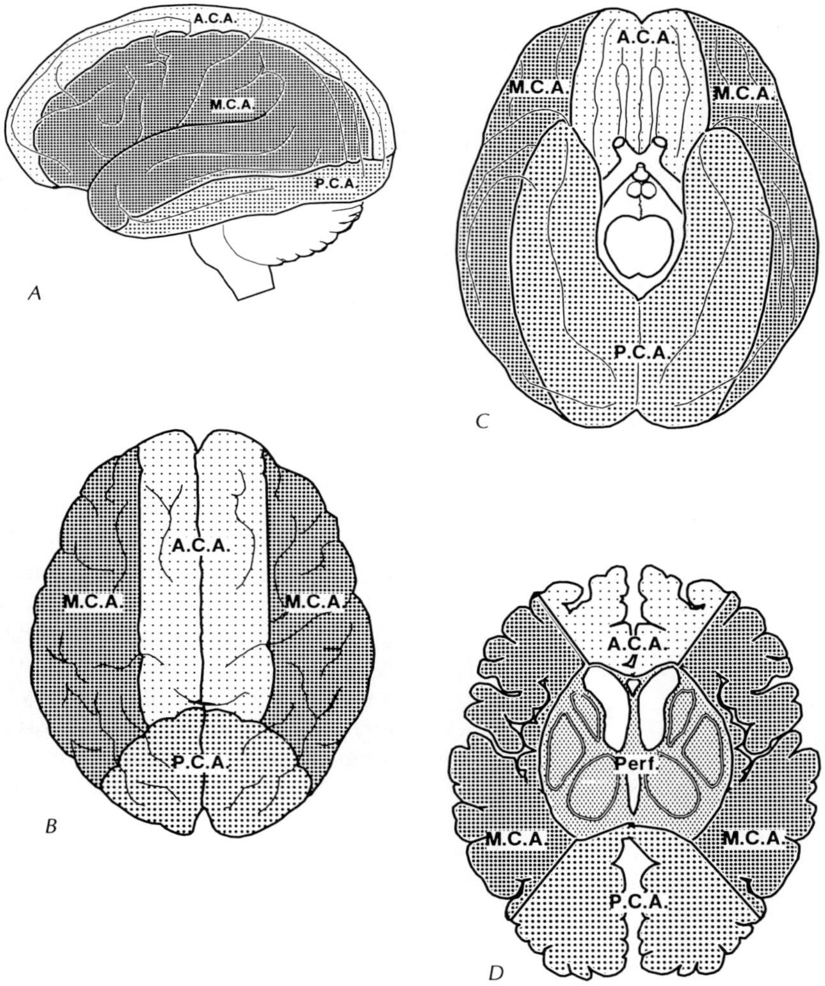

Figure 2-10. Cerebral distribution of the internal carotid artery branches. *A.* Lateral view. *B.* Superior view. *C.* Basal view. *D.* Horizontal section through the basal ganglia and thalamus. Lines bordering adjacent vascular territories represent watershed zones. ACA = anterior cerebral artery; MCA = middle cerebral artery; PCA = posterior cerebral artery; Perf = perforators from the carotid and basilar arteries.

parietal, occipital, and temporal lobes (Fig. 2-10).

VERTEBRAL ARTERIES

The paired vertebral arteries are the largest and most proximal branches of the subclavian arteries (Fig. 2-4). Variations in size between the two vertebral arteries are quite common.[14] Branches of the vertebral arteries supply the upper part of the spinal cord, the brain stem, the cerebellum, and a large portion of the posterior-inferior aspect of the cerebral cortex (Fig. 2-10). As illustrated in Fig. 2-13, the vertebral artery can be divided into four anatomic segments: initial soft tissue or cervical: inter-

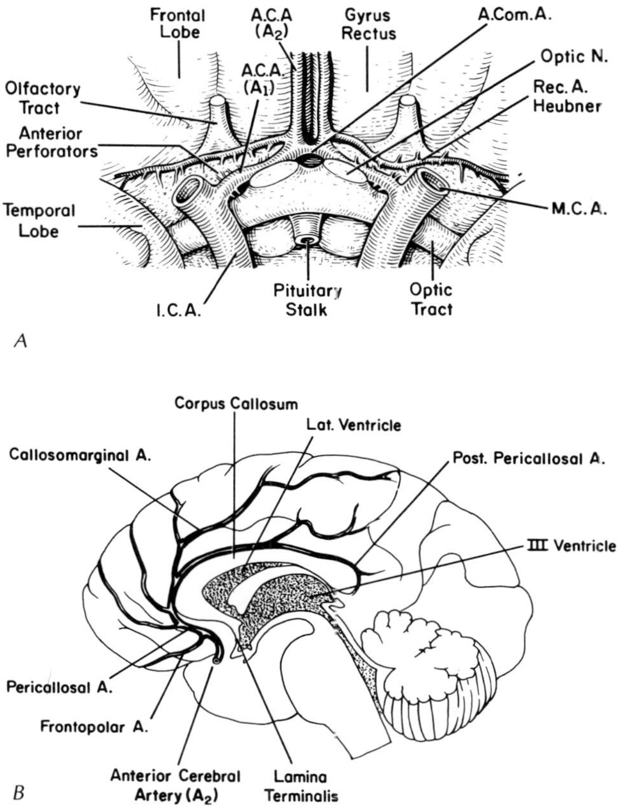

Figure 2-11. Distribution and branches of the anterior cerebral artery (ACA). *A.* Basal-frontal view. *B.* Midsagittal view. AComA = anterior communicating artery; A_1 = precommunicating segment of ACA; A_2 = postcommunicating segment of the ACA; MCA = middle cerebral artery; ICA = internal carotid artery.

vertebral; horizontal or suboccipital; and intracranial or subarachnoid.

The initial soft tissue segment of the vertebral artery passes superiorly and posteriorly from its origin, behind the common carotid artery and in front of the transverse process of the seventh cervical vertebra. There are no major branches from this segment, although there may be a few small branches to the muscles of the neck. The intervertebral segment begins where the artery enters the foramen transversarium of the sixth (or occasionally the fifth) cervical vertebra. The artery then follows a straight course through the foramina transversaria of the remaining upper cervical vertebrae anterior to the ventral rami of the cervical nerves and accompanied by a venous plexus. In addition to spinal branches to the adjacent spinal cord and vertebrae, this segment gives off numerous muscular branches that form connections with branches of the subclavian and external carotid arteries. At the upper end of the intervertebral segment, the vertebral artery turns laterally to reach the foramen transversarium of the atlas.

The horizontal segment begins where the vessel emerges from the foramen transversarium of the atlas. The vertebral artery then bends sharply backward and medially around the lateral mass of the atlas before turning anteriorly to enter the spinal canal. This segment is contained within the suboccipital triangle and is covered by the semispinalis capitis muscle. Branches arising from the horizontal seg-

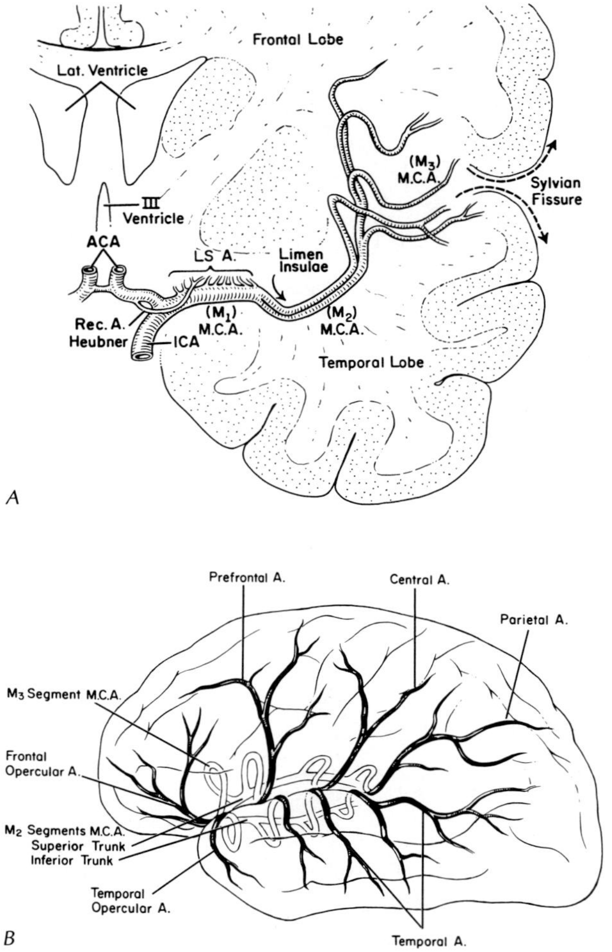

Figure 2-12. Distribution and branches of the middle cerebral artery (MCA). *A.* Anterior view. *B.* Lateral view. M_1 = main MCA trunk to limen insulae; M_2 = MCA trunk to overlying insular surface; M_3 = segments of MCA to external cortical surface; LSA = lenticulostriate arteries; ACA = anterior cerebral artery; ICA = internal carotid artery.

ment include muscular branches to the suboccipital muscles and meningeal branches to the posterior cranial fossa. The intracranial segment of the vertebral artery begins as the artery perforates the dura at the base of the skull and passes through the foramen magnum. The vertebral arteries then ascend medially in front of the medulla oblongata, uniting at the level of the pontomedullary junction to form the basilar artery. Important branches of the intracranial segment are the anterior spinal and posterior inferior cerebellar arteries. The anterior spinal artery (Fig. 2-13) is formed by branches from both vertebral arteries, which join at the midline and descend in the anteromedian fissure to supply the medulla and spinal cord. Extension of the anterior spinal artery down the spinal cord is dependent on numerous contributions from segmental vessels. The posterior inferior cerebellar artery (Figs. 2-13 and 2-14) is typically the largest branch of the vertebral. It supplies the me-

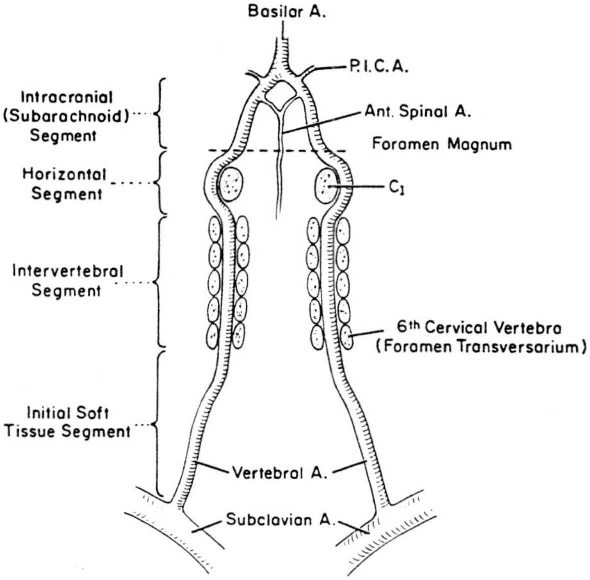

Figure 2-13. Segments and branches of the vertebral artery. PICA = posterior inferior cerebellar artery; C_1 = first cervical vertebra.

dulla and the inferior surface of the cerebellum. The posterior spinal arteries are usually branches of the posterior inferior cerebellar arteries, but they also may originate directly from the vertebrals.

Basilar Artery

From the junction of the two vertebral arteries in front of the lower border of the pons, the basilar artery ascends in the midline to the upper border of the pons. It provides the blood supply to the upper brainstem, the cerebellum, the occipital lobes, and portions of the temporal lobes. The major branches of the basilar artery are three sets of paired vessels (Fig. 2-14). The anterior inferior cerebellar arteries are the first and smallest of these branches; they supply the upper medulla, lower pons, and adjacent cerebellum. The superior cerebellar arteries arise from the distal basilar artery and supply the upper aspect of the cerebellum. The posterior cerebral arteries are the terminal branches of the basilar artery. Branches of the posterior cerebrals supply the thalamus and midbrain, the choroid plexus, and the posterior portions of the occipital and temporal lobes (Fig. 2-10). As previously mentioned, the posterior cerebral arteries are joined to the internal carotid circulation by the posterior communicating arteries during embryologic development; however, this fetal arrangement usually does not persist (Fig. 2-9).[12]

COLLATERAL CIRCULATION

The collateral circulation to the brain and related structures depends on connections between the carotid and vertebral circulation of the two sides, as well as anastomotic channels between the ipsilateral carotid and vertebrobasilar systems and the internal and external carotid arteries. The most critical feature of the collateral pathways to the cerebral hemispheres is the circle of Willis, a ring of arteries surrounding the pituitary stalk in the sub-

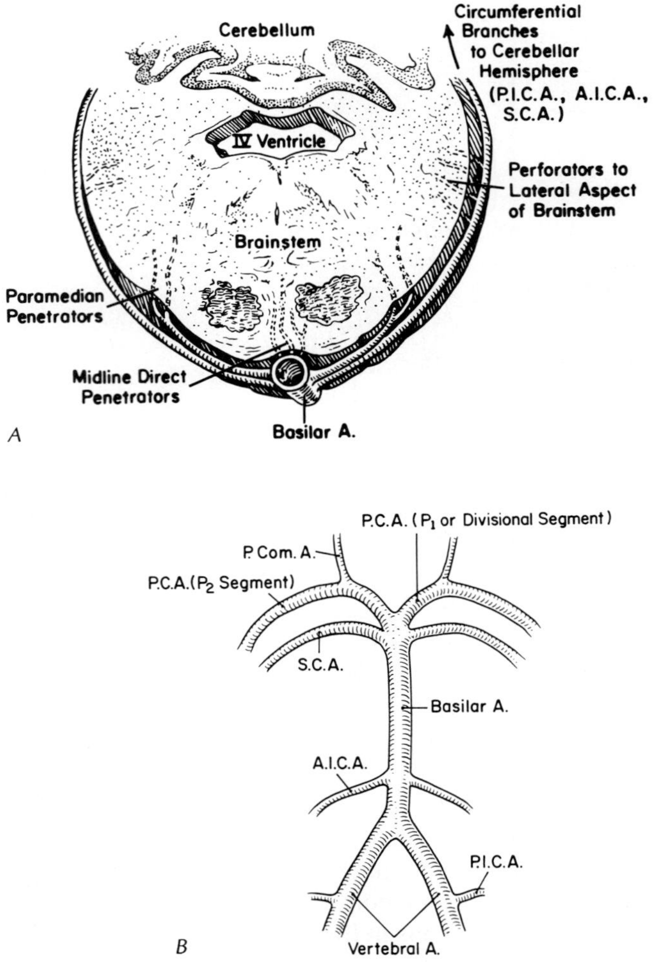

Figure 2-14. Basilar artery and vertebral arteries. *A.* Typical distribution of branches to the brainstem, cerebellum, and occipital lobes. *B.* Major paired branches include the: posterior inferior cerebellar arteries (PICA); anterior inferior cerebellar arteries (AICA); superior cerebellar arteries (SCA); and posterior cerebral arteries (PCA). PComA = posterior communicating artery; P_1 = precommunicating segment PCA; P_2 = postcommunicating segment PCA.

arachnoid space at the base of the brain (Fig. 2-9). The terminal ends of the internal carotid arteries are located along the lateral portions of this ring. Anteriorly, the circle is formed by the A_1 segments of the two anterior cerebral arteries and the anterior communicating artery (Fig. 2-11*A*); posteriorly, the circle consists of the two posterior communicating arteries and the proximal segments of the posterior cerebral branches of the basilar artery (Fig. 2-14*B*).

A functionally intact circle of Willis provides a route for collateral flow between both the anterior and posterior circulations and the two cerebral hemispheres. When this situation is present, compensatory flow can occur in response to unilateral internal carotid occlusion or stenotic lesions in multiple extracranial cerebral arteries. However, hypoplasia of the anterior or posterior communicating arteries is relatively common, and an ideal functionally intact circle of Willis is found in less than half of individuals.[15,16] In the normal cerebral circulation there appears to be no significant flow through the communicating segments of the circle of Willis, and each internal carotid or vertebral artery perfuses only the appropriate ipsilateral territory.

As illustrated in Fig. 2-15, there are a variety of potential anastomotic channels between the carotid and vertebrobasilar systems. Except for the posterior communicating arteries, all are rare and probably represent persistent developmental anomalies. The presence of one or more of these collateral routes explains how distal patency of a vertebral artery can be maintained with more proximal vertebral artery occlusion and how an internal carotid artery can remain patent following ipsilateral common carotid occlusion.

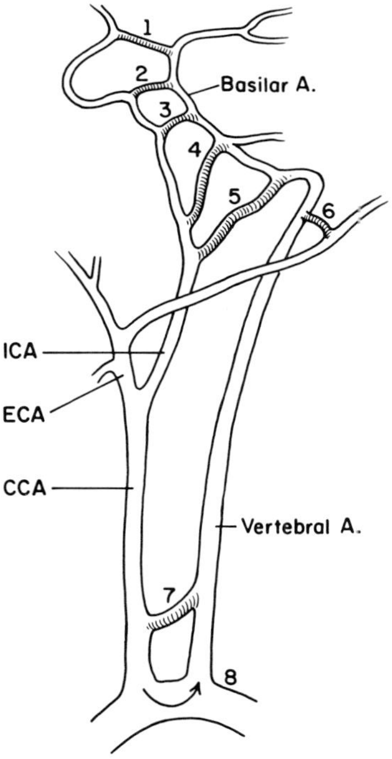

Figure 2-15. Anastomoses between the carotid and vertebral systems. Shaded segments represent potential collateral routes. 1, Posterior communicating artery; 2, trigeminal artery; 3, otic artery; 4, hypoglossal artery; 5, proatlantal intersegmental artery; 6, occipital-vertebral arterial anastomoses; 7, cervical intersegmental artery; and 8, retrograde filling into the subclavian artery. CCA = common carotid artery; ECA = external carotid artery; ICA = internal carotid artery.

Potential anastomoses between the internal and external carotid arteries have already been mentioned, and the ophthalmic artery is the most significant of these collateral routes (Fig. 2-5). The ophthalmic artery provides connections between the facial and superficial temporal branches of the external carotid and the supraclinoid segment of the internal carotid. In the presence of arterial lesions that reduce pressure or flow in the distal internal carotid circulation, the ophthalmic artery becomes a collateral vessel, and reversed flow is observed in the ophthalmic artery and its periorbital branches.

The potential for collateral flow at the cortical level is limited, although some connections exist along the "watershed" areas between the territories of the anterior and middle cerebral arteries and the middle and posterior cerebral arteries (Fig. 2-10). These watershed areas are particularly susceptible to anoxic injury following occlusion of the major proximal artery or generalized low-flow states.[17]

REFERENCES

1. Sadler TW: *Langman's Medical Embryology*, 6th ed. Baltimore, Williams & Wilkins, pp 179–227, 1990.
2. Padget DH: The development of the cranial arteries in the human embryo. *Contrib Embryol* 32:205, 1948.
3. Barry A: The aortic arch derivatives in the human adult. *Anat Rec* 111:221, 1951.
4. Ekstrom G, Sandblom P: Double aortic arch: Embryonic development. *Acta Chir Scand* 102:183, 1951.
5. McDonald JJ, Anson BJ: Variations in origin of arteries derived from the aortic arch in Ameri-

can whites and negroes. *Am J Phys Anthropol* 27:91, 1940.
6. Austin EH, Wolfe WG: Aneurysm of aberrant subclavian artery with review of the literature. *J Vasc Surg* 2:571, 1985.
7. Valentine RJ, Carter DJ, Clagett GP: A modified extrathoracic approach to the treatment of dysphagia lusoria. *J Vasc Surg* 5:498, 1987.
8. McCallen AM, Schaff B: Aneurysm of an anomalous right subclavian artery. *Radiol* 66:561, 1956.
9. Liechty JD, Shields TW, Anson BJ: Variations pertaining to the aortic arches and their branches. *Quart Bull Northw Univ Med Sch* 31:136, 1957.
10. Sarkari NBS, Holmes JM, Bickerstaff ER: Neurological manifestations associated with internal carotid loops and kinks in children. *J Neurol Neurosurg Psychiat* 33:194, 1970.
11. Weibel J, Fields WS: Tortuosity, coiling, and kinking of the internal carotid artery: Etiology and radiographic anatomy. *Neurology* 15:7, 1965.
12. Saeki N, Rhoton AL Jr: Microsurgical anatomy of the upper basilar artery and the posterior circle of Willis. *J Neurosurg* 46:563, 1977.
13. Perlmutter D, Rhoton AL Jr: Microsurgical anatomy of the anterior cerebral—anterior communicating—recurrent artery complex. *J Neurosurg* 45:259, 1976.
14. Stopford SB: The arteries of the pons and medulla oblongata. *J Anat Physiol* 50:131, 1915.
15. Pallie W, Samarasinge DD: A study in the qualification of the circle of Willis. *Brain* 85:569, 1962.
16. Stehbens W: Aneurysms and anatomical variations of the cerebral arteries. *Arch Pathol* 75:45, 1963.
17. Meyer JS: Circulatory changes following occlusion of the midline cerebral artery and their relationship to function. *J Neurosurg* 15:653, 1958.

3

Cerebrovascular Atherosclerosis

Ted R. Kohler
David Gordon

Cerebrovascular atherosclerosis causes the majority of ischemic strokes. Most symptomatic lesions occur at the carotid bifurcation, although the aortic arch and carotid siphon also may be affected. This chapter will focus on the development of cerebrovascular atherosclerosis, exploring what is known about its pathophysiology at the cellular level and why these lesions have a propensity for the carotid bulb. It is intended to lay the groundwork for Chap. 4, which describes how complex carotid plaques cause ischemic neurologic events.

RISK FACTORS

The risk factors for atherosclerosis are well known and are abundant in our culture. While the influences of gender, diabetes, and genetic predisposition cannot yet be modified, the powerful effects of cigarette smoking, hypertension, and elevated lipid levels can. Smoking undoubtedly is the most important modifiable risk factor, but hypertension also plays a major role. Hypertension affects approximately 20 percent of the adult population and is now readily treated in most patients. Elevated blood pressure appears to be a more significant risk factor for atherosclerosis in the carotid arteries than elsewhere in the arterial tree.

High plasma levels of the low-density lipoproteins (LDL) clearly increase the risk for atherosclerosis, while increased levels of the high-density lipoproteins (HDL) are protective. Intensive lipid-lowering regimens can slow progression of atherosclerosis in the coronary circulation and can even cause lesion regression.[1] The cost-effectiveness of the large-scale public health efforts currently contemplated to modify lipid levels in the general population is controversial.

DEVELOPMENT OF ATHEROSCLEROTIC LESIONS

Large complex atherosclerotic plaques that can restrict blood flow or produce emboli are the result of decades of growth involving intimal lesions that began as fatty streaks. Our knowledge of the progression of atherosclerosis is based on autopsy studies and animal models using either fat feeding or atherosclerosis-prone strains. One such animal strain is the Wantanabe heritable hyperlipidemic rabbit, which lacks LDL receptors, a condition similar to humans with familial hypercholesterolemia. The development of these lesions is similar in man and in animal models. However, development of complex plaques with thrombosis, like those that cause symptoms in man, is rare in experimental atherosclerosis.

Animal Models of Atherosclerosis

In animal models, the earliest arterial finding after the beginning of fat feeding is increased adherence of circulating monocytes to the luminal surface.[1] Occasionally these cells can be seen on scanning electron microscopy as they penetrate the endothelium and enter the intima, where they undergo phenotypic changes to become resident arterial macrophages. Macrophages take up oxidized LDL, transforming themselves into foam cells.[1] LDL moves freely across the endothelium to enter the intima from the plasma and can be oxidized by endothelium, smooth muscle cells, or macrophages. HDL also freely enters the arterial wall, where it removes cholesterol from macrophages in the intima. This cholesterol is transferred to LDL and very low-density lipoprotein (VLDL) particles in the plasma. These particles subsequently are taken up by the liver.[2]

Uptake of oxidized LDL occurs through the acetyl LDL receptor and various other "scavenger" receptors. Arterial macrophages have an increased expression of these acetyl LDL receptors. Oxidized LDL can contribute to the accumulation of monocytes in the intima because it is chemotactic for circulating monocytes and inhibits the motility of tissue macrophages; it is also cytotoxic and can cause cell injury, further stimulating atherogenesis. In addition, oxidized LDL may contribute to vascular wall dysfunction by inhibiting the release of endothelium-derived relaxing factors and stimulating the release of chemotactic and mitogenic factors from endothelial cells.[1] A schematic representation of the possible events leading from elevated plasma LDL levels to the development of atherosclerotic plaques is given in Fig. 3-1.

Human Atherosclerosis

Stary has described the evolution of human atherosclerotic lesions from birth to adulthood based on autopsy studies of the coronary arteries and aorta.[3] Adaptive, eccentric intimal thickening is present from birth, typically occurring in low-flow regions opposite flow-dividers (Fig. 3-2). This intimal thickening consists of two distinct layers that differ in density and in the nature of their smooth muscle cells and matrix. The inner layer is rich in proteoglycan matrix and has very few elastic fibers or cells. Smooth muscle cells in this re-

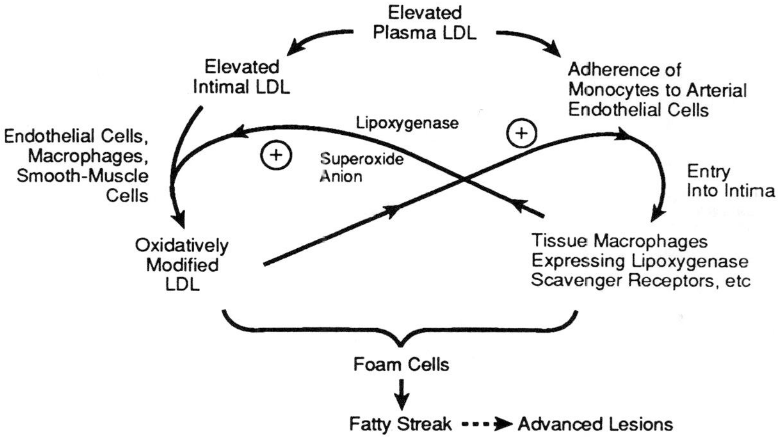

Figure 3-1. Elevated plasma LDL results in increased intimal LDL, which is then transformed by cells in the vascular wall to its oxidized form. Oxidized LDL contributes to cell migration and proliferation, as well as to cellular damage. Plasma LDL also stimulates adherence of monocytes to the endothelium and entry of these cells into the intima, where they become tissue macrophages that take up modified LDL. (*From Steinberg.*[1] *Reproduced with permission.*)

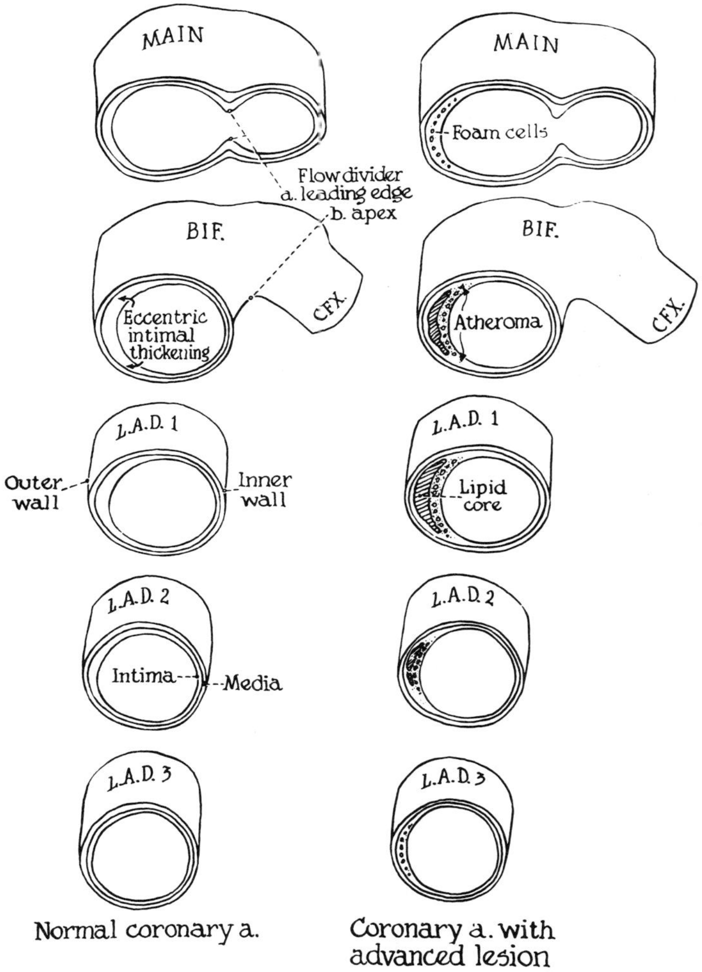

Figure 3-2. Eccentric intimal thickening in a normal coronary artery and a coronary artery with advanced atherosclerosis. The atheroma evolves through several progressive stages in the area of eccentric thickening. (*From Stary.*[3] *Reproduced with permission.*)

gion are loosely arranged and are of the synthetic phenotype, lacking myofilaments and rich in rough endoplasmic reticulum. Macrophages are found immediately below the endothelium in this layer. The deeper, musculoelastic layer is rich in elastic fibers and cells. Smooth muscle cells in this deep layer are densely packed in an orderly array and are of the contractile phenotype, rich in myofilaments.

Five types of lesions have been described, ranging from minimal, microscopic collections of macrophages to complex, advanced atherosclerotic plaques (Table 3-1).[3] These lesions represent the progression of atherosclerosis, which begins in the first decade of life. The earliest lesions (Type I) are isolated macrophage-derived foam cells, sometimes occurring in clusters, with only occasional lipid-laden smooth muscle cells. Macrophages are located in the subendothelial region and are much more numerous in areas of eccentric thickening. Macrophage-derived foam cells, on the other hand, are more commonly seen in the deep part of the proteoglycan layer. Type I lesions have very little extracellular lipid and can be seen only on microscopic examination. These lesions were found in 45 percent of infants during the first eight months of life and became less frequent after that age.

At puberty, more substantial accumulations of macrophage-derived foam cells appear as fatty streaks in over half of children. These lesions (Type II) are visible grossly in regions where the proteoglycan layer is relatively thin. Type II lesions contain layers of foam cells, some lipid in the intercellular matrix, and some lipid-containing smooth muscle cells. Smooth muscle cells in these lesions are mostly of the synthetic phenotype, and their number is not increased compared to normal intima. However, the number of macrophage-

Table 3-1 Classification and Description of Types of Atherosclerotic Lesions in Human Coronary Arteries

Type of lesion	Description	Characteristics	Age of onset
I	Isolated macrophage foam cells	Increase in macrophages and presence of isolated foam cells in proteoglycan layer; no change in intimal smooth muscle oells; lipid particles do not accumulate extracellularly	From first week of life; decreased after first year
II	Fatty streak	Increase in macrophages and presence of layers of macrophage foam cells and lipid-laden smooth muscle cells; extracellular lipid particles are present but thinly dispersed	From late first decade on (early puberty)
III	Preatheroma	All Type II changes plus multiple deposits of pooled extracellular lipid in musculoelastic layer	From mid-second decade on
IV	Atheroma	All Type III changes plus enlargement and change of musculoelastic layer by confluent extracellular lipid (lipid core); in core region, structural intimal smooth muscle cells are dispersed and decreased	From mid-second decade on
V	Fibroatheroma	All Type IV changes plus enlargement and change of upper intima by development of "collagenous cap"; increase and layering of secretory phenotype smooth muscle cells in a massive matrix of collagen	From mid-third decade on

Source: Modified from Stary.[3]

derived foam cells is increased. These cells tend to be deep in the proteoglycan layer.

More advanced, Type III lesions (preatheroma) begin to appear during the middle of the second decade of life, usually in areas of eccentric thickening. These lesions are transitional between the fatty streak and an atheroma (Type IV), and they contain substantially more extracellular lipid droplets and particles, which form aggregates in the musculoelastic layer below the layers of macrophage-derived foam cells. Most extracellular lipid is in the form of cholesterol crystals, while the foam cells contain cholesterol ester. These lipid collections replace matrix and disrupt the intimal structure, dispersing smooth muscle cells. On gross inspection, these lesions look like small white elevations, although they do not compromise the lumen.

Type IV lesions are atheromas. They appear at the end of puberty and can cause ischemic symptoms. These lesions have the same general features as preatheromas, but the lipid accumulations fuse into large lipid cores that are more destructive. These are often called necrotic cores, although the major component is lipid. Only a few scattered smooth muscle cells, some of which are dead, remain in this region. Macrophages border the lipid cores on the luminal side.

Type V lesions are referred to as fibroatheromas. They have developed a fibrous cap that consists of smooth muscle cells rich in rough endoplasmic reticulum and a dense matrix of collagen and capillaries. Thickening of this cap is accelerated by deposition of platelets and fibrin, which may be incorporated into the intima. Type V lesions appear in the third or fourth decade of life. These lesions have a lipid core that contains thick layers of newly-formed collagen. More advanced forms of Type V lesions (sometimes called Type VI lesions) contain fissures, hematomas, and thin deposits of surface thrombus. About 60 percent of persons between 30 and 39 years of age have Type III, IV, or V lesions in their coronary arteries. Stary found that lesions in the aorta are fundamentally the same as those in the coronary circulation. Carotid atherogenesis probably follows a similar pattern.

THEORIES OF ATHEROGENESIS

There are several theories of atherogenesis, each focusing on one of the principal components of the process—thrombus organization, fatty infiltration, and cellular proliferation. The encrustation theory, put forth by von Rokitansky in 1852 and subsequently modified by Duguid, focuses on the intimal thickening that results from successive layering and organization of fibrin deposits on the luminal surface. Deposited fibrin undergoes organization by fibroblasts with secondary accumulation of lipid. Virchow proposed the lipid hypothesis in 1856. He viewed the accumulation of lipid in the intima as a consequence of altered permeability of the vessel lining, resulting in transduction of blood lipid into the arterial wall.

The injury and cellular response hypothesis focuses on cellular proliferation during atherogenesis. This theory was formally proposed by Ross and Glomset in 1973[4,5] and has undergone many modifications.[6] It was based on the observation that smooth muscle cell proliferation is a prominent feature of both early atherogenesis and intimal hyperplasia following injury. The central hypothesis is that dysfunctional endothelium interacts with macrophages, platelets, and smooth muscle cells to initiate the formation of intimal lesions. The underlying endothelial injury could be caused by local hemodynamic forces, increased exposure to blood-borne atherogenic elements in regions of low shear, or cell damage caused by viral infection, immune complexes, or exposure to toxins such as oxidized LDL or components of tobacco smoke. Macrophages and T lymphocytes adhere more avidly to injured endothelium. These cells then migrate into the intima, where they take up oxidized LDL through the acetyl LDL receptor, becoming macrophage-derived foam cells.

Endothelial cell loss has been detected in areas rich in lipid-laden foam cells in fat-fed swine and monkey lesions.[1] Platelet thrombi may form where these macrophages migrate back into the vessel lumen or where endothelial injury has caused gaps in the endothelial lining.[6] Activated platelets may release many growth and migratory factors, such as platelet-derived growth factor (PDGF), that influence underlying smooth muscle cells. In addition, such products of thrombosis as thrombin may be strong stimulators of smooth muscle cell growth. T cell production of mediators such as interferon-γ may play an important regulatory role for type I collagen.[7] This cytokine may affect smooth muscle cells in the lesion, causing them to become activated and express receptors for PDGF.

In the initial response to injury hypothesis, smooth muscle cell proliferation was attributed largely to release of PDGF and other growth factors from aggregating platelets on the injured surface. However, several findings suggest a more limited role for platelet-stimulated smooth muscle cell proliferation in atherogenesis. For example, it is now known that fibroblast growth factor (FGF) released from damaged smooth muscle cells is a more important mitogen than PDGF in the early phase following traumatic arterial injury. Furthermore, endothelial disruption has not been detected in regions where early atherosclerotic lesions develop. Finally, foam cells in fatty streaks are derived primarily from macrophages rather than smooth muscle cells.[1]

ARTERIAL INJURY AS A MODEL OF PLAQUE DEVELOPMENT

Smooth muscle cells and the matrix they produce are significant components of atherosclerotic plaque. It is likely that the factors that control accumulation of these cells in the intima are similar in lesions of atherosclerosis and intimal hyperplasia following injury to normal vessels. The cellular and molecular events following arterial injury have been studied extensively in animal models.[8] This work has greatly advanced our understanding of the cellular interactions that control smooth muscle cell proliferation and function. Perhaps the best characterized model is balloon injury of the rat carotid artery. This form of injury completely denudes the endothelium and causes loss of approximately 20 percent of the smooth muscle cells in the media. Similar injuries are likely to result from endarterectomy or balloon angioplasty in human arteries. A more limited endothelial cell loss without underlying smooth muscle cell damage occurs during development of atherosclerotic lesions.

Within minutes of arterial injury, the denuded vessel surface is covered with a sheet of platelets which adhere, spread, and degranulate, releasing smooth muscle cell mitogens and chemoattractants, such as transforming growth factor β, PDGF, and an epidermal growth factor-like protein. However, thrombosis is a limited phenomenon; after one day, very little further platelet accumulation occurs, perhaps because plasma proteins coat the surface and prevent platelet adhesion. Smooth muscle cells synchronously enter the cell cycle within hours of the injury.[9] Thereafter, the number of nondividing cells remains constant, suggesting that these cells either proliferate within the first 48 h after injury or not at all.

Both proliferating and nonproliferating cells may migrate across the internal elastic lamina onto the luminal surface, where proliferation continues. Rates of cell division reach a peak by 48 h after injury, at which time 40 percent have entered the cell cycle. Proliferation rates drop to 20 percent by one week and reach quiescent levels (0.05 percent) by four weeks.

In this early phase, the arterial wall thickens, owing to both smooth muscle cell proliferation and matrix production (collagen, elastin, and proteoglycans) by these cells. Wall thickening continues for up to three months, well after proliferation has ceased, owing to continued matrix production (Fig. 3-3).

This hyperplastic process consists of two distinct smooth muscle cell responses—proliferation and migration from the media across the internal elastic lamina to the intima. Recent studies suggest that proliferation is stimulated primarily by smooth muscle cell damage at the time of the injury, whereas migration is caused by the release of platelet products. An important role for platelets in stimulating cellular proliferation was suggested by the early work of Friedman and coworkers, who demonstrated reduced intimal hyperplasia following balloon injury in rabbits rendered thrombocytopenic with antiplatelet antibodies.[10] More recent studies using thrombocytopenic rats indicate that the primary role of platelets is stimulation of migration rather than proliferation.[11] This is consistent with the finding that very little smooth muscle cell proliferation takes place when the endothelium is gently denuded using a fine nylon loop that does not injure smooth muscle cells in the media.[12,13] Finally, studies using direct infusion of PDGF or antibodies to it reveal that the main role of this growth factor is to stimulate smooth muscle cell migration rather than proliferation.[14,15]

Smooth muscle cells are capable of synthesizing many growth factors, and these may be secreted at an increased rate following injury, thus stimulating proliferation in a paracrine fashion. When grown in culture, smooth muscle cells derived from injured arterial media produce up to five times more PDGF than do cells from uninjured arteries.[16] Smooth mus-

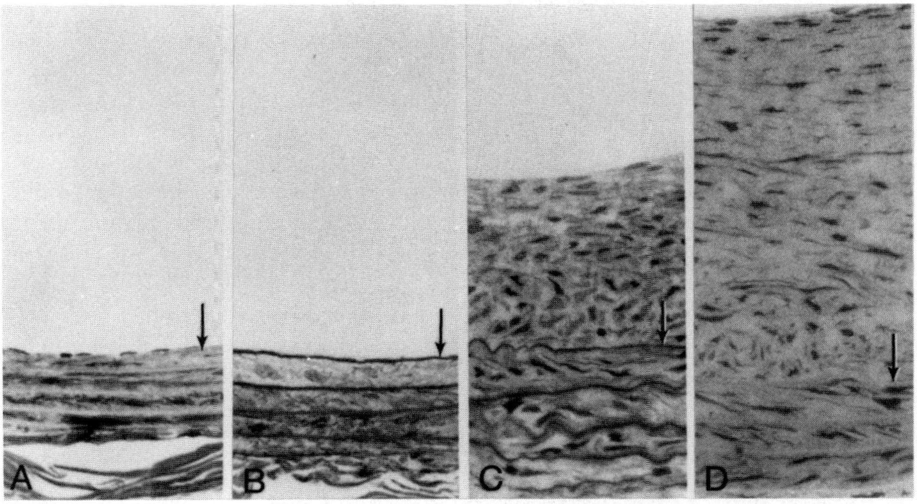

Figure 3-3. Histologic cross-sections of the region lacking endothelium from injured carotid arteries: *A.* Normal vessel. Note single layer of endothelium in intima. *B.* Denuded vessel at 2 days. Note loss of endothelium. *C.* Denuded vessel at 2 weeks. Intima is now markedly thickened because of smooth muscle proliferation. *D.* Denuded vessel at 12 weeks. Further intimal thickening has occurred. Internal elastic lamina is indicated by arrow. Lumen is at the top. Original magnification × 260. (*From Clowes.*[55] *Reproduced with permission.*)

cle cells from balloon-injured carotid arteries also express mRNA for insulin-like growth factor[17] and transforming growth factor β (unpublished data), which are mitogenic for smooth muscle cells in culture. Basic fibroblast growth factor (bFGF) is synthesized by the arterial wall and may be released when smooth muscle cells are injured.[18] Infusion of bFGF following gentle denudation of the rat carotid artery markedly increases smooth muscle cell proliferation.[18] Conversely, systemic injection of a neutralizing antibody against bFGF before balloon injury decreases the induced smooth muscle cell proliferation by approximately 80 percent.[19] These data suggest that endogenous bFGF is the major mitogen controlling the growth of vascular smooth muscle cells following injury.

In the balloon injury model, smooth muscle cells stop proliferating after several weeks. This may occur because mitogens such as bFGF released after injury become depleted or from active inhibition of proliferation. Cytokines released from lymphocytes in the vessel wall may inhibit smooth muscle cell growth. Hansson and associates demonstrated that interferon-γ, a secretory product of activated T lymphocytes, inhibits smooth muscle cell proliferation in vitro and induces the expression of class II major histocompatibility complex antigens (Ia).[20] These workers found a strong negative correlation in vivo between Ia expression and proliferation of intimal smooth muscle cells following balloon injury, suggesting that interferon-γ regulates smooth muscle cell growth following injury.

The endothelium also can produce factors that inhibit smooth muscle cell growth. In the rat balloon injury model, smooth muscle cells stop proliferating much sooner in regions where the endothelium has regrown. This may be because luminal smooth muscle cells, unlike endothelial cells, form loose junctions that allow nutrients and mitogens to enter the arterial wall. Alternatively, the endothelium may secrete molecules that inhibit smooth muscle cell growth, such as heparan sulfate. The endothelium is capable of producing both growth promoters (transforming growth factor β, PDGF, FGF, and interleukin-1) and growth inhibitors (heparan sulfate and endothelium-derived relaxing factor).[21–25] Heparan sulfate, when released from its proteoglycan, can inhibit smooth muscle cell growth. The anticoagulant drug heparin is a related molecule and is a potent inhibitor of neointimal growth in the rat injury model.

ATHEROSCLEROSIS AT THE CAROTID BIFURCATION

Shear is an important determinant of wall thickening in atherosclerosis, as it is in intimal hyperplasia in vein grafts and injured arteries. Atherosclerosis tends to occur in areas of reduced or oscillating shear, such as the lateral aspect of the carotid bulb (Fig. 3-4).[26–29] This arterial segment is unique in that the internal carotid branch of the common carotid artery is normally wider than the parent vessel. Flow studies using Plexiglas models and duplex scanning of human carotid bifurcations reveal flow separation and secondary vortex formation in the region of the lateral bulb where intimal thickening and plaque formation are most prominent (Figs. 3-5 and 3-6). In contrast, the medial region of the bulb, which contains the flow divider, has high and unidirectional shear forces and is relatively spared of atherosclerosis.

A similar pattern of plaque formation occurs in other regions of low shear, such as the proximal rim of the origins of lumbar and visceral aortic branches and the lateral walls of the aortic bifurcation.[29] Several possible mechanisms for this propensity for atherosclerosis in regions of low shear have been outlined in the review by Glagov and associates.[29]

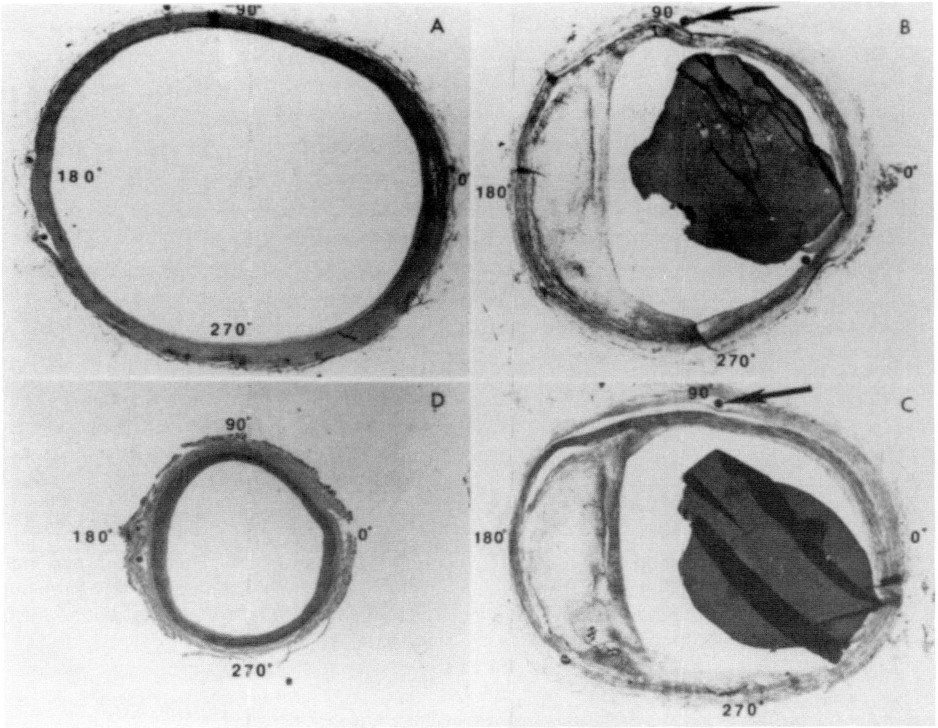

Figure 3-4. Serial histologic preparations of transverse sections though a typical carotid bifurcation. *A.* Common carotid artery. *B.* Proximal internal carotid artery. *C.* Midpoint of carotid bulb. *D.* Distal internal carotid artery. Note that plaque develops in a crescentic pattern along the lateral aspect of the carotid bulb (180° location), where flow separation causes low and oscillating shear. (*From Zarins.*[27] *Reproduced with permission.*)

Low shear causes increased residence time of blood particles adjacent to the luminal surface. Model flow systems demonstrate prolonged residence of bubbles in the carotid bulb after the mainstream bubbles have cleared (Fig. 3-7). Thus, the endothelium in this region has increased exposure to platelets, lipids, and any other blood-borne factors that may enhance plaque development. Endothelial cell function is also influenced by shear, and flow-induced changes in intercellular attachments or cellular metabolism could enhance atherogenesis. The barrier between the blood and the vessel wall may become leaky in regions of low shear. Atherosclerosis-prone arterial segments have increased permeability for entry of albumin into the intima. Low shear conditions may also interfere with the supply of nutrients to the endothelium and could enhance margination and attachment of monocytes and platelets to the luminal surface. Specific leukocyte-endothelial adhesion molecules are thought to mediate this attachment, and recently the endothelial expression of at least one of these ligands, intercellular adhesion molecule-1, has been found to be affected by flow in a manner that correlates with mononuclear inflammatory cell adhesion.[30,31]

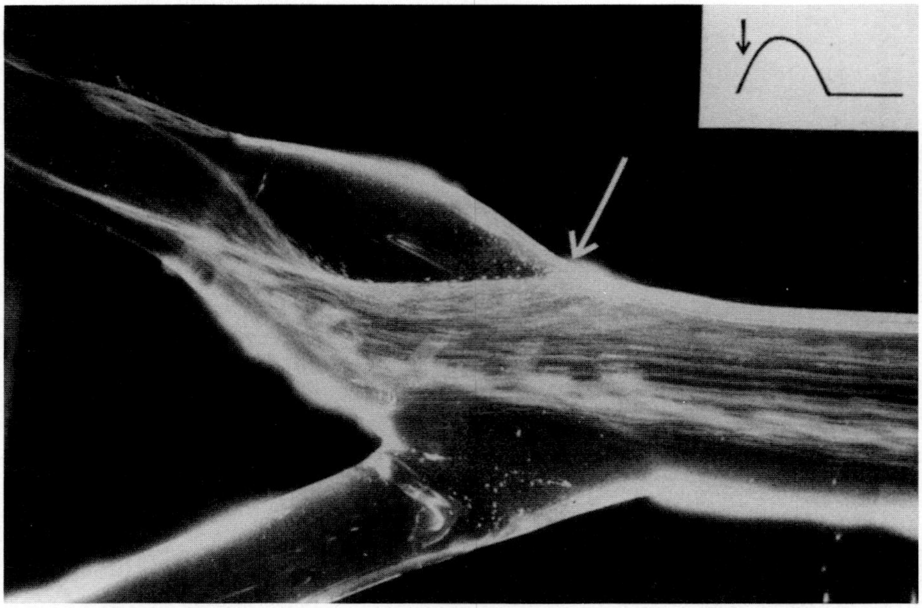

Figure 3-5. Hydrogen bubble flow visualization study in a Plexiglas model of the carotid bifurcation using a pump that simulates pulsatile carotid flow. The flow pattern is typical of early systole (insert indicates the time during the pulse cycle). The white arrow indicates the proximal point of flow separation along the outer wall of the carotid bulb. (*From Ku.*[56] *Reproduced with permission.*)

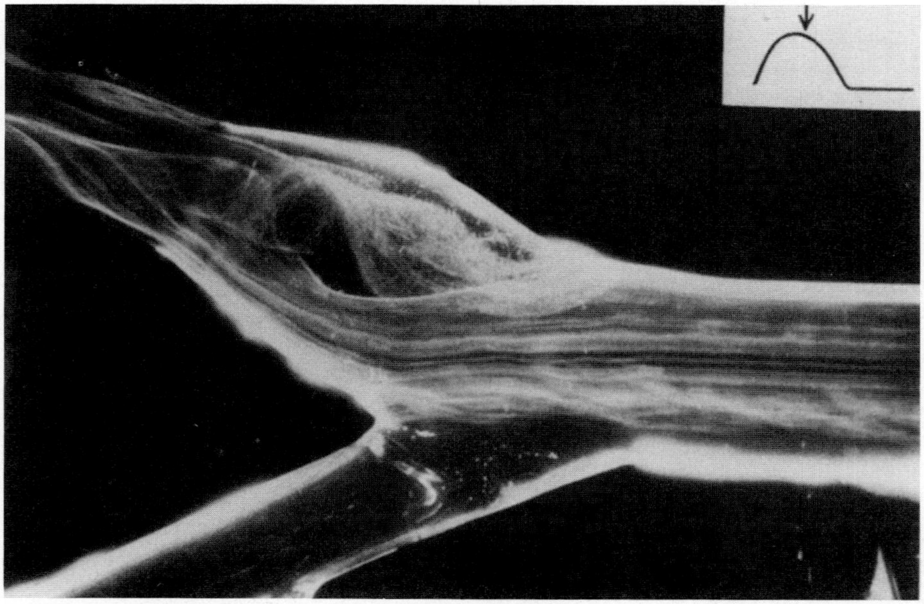

Figure 3-6. Flow visualization study, as in Fig. 3-5, demonstrating helical flow patterns during diastole. (*From Ku.*[56] *Reproduced with permission.*)

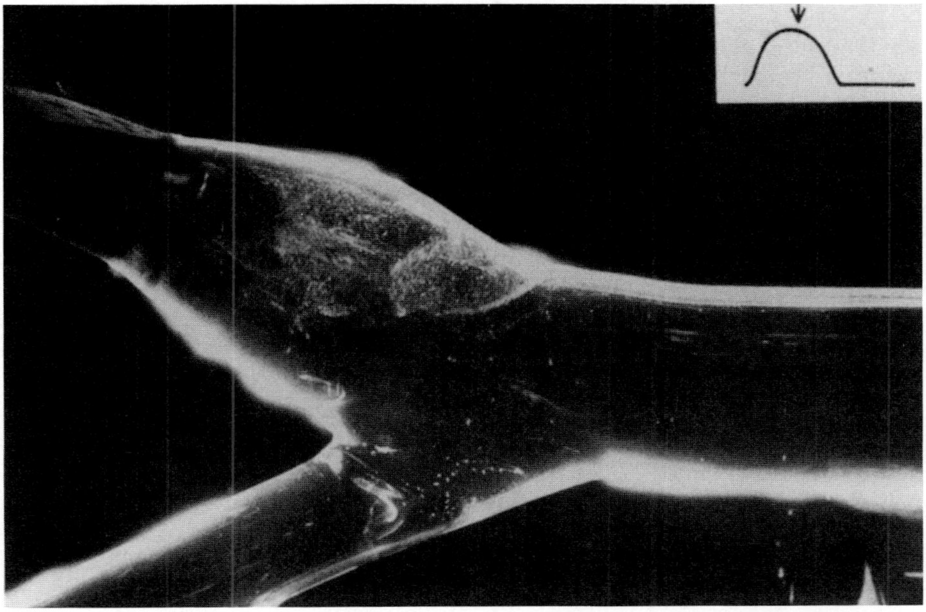

Figure 3-7. Flow visualization study, as in Fig. 3-5 and 3-6, demonstrating prolonged residence time of bubbles in the sinus region, where atherosclerosis begins. (*From Ku.*[56] *Reproduced with permission.*)

CELLULAR INTERACTIONS IN ATHEROGENESIS

Smooth muscle cells are the most abundant cell type in atherosclerotic lesions. These cells may accumulate cholesterol or other lipids, producing the vacuolated appearance of smooth muscle-derived foam cells which is characteristic of atherosclerotic plaque. Quiescent smooth muscle cells are well-differentiated, containing contractile cytoplasmic filaments and expressing smooth muscle actin, myosin, and desmin. Proliferating smooth muscle cells may lose most or all of these differentiated features. The bulk of plaque volume is composed of extracellular matrix, especially collagen, produced by smooth muscle cells.

The importance of smooth muscle cell proliferation in plaque development is now well accepted, and many growth factors have been identified that stimulate this process. Some of these, such as PDGF and FGF, have been demonstrated in human arterial lesions. PDGF has been found in regions of human carotid plaques where cells are proliferating.[32–34] Growth-promoting activities associated with penetrating microvessels in these plaques also appear to be important. Studies using the proliferating cell nuclear antigen as a marker of cell proliferation in carotid plaques reveal that smooth muscle cell proliferation occurs at a much lower rate than that observed after acute arterial injury in animal models, where there is a large but brief period of cell growth. Cell proliferation in human atherosclerotic plaques is more similar to that found in animal models of hypercholesterolemia.[35–41] This suggests that cell growth in atherogenesis is slow and indolent.

Serial angiographic and ultrasound studies have indicated that individual human plaques may differ in their rates of growth.[42,43] At least three patterns of human atherosclerotic plaque growth are theoretically possible: (1) a single, brief proliferative burst associated with some unspecified injury, followed by a long, minimally proliferative phase analogous to models of acute arterial injury; (2) several such episodes of brief proliferative activity due to repeated injuries, causing plaques to grow in an intermittent fashion; and (3) slow, indolent growth similar to animal models of hypercholesterolemia.

Macrophages are a potentially important source of growth factors that may contribute to smooth muscle cell proliferation and matrix production. Macrophages and T cells in the arterial wall are in various states of cell activation.[44,45] Activated macrophages produce more factors that stimulate smooth muscle cell growth and influence matrix deposition and composition. Macrophages also can cause endothelial injury by production of such cytotoxins as the superoxide anion and proteolytic or lipolytic enzymes.[1] Along with macrophages, plaques contain T cells and a few scattered B cells. The role of these latter cell types in atherogenesis, if any, is not yet understood. However, they clearly play an important part in transplant arteriosclerosis, which is immune-mediated, and their presence in carotid plaques suggests that they may have a similar role in standard atherogenesis.

In addition to smooth muscle cells, proliferation occurs in monocytes, macrophages, and possibly lymphocytes and endothelial cells in the process of neovascularization.[46] Thymidine labeling studies have shown that much of the proliferation occurs in foam cells, and up to one-quarter of these cells are macrophages. Plaque development proceeds under the influence of growth inhibitors and promoters released during complex interactions between endothelium, smooth muscle cells, macrophages, platelets, and lymphocytes.[47] There are many possible feedback loops (Fig. 3-8). These include production of PDGF, endothelial cell growth factor (ECGF), FGF, cytokines such as interleukin, and vasoactive molecules such as serotonin, endothelin, and endothelium-derived relaxation factor that also regulate growth. Cell injury may be caused by LDL, oxygen radicals, or hemodynamic forces. Such injury may cause the release of intracellular FGF or may modify the production of other growth regulators. Regulation of adhesion molecules also can influence the interaction of endothelium and white blood cells.

Control of matrix synthesis is a very important aspect of overall plaque growth, since the bulk of the plaque volume is extracellular matrix. The intimal matrix is composed of several proteoglycan species as well as several types of collagen. In one study, collagen constituted roughly half of total plaque protein and was a particularly prominent component of advanced, calcified atherosclerotic plaques.[48] Collagen breakdown may be an important precursor of plaque instability because it provides much of the tensile strength of the intima and the fibrous cap.

PATHOLOGY OF ADVANCED ATHEROSCLEROTIC LESIONS

Atherosclerotic vessels appear to adjust their diameter in response to blood flow conditions. Glagov and coworkers found that when human coronary arteries are moderately constricted by atherosclerotic plaque, the vessels dilate in a manner that maintains normal shear.[49] However, this process is limited, and luminal narrowing occurs when lesions become larger than 40 percent of the cross-sectional vessel area. Thus, plaques produce symptoms when they enlarge beyond the ability of the vessel to compensate or when the surface becomes unstable and thrombus forms.

Carotid plaques usually are present for decades before they become unstable and produce symptoms. The transition from a stable

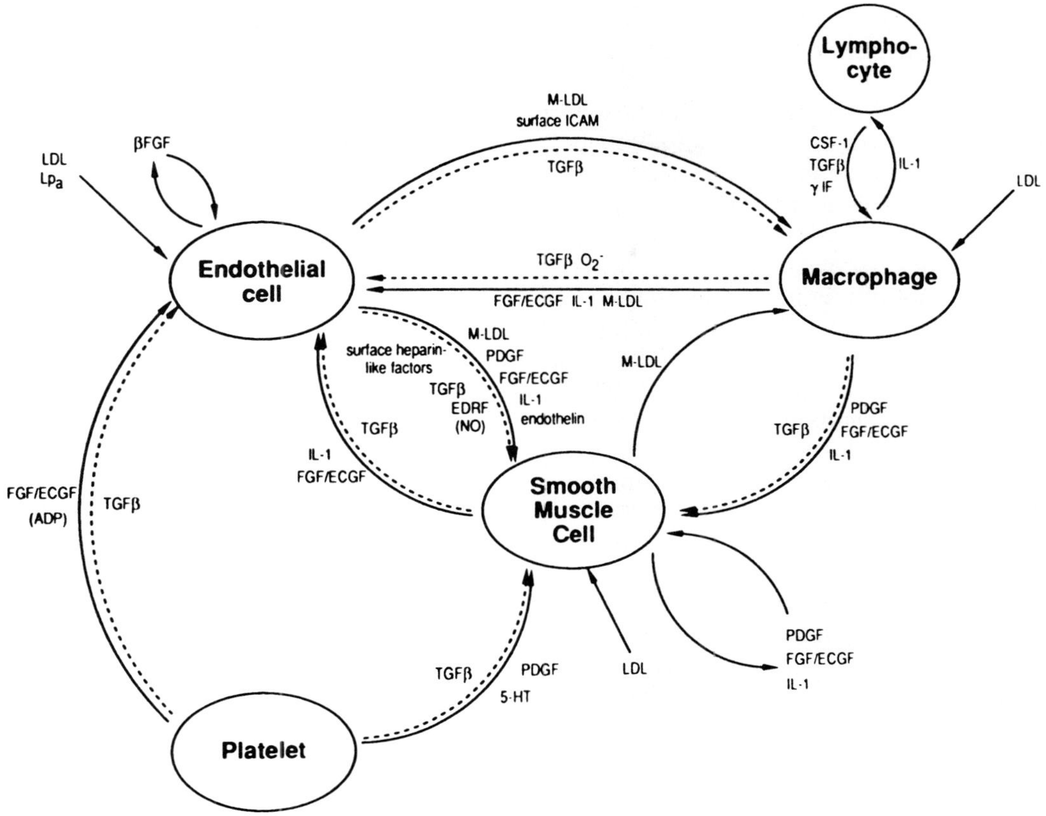

Figure 3-8. Interactions between cell types involved in progression of atherosclerosis. Cells release factors that may influence their own growth (autocrine interactions) as well as the growth of surrounding cells (paracrine interactions). Molecules with mainly stimulatory function for growth, contraction, adhesion, secretion, or gene expression are depicted with solid lines. Those with mainly inhibitory function are depicted with broken lines, except for autocrine and lymphocyte interactions, which are depicted with only solid lines for simplicity. Abbreviations: platelet-derived growth factor (PDGF), endothelial cell growth factor group (FGF/ECGF), interleukin (IL-1), transforming growth factor (TGF), serotonin (5-HT), endothelial-derived relaxation factor (EDRF), nitric oxide (NO), adenosine-5 diphosphate (ADP), low density lipoproteins (LDL Lp(a), M-LDL), colony stimulating factor (CSF), intercellular adhesion molecules (ICAM). (*From Hathaway.*[47] *Reproduced with permission.*)

to an unstable state is likely to involve such factors as disruption of the fibrous cap, local hemodynamic patterns, and certain plaque characteristics such as intraplaque hemorrhage, the extent of central necrosis, and the composition of the matrix. Noninvasive determination of plaque composition with ultrasound, magnetic resonance imaging, or other techniques may enhance our ability to predict which lesions will produce symptoms. Unfortunately, efforts to relate the plaque characteristics noted on imaging studies with the plaque morphology seen on histologic examination have been difficult, and definite correlation with the clinical course is also lacking.[50,51] These efforts are continuing, however, and may be aided by improvements in imaging techniques and better understanding of the pathologic process.

Advanced lesions are typically eccentric with a central core consisting of free lipid, cholesterol crystals, and areas of calcification. Focal calcification is commonly seen in the necrotic cores and frequently involves other acellular fibrous regions of the plaque as well. Calcification usually is considered to be dystrophic, with dead cellular debris forming a nidus for calcium phosphate crystal formation. However, the recent demonstration of specific proteins such as osteopontin and morphogenic bone protein in such lesions suggests that the biology of plaque calcification is similar to early bone formation.[52]

Cholesterol in advanced atherosclerotic plaques is derived from dying foam cells or conversion of LDL within the matrix. The arterial media is not typically involved, but it may become thin in regions of marked intimal thickening. Although capillaries grow into these lesions, they may not provide adequate nutrient supply to the central core, leading to necrosis. The fibrous cap overlying the plaque is composed of dense connective tissue with some smooth muscle cells. Rupture of this cap, possibly as a result of local hemodynamic stresses, is accompanied by release of necrotic debris that may embolize to the cerebral circulation.

Most intraplaque hemorrhage is due to disruption of the fibrous cap. This intraplaque hemorrhage is rich in platelets and fibrin, and therefore actually represents thrombosis rather than hemorrhage. Factors contributing to cap disruption include hypertension, arterial stenosis, decreased collagen content in the cap, decreased width of the cap, and the presence of a large, soft lipid core. Macrophage infiltration near the shoulder region of the plaque, where disruption most commonly occurs, may contribute to weakening of the cap through release of proteases (elastase and collagenase) that break down the extracellular matrix. Analysis of plaques that have undergone disruption and thrombosis has revealed the presence of both macrophages and T lymphocytes.[53] Macrophages contribute to thrombosis by releasing tissue factor and possibly plasminogen activator inhibitor-1.[53] Large amounts of mRNA for tissue factor are located in the plaque core around cholesterol crystals.[54] Surface thrombosis also occurs as the blood is exposed to the necrotic core with its highly thrombogenic interstitial collagen and tissue factor. Plaque fissuring is common, and healing of these lesions may contribute to plaque enlargement.[53]

Hemorrhage is often a prominent feature in unstable plaques. Bleeding may result from either rupture of the overlying fibrous cap or rupture of one of the thin-walled, capillary-like vessels prevalent in these plaques. This latter mechanism is the most likely explanation for the hemorrhage seen beneath an intact fibrous cap. These penetrating vessels appear to be derived from the vasa vasorum in the adventitia, although some may arise directly from the arterial lumen. Penetrating vessels may play an important role in supporting the growth of the developing plaque. Thrombus or hemosiderin often is found in the vicinity of these vessels, suggesting that they are prone to disrupt and cause hemorrhage. However, it may be that organizing blood components stimulate the growth of these vessels into the plaque. Angiogenic activity has been demonstrated in atherosclerotic plaques.

The pathogenesis of cerebral ischemic events resulting from atherosclerotic plaques and the mechanism of disruption of the fibrous cap are discussed in greater detail in Chap. 4.

REFERENCES

1. Steinberg D, Witztum JL: Lipoproteins and atherogenesis. *JAMA* 264:3047–3052, 1990.
2. Davies MJ, Krikler DM, Katz D: Atheroscle-

rosis: Inhibition of regression as therapeutic possibilities. *Br Heart J* 65:302–310, 1991.

3. Stary HC: Evolution and progression of atherosclerotic lesions in coronary arteries of children and young adults. *Arteriosclerosis* 9:119–132, 1989.
4. Ross R, Glomset JA: The pathogenesis of atherosclerosis (first of two parts). *N Engl J Med* 295:369–377, 1976.
5. Ross R, Glomset JA: The pathogenesis of atherosclerosis (second of two parts). *N Engl J Med* 295:420–425, 1976.
6. Ross R: The pathogenesis of atherosclerosis: A perspective for the 1990's. *Nature* 362:801–809, 1993.
7. Rekhter MD, Jhang K, Narayanan AS, et al: Type I collagen gene expression in human atherosclerosis: localization to specific plaque regions. *Am J Pathol* 143:1634–1648, 1993.
8. Clowes AW, Reidy MA, Clowes MM: Mechanisms of stenosis after arterial injury. *Lab Invest* 49:208–215, 1983.
9. Majesky MW, Schwartz SM, Clowes MM, Clowes AM: Heparin regulates smooth muscle S phase entry in the injured rat carotid artery. *Circ Res* 61:296–300, 1987.
10. Friedman RJ, Stemerman MB, Wenz B, et al: The effect of thrombocytopenia on experimental arteriosclerotic lesion formation in rabbits. Smooth muscle cell proliferation and reendothelialization. *J Clin Invest* 60:1191–1201, 1977.
11. Fingerle J, Johnson R, Clowes AW, et al: Role of platelets in smooth muscle cell proliferation and migration after vascular injury in rat carotid artery. *Proc Natl Acad Sci USA* 86:8412–8416, 1989.
12. Tada T, Reidy MA: Endothelial regeneration. IX. Arterial injury followed by rapid endothelial repair induces smooth-muscle cell proliferation but not intimal thickening. *Am J Pathol* 129:429–433, 1987.
13. Fingerle J, Au YPT, Clowes AW, Reidy MA: Intimal lesion formation in rat carotid arteries after endothelial denudation in absence of medial injury. *Arteriosclerosis* 10:1082–1087, 1990.
14. Jawien A, Bowen-Pope DF, Lindner V, et al: Platelet-derived growth factor promotes smooth muscle migration and intimal thickening in a rat model of balloon angioplasty. *J Clin Invest* 89:507–511, 1992.
15. Ferns GAA, Raines EW, Sprugel KH, et al: Inhibition of neointimal smooth muscle accumulation after angioplasty by an antibody to PDGF. *Science* 253:1129–1132, 1991.
16. Walker LN, Bowen-Pope DF, Reidy MA: Production of platelet-derived growth factor-like molecules by cultured arterial smooth muscle cells accompanies proliferation after arterial injury. *Proc Natl Acad Sci USA* 83:7311–7315, 1986.
17. Cercek B, Fishbein MC, Forrester JS, et al: Induction of insulin-like growth factor I messenger RNA in rat aorta after balloon denudation. *Circ Res* 66:1755–1760, 1990.
18. Lindner V, Lappi DA, Baird A, et al: Role of basic fibroblast growth factor in vascular lesion formation. *Circ Res* 68:106–113, 1991.
19. Lindner V, Reidy MA: Proliferation of smooth muscle cells after vascular injury is inhibited by an antibody against basic fibroblast growth factor. *Proc Natl Acad Sci USA* 88:3739–3743, 1991.
20. Hansson GK, Jonasson L, Holm J, et al: Gamma-interferon regulates vascular smooth muscle proliferation and Ia antigen expression in vivo and in vitro. *Circ Res* 63:712–719, 1988.
21. Castellot JJ Jr, Addonizio ML, Rosenberg R, Karnovsky MJ: Cultured endothelial cells produce a heparin-like inhibitor of smooth muscle cell growth. *J Cell Biol* 90:372–379, 1981.
22. Cooke JP, Stamler J, Andon N, et al: Flow stimulates endothelial cells to release a nitrovasodilator that is potentiated by reduced thiol. *Am J Physiol Heart Circ Physiol* 259:H804–H812, 1990.
23. Buga GM, Gold ME, Fukuto JM, Ignarro LJ: Shear stress-induced release of nitric oxide from endothelial cells grown on beads. *Hypertension* 17:187–193, 1991.
24. Ralevic V, Milner P, Hudlicka O, et al: Substance P is released from the endothelium of normal and capsaicin-treated rat hind-limb vasculature, in vivo, by increased flow. *Circ Res* 66:1178–1183, 1990.
25. Hsieh H-J, Li N-Q, Frangos JA: Shear stress increases endothelial platelet-derived growth

factor mRNA levels. *Am J Physiol Heart Circ Physiol* 260:H642–H646, 1991.

26. Ku DN, Giddens DP, Zarins C, Glagov S: Pulsatile flow and atherosclerosis in the human carotid bifurcation. *Arteriosclerosis* 5:293–302, 1985.
27. Zarins CK, Giddens DP, Bharadvaj BK, et al: Carotid bifurcation atherosclerosis: Quantitative correlation of plaque localization with flow velocity profiles and wall shear stress. *Circ Res* 53:502–514, 1983.
28. Friedman MH, Hutchins GM, Bargeron CB, et al: Correlation between intimal thickness and fluid shear in human arteries. *Atherosclerosis* 39:425–436, 1981.
29. Glagov S, Zarins C, Giddens DP, Ku DN: Hemodynamics and atherosclerosis. Insights and perspectives gained from studies of human arteries. *Arch Pathol Lab Med* 112:1018–1031, 1988.
30. Resnick N, Collins T, Atkinson W, et al: Platelet-derived growth factor B chain promoter contains a cis-acting fluid shear-responsive element. *Proc Natl Acad Sci USA* 90:4591–4595, 1993.
31. Walpola PL, Gotlieb AI, Langille BL: Monocyte adhesion and changes in endothelial cell number, morphology, and F-actin distribution elicited by low shear stress in vivo. *Am J Pathol* 142:1392–1400, 1993.
32. Wilcox JN, Smith KM, Williams LT, et al: Platelet-derived growth factor mRNA detection in human atherosclerotic plaques by in situ hybridization. *J Clin Invest* 82:1134–1143, 1988.
33. Brogi E, Winkles JA, Underwood R, et al: Distinct patterns of expression of fibroblast growth factors and their receptors in human atheroma and nonatherosclerotic arteries: Association of acidic FGF with plaque microvessels and macrophages. *J Clin Invest* 92:2408–2418, 1993.
34. Ross R, Masuda J, Raines EW, et al: Localization of PDGF-B protein in macrophages in all phases of atherogenesis. *Science* 248:1009–1012, 1990.
35. Katsuda S, Coltrera MD, Ross R, Gown AM: Human atherosclerosis: IV. Immunocytochemical analysis of cell activation and proliferation in lesions of young adults. *Am J Pathol* 142:1787–1793, 1993.
36. O'Brien ER, Alpers CE, Stewart DK, et al: Proliferation in primary and restenotic coronary atherectomy tissue: Implications for antiproliferative therapy. *Circ Res* 73:223–231, 1993.
37. Kim DN, Schmee J, Lee KT, Thomas WA: Atherosclerotic lesions in the coronary arteries of hyperlipidemic swine. *Atherosclerosis* 64:231–242, 1987.
38. Kim DN, Imai H, Schee J, et al: Intimal cell mass-derived atherosclerotic lesions in the abdominal aorta of hyperlipidemic swine. Part I. Cell of origin, cell divisions, and cell losses in the first 90 days on diet. *Atherosclerosis* 56:169–188, 1985.
39. Kim DN, Schmee J, Ho HT, Thomas WA: The "turning off" of excessive cell replicative activity in advanced atherosclerotic lesions of swine by a regression diet. *Atherosclerosis* 71:131–142, 1988.
40. Rosenfeld ME, Ross R: Macrophage and smooth muscle cell proliferation in atherosclerotic lesions of WHHL and comparably hypercholesterolemic fat-fed rabbits. *Arteriosclerosis* 10:608–687, 1990.
41. Walker LN, Reidy MA, Bowyer DE: Morphology and cell kinetics of fatty streak lesion formation in the hypercholesterolemic rabbit. *Am J Pathol* 125:450–459, 1986.
42. Roederer GO, Langlois YE, Lusiani L, et al: Natural history of carotid artery disease on the side contralateral to endarterectomy. *J Vasc Surg* 1:62–72, 1984.
43. Brunel P, Bourassa MG, Wiseman A: Different rates of coronary artery disease progression in patients with normal and mildly diseased coronary arteries. *Coronary Artery Dis* 2:449–454, 1991.
44. Hansson GK, Jonasson L, Seifert PS, Stemme S: Immune mechanisms in atherosclerosis. *Arteriosclerosis* 9:567–578, 1989.
45. Libby P, Hansson GK: Involvement of the immune system in human atherogenesis: Current knowledge and unanswered questions. *Lab Invest* 64:5–15, 1991.
46. Villaschi S, Spagnoli LG: Autoradiographic

and ultrastructural studies on the human fibroatheromatous plaque. *Atherosclerosis* 48:95–100, 1983.

47. Hathaway DR, March KL: Molecular cardiology: New avenues for the diagnosis and treatment of cardiovascular disease. *J Am Coll Cardiol* 13:265–282, 1989.
48. Smith EB: The influence of age and atherosclerosis on the chemistry of aortic intima. *J Atheroscler Res* 55:241–248, 1965.
49. Glagov S, Weisenberg E, Zarins CK, Stankunavicius R: Compensatory enlargement of human atherosclerotic coronary arteries. *N Engl J Med* 316:1371–1375, 1987.
50. Bassiouny HS, Davis H, Massawa N, et al: Critical carotid stenosis: Morphological and chemical similarity between symptomatic and asymptomatic plaques. *J Vasc Surg* 9:202–212, 1989.
51. Imparato AM, Riles TS, Gorstein F: The carotid bifurcation plaque: Pathologic findings associated with cerebral ischemia. *Stroke* 10:238–245, 1979.
52. Bostrom K, Watson KE, Horn S, et al: Bone morphogenetic protein expression in human atherosclerotic lesions. *J Clin Invest* 91:1800–1809, 1993.
53. Fuster V, Badimon L, Badimon JJ, Chesebro JH: The pathogenesis of coronary artery disease and the acute coronary syndromes. *N Engl J Med* 326:242–250, 1992.
54. Haudenschild CC: Pathogenesis of atherosclerosis: State of the art. *Cardiovasc Drug Ther* 4(suppl 5):993–1004, 1990.
55. Clowes AW, Reidy MA, Clowes MM: Kinetics of cellular proliferation after arterial injury. I. Smooth muscle growth in the absence of endothelium. *Lab Invest* 49:327–333, 1983.
56. Ku DN, Giddens DP: Pulsatile flow in a model carotid bifurcation. *Arteriosclerosis* 3:331–339, 1983.

4

Mechanisms of Cerebral Ischemia

Ted R. Kohler

Cerebral ischemic events may be considered as either hemorrhagic or ischemic. Purely ischemic events result from intrinsic vessel occlusion (thrombotic infarction) or embolization from the heart or ulcerated atherosclerotic plaques in the arteries supplying the brain. The relative incidence of hemorrhagic and ischemic events varies among different ethnic groups. The percentage of ischemic strokes is higher in Caucasians than in Asians, and primary intracerebral or subarachnoid hemorrhage is much more common in blacks than in whites.[1] Embolism from atherosclerotic plaques in the extracranial cerebrovascular system is the most common cause of cerebral infarction, and cardiogenic emboli are the second most common cause.[2,3] Approximately 60 percent of ischemic strokes are thrombotic or thromboembolic in association with large artery atherosclerosis, 20 percent are due to penetrating artery disease (lipohyalinosis—hyalin changes in small arteries and arterioles resulting in thickened, fibrotic vessels prone to thrombosis), 15 percent are related to cardiovascular emboli, and the remaining 5 percent are due to miscellaneous other causes.[1] Altogether, thromboembolism is responsible for over 80 percent of strokes.[4] This chapter will focus on cerebral ischemia caused by extracranial cerebrovascular disease.

CEREBRAL EVENTS RESULTING FROM ATHEROSCLEROTIC LESIONS

The problem with all studies of stroke etiology is the difficulty in distinguishing between the various causes of stroke. Even at autopsy it may be difficult to differentiate embolism from primary thrombosis as the cause of occlusion in a cerebral vessel. For example, the National Survey of Stroke reported the distribution of strokes to be 82.4 percent thrombotic, 12.2 percent hemorrhagic, and only 5.4 percent embolic.[5] However, strokes were considered thrombotic if arteriography revealed stenosis or obstruction of cerebral, carotid, or vertebral arteries, and embolic if a likely source of emboli was present, including cardiac or carotid atherosclerosis. Based on this classification, many strokes caused by emboli arising in the carotid circulation would be inappropriately categorized as thrombotic.

The importance of the carotid bifurcation as a source for cerebral emboli was evident in the findings of the Joint Study of Extracranial Arterial Occlusion. This study began in 1959, when DeBakey organized 24 institutions to assess prospectively the role of arteriography and extracranial arterial surgery in the evaluation and treatment of patients with cerebral ischemia.[6] Between 1961 and 1965 a total of 4748 patients were entered into the study. Although a few asymptomatic patients were included, most had ischemic symptoms. Patients with bloody cerebrospinal fluid were specifically excluded. Arterial lesions at surgically accessible sites were noted in 74.5 percent of the patients (Fig. 4-1).[7] The carotid bifurcation was by far the most common site of disease. Approximately one-third of the patients had lesions adjacent to or within the origin of the internal carotid artery.

In 1988 Bogousslavsky and associates reported on 1000 patients with a first stroke who were entered into the Lausanne Stroke Registry.[2] This registry was not population-based but included all patients referred to the Centre Hospitalier Universitaire Vaudois, which is the only public hospital serving Lausanne's 200,000 inhabitants. Consequently, this study tended to exclude strokes that were immediately fatal or rapidly reversible. All patients underwent computed tomography (CT) of the head and Doppler ultrasonography of the ca-

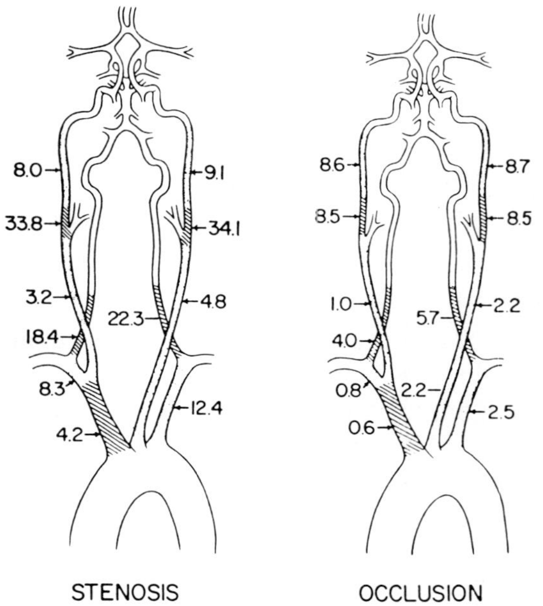

Figure 4-1. Distribution of extracranial arterial lesions (percent) at surgically accessible sites in 4748 patients in the Joint Study of Extracranial Arterial Occlusion. (*Modified from Hass.*[7])

rotid arteries, as well as electrocardiography and routine blood and urine tests. Strokes in these 1000 patients were due to infarction in 89.1 percent and hemorrhage in 10.9 percent. The presenting clinical features of a stroke did not correlate with the cause. Smoking and hypertension were the most common risk factors. Infarcts were located in the carotid territory in 71 percent and in the vertebrobasilar territory in 29 percent. The Harvard Cooperative Stroke Registry reported that approximately 75 percent of embolic strokes occurred in the distribution of the middle cerebral artery, whereas only 3 percent were in the anterior cerebral artery circulation.[4] This is most likely due to the greater amount of blood flow carried by the middle cerebral artery.

Table 4-1 summarizes the etiology of carotid territory infarcts in the Lausanne Stroke Registry. Atherosclerosis was the cause in nearly half of the patients (45.4 percent); only about 20 percent were cardioembolic. Most strokes were related to atherosclerosis, cardioembolic disease, or hypertension. While strokes involving the deep cerebral structures were more likely to be hemorrhagic, the majority of superficial territory strokes were due to atherosclerosis. A transient ischemic attack (TIA) more often preceded an infarct than a hemorrhage. Doppler studies or arteriography revealed a 50 percent or greater diameter stenosis or a total occlusion in 55 percent of patients with internal carotid artery territory infarcts. One-third of the strokes in the territory of a deep penetrating artery occurred in the absence of hypertension and in association with atherosclerotic lesions, suggesting that many lacunar infarcts may be caused by atheroembolism. The authors reviewed the results of 15 prior studies involving 11,230 patients with stroke. Overall, 59 percent of these patients had atherosclerosis and 17 percent had embolic heart disease. The Lausanne group attributed the lower rate of stroke due to atherosclerosis in their study to misclassification of hypertensive lacunar infarcts in the other studies and more accurate diagnosis of cardioembolic disease in their study.

Table 4-1 Etiology of Carotid Territory Cerebral Infarcts from the Lausanne Stroke Registry[a]

Etiology	Entire MCA (*n* = 77)	Deep MCA (*n* = 193)	Superficial MCA (*n* = 311)	ACA (*n* = 20)	Entire ICA (*n* = 8)	Watershed (*n* = 23)	Total
Atherosclerosis with stenosis	38	16	35	0	12.5	75	29.6
Atherosclerosis without stenosis	12	9	20	50	0	4	15.8
Total atherosclerosis	50	25	55	50	12.5	79	45.4
Emboligenic heart disease	25	8	24	35	0	9[b]	18.7
Combined atherosclerosis and emboligenic	5	2	4	0	12.5	4	3.5
Hypertensive	0	47	0	0	0	0	14.4
Combined hypertensive and emboligenic	0	6	0	0	0	0	1.8
Arterial dissection	15	1	3	5	25	4	4.2
Other etiologies	0	4	5	0	37.5	0	4.2
Undetermined	5	7	9	10	12.5	4	7.8

[a]Data are percent of column. MCA = middle cerebral artery; ACA = anterior cerebral artery; ICA = internal carotid artery; PCA = posterior cerebral artery.

[b]Hemodynamic cardiac cause (no embolism): hypotension due to acute bradycardia.

SOURCE: Modified from Bogousslavsky.[2]

ASSOCIATION OF CEREBRAL ISCHEMIA WITH CAROTID DISEASE

In the 1800s most physicians thought that strokes were caused by intracranial arterial disease, either vessel spasm or thrombosis. This belief was due in part to the early focus of neurologists and neuropathologists on cerebral pathology and its relationship to symptoms. In addition, during that period the extracranial carotid arteries were not studied at autopsy because they were preserved for use in embalming the head and neck. Furthermore, diagnosis of carotid occlusive disease during life was not possible until the development of cerebral arteriography, which followed the initial report by Moniz in 1927.[8]

Gowers was the first to link stroke with extracranial vascular disease when in 1875 he reported a patient with right hemiplegia and blindness in the left eye associated with occlusion of the left carotid artery.[9] This report was largely ignored until the early 1900s, when several reports appeared describing optic atrophy and contralateral hemiplegia in association with carotid occlusion.[10,11] In 1914 Hunt emphasized the importance of cervical artery obstructive disease as a cause of "softening of the brain."[12] He drew the analogy between cerebral and lower extremity arterial occlusive disease and urged that all patients with cerebral symptoms of vascular origin have a detailed arterial examination. However, routine cerebral arteriography was still not to be available for several decades.

In 1937, ten years after his first report, Moniz documented carotid artery occlusion by arteriography. Subsequently, Johnson and Walker described the association between internal carotid artery thrombosis and cerebral symptoms in 500 arteriograms of patients suspected of having brain tumor or aneurysm.[13] They pointed out that patients with carotid occlusion may present with transient attacks of headache, hemiparesis, paresthesias, and aphasia, usually of sudden onset and lasting only minutes to an hour.

After the association between extracranial carotid artery disease and cerebral ischemia was recognized, it was still not known how these fixed arterial lesions might cause intermittent symptoms. For decades it was assumed that vasospasm played an important role in cerebral ischemia. This was suggested by Fisher in 1951 in his description of intermittent neurologic symptoms in four patients with carotid occlusion.[14] Treatment aimed at relieving symptoms by reducing spasm with vasodilating drugs, segmental carotid artery resection, or cervical sympathectomy was unsuccessful. These findings, and experimental data suggesting that cerebral vessels are not prone to spasm, stimulated a search for other mechanisms to explain transient cerebral ischemic events.[15]

The "hypotensive crisis" theory gained popularity in the 1950s. This theory proposed that brief episodes of hypotension, together with cerebrovascular occlusive disease, caused vascular insufficiency and cerebral symptoms. In 1957 Hutchinson and Yates advanced this theory in their report on the association between carotid occlusion and cerebral infarction in 83 patients who died of stroke.[16] In the same year, Denny-Brown and Meyer demonstrated that hypotension induced temporary hemiplegia in monkeys with experimental carotid occlusion.[17] Corday, Rothenberg, and Weiner were also proponents of the hypotensive crisis theory, and in 1956 they published clinical and experimental observations to support it.[18] They produced hemorrhagic shock in monkeys with right internal carotid artery stenosis and demonstrated more profound EEG changes on the side of the compromised carotid artery.

By the early 1960s the importance of embolism from carotid plaques was becoming recognized. However, hypotension was still considered a significant cause of ischemic cerebral events.[19] Several important clinical observations that contradicted the hypotensive crisis theory eventually caused it to be abandoned. Fazekas and Alman reported nine patients with TIA who inadvertently had acute hypotension induced by vagal stimulation during carotid puncture.[20] These patients were noted to have marked decreases in cerebral blood flow associated with generalized cerebral ischemia but did not develop focal neurologic symptoms. Millikan observed that transient hypotension is rarely found in patients with intermittent cerebrovascular insufficiency.[21] In fact, focal ischemic symptoms tend not to be related to position or postural hypotension. Drake and Drake noted that posturally-related transient ischemic events are much more likely to be caused by vascular insufficiency of the brain stem.[22] Furthermore, although medical treatment of hypertension is often associated with transitory positional light-headedness, focal ischemic symptoms are rare. As further evidence against the hypotensive crisis theory of cerebral symptoms, Russell and Cranston measured ophthalmic artery pressures and observed low pressures in asymptomatic patients with complete internal carotid artery occlusion and normal pressures in symptomatic patients with carotid stenosis.[23] Many authors have noted that intermittent cerebral symptoms usually stop after the internal carotid artery occludes. This obviously would not be the case if decreased blood flow were the primary mechanism of these symptoms.

Several workers unsuccessfully attempted to reproduce cerebral symptoms in patients by deliberately reducing blood pressure using a combination of drugs and a tilt table. Kendall and Marshall studied 37 patients with TIA. Blood pressure was reduced until signs of generalized cerebral ischemia or loss of consciousness occurred.[24] About half the patients developed focal signs, but most did so only after developing signs of generalized ischemia. The authors concluded that the then popular "haemodynamic crisis" hypothesis should be abandoned. They argued against the prevailing reluctance of physicians to treat hypertension and against the practice of treating cerebrovascular disease with pressor agents.

THE EMBOLIC THEORY

Chiari is credited with the first observation, made in 1905, that cerebral emboli may arise from arterial ulceration and thrombosis at the carotid bifurcation.[25] The embolic theory of cerebrovascular ischemia gained acceptance in the mid-1900s as many studies demonstrated the common occurrence of atherosclerotic disease in the extracranial cerebrovascular system. Several authors noted that patients with cerebral ischemic symptoms had a much higher prevalence of high-grade stenoses and occlusions than did asymptomatic patients.

In 1951 Fisher noted that study of the cervical portions of the carotid arteries at autopsy frequently could explain the cause of premortem cerebrovascular events.[14] He found a 9.5 percent prevalence of advanced carotid disease in 432 routine autopsies. This was about the same frequency as that of cerebral hemorrhage and hypertensive atherosclerotic cerebral disease, and slightly less than cerebral embolism. He noted that most of the arterial disease was atherosclerotic and was confined to the carotid bulb, with remarkable sparing of the more distal internal carotid artery. Fisher described ulceration of the plaque, hemorrhage within the plaque, mural thrombus, and thrombus formation distal to extremely tight carotid lesions, presumably due to slow flow beyond the stenosis. He observed that thrombosis of the carotid bulb often was followed by distal progression of thrombosis to the level of the ophthalmic or cerebral branches of the internal carotid artery. While he noted that total occlusion of the internal carotid artery may be clinically silent, hemiplegia was the most common presentation. This neurologic deficit usually developed slowly in a stuttering fashion over days or was preceded by prodromal symptoms consisting of fleeting attacks of paralysis, paresthesia, dysphasia, or monocular blindness. Because cerebral arteriography was still not widely available at the time Fisher wrote this article, diagnosis of carotid artery disease depended on palpation of the neck vessels, and the association between the arterial and clinical findings was circumstantial. Fisher noted the dubious value of cervical sympathetic block, which was then popular, and postulated that ". . . it is even conceivable that some day vascular surgery will find a way to by-pass the occluded portion of the artery during the period of ominous fleeting symptoms."

It was also recognized in the mid-1900s that advanced atherosclerosis can cause cholesterol emboli to the kidneys, spleen, and pancreas.[26,27] Compelling evidence for embolization in the territory of the carotid artery came from the finding of atherosclerotic debris in the ocular fundi of patients with cerebrovascular symptoms. In 1958 Hollenhorst first reported his observations of bright plaques in the retinal vessels. He later reported similar findings in 27 of 235 patients with carotid artery occlusive disease.[28,29] Many of these plaques had the optical characteristics of crystals. He observed that the plaques could remain stationary or could break up and lodge at successively smaller bifurcations until they finally disappeared. Similar lesions were noted in six of 35 patients who had recently undergone carotid endarterectomy. Cholesterol debris from human atherosclerotic lesions injected into the carotid arteries of monkeys produced retinal findings very similar to those seen in patients with carotid artery disease.[30] Most of these emboli tended to pass rapidly through the retinal vessels and disappear. Hollenhorst found that 63 percent of patients with retinal emboli had symptoms or signs of cerebral ischemia. The association between retinal emboli and emboli to the cerebral circulation was emphasized by noting that in 79 percent of the patients with both cerebral symptoms and retinal findings, crystals were lodged in the ipsilateral eye.

In 1959 Fisher reported his observation of emboli in the ocular fundus of a patient during two episodes of amaurosis fugax.[31] Arteriography demonstrated an ipsilateral carotid bulb narrowing. Fisher remarked that in the past transient neurologic deficits were attributed to ". . . vasospasm, fluctuation in the systemic blood pressure, progressive thrombosis, multiple embolism, or a reduction in intracranial circulation related to upright posture." From his observations he concluded that ". . . intracranial transient ischaemic episodes—at least in some instances—will also find their explanation in the occurrence of local cerebral embolism or microembolism analogous to the process witnessed in the retinal circulation of our patient."

In 1972 Kollarits and coworkers reported that arteriography identified carotid bifurcation disease as the source of emboli in nearly 100 percent of patients with retinal strokes.[32] They suggested that carotid surgery may prevent progressive ocular and cerebral events in these patients. Gunning and colleagues described two patients who were observed to have white plugs passing through retinal arteries during an attack of blindness.[33] They pointed out the similarity between this phenomenon and their previous description of embolism to the upper extremity in patients with cervical rib and mural thrombus in the subclavian artery. They further noted an association between ischemic cerebral symptoms or temporary blindness and arteriographic evidence of internal carotid artery stenosis. Examination of the operative specimens from several patients undergoing carotid endarterectomy identified fresh thrombus in cases where symptoms had occurred within the preceding seven weeks, suggesting that embolic material from these mural thrombi might be the source of symptoms. They also described several cases of TIAs that could not be ascribed to hypotension or cerebral vasospasm but were associated with evidence of retinal emboli or relief of symptoms with anticoagulation.

In 1963 McBrien and coworkers provided pathologic confirmation of the nature of retinal emboli. They described the appearance of emboli in retinal vessels in a patient who became symptomatic after an ipsilateral carotid endarterectomy and eventually died.[34] At postmortem, these vessels were found to contain platelet aggregates with some leukocytes. Russell reported two cases of carotid disease associated with monocular blindness that had ophthalmoscopic or postmortem evidence of embolization.[35] He suggested that "if a localized source of emboli can be identified it may be removed." In one of the cases he presented, thromboendarterectomy of an occluded internal carotid artery was followed by massive stroke and death.

The observation of embolic material in the retinal vessels gave strong support to the embolic theory of cerebral ischemic events. Similar observations were made when it became possible to detect evidence of cerebral infarction noninvasively with CT scanning. Zukowski and colleagues reported that 88 percent of patients presenting with transient neurologic events had evidence of ipsilateral cerebral infarction by CT scan.[36] Infarcts were particularly common in patients with ulcerated carotid lesions.

One of the main problems with the embolic theory is the fact that an individual patient's repeated attacks usually involve the same symptoms. Intuitively, it would seem that emboli from an extracranial source would tend to lodge in various cerebral vessels and therefore cause varying symptoms. Kollarits and coworkers proposed that ". . . if thrombi repeatedly arise from a single focus then they may follow precisely the same anatomical course, thus giving rise to a succession of quite identical attacks of ischaemia."[32] They cited the experiments of Honour and Russell showing that injury of an artery can cause platelet emboli that follow the same path into identical peripheral arterial branches.[37] This concept was dramatically demonstrated in an experiment by Millikan and associates in which microbeads were injected at ten-minute intervals into the origin of the internal carotid artery of a monkey.[38] Figure 4-2 shows eight of these beads lined up in the same artery on the surface of the brain (Millikan CH, personal communication). Millikan and colleagues proposed that thrombi form on areas of endothelial injury, embolize, travel to a branch where they lodge for a few minutes causing symptoms, and then fragment and are carried away.[39] The location of the endothelial injury determines which vessel branch point will be temporarily occluded and therefore what symptoms will occur. They noted that while the gross characteristics of each TIA are gen-

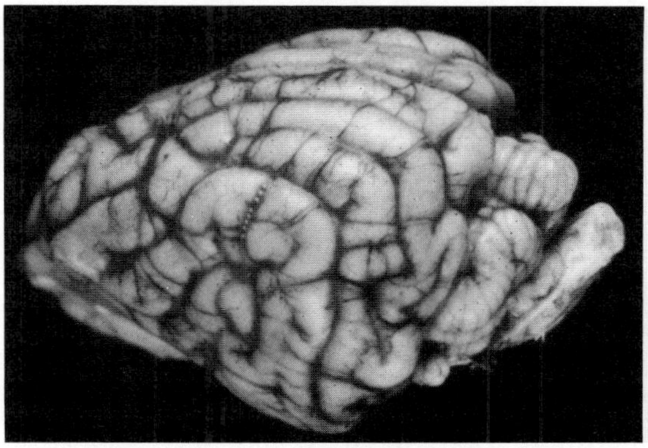

Figure 4-2. Eight microbeads injected at ten-minute intervals from the same point at the origin of the internal carotid artery lined up in a single surface vessel of the monkey brain. (*Photograph courtesy of C. H. Millikan, M.D.*)

erally the same, a careful history will often reveal slight differences from one episode to another.

The fact that anticoagulation often ameliorates neurologic symptoms supports the embolic theory. Millikan and associates stressed the importance of TIA as a precursor of cerebral infarction and first described the successful use of anticoagulation for treatment of intermittent ischemic attacks.[39] They pointed out that the previous failures of anticoagulation resulted from instituting treatment after internal carotid artery occlusion had caused a permanent deficit, rather than when the patient was suffering from intermittent symptoms and the internal carotid was still patent. Other authors described similar successes with anticoagulant therapy. Fisher reported that anticoagulants can abolish TIA and "prevent or postpone" strokes.[40]

CAROTID ENDARTERECTOMY AND CEREBRAL ISCHEMIA

The prevalence of ulceration in carotid artery plaques was pointed out by Julian and coworkers in 1963. They also noted that the presence of ulceration is often difficult to detect by arteriography.[41] Drake and Drake found that 90 percent of patients with cerebrovascular insufficiency had stenotic arterial lesions that presumably gave rise to their symptoms.[22] In a study of carotid endarterectomy specimens, Sterpetti and colleagues found that ulceration and mural thrombus were the only morphologic findings that correlated statistically with the presence of hemispheric symptoms.[42] However, during the early development of carotid endarterectomy it was thought that the principal benefit of the operation was related to an improvement in blood flow rather than removing a source of emboli.

Crawford and coworkers reported an early experience with carotid endarterectomy and noted that the most severe symptoms were associated with carotid lesions that caused a reduction in pressure.[43] This level of obstruction generally occurred when the arterial diameter was reduced by 50 percent or more. They suggested that symptoms were related to a reduction in blood flow, although flow was not directly measured. These authors measured carotid pressures at the time of operation and did not perform revascularization unless there was a significant reduction in pressure across the lesion. However, if reduced carotid blood flow were an important mechanism of cerebral ischemia, very few patients would benefit from carotid endarterectomy, since flow is not significantly reduced until lesions approach 90 percent diameter reduction. Brice, Dowsett, and Lowe studied the hemodynamic effect of acute carotid artery stenosis in patients undergoing common carotid artery ligation for berry aneurysm.[44] They found that stenoses did not reduce cerebral blood flow until they narrowed the lumen to less than two square millimeters.

Moore and Hall emphasized the importance of emboli rather than flow reduction as a cause of cerebral events. They reported the results of carotid endarterectomy in 49 symptomatic patients with irregular or ulcerated carotid plaques but no significant luminal narrowing.[45,46] The observation that most of the patients had no further neurologic symptoms following surgery was taken as evidence supporting the embolic theory of cerebral ischemia. Further evidence that symptoms of carotid disease are not caused by reduced flow comes from the observation that clamping of the carotid artery is generally well tolerated. Less than 20 percent of patients require shunting for EEG changes or neurologic symptoms (in the case of local anesthesia) during cross clamping.[47] Furthermore, cerebral blood flow is remarkably normal in patients with extracranial arterial stenoses and typically does not change after carotid endarterectomy.[48]

Perhaps the most compelling evidence for the importance of carotid bifurcation disease in cerebral ischemia is the documented efficacy of carotid endarterectomy in preventing strokes in symptomatic patients with high-grade carotid stenosis. In 1953 Strully, Hurwitt, and Blankenberg reported the feasibility of removing thrombus from the carotid artery.[49] They attempted a thrombectomy of an occluded internal carotid artery in a patient who had suffered an ipsilateral stroke, but they were unable to retrieve thrombus from the distal artery and therefore ligated it. They concluded that "A by-passing arterial anastomosis or thrombo-endarterectomy should be successful when the occlusion is localized to the cervical portion of the internal carotid artery. Early diagnosis and removal of a localized thrombus can probably result in reducing cerebral damage and prevent further insult caused by vascular insufficiency."

Early surgical treatment of cerebrovascular disease included cervical sympathectomy and arterectomy in an attempt to reduce arterial spasm. During the mid-1950s several groups reported their experience with carotid revascularization. In their 1955 report of an operation performed in 1951, Carrea, Molins, and Murphy were among the first to advocate resection of a highly stenotic or occluded internal carotid artery with reestablishment of flow by end-to-end anastomosis to the divided external carotid artery.[50] In 1954 Eastcott, Pickering, and Rob reported reconstruction of the internal carotid artery in a patient who had 32 intermittent attacks of right-sided hemiplegia, aphasia, and left eye blindness.[51] Arteriography revealed a presumed thrombus nearly occluding the origin of the left internal carotid artery. It also was noted that most of the attacks occurred at night in association with episodes of palpitations, rapid heart rate, and chest tightness. Surgery was performed with the intent of replacing the diseased segment with a graft, and the involved segment of internal carotid artery was resected under hypothermia without anticoagulation. However, the remaining vessel was sufficiently redundant to allow reconstruction by direct reanastomosis of the internal and common carotid arteries. The patient had no further cerebral symptoms. The authors noted that symptoms of this nature had previously been called "hypertensive encephalopathy" and attributed to cerebral vascular spasm, but in their opinion "to imagine that on 32 different occasions, and without any obvious cause, the arteries to the left eye and left hemisphere suddenly contracted enough to produce ischæmia while other arteries did not would constitute a considerable exercise in credulity." They noted that similar syndromes also occur with mitral stenosis and atrial fibrillation, and in these circumstances the symptoms could only be attributed to embolization; however, they failed to realize that carotid atherosclerotic plaque could be a source of embolism. In fact, the appearance of the obstructing plaque in the surgical specimen was not even described. The authors commented that "it is not easy to see how a stable obstruction, such as this was, could give rise to intermittent ischæmia unless there were periods in which arterial pressure fell low enough for long enough." They attributed the symptoms to decreased flow across the obstructing lesion during episodes of paroxysmal tachycardia and attempted to prove this by deliberately reducing the patient's blood pressure to reproduce the symptoms. Failure of this experiment was attributed to inadequate blood pressure reduction.

During the 1980s, the increasing use of carotid endarterectomy made it the most rapidly growing operation done in the United States. In 1987 an estimated 150,000 procedures were performed at an average cost of $13,000 per operation.[52] However, the dramatic increase in the number of procedures, combined with reports of unusually high complication rates, led many physicians to question the role of carotid endarterectomy in the prevention of stroke.[53,54] As a result, several randomized clinical trials were initiated to address this issue (Chaps. 16 and 17). Both the North American Symptomatic Carotid Endarterectomy Trial (NASCET) and the European Carotid Surgery Trial (ECST) demonstrated the efficacy of carotid endarterectomy for stroke prevention in patients with TIA or mild stroke and an ipsilateral 70 percent or greater diameter-reducing internal carotid stenosis by arteriography.[55–57] In the NASCET, surgery reduced the cumulative risk of stroke at two years from 26 to 9 percent in this group of patients. The NASCET data did not permit any definitive recommendations for patients with 30 to 69 percent carotid stenosis because too few patients with this degree of narrowing were entered in the study. The ECST demonstrated that patients with less than 30 percent narrowing did not benefit from surgery.

Two major prospective trials examining the role of carotid endarterectomy in asymptomatic patients also were undertaken. The Veterans Affairs Cooperative Study Group randomized 444 asymptomatic male patients with carotid stenoses of 50 percent or greater diameter reduction to either aspirin alone or aspirin plus carotid endarterectomy.[58] The incidence of all ipsilateral neurologic events (TIA, amaurosis fugax, or stroke) was significantly reduced in the surgical group (8.0 percent) compared with the medical group (20.6 percent) ($p < .001$). Although the reduction in ipsilateral stroke alone did not reach statistical significance (4.7 percent vs. 9.4 percent, $p < .06$), three of the ten strokes in the surgical group were a result of arteriography and could have been prevented by a diagnostic routine that eliminated this test (Chap. 21). Because the two groups had equivalent rates of stroke and death combined, the debate over the role of carotid endarterectomy in asymptomatic patients continues. The efficacy of carotid endarterectomy in stroke prevention appears to be less in patients who have not had symptoms. Therefore, large numbers of patients are needed to achieve adequate statistical power in clinical trials. It is hoped that the larger Asymptomatic Carotid Atherosclerosis Study sponsored by the National Institutes of Health will help settle this controversy.

CEREBRAL ISCHEMIA FOLLOWING CAROTID OCCLUSION

About one-third of patients experience a significant cerebral event at the time of internal carotid artery occlusion from either an acute reduction in blood flow or embolization from the column of fresh thrombus. Following internal carotid occlusion the risk of ipsilateral stroke remains increased. Nicholls and coworkers studied 212 patients with internal carotid artery occlusion and reported a five-year cumulative stroke rate of 25 percent and death rate of 38 percent.[59]

There are at least four possible mechanisms for these ipsilateral events. First, blood flow is reduced beyond the occlusion, making this territory more susceptible to hypoperfusion. Connolly and Stemmer have advocated endarterectomy of the external carotid artery in symptomatic patients with ipsilateral internal carotid artery occlusion in order to improve cerebral blood flow.[60] They reported symptomatic improvement in 45 such cases. The second mechanism for ipsilateral events following internal carotid occlusion is embolization from the top of the thrombus column. Carotid occlusion typically originates at the common carotid artery bifurcation and may involve only the proximal internal carotid or both the internal and common carotid arteries. The stagnant column of blood in the distal internal carotid artery eventually thromboses up to the level of the first branch supplying flow into the lumen. This is most often at the level of the ophthalmic artery, which normally carries blood from the internal carotid artery to the eye. In the case of internal carotid artery occlusion, flow is reversed in the ophthalmic artery as "the face feeds the brain." Blood flowing through the ophthalmic artery encounters thrombus in the internal carotid and may carry fragments of this thrombotic material into the brain. A third source of emboli is atherosclerotic plaque in the contralateral carotid artery that supplies the brain through cross-filling collaterals in the circle of Willis. It has been noted that carotid occlusion is more often symptomatic in the presence of untreated contralateral carotid stenosis. The ability of platelet aggregates to embolize from one carotid artery to the circulation of an occluded contralateral carotid artery has been demonstrated in rodents.[61] The fourth source of emboli is the nonobliterated stump of the occluded internal carotid artery. Emboli originating in an internal carotid stump can pass through the external carotid branches into the retinal or cerebral circulation.[62]

PLAQUE DISRUPTION AND HEMORRHAGE

Although carotid atherosclerosis is a very common cause of cerebral ischemia, the majority of patients with atherosclerotic carotid lesions are asymptomatic. In 1960 Martin and associates reported that 40 percent of patients over 50 years had at least a 50 percent stenosis of one or more extracranial cerebral vessels at autopsy, and most of these lesions had been asymptomatic.[63] Atherosclerotic plaques usually produce symptoms when they become unstable owing to fissuring or cracking of the fibrous cap. When this occurs, release of necrotic debris from the lipid core exposes blood to lipid, tissue factor, and collagen, resulting in further thrombosis (Fig. 4-3).

This phenomenon has been particularly well studied in coronary artery disease, where it is assumed to initiate unstable angina and acute myocardial infarction. Fuster and colleagues have reviewed the role of plaque rupture in coronary artery disease.[64] Rupture of plaques is a principle cause of ischemic coronary syndromes, and plaques with large lipid collections are particularly prone to rupture. Thrombus that forms after plaque disruption may lead to decreased perfusion and an unstable coronary syndrome or may organize and cause accelerated luminal narrowing. The extent of myocardial damage depends on the size of the vessel affected, the duration of occlusion, the extent of collateral flow, and the ability of the fibrinolytic system to clear the thrombus. Plaque disruption is particularly prevalent in coronary arteries of patients who have died from myocardial infarction.

Breakdown of the fibrous cap in carotid lesions undoubtedly is also an important factor in producing cerebral ischemic symptoms. Plaque hemorrhage and disruption are more frequent in carotid endarterectomy specimens from patients who had symptoms than from those who were asymptomatic.[65,66] The plaque cap consists mainly of connective tissue matrix, smooth muscle cells, and lipid-laden macrophages. The concentration of macrophages appears to be higher in caps of plaques that ulcerate and in regions where fissures occur, perhaps because of local breakdown of collagen and other matrix components by proteolytic enzymes released from activated macrophages.[67–69] Eccentric plaques with soft lipid cores are more prone to rupture. Finite-element analysis of stress forces on plaques reveals increased force in the shoulder region of the plaque (Fig. 4-4).[69] The source of blood in intraplaque hemorrhage may be from the arterial lumen through fissures in the plaque or from capillaries that grow into the plaque substance. The high velocity of blood flow at the site of severe arterial narrowing causes a reduction in intraluminal blood pressure by the Bernoulli effect. This reduction of intraluminal pressure may contribute to bleeding from vessels within the plaque.[70]

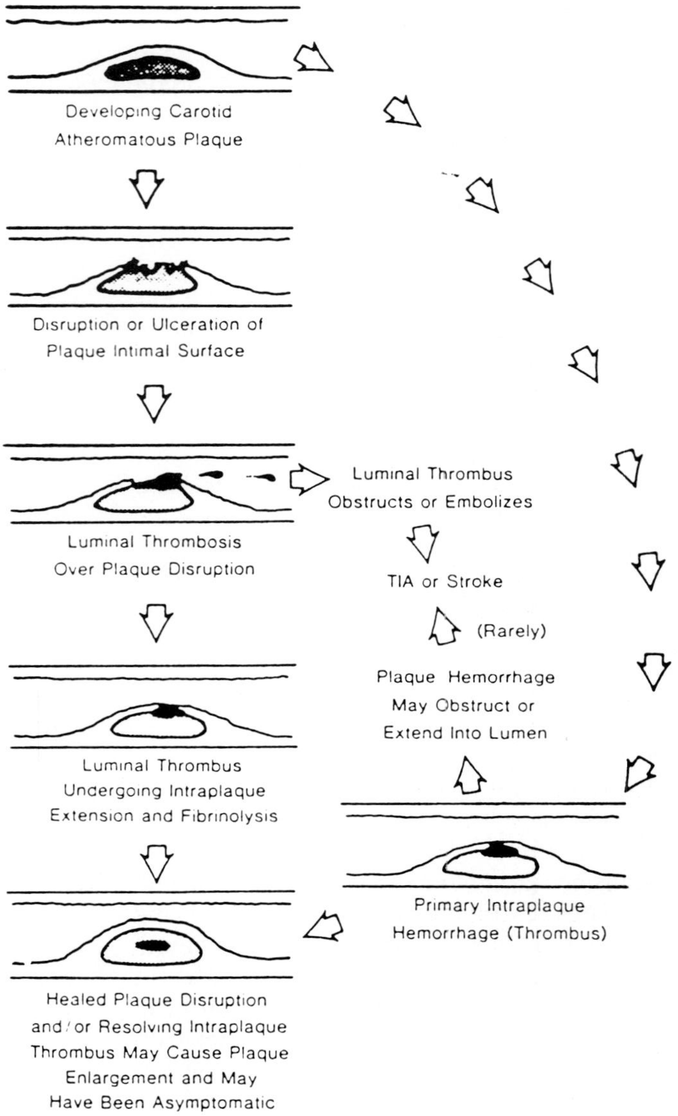

Figure 4-3. Mechanism by which carotid plaque can cause symptoms by disruption and embolization or by obstruction of the lumen. Either intraplaque hemorrhage or thrombus on the surface of the disrupted plaque can contribute to this process by causing the plaque to enlarge. TIA = transient ischemic attack. (*Modified from Fisher.*[65])

CELLULAR MECHANISMS OF INJURY

When perfusion pressure is reduced, cerebral blood flow is maintained by vasodilatation. This mechanism of autoregulation can maintain a steady level of cerebral blood flow for blood pressures ranging between 60 and 130 mmHg.[71] Below this level, arterial supply is insufficient to meet metabolic demands, and tissue ischemia results. Low perfusion pressures may occur with severe systemic hypotension or when terminal arteries are blocked by embolism or thrombosis.

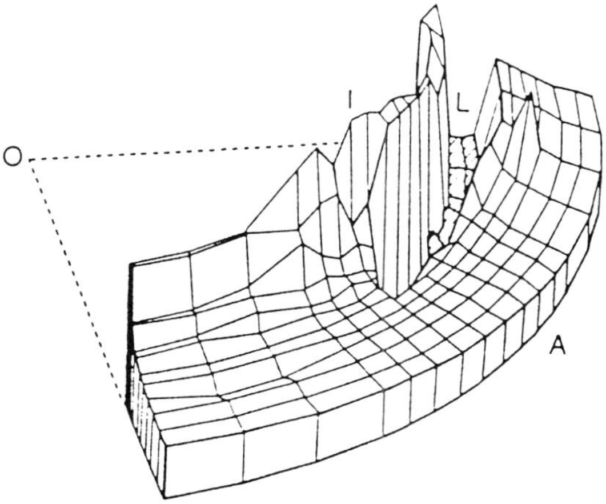

Figure 4-4. Three-dimensional stress map from finite-element analysis of a coronary artery plaque. Note that the maximum stress occurs at the center of the plaque cap and at the shoulder of the lipid core. L = lipid core; A = adventitia; I = intima; O = center of lumen. (*Modified from Richardson.*[69])

When ischemia is profound, cell death occurs rapidly. Mild to moderate perfusion deficits may cause neurons to fail before cell death occurs. After several hours of marginal perfusion, membrane function is impaired, potassium leaks out of the cells, synthesis of neurotransmitters stops, and blood flow is further hampered by the release of vasoactive substances and intravascular coagulation.[1] Incomplete ischemia may cause more tissue loss than a brief period of complete ischemia. Lactic acid generated by anaerobic metabolism during incomplete ischemia exacerbates tissue injury after reperfusion. Following embolization or thrombosis of cerebral vessels, central areas of necrosis may be surrounded by regions of moderate ischemia, referred to as penumbra regions. Restoration of blood flow to these regions before irreversible damage occurs potentially can salvage areas that otherwise would go on to necrosis.

Table 4-2 Composition of Cardiogenic Emboli

Platelets (nonbacterial thrombotic endocarditis)
Laminated fibrin-rich thrombi (ventricular aneurysms)
Calcific material (aortic stenosis)
Tumor (myxoma)

SOURCE: Modified from Cerebral Embolism Task Force.[73]

CARDIOGENIC BRAIN EMBOLISM

The task force on cerebral embolism determined that about one in six ischemic strokes is caused by emboli from the heart.[72,73] Cardiac emboli may arise from the wall of the heart, from diseased valves, or from tumors (Table 4-2). Bogousslavsky and coworkers reviewed the cardiac sources of stroke in 305 patients who had recent neurologic events.[3] Their findings are summarized in Table 4-3.

Table 4-3 Cardiac Sources of Embolism (%)

Myocardial Abnormalities	27.6
Focal left ventricular akinesis	20
Focal left ventricular akinesis with thrombus	2.3
Global hypokinesis	2.3
Patent foramen ovale	2
Left atrial myxoma	0.7
Left ventricular thrombus	0.3
Isolated valvular abnormalities	23.3
Mitral valve prolapse	16.7
Mitral stenosis or insufficiency (rheumatic or endocarditis)	3.3
Prosthetic valves	3.3
Isolated arrhythmias	41.6
Atrial fibrillation	38.7
Sick sinus syndrome	2.9
Arrhythmias and myocardial abnormalities	**3.9**
Arrhythmias and valvular abnormalities	**3.6**

SOURCE: Modified from Bogousslavsky.[3]

Concomitant large vessel arterial disease (either intracranial or extracranial) ipsilateral to the involved hemisphere was present in 10.8 percent of cases. Embolic stroke may result from almost any disease of the heart. The less common sources of emboli are listed in Table 4-4. Treatment of cardiogenic embolism is discussed in Chap. 15.

VERTEBROBASILAR SYMPTOMS

Disease affecting the vertebrobasilar or posterior circulation tends to produce nonfocal symptoms such as dizziness, diplopia, ataxia, drop attacks, and crossed motor deficits (Chap. 7). Unlike deficits caused by embolism from plaques in the carotid circulation, vertebrobasilar symptoms often are related to postural changes or head position. These symptoms presumably are due to diminished blood supply to the brain stem or posterior cerebral circulation. Because the vessels of the vertebrobasilar system are much smaller than those of the carotid system, plaques tend to cause occlusion before they become large enough to ulcerate and embolize.

Table 4-4 Uncommon Sources of Cardiogenic Emboli

Nonischemic cardiomyopathies
Ventricular thrombi without underlying heart disease
Polycystic disease
Myeloproliferative disorders/thrombocythemia
Systemic lupus
Malignancy
Idiopathic
Mitral valve prolapse
Mitral annulus calcification
Nonbacterial thrombotic endocarditis
Infective endocarditis
Inflammatory valvulitis
Calcific aortic stenosis
Atrial septal aneurysms
Aortic aneurysms
Paradoxical emboli
Atrial septal defects
Patent foramen ovale
Ventricular septal defects
Pulmonary arteriovenous fistulas
Cardiac tumors

SOURCE: Modified from The Cerebral Embolism Task Force.[73]

The subclavian steal syndrome is a special case of low flow causing vertebrobasilar symptoms. Stenosis or occlusion of the subclavian or innominate arteries proximal to the origin of the vertebral can result in reversal of flow in the vertebral artery, which then serves as a source of collateral blood supply to the upper extremity on the side of the proximal lesion. Flow reversal occurs with blood pressure reductions of as little as 20 mmHg. Contorni's 1960 report is credited as the first to describe cerebral symptoms related to subclavian artery disease.[74] A year later, Reivich reported two patients with this syndrome and described experiments in dogs demonstrating that vertebral flow stops when mean pressure in the distal subclavian artery is reduced by about 10 percent.[75] An accompanying editorial in the *New England Journal of Medicine* coined the term "subclavian steal syndrome."[76] In 1967 McLaughlin and associates reported eight patients who underwent various forms of vascular reconstruction for this syndrome with relief of symptoms.[77]

Exercise of the arm on the affected side often brings on or exacerbates symptoms, and arm claudication may be a prominent clinical feature of the subclavian steal syndrome. Cerebral symptoms may be hemispheric or nonhemispheric; however, these patients often have concomitant disease of the carotid system that may be the cause of hemispheric symptoms. A widely patent carotid system generally can supply all of the brain as well as collateral flow to the upper extremity.[78] In experiments using dogs, Eklöf and Schwartz found that retrograde vertebral flow due to subclavian artery occlusion did not interfere with cerebral blood flow, even when one carotid artery and the contralateral vertebral artery also were occluded.[79] Cerebral blood flow was reduced only when both carotid arteries were occluded.

It is now recognized that flow reversal in the vertebral artery is relatively common and usually asymptomatic. Nicholls and colleagues reported the benign nature of retrograde vertebral artery flow in 43 patients diagnosed by duplex ultrasound.[80] Less than 20 percent of these patients had typical symptoms of the subclavian steal syndrome. Nearly one-third were asymptomatic, 30 percent had nonhemispheric symptoms, and 20 percent had hemispheric symptoms. During the 19-month follow-up period, none of the asymptomatic patients became symptomatic, and there were no strokes or stroke-related deaths. While surgical procedures that restored antegrade vertebral artery flow did not necessarily improve symptoms of posterior circulation ischemia, symptoms improved in some patients following carotid endarterectomy.

Moran and coworkers reported that patients with subclavian steal syndrome are more likely to experience a TIA or stroke involving the carotid circulation than the vertebrobasilar circulation.[81] During a four-year follow-up of 55 patients, 70 percent had progression of disease in the carotid arteries, and none had a vertebrobasilar stroke. Only three patients required revascularization for arm ischemia. Most patients with vertebral artery disease also will have significant carotid artery disease, which is much more likely to be the cause of cerebral ischemia. In general, vertebral or subclavian artery stenoses should not be addressed unless symptoms persist after any significant carotid stenoses are repaired. The indications for vertebral artery surgery are discussed in Chap. 19; the surgical management of subclavian steal syndrome and vertebral artery disease are covered in Chaps. 29 and 30.

REFERENCES

1. Rogers SJ, Sherman DG: Pathophysiology and treatment of acute ischemic stroke. *Clin Pharm* 12:359, 1993.
2. Bogousslavsky J, van Melle G, Regli F: The Lausanne Stroke Registry: Analysis of 1,000 consecutive patients with first stroke. *Stroke* 19:1083, 1988.
3. Bogousslavsky J, Cachin C, Regli F, et al: Cardiac sources of embolism and cerebral infarction—clinical consequences and vascular concomitants: The Lausanne Stroke Registry. *Neurology* 41:855, 1991.
4. Mohr JP, Caplan LR, Melski JW, et al: The Harvard Cooperative Stroke Registry: A prospective registry. *Neurology* 28:754, 1978.
5. Walker AE, Robins M, Weinfeld FD: The National Survey of Stroke. Clinical findings. *Stroke* 12:113, 1981.
6. Fields WS, North RR, Hass WK, et al: Joint study of extracranial arterial occlusion. I. Organization of study and survey of patient population. *JAMA* 203:153, 1968.
7. Hass WK, Fields WS, North RR, et al: Joint study of extracranial arterial occlusion. II. Arteriography; techniques; sites; and complications. *JAMA* 203:159, 1968.
8. Moniz E: L'encephalographie arterielle son importance dans la localisation des tumeurs cerebrales. *Revue Neurologique (Paris)* 2:72, 1927.
9. Gowers WR: On a case of simultaneous embolism of central retinal and middle cerebral arteries. *Lancet* 2:794, 1875.
10. Cadwalader WB: Unilateral optic atrophy and contralateral hemiplegia consequent on occlusion of the cerebral vessels. *JAMA* 59:2248, 1912.
11. Guthrie LG, Mayou S: Right hemiplegia and atrophy of left optic nerve. *Proc R Soc Med* 1:180, 1908.
12. Hunt JR: The role of the carotid arteries in the causation of vascular lesions of the brain, with remarks on certain special features of the symptomatology. *Am J Med Sci* 147:704, 1914.
13. Johnson HC, Walker AE: The angiographic diagnosis of spontaneous thrombosis of internal

and common carotid arteries. *J Neurosurg* 8:631, 1951.
14. Fisher CM: Occlusion of the internal carotid artery. *Arch Neurol Psychiat* 65:346, 1951.
15. Rothenberg SF, Corday E: Etiology of transient cerebral stroke. *JAMA* 164:2005, 1957.
16. Hutchinson EC, Yates PO: Caroticovertebral stenosis. *Lancet* 1:2, 1957.
17. Meyer JS, Denny-Brown D: The cerebral collateral circulation. II. Production of cerebral infarction by ischemic anoxia and its reversibility in early stages. *Neurology* 7:567, 1957.
18. Corday E, Rothenberg S, Weiner SM: Cerebral vascular insufficiency: An explanation of the transient stroke. *Arch Intern Med* 98:683, 1956.
19. Meyer JS: Occlusive cerebrovascular disease. Pathogenesis and treatment. *Am J Med* 30:577, 1961.
20. Fazekas JF, Alman RW: The role of hypotension in transitory focal cerebral ischemia. *Am J Med Sci* 248:567, 1964.
21. Millikan CH: The pathogenesis of transient focal cerebral ischemia. *Circulation* 32:438, 1965.
22. Drake WEJ, Drake MAL: Clinical and angiographic correlates of cerebrovascular insufficiency. *Am J Med* 45:253, 1968.
23. Russell RW, Cranston WI: Ophthalmodynamometry in carotid artery disease. *J Neurol Neurosurg Psychiat* 24:281, 1961.
24. Kendall RE, Marshall J: Role of hypertension in the genesis of transient focal cerebral ischemic attacks. *Br Med J* 2:344, 1963.
25. Chiari H: Ueber das Verhalten des Teilungswinkels der Carotid communis bei der Endarteriitis chronica deformans. *Verh Dtsch Ges Pathol* 9:326, 1905.
26. Handler FP: Clinical and pathological significance of atheromatous embolization, with emphasis on an etiology of renal hypertension. *Am J Med* 20:366, 1956.
27. Flory CM: Arterial occlusions produced by emboli from eroded aortic atheromatous plaques. *Am J Pathol* 21:549, 1945.
28. Hollenhorst RW: Ocular manifestations of insufficiency or thrombosis of the internal carotid artery. *Am Opth Soc* 56:474, 1958.
29. Hollenhorst RW: Significance of bright plaques in the retinal arterioles. *JAMA* 178 (1):123, 1961.
30. Hollenhorst RW: Vascular status of patients who have cholesterol emboli in the retina. *Am J Ophthalmol* 61:1159, 1966.
31. Fisher CM: Observations of the fundus oculi in transient monocular blindness. *Neurology* 9:333, 1959.
32. Kollarits CR, Lubow M, Hissong SL: Retinal Strokes. I. Incidence of carotid atheromata. *JAMA* 222:1273, 1972.
33. Gunning AJ, Pickering GW, Robb-Smith AHT, Russell RR: Mural thrombosis of the internal carotid artery and subsequent embolism. *Q J Med* 33:155, 1964.
34. McBrien DJ, Bradley RD, Ashton N: The nature of retinal emboli in stenosis of the internal carotid artery. *Lancet* 1:697, 1963.
35. Russell RWR: Observations on the retinal blood-vessels in monocular blindness. *Lancet* 2:1422, 1961.
36. Zukowski AJ, Nicolaides AN, Lewis RT, et al: The correlation between carotid plaque ulceration and cerebral infarction seen on CT scan. *J Vasc Surg* 1:782, 1984.
37. Honour AJ, Russell RWR: Experimental platelet embolism. *Br J Exp Pathol* 43:350, 1962.
38. Moore WS: Fundamental considerations in cerebrovascular disease, in Rutherford RB: *Vascular Surgery,* 3d ed. Philadelphia, WB Saunders, p. 1291, 1989.
39. Millikan CH, Siekert RG, Shick RM: Studies in cerebrovascular disease. V. The use of anticoagulant drugs in the treatment of intermittent insufficiency of the internal carotid system. *Proc Staff Meet Mayo Clin* 30:578, 1955.
40. Fisher CM: The use of anticoagulants in cerebral thrombosis. *Neurology* 8:311, 1958.
41. Julian OC, Dye WS, Javid H, Hunter JA: Ulcerative lesions of the carotid artery bifurcation. *Arch Surg* 86:803, 1963.
42. Sterpetti AV, Hunter WJ, Schultz RD: Importance of ulceration of carotid plaque in determining symptoms of cerebral ischemia. *J Cardiovasc Surg* 32:154, 1991.
43. Crawford ES, DeBakey ME, Blaisdell FW, et al: Hemodynamic alterations in patients with cerebral arterial insufficiency before and after operation. *Surgery* 48:76, 1960.
44. Brice JG, Dowsett DJ, Lowe RD: Hemody-

namic effects of carotid artery stenosis. *Br Med J* 2:1363, 1964.
45. Moore WS, Hall AD: Importance of emboli from carotid bifurcation in pathogenesis of cerebral ischemic attacks. *Arch Surg* 101:708, 1970.
46. Moore WS, Hall AD: Ulcerated atheroma of the carotid artery. *Am J Surg* 237:242, 1968.
47. Whittemore AD, Kauffman JL, Kohler TR, Mannick JA: Routine electroencephalographic (EEG) monitoring during carotid endarterectomy. *Ann Surg* 197:707, 1983.
48. Adams JE, Smith MC, Wylie EJ: Cerebral bloodflow and hemodynamics in extracranial vascular disease: Effect of endarterectomy. *Surgery* 53:449, 1963.
49. Strully KJ, Hurwitt ES, Blankenberg HW: Thrombo-endarterectomy for thrombosis of the carotid artery in the neck. *J Neurosurg* 10:474, 1953.
50. Carrea R, Molins M, Murphy G: Surgical treatment of spontaneous thrombosis of the internal carotid artery in the neck. Carotid-carotid anastomosis: Report of a case. *Acta Neurol Latinoam* 1:71, 1955.
51. Eastcott HHG, Pickering GW, Rob CG: Reconstruction of internal carotid artery in a patient with intermittent attacks of hemiplegia. *Lancet* 2:994, 1954.
52. Pokras R, Dyken ML: Dramatic changes in the performance of endarterectomy for diseases of the extracranial arteries of the head. *Stroke* 19:1289, 1988.
53. Chambers BR, Norris JW: The case against surgery for asymptomatic carotid stenosis. *Stroke* 15:964, 1984.
54. Barnett HJ, Plum F, Walton JN: Carotid endarterectomy—an expression of concern. *Stroke* 15:941, 1984.
55. North American Symptomatic Carotid Endarterectomy Trial Collaborators: Beneficial effect of carotid endarterectomy in symptomatic patients with high-grade carotid stenosis. *N Engl J Med* 325:445, 1991.
56. European Carotid Surgery Trialists' Collaborative Group: European carotid surgery trial: Interim results for symptomatic patients with severe (70–99%) or with mild (0–29%) carotid stenosis. *Lancet* 337:1235, 1991.
57. Mayberg MR, Wilson SE, Yatsu F, et al: Carotid endarterectomy and prevention of cerebral ischemia in symptomatic carotid stenosis. Veterans Affairs Cooperative Studies Program 309 Trialist Group. *JAMA* 266:3289, 1991.
58. Hobson RW, Weiss DG, Fields WS, et al: Efficacy of carotid endarterectomy for asymptomatic carotid stenosis. *N Engl J Med* 328:221, 1993.
59. Nicholls SC, Kohler TR, Bergelin RO, et al: Carotid artery occlusion: Natural history. *J Vasc Surg* 4:479, 1986.
60. Connolly JE, Stemmer EA: Endarterectomy of the external carotid artery. *Arch Surg* 106:799, 1973.
61. Tietjen GE, Futrell N, Garcia JH, Millikan C: Platelet emboli in rat brain cross when the contralateral carotid artery is occluded. *Stroke* 22:1053, 1991.
62. Barnett HJ, Peerless SJ, Kaufmann JC: "Stump" on internal carotid artery—a source for further cerebral embolic ischemia. *Stroke* 9:448, 1978.
63. Martin MJ, Whisnant JP, Sayre GP: Occlusive vascular disease in the extracranial cerebral circulation. *Arch Neurol* 3:530, 1960.
64. Fuster V, Stein B, Ambrose JA, et al: Atherosclerotic plaque rupture and thrombosis. Evolving concepts. *Circulation* 82:II47, 1990.
65. Fisher M, Blumenfeld AM, Smith TW: The importance of carotid artery plaque disruption and hemorrhage. *Arch Neurol* 44:1086, 1987.
66. Imparato AM, Riles TS, Mintzer R, Baumann FG: The importance of hemorrhage in the relationship between gross morphologic characteristics and cerebral symptoms in 376 carotid artery plaques. *Ann Surg* 197:195, 1983.
67. Davies MJ, Richardson PD, Woolf N, et al: Risk of thrombosis in human atherosclerotic plaques: Role of extracellular lipid, macrophage, and smooth muscle cell content. *Br Heart J* 69:377, 1993.
68. Lendon CL, Davies MJ, Born GV, Richardson PD: Atherosclerotic plaque caps are locally weakened when macrophages density is increased. *Atherosclerosis* 87:87, 1991.
69. Richardson PD, Davies MJ, Born GV: Influence of plaque configuration and stress distri-

bution of fissuring of coronary atherosclerotic plaques. *Lancet* 2:941, 1989.

70. Beach KW, Hatsukami T, Detmer PR, et al: Carotid artery intraplaque hemorrhage and stenotic velocity. *Stroke* 24:314, 1993.
71. James IM, Millar RA, Purves MY: Observations on the intrinsic neural control of cerebral blood flow in the baboon. *Circ Res* 25:77, 1969.
72. Cerebral Embolism Study Group: Cardioembolic stroke, immediate anticoagulation, and brain hemorrhage. *Arch Intern Med* 147:636, 1987.
73. Cerebral Embolism Task Force: Cardiogenic brain embolism: The second report of the Cerebral Embolism Task Force. *Arch Neurol* 46: 727, 1989.
74. Contorni L: Cirolo collaterale vertebro-vertebrale nella obliterazione dell arteria subclavia alla sur origine. *Minerva Chir* 15:268, 1960.
75. Reivich M: Reversal of blood flow through vertebral artery and its effect on cerebral circulation. *N Engl J Med* 265:878, 1961.
76. New vascular syndrome—"The Subclavian Steal," editorial. *N Engl J Med* 265:912, 1961.
77. McLaughlin JS, Linberg E, Attar A: Cerebral vascular insufficiency. Syndromes of reversed blood flow in vessels supplying the brain. *Am Surg* 33:317, 1967.
78. Mozersky DJ, Barnes RW, Sumner DS, Strandness DE Jr: Hemodynamics of innominate artery occlusion. *Ann Surg* 178:123, 1973.
79. Eklof B, Schwartz SI: Effects of subclavian steal and compromised cephalic blood flow on cerebral circulation. *Surgery* 68:431, 1969.
80. Nicholls SC, Koutlas TC, Strandness DE: Clinical significance of retrograde flow in the vertebral artery. *Ann Vasc Surg* 5:331, 1991.
81. Moran KT, Zide RS, Persson AV, Jewell ER: Natural history of subclavian steal syndrome. *Am Surg* 54:643, 1988.

5

Nonatherosclerotic Disorders of the Cerebral Circulation

Thomas S. Hatsukami

Atherosclerosis is the most common arterial disease process responsible for ischemic neurologic events. In this chapter, the less prevalent disorders of the extracranial carotid and vertebral arteries will be reviewed. These include carotid dissection, fibromuscular dysplasia, Takayasu's and giant cell arteritis, internal carotid coils and kinks, aneurysms, and radiation-induced arterial disease.

CAROTID DISSECTION

Arterial dissection is defined as intimal disruption and extravasation of blood into the layers of the arterial wall, resulting in luminal stenosis, occlusion, or aneurysm formation. Carotid dissections typically involve the cervical and occasionally the intracranial segments of the internal carotid artery (ICA). Common carotid and external carotid artery dissections have been reported but are rare.[1]

Epidemiology

Carotid artery dissection was first described by Jentzer in 1954.[2] Since that time, over 260 cases have been reported; however, the true incidence is difficult to determine because the diagnosis is easily missed in patients who have minimal symptoms.[1] Internal carotid dissection occurs in all age groups, but is more common in young adults. The mean age ranges from 41 to 45 years for spontaneous carotid dissection, but tends to be lower in trauma victims.[3,4] A predilection for one gender or side has not been clearly demonstrated.[5,6] Arterial dissections occurring at multiple sites are relatively frequent. In a review of 42 patients with ICA dissections from the Mayo Clinic, 13 (31 percent) of the patients had multiple dissections.[7]

Pathophysiology

Internal carotid artery dissections can be considered as either traumatic or spontaneous. In addition to penetrating trauma (stab and gunshot wounds) and iatrogenic injuries (angiography), ICA dissections can occur in association with blunt trauma—most commonly motor vehicle accidents. Several mechanisms have been proposed for carotid dissections secondary to blunt injuries. Zelenock and coworkers postulated that cervical hyperextension and rotation results in intimal injury as the vessel is stretched on the upper cervical vertebrae (C2/C3) or styloid process (Fig. 5-1).[8] They also noted that fractures or posterior dislocations of the mandible may result in transmural injury to the ICA as it is crushed between the angle of the mandible and the up-

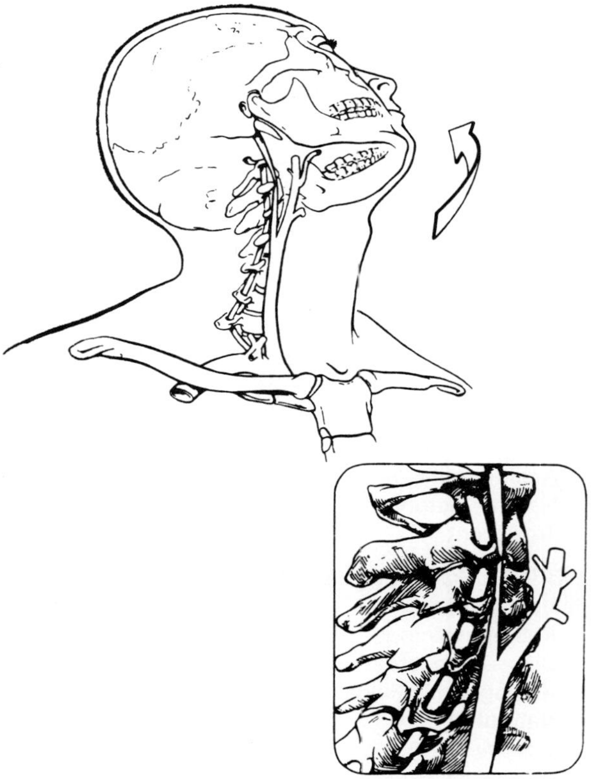

Figure 5-1. A proposed mechanism for the development of carotid dissection secondary to blunt trauma. Intimal injury is caused by cervical hyperextension and rotation with stretching of the vessel over the transverse processes of the second and third cervical vertebrae. (*From Zelenock et al.*[8] *Reproduced by permission.*)

per cervical transverse processes (Fig. 5-2). Other mechanisms include direct blows to the neck, intraoral trauma, and basilar skull fractures.

Controversy exists over whether carotid dissections truly occur spontaneously. A number of reports suggest a role for such trivial forms of trauma as paroxysms of coughing, retching, or vomiting[9]; cervical hyperextension associated with "bottoms up" drinking[10]; turning the head while leading a parade, old whiplash injuries,[4] diving into water[11]; childbirth,[12] and "head banging" during punk-rock dancing.[13] However, in most patients the cause of spontaneous carotid dissection is unknown.

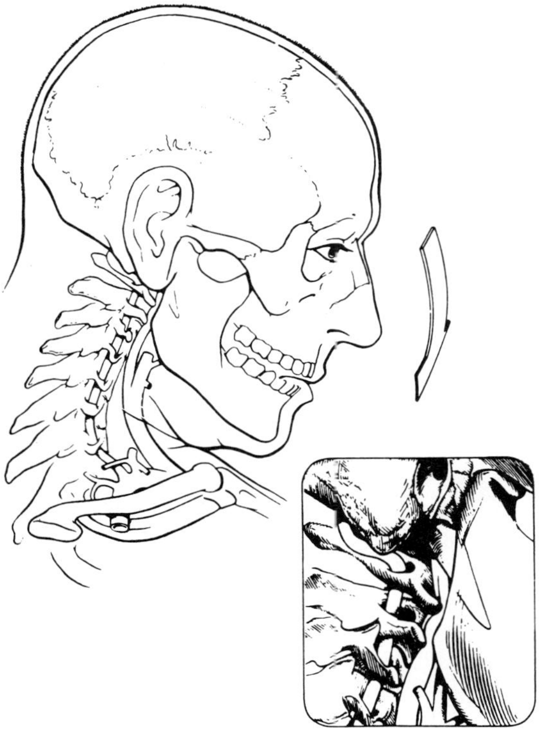

Figure 5-2. An alternative mechanism for the development of carotid dissection secondary to blunt trauma (see Fig. 5-1). Intimal injury is caused by direct compression of the carotid artery between the angle of the mandible and the upper cervical vertebrae. (*From Zelenock et al.*[8] *Reproduced by permission.*)

Dissections that occur in the subintimal or superficial medial plane typically compress the true lumen and result in vessel narrowing or occlusion. Alternatively, deeper dissections into the subadventitial plane may result in vessel enlargement, sometimes referred to as a "dissecting aneurysm." The involved artery is often normal histologically, but a number of arteriopathies have been associated with dissection. Fibromuscular dysplasia (FMD) has been identified in 15 to 20 percent of patients.[3,4,14,15] Cystic medial necrosis was described in earlier reports of autopsy specimens, but is less common in more recent reports based on surgical specimens.[16–19] Internal carotid dissection also has been observed in association with Marfan's syndrome.[20]

Clinical Presentation

There are no pathognomonic symptoms and signs for carotid dissection. The multiplicity of presentations makes the diagnosis difficult, and the condition easily can be missed in trauma patients who have an altered level of consciousness. The presence of significant facial trauma or cervical spine injury should raise the level of suspicion.

The literature suggests that approximately 35 to 75 percent of patients with carotid dissection present with ischemic neurologic events, either transient ischemic attack (TIA), stroke, or both.[3,4,21,22] Other common manifestations include unilateral headache, ipsilateral partial Horner's syndrome (oculosympathetic palsy), and subjective (detected by the patient) or objective (detected by the examiner) carotid bruits. Other less common findings include scalp tenderness, neck swelling, dysgeusia (involvement of the chorda tympani branch of cranial nerve VII), slurred speech (ipsilateral involvement of cranial nerve XII), and dysphagia (involvement of cranial nerves IX and X).[9,23] The most common combination of symptoms associated with spontaneous carotid dissection is unilateral headache followed after a delay by cerebral ischemic symptoms.[15] The second most common combination is unilateral headache and oculosympathetic palsy ipsilateral to the headache.[24]

The headache associated with carotid dissection is usually unilateral and focal, frequently in the frontal, orbital, and periorbital regions.[6] Oculosympathetic palsy is manifested by ptosis and miosis, but not by anhydrosis. Sympathetic fibers supplying the sweat glands of the face accompany the external carotid artery, which is rarely affected by dissection, whereas the sympathetic fibers for the eyes follow the internal carotid.[24] Mechanisms for hemispheric neurologic deficits include embolic events secondary to platelet aggregation and thrombus formation at sites of intimal tears or aneurysms and flow reduction from luminal stenosis. Intracranial dissection, in addition to causing ischemic or embolic events, also may produce symptoms secondary to subarachnoid hemorrhage.[25–27] The mechanism of lower cranial nerve palsies has not been precisely defined, but proposed causes include direct compression or compromise of the vascular supply to the nearby cranial nerves.[28]

Angiographic Findings

Diagnostic studies used to detect carotid artery dissection include ocular pneumoplethysmography (OPG), ultrasonic duplex scanning, computed tomography (CT), and magnetic resonance imaging; however, contrast angiography is the gold standard. In addition to showing the origin of the dissection, angiography documents the extent of dissection, the presence of distal embolization, and the status of collateral flow. Duplex scanning and OPG will detect the presence of stenosis or occlusion and typically have been used for follow-up testing. Computed tomography has been used to provide information on vessel wall thickness, extent of dissection, and pseudoaneurysm formation.[29] Magnetic resonance imaging may show a flow void when there is occlusion or a hyperintense signal related to hemorrhage within the arterial wall.

The most classic angiographic finding associated with carotid dissection is the "string sign" first described by Ojemann: an elongated, tapered narrowing of the lumen with irregularity of the luminal wall (Fig. 5-3).[30] Dissections most commonly originate in the carotid bulb, 2 to 4 cm distal to the origin of the ICA. They usually extend to the level of the petrous temporal bone, but occasionally continue intracranially. In a review by Meissner and Mokri of 80 patients with spontaneous ICA dissections, the most common angiographic finding was luminal stenosis.[6] Abrupt reconstitution of the lumen was the second

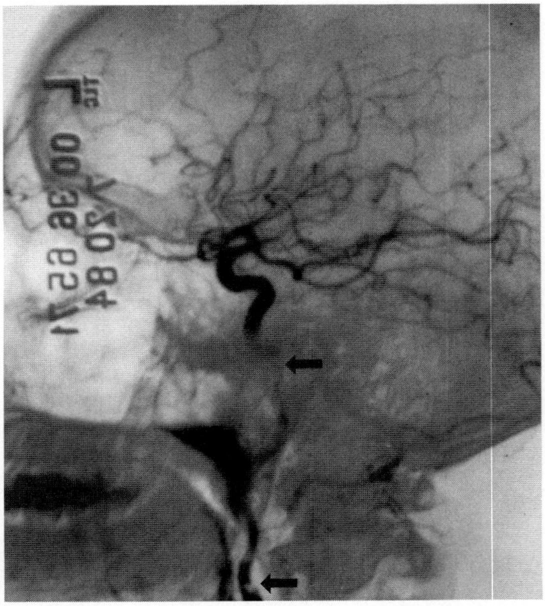

Figure 5-3. Characteristic tapered narrowing or "string sign" associated with internal carotid artery dissection. The dissection originates in the region of the carotid bulb and extends into the petrous segment of the internal carotid artery where there is abrupt reconstitution of the lumen (*arrows*).

most common finding, usually occurring at the base of the skull. Aneurysms were noted in approximately one-third of the patients. Occlusions of the ICA typically were noted distal to the bulb and had a tapered appearance, resembling a candle flame. Distal occlusions from embolization were found in approximately 10 percent of the patients.

Natural History

In general, the clinical outcome of carotid dissection appears to be favorable. Several studies have shown a 78 to 92 percent rate of recovery when patients were either asymptomatic or had only mild symptoms at the time of presentation.[4,6,21] On the other hand, patients who presented with a fixed neurologic deficit showed only a 40 percent rate of good recovery.[3] Traumatic dissections appear more likely to result in fixed neurologic deficits.[21]

Angiographic follow-up studies also report favorable outcomes. In 1986, Mokri and colleagues reported on 23 patients with 29 spontaneous ICA dissections who underwent follow-up angiography.[15] Stenosis of the ICA either completely resolved or substantially improved in more than 85 percent of the dissected vessels. Over 60 percent of dissecting aneurysms either resolved or decreased in size. Recurrence of the dissection or rupture of a dissecting aneurysm were not noted.

Treatment

Absolute guidelines for optimal treatment of carotid artery dissections have not been established. In many cases, surgical therapy is limited by the technical difficulties involved in obtaining distal control and the risk of converting an ischemic infarct into a hemorrhagic infarct following revascularization. The discouraging early surgical experience, coupled with the relatively favorable results of nonoperative therapy, has led to the current recommendation for initial medical management. Surgical intervention is reserved for patients who fail medical therapy and have an accessible lesion.[3] Anecdotal reports suggest that anticoagulation with warfarin for three to four months may reduce the risk for subsequent stroke.[15,31] However, anticoagulant therapy may not be an option in trauma patients. Anticoagulation is also contraindicated in cases of intracranial ICA dissection, which often are associated with subarachnoid hemorrhage.[3,32,33] Antiplatelet agents may be considered in these patients.[4]

Surgical options that have been described include thrombectomy, progressive dilatation, endarterectomy, and intimectomy. In most cases, however, the dissected artery is extremely friable, and the extent of dissection precludes the use of these techniques. For such patients, carotid resection and replacement or carotid ligation may be necessary. Extracranial–intracranial bypass can be considered in individuals without adequate collateral flow.

FIBROMUSCULAR DYSPLASIA

Fibromuscular dysplasia has been described as a heterogeneous group of nonatherosclerotic, noninflammatory vascular diseases of unknown cause.[34] The lesions of FMD were first observed in the renal arteries in 1938 by Leadbetter and Burkland.[35] Twenty-five years later, Palubinskas and Ripley first reported FMD of the ICA.[36]

Epidemiology

The true incidence of FMD is not known because many patients are asymptomatic. It is a relatively uncommon condition, with approximately 700 cases reported in the literature.[34] In a review of 13,955 cerebral angiograms performed at the Mayo Clinic from1962 through 1979, Corrin and coworkers identified internal carotid FMD in 82 (0.6 percent) of the cases.[37] This prevalence is similar to the 0.9 percent rate reported by Mettinger and Ericson in their review of 4000 consecutive cerebral angiograms performed at the Karolinska Institute.[38] There is a marked preponderance of females in the reported series, and the disease tends to occur in the fourth and fifth decades of life.[9]

Pathophysiology

Fibromuscular dysplasia has been noted in renal, mesenteric, iliac, carotid, vertebral, and intracranial arteries, but the lesions most commonly are found in the renal and extracranial internal carotid arteries. Common and external carotid artery involvement have been reported but are rare.[39] Bilateral ICA involvement occurs in up to 86 percent of individuals.[40] The vertebral arteries are affected in approximately 17 percent of cases.[41]

The exact pathogenesis of FMD is unknown. Some investigators speculate that the predominance in women suggests possible hormonal influences on the development of FMD. Others propose that the involved segments are deficient in medial blood supply from the vasa vasorum.[42–44]

Stanley and colleagues describe four types of arterial fibroplasia: intimal fibroplasia; medial fibroplasia; medial hyperplasia; and perimedial dysplasia.[45] Intimal and medial fibroplasia are the principal forms of carotid and vertebral fibroplasia, with medial fibroplasia being the most common.[34] Histologic findings consist of smooth muscle cell hyperplasia, destruction of elastic fibers with proliferation of fibroblasts, and general disorganization of the arterial wall.[40] Constrictions caused by the hyperplastic and fibrotic media, and dilatations representing hypoplastic or absent media, result in a "string of beads" appearance on angiography (Fig. 5-4).

Conditions associated with carotid FMD include spontaneous carotid dissection and intracranial aneurysm formation. Intracranial aneurysms have been reported in 15 to 50 percent of individuals with FMD.[38,46] In a review of 284 cases of aortocranial FMD, Mettinger noted that 61 (21 percent) of the patients had an intracranial aneurysm.[41]

Clinical Presentation

Most patients with carotid FMD probably are asymptomatic, and the clinical diagnosis is made more difficult by the nonspecific nature of the presenting symptoms and signs. In a series of 101 patients treated at the University of California at San Francisco, 77 percent had a carotid bruit, 37 percent had hypertension, 17 percent had electrocardiographic abnormalities, and 9 percent had neurologic deficits.[46] In a series of 49 patients with angiographically documented FMD, Stewart and coworkers noted that 11 (22 percent) of the patients were asymptomatic, 20 (41 percent) presented with focal cerebral or retinal ischemic symptoms, and three (6 percent) presented with an intracranial hemorrhage.[47] The remaining patients had nonlateralizing or nonischemic symptoms.

Angiographic Findings

Internal carotid arteries affected by FMD have been described as being longer than normal.[42,48] The middle and distal thirds of the cervical ICA segment are most commonly involved (Fig. 5-4).[46] As noted above, the irregularly spaced constrictions of the arterial lumen alternating with dilatations result in the appearance of a "string of beads." Less common angiographic features of FMD include tubular stenosis, a diverticulum of the arterial wall, or a noncircumferential, weblike stenosis.[9,38]

Natural History

The natural history of carotid FMD is not well documented because many asymptomatic patients with the disease remain undiagnosed and most symptomatic patients receive some type of treatment or intervention. Stewart and colleagues reviewed the Emory University Hospital experience from 1969 through 1985.[47] Seventy-three nonoperated arteries in 42 patients were followed for up to 16 years (mean 6.8 years). Three patients required surgical intervention, but the remainder had no new neurologic symptoms develop during follow-up.

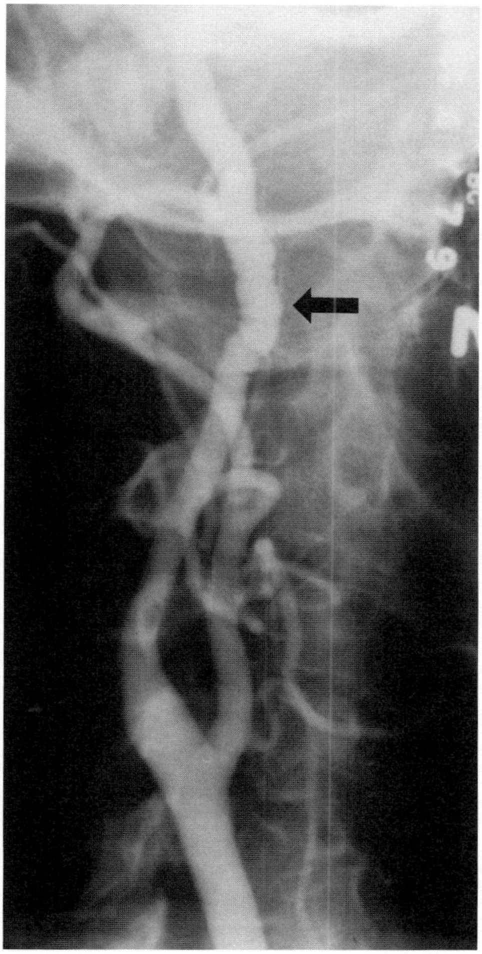

Figure 5-4. Alternating luminal constrictions and dilatations resulting in the characteristic "string of beads" appearance associated with fibromuscular dysplasia of the internal carotid artery (*arrow*). The most distal portion of the extracranial internal carotid artery is involved.

Among the three patients who had an operative procedure, one had a carotid endarterectomy for an asymptomatic 80 percent atherosclerotic stenosis; the other two underwent graduated operative dilatation for "nonfocal ischemia" (syncope, dizziness, and bilateral blurred vision).

In another series of 82 patients with carotid FMD, Corrin and coworkers also noted a benign natural history.[37] Only three cerebral ischemic events occurred during follow-up periods extending to 231 months (mean of 60 months). One of the patients had bilateral carotid FMD and had a left hemispheric stroke at 216 months. The second patient had a right carotid territory infarct 50 months after identification of left carotid FMD; the third patient had a brain stem infarct 136 months after identification of bilateral carotid FMD without vertebral artery involvement. The authors noted that in all three patients, associated intracranial mass lesions were present. They also noted that among 13 patients who presented with focal cerebral ischemia, none had a subsequent cerebral ischemic event during a mean follow-up of 75 months.

Treatment

The treatment of carotid FMD is controversial, as there are no therapeutic trials to guide clinical decision-making. Based on reports that indicate a benign natural history, some authors recommend initial treatment of symptomatic patients with aspirin or dipyridamole.[9,37,47] Oral anticoagulants are suggested for patients with persistent symptoms. Operative procedures such as graduated arterial dilatation, endarterectomy, or bypass grafting are reserved for patients at high risk for stroke whose disease is refractory to medical management.

Effeney and associates contend that a significant proportion of patients referred to their center present with neurologic deficits and that intraluminal dilatation of symptomatic FMD can be performed with minimal risk.[46] In 150 operations performed on 101 patients there were no deaths, three early postoperative strokes, nine transient neurologic deficits, and one vessel perforation. They also concluded that the operation is durable and provides long-lasting benefits. Patients were studied serially for up to five years; only one patient developed an occlusion, and two patients required reoperation. During a follow-up period of up to 17 years, two patients had strokes. Based on this experience, Effeney and associates recommended treating patients with carotid FMD and ischemic neurologic symptoms by graduated intraoperative arterial dilatation. However, prophylactic surgery is not warranted in asymptomatic patients, as the natural history of these patients is unknown.[46]

Percutaneous transluminal angioplasty has been used successfully with renal artery FMD and has been suggested as an alternative to operative intervention for similar lesions in the carotid artery.[49–52] However, the experience reported with this approach is limited. Valid concerns have been raised about the potential risks, which include distal embolization, intimal dissection, carotid-cavernous fistula formation, and technical difficulties due to the ICA tortuosity common in these patients.[44,53,54]

ARTERITIS

Giant Cell Arteritis

Giant cell arteritis (GCA) is a generalized vasculitis that typically affects the medium- and large-sized arteries in elderly patients, more commonly in women than men. Classically, GCA presents as temporal arteritis with headache, scalp tenderness, jaw claudication and visual disturbances, or as polymyalgia rheumatica.

Epidemiology Giant cell arteritis appears to be a disease that is nearly exclusive to the Caucasian population.[55] In a Swedish study performed between 1977 and 1986, the average annual incidence of biopsy proven GCA was noted to be 6.7 per 100,000 inhabitants. In individuals aged 50 years or older, the average incidence was 18.3 per 100,000 inhabitants, with values of 25 cases/100,000 per year for women and 9.4 cases/100,000 per year for men.[56] These figures are similar to those reported from Olmsted County in Minnesota,[57] where the incidence of GCA in individuals over 50 years of age was 17.0 cases/100,000 per year (95 percent confidence interval 13.6–20.5). There was also a threefold greater incidence in women (23.4, 95 percent confidence interval 18.2–28.7) than in men (7.4, 95 percent confidence interval 3.7–11.0). Both series noted that the incidence in women appears to be increasing, whereas in men the rate is stable or dropping.

Pathophysiology The pathogenesis of GCA is unknown, although it has been suggested that an autoimmune response directed against the vascular wall or its constituents may be involved.[55] Typical histologic features include granulomatous inflammation with infiltration of histiocytes and multinucleated giant cells and fragmentation of the internal elastic lamina.[58] The carotid artery branches are the vessels most frequently involved with GCA, followed by the large- and medium-sized arteries of the upper and lower extremities.

Clinical Presentation The typical clinical presentation begins with a one- to three-week period of flu-like symptoms, low-grade fever, malaise, and headache. Following this initial phase, the patient may present with jaw claudication, polymyalgia rheumatica, and abnormal temporal arteries. Visual symptoms such as amaurosis fugax, permanent visual loss, scintillating scotomata, and diplopia tend to occur in the second or third month in 20 to 60 percent of patients.[48]

Laboratory findings are nonspecific and include an elevated erythrocyte sedimentation rate (ESR), mild normocytic anemia, mild thrombocytosis, leukocytosis, and elevations of prothrombin time, alkaline phosphatase, and transaminase. Rarely, patients with active disease will have a normal ESR. In some of these patients, ESR elevation will be unmasked once anti-inflammatory agents are discontinued.[48]

Temporal artery biopsy of the most clinically abnormal site should be performed in all cases. A 4- to 7-cm specimen is recommended, particularly when the artery is grossly normal, because of the intermittent distribution of lesions. Some authors recommend contralateral biopsy when the first biopsy is negative and the clinical suspicion is strong.[59,60] In a study from the Mayo clinic, positive contralateral biopsies were noted in an additional 14 percent of cases.[61] However, other studies report that when bilateral biopsies are performed it is unusual to find unilateral temporal artery involvement. In a series of 60 patients who underwent bilateral biopsies, Klein and coworkers found only three cases of unilateral involvement.[62]

Characteristic angiographic findings include long, tapered narrowings with poststenotic dilatation, occlusion, and collateral vessel formation. Branches of the carotid artery, the subclavian-axillary-brachial vessels, and the superficial femoral and deep femoral arteries most commonly are affected (Fig. 5-5). The coronary, visceral, cerebral, and vertebral arteries are involved less commonly. Thoracic aortic dissection and aneurysm formation in the thoracic and abdominal aorta have also been reported.[48,63]

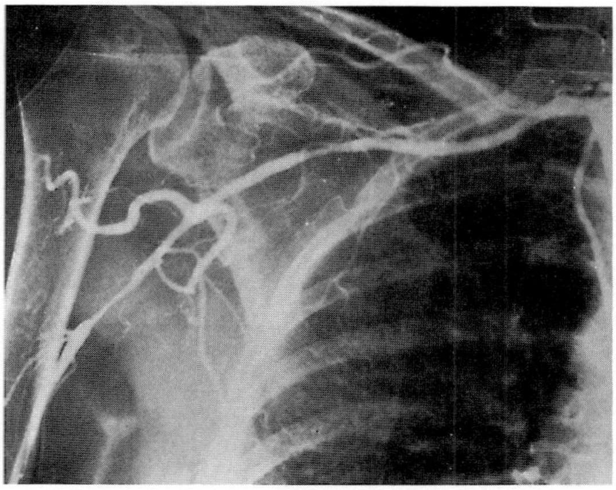

Figure 5-5. Subclavian-axillary-brachial angiogram of a 77-year-old woman with temporal arteritis confirmed by biopsy. Note the long, tapered areas of narrowing. (*Courtesy of Kaj H. Johansen, M.D., Ph.D.*)

Treatment Temporal arteritis is considered to be a medical emergency, and delay in therapy may result in permanent loss of vision. Blindness occurs in 10 to 60 percent of patients not treated promptly.[48] Steroids should be started immediately, followed by temporal artery biopsy. Several authors have noted that the biopsy results will not be affected by two or three days of steroid therapy.[48,59,64] However, Allison and colleagues reported that after one week of steroid therapy the positive biopsy rate fell from 60 percent to less than 10 percent.[65]

Vascular reconstruction is rarely required for GCA. Typical indications include persistent limb ischemia following an adequate trial of medical therapy, aneurysm formation, aortic valvular incompetence, and aortic dissection. Elective procedures should be delayed until the disease becomes quiescent, since graft occlusion is common when operation is performed during the active phase of the disease.[48]

Giant cell arteritis is generally self-limited, and with appropriate medical therapy it should not adversely influence life expectancy. In a European series of 90 patients with GCA followed for nine to 16 years, the survival rate was similar to the general population.[66]

Takayasu's Arteritis

Takayasu was an ophthalmologist who in 1908 first described the finding of unusual retinal arteriovenous anastomoses in a young woman.[67] Onishi noted that these retinal changes were associated with absent pulses in the upper extremities. However, the first clinical case description may have been as early as 1761, when Margagni described the autopsy findings in a 40-year-old woman with absent radial pulses, a thickened ectatic proximal aorta, lower thoracic aortic stenoses, cardiac hypertrophy, and pulmonary edema.[68]

Epidemiology Takayasu's arteritis is an inflammatory arteriopathy of unknown etiology that primarily affects the aorta and its major branches, and less commonly the pulmonary arteries. Although it traditionally has been regarded as a disease of young Asian women, more recent experience demonstrates that Takayasu's arteritis can occur in all races and age groups; however, it is most common in women in the second and third decades of life.[69] There are few reliable data on the actual incidence of Takayasu's arteritis. In a 13-year population study of Olmsted County, Minnesota, three cases were noted, giving an incidence of 2.6 cases/million per year.[70]

Pathophysiology The clinical course of Takayasu's arteritis has been divided into three phases.[69] The first is characterized by systemic inflammatory involvement with arthralgias, myalgias, malaise, night sweats, fever, and weight loss. The second phase is described as a vessel inflammatory stage, in which discomfort in the region of the involved arteries is noted. Patients in the third or "burned-out" phase present with signs and symptoms of ischemia caused by arterial stenosis or occlusion.

Histologic findings initially consist of inflammatory cells invading the adventitia and media but not the intima. In the latter stages of the disease, fibrous scarring of the media and adventitia occurs along with disruption of the elastic laminae, degeneration of the media, and an increase in ground substance in the intima.[69,71,72] The end-result is vessel stenosis and occlusion. Less commonly, aneurysms develop, typically in the ascending aorta.

Clinical Presentation The clinical presentation can vary considerably among individual patients. Some patients will not exhibit all three of the phases described. In others, the phases may overlap. Signs and symptoms of ischemia may occur early in the clinical course or may not appear until years after the onset of systemic inflammatory symptoms.

Ischemic sequelae of Takayasu's arteritis include stroke, renovascular hypertension, upper and lower extremity ischemia, mesenteric ischemia, and myocardial infarction. The classic clinical findings are the absence of upper extremity pulses and the presence of multiple vascular bruits. In a series of 32 patients from the Mayo Clinic, Hall and coworkers noted that 14 (45 percent) had symptoms of upper extremity vascular insufficiency and 30 (94 percent) had multiple bruits.[70] Visual symptoms, including blurred vision, diplopia, or amaurosis fugax, were noted in approximately 30 percent of patients.[73] The disease may involve the pulmonary arteries in some patients, resulting in pulmonary hypertension, shortness of breath, and pleuritic chest pain. With involvement of the ascending aorta, patients may present with symptoms and signs of aortic valvular insufficiency secondary to aneurysm formation.

Angiography in patients with Takayasu's arteritis frequently shows stenosis or occlusion of the proximal extracranial cerebral arteries in the vicinity of the aorta (Fig. 5-6). Among 244 angiograms reviewed by Liu, 85 percent of the lesions were purely stenotic, 2 percent were aneurysmal, and the remainder were a combination of both.[74]

Natural History In a large group of Japanese patients, Ishikawa noted that the prognosis of Takayasu's arteritis was dependent on the presence of complications and the severity of disease.[75,76] Those with complications such as hypertension, retinopathy, aortic valvular insufficiency, and aneurysm formation, to-

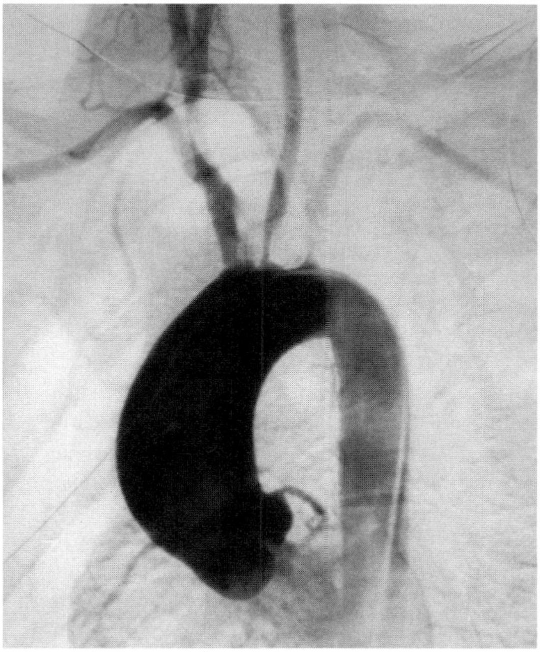

Figure 5-6. Arch aortogram of a patient with Takayasu's arteritis. Severe stenoses of the proximal left common carotid and left subclavian arteries are present. (*Courtesy of Joseph Eskridge, M.D.*)

gether with a progressive clinical course, had a six-year survival of only 55 percent. On the other hand, patients without complications and with stable disease had a six-year survival of 98 percent.

In studies of patients in North America, the survival rates approximate the latter group in Ishikawa's study.[70,77] Hall and colleagues, in a series from the Mayo Clinic, reported a five-year survival of 94 percent.[70] Death was most commonly due to congestive heart failure, cerebrovascular accident, myocardial infarction, or renal failure.

Treatment Corticosteroids are the initial treatment of choice for patients with active disease.[70,77] In the Mayo Clinic series, 29 patients with active Takayasu's arteritis were treated with oral prednisone.[70] Dramatic improvement of systemic inflammatory symptoms occurred in all patients within days to weeks. Eight of 16 patients with absent pulses had return of pulses, and 13 patients were able to discontinue corticosteroids after a median treatment period of 22 months.

Adjuvant immunosuppressive therapy has been recommended in patients refractory to daily corticosteroid therapy. In a prospective study performed at the National Institutes of Health Clinical Center, six of 16 patients with evidence of disease progression while on daily corticosteroid therapy were treated with cyclophosphamide.[77] Four of the six responded favorably with remission of their disease.

Vascular reconstruction has been successfully performed in selected patients who continue to have ischemic symptoms despite medical therapy. However, the role of surgical intervention in asymptomatic patients is uncertain owing to the uncommon nature of the disease. Giordano and coworkers argue that multiple brachiocephalic vessels are frequently involved, severely compromising cerebral blood flow, and that stroke is a common presenting symptom.[69] Furthermore, in their experience, bypass procedures can be performed with little morbidity and mortality in these patients and are effective in preventing stroke. In 21 vascular surgical procedures performed on ten patients with Takayasu's arteritis, there were no deaths. Seven of these procedures were for cerebral revascularization, and during an average follow-up of five years no strokes occurred.

In general, most authors recommend avoiding surgery during the active phase of the disease.[69,70] Hall and associates observed that three of 12 patients developed graft stenosis or occlusion and that all three appeared to have active disease at the time of surgery.[70] In a series of 36 vascular grafts placed in 29 patients, Pajari and coworkers reported a five-year patency rate of 53 percent when the initial operation was performed while the disease was active, compared with 88 percent in patients who had inactive disease at the time of surgery.[78]

Endarterectomy and patch angioplasty are not considered good surgical options because of the transmural inflammatory nature of Takayasu's arteritis. Bypass with placement of anastomoses in unaffected arteries is generally the procedure of choice. Furthermore, Giordano and colleagues suggest that the subclavian or axillary arteries should not be used as inflow sources, even if they are normal at the time of surgery, because of the high incidence of subsequent involvement of these vessels.[69] They prefer to place proximal anastomoses in the ascending aorta, which is less frequently affected. Regardless of the approach used, all these patients require close postoperative surveillance because of the frequent development of anastomotic stenoses, which can occur as early as one or two years after the initial operation.

KINKS AND COILS

Kinks and coils of the ICA are the result of abnormal elongation of the vessel and probably have both congenital and acquired causes. As early as 1898, Kelly reported finding large pulsating vessels in the pharynx in the proximity of tortuous internal carotid arteries.[79] Shortly after 1900, numerous papers were published describing fatal hemorrhagic complications following injury to tortuous carotid arteries during tonsillectomy or adenoidectomy.[80–82] One of the first reports of neurologic symptoms associated with kinked carotid arteries was by Quattlebaum and associates in 1959.[83] They described three patients with hemiplegia and kinked carotid arteries who were treated by resection of the abnormal segment.

Epidemiology

The true incidence of kinks and coils is unknown because most patients with tortuosities and coiling of the carotid artery are asymptomatic. Furthermore, most reports are based on angiographic studies performed in elderly patients with cerebrovascular disorders. One of the largest series comes from the Methodist Hospital in Houston, Texas, where 2453 carotid angiograms were performed in 1407 patients.[84] Tortuosity of the carotid artery was found in 489 (35 percent), coiling in 88 (6 percent), and kinking in 65 (5 percent). Among 76 patients with coiled carotid arteries, 40 (53 percent) had bilateral involvement. Fifteen (28 percent) of 53 patients with kinked carotid arteries had bilateral disease.

In another review of 1000 consecutive carotid angiograms, Metz and coworkers noted ICA kinking in 161 cases (16 percent).[85] Kinking was considered present when the angle between the two segments of vessel forming the kink was 90° or less, or when the vessel formed a complete loop (Fig. 5-7, see also Figs. 2-7 and 2-8). Kinked carotid vessels were present in every decade examined (the first through the eighth), but most cases occurred between ages 41 and 70 years.

Pathophysiology

Several theories on the cause of carotid kinking have been proposed. In 1925, Kelly suggested two: failure of a developmental process and vessel wall changes caused by atherosclerosis.[86] As discussed in Chap. 2, the carotid artery is formed by the third aortic arch and the dorsal aorta. During embryologic development, there is a prominent bend at the junction of these vessels which straightens as the heart descends into the thorax. Kinking of the carotid artery may occur if this straightening process is incomplete. Support for this hypothesis is provided by the relatively common occurrence of bilateral carotid tortuosity in young individuals. The second hypothesis is based on the presence of concomitant atherosclerosis, hypertension, and tortuosity in older individuals. Degeneration of the arterial

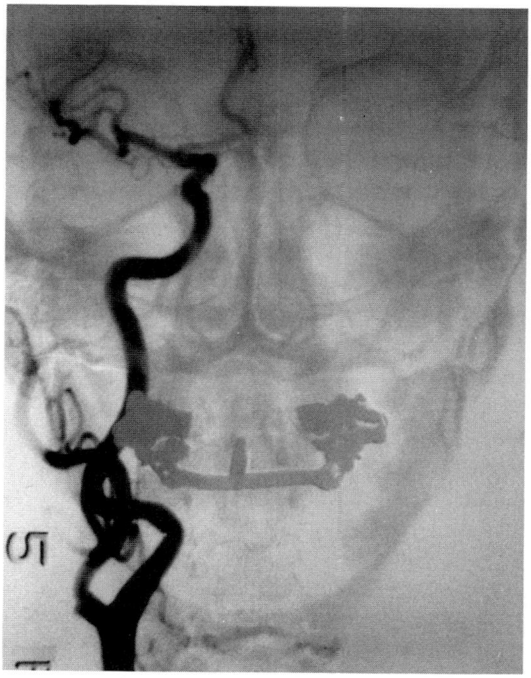

Figure 5-7. Angiogram of a carotid bifurcation showing a kink in the internal carotid artery. There does not appear to be any significant stenosis associated with this particular lesion.

wall, loss of elasticity, and increased intraluminal pressure are believed to result in elongation and consequent tortuosity of the vessel.

Clinical Presentation

If cerebral blood flow is not compromised, as is typical of carotid loops or coils, the finding may be of no clinical significance. Kinks in the carotid artery are more likely to produce luminal narrowing and flow restriction. Depending on the patient's ability to compensate by autoregulation and collateral flow through the circle of Willis, this reduction in flow may or may not result in ischemic neurologic symptoms. In addition, vessel kinking may cause local turbulence and intimal ulceration.[87] Thrombus and platelet aggregates from such sites may subsequently embolize. Thus, symptoms are generally similar to those caused by atherosclerotic disease of the carotid bifurcation: hemispheric TIA; stroke; or amaurosis fugax. When kinking of the vertebral artery occurs, patients may present with symptoms of vertebrobasilar insufficiency: vertigo; ataxia; diplopia; bilateral paresthesias; dysarthria; or drop attacks.

There are few physical findings associated with carotid kinks and coils, none of which are pathognomonic. A pulsatile mass or a bruit may be noted, as well as a prominent pulsation adjacent to the tonsils. Although noninvasive tests such as OPG and duplex scanning are useful, the diagnosis is typically made by angiography.

Treatment

The natural history of these lesions is not precisely known because of the relatively small numbers of patients identified with carotid kinks or coils. Conservative or nonoperative management is generally recommended for asymptomatic patients. In symptomatic patients with hemodynamically significant kinking and no other apparent cause for ischemic neurologic events, surgical correction is indicated.[88–90]

Surgical options include transection of the ICA and reimplantation more proximal into the common carotid artery, segmental resection and end-to-end anastomosis of the ICA, and segmental resection and end-to-end anastomosis of the common carotid artery.[88,91–94] Many authors note that ligation and division of the external carotid artery is required when performing common carotid artery resection; however, Poindexter and colleagues advocate mobilization and preservation of this potential collateral vessel.[88] When concomitant carotid endarterectomy is performed, patch angioplasty has been recommended for arterial closure because the ICA is frequently small.[91,94] Smith and coworkers described a technique for patch angioplasty using a portion of the resected ICA.[94]

Although published series are small, operative interventions for kinked carotid arteries appear to be associated with little morbidity or mortality. Collins and associates reported no perioperative strokes or deaths in 19 patients who underwent carotid resection and patch angioplasty.[91] One patient developed a hypoglossal nerve palsy and required reintubation for upper airway obstruction. During an average follow-up of 25 months (range 4 to 58 months), two patients had ischemic neurologic events contralateral to the reconstruction, and one patient suffered an ipsilateral stroke 41 months postoperatively but had a normal OPG examination. All seven patients in the series reported by Poindexter and colleagues became asymptomatic, and there were no deaths or complications during a follow-up period of up to four years.[88]

ANEURYSMS

Epidemiology

Extracranial carotid artery aneurysms are rare. In 1979, Schechter found 853 carotid aneurysms in a review of the literature published since 1687.[95] Males appear to be affected more often than females (male:female ratio 2.5:1), and associated aneurysms in the aorta or other peripheral arteries are noted in approximately 14 to 20 percent of patients.[96] The bifurcation of the common carotid artery is the most common site for extracranial carotid aneurysms; the internal carotid is the next most common, followed by the external carotid artery.

Pathophysiology

Atherosclerosis frequently is associated with carotid aneurysms, but it is unclear whether this is a coincidental finding in this age group or whether it is a causative factor. Other causes include trauma or infection, and less frequently FMD, dissection, cystic medial necrosis, Marfan's syndrome, polyarteritis nodosa, arteritis, and previous radiation therapy.[95,97–99]

Trauma typically results in the formation of pseudoaneurysms, which can occur following both blunt and penetrating injuries (Chap. 31). Iatrogenic injuries also may be responsible for pseudoaneurysm formation, including previous carotid endarterectomy, tonsillectomy, dental extraction, neck dissection for malignancy, carotid clamping or ligation, and direct puncture either during carotid angiography or during attempted cannulation of the internal jugular vein.[95]

Mycotic carotid aneurysms occur as a result of hematogenous bacterial seeding, direct extension from nearby tissues (peritonsillar abscess, mastoiditis, pharyngitis, or dental abscess), following carotid endarterectomy, or from cervical injection of illicit drugs (Figs. 5-8, 5-9). In the latter group, extension of the infectious process into the mediastinum may further complicate management.[100] Mycotic aneurysms caused by syphilis and tuberculosis were reported frequently in the first half of the 20th century.[101,102] In contemporary series, *Staphylococcus aureus* and *Streptococcus pyogenes* have been the most common organisms.[101,103] Other responsible organisms include Salmonella, Klebsiella, *Escherichia coli,* Pseudomonas, *Streptococcus viridans, Proteus mirabilis,* Corynebacterium, and *Yersinia enterocolitica.*[101,103,104]

Clinical Presentation

As with aneurysmal disease in other locations, many patients with carotid aneurysms are completely asymptomatic, and the diagnosis is suspected after detection of a pulsatile mass on physical examination. However, some patients present with nonspecific complaints of neck pain, tinnitus, headache, or dizziness. Others may have neurologic symptoms, including amaurosis fugax, hemispheric TIA, stroke, Horner's syndrome, and deficits from

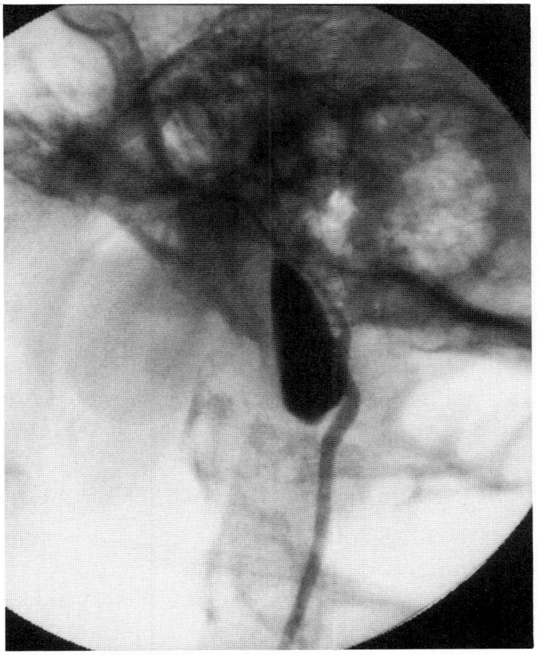

Figure 5-8. Internal carotid angiogram in a 10-year-old boy showing a mycotic pseudoaneurysm secondary to a peritonsillar abscess. This was treated by intraluminal occlusion of the internal carotid artery. (*Courtesy of Joseph Eskridge, M.D.*)

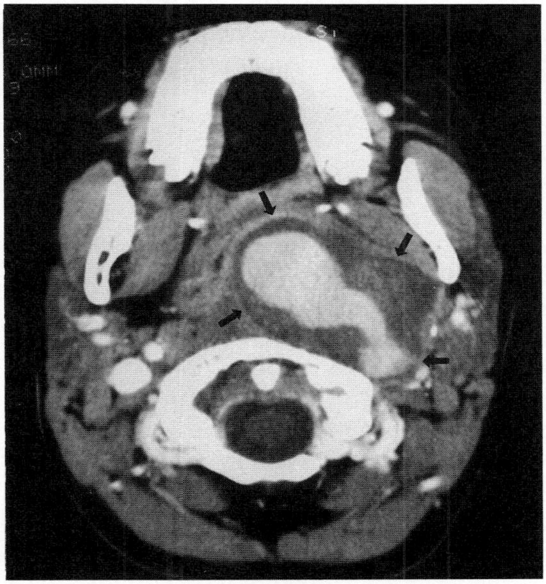

Figure 5-9. Contrast-enhanced CT scan of the patient shown in Fig. 5-8. The large mycotic pseudoaneurysm of the left internal carotid artery is partially filled with thrombus (*arrows*). (*Courtesy of Joseph Eskridge, M.D.*)

compression of cranial nerves V, VII, IX, XI, or XII. In a series of 24 extracranial carotid aneurysms found in 21 patients at the University of Michigan, 50 percent of the patients presented with neurologic symptoms, including amaurosis fugax, TIA, and stroke.[96] In another series of 37 aneurysms in 34 patients from the Methodist Hospital in Houston, Texas, only five patients (15 percent) presented with cerebrovascular symptoms.[99]

Patients with rupture of a carotid aneurysm may have airway compromise due to compression or exsanguinating hemorrhage from the nose, mouth, or ear. Rupture is unusual with true aneurysms of the carotid artery but is more common with mycotic carotid aneurysms and pseudoaneurysms. None of the 24 atherosclerotic carotid aneurysms described in the Michigan series presented with aneurysm rupture.[96] In a series of 22 carotid aneurysms in 21 patients from the University of California at San Francisco, spontaneous hemorrhage did not occur in any of the eight patients with atherosclerotic aneurysms; however, five of ten patients with carotid artery pseudoaneurysms presented with this complication.[104] All five of these patients had an infectious etiology for their pseudoaneurysms.

The differential diagnosis includes tortuous, coiled, or kinked carotid arteries, carotid body tumors, and other neck masses such as enlarged lymph nodes, salivary gland tumors, branchial cleft cysts, or peritonsillar abscesses. The diagnosis can be confirmed with duplex ultrasonography or CT. Angiography is performed for preoperative planning to determine the site, configuration, and the proximal and distal extent of the aneurysm, as well as the status of collateral circulation.

Treatment

In patients with neurologic symptoms in whom other causes have been excluded, the need for operative intervention is clear. The optimal treatment for small asymptomatic aneurysms is less obvious, as there are few natural history data to guide therapy. Zwolak and coworkers observed three strokes among six previously asymptomatic patients with angiographically documented carotid aneurysms who were followed for a mean of 6.3 years.[96]

Surgical options include aneurysmectomy or aneurysmorrhaphy, with either primary anastomosis, patch closure, or reconstruction using a saphenous vein graft or transposition of the external carotid artery. With saccular aneurysms, aneurysmorrhaphy with primary or patch closure frequently is possible. Smaller fusiform aneurysms may be amenable to aneurysmectomy, but larger lesions may best be managed with aneurysmorrhaphy to reduce the likelihood of cranial nerve injury. In cases where distal control is not obtainable, carotid ligation with or without extracranial-to-intracranial bypass may be the only option.

In addition to the risk of ischemic hemispheric complications, cranial nerve injuries occur with increased frequency, particularly in patients with distal internal carotid aneurysms. In the Michigan series previously described, 14 aneurysmectomies and four aneurysmorrhaphies were performed for atherosclerotic carotid aneurysms.[96] There were no surgical deaths, but three patients developed transient neurologic deficits, and one patient suffered a permanent deficit. In addition, transient cranial nerve deficits occurred in three patients, and one patient developed a permanent cranial nerve deficit. No late strokes were noted in the surgically treated patients during a 7.6-year follow-up period. In a review by Sundt and coworkers from the Mayo Clinic, it was concluded that injuries to the facial, hypoglossal, spinal accessory, and main trunk of the vagus nerves were usually avoidable; however, injuries to the glossopharyngeal nerve and the pharyngeal and superior laryngeal branches of the vagus nerve presented more of a problem.[105] Sundt and coworkers reported that damage to the pharyngeal and superior laryngeal branches resulted in considerable dysphagia, even in the presence of a normally innervated contralateral side. Of note, all the patients in the Mayo Clinic series had aneurysms of the distal ICA.

RADIATION-INDUCED ARTERIAL DISEASE

As early as 1899, Gassman described swelling and proliferation of the vascular endothelium and luminal narrowing associated with radiodermatitis.[106] Radiation-induced atheromatous disease in larger vessels was first reported by Thomas and Forbus in 1959.[107] The less frequent complication of rupture in irradiated arteries was documented in 1940 by Cade.[108]

Reports of the association between ischemic cerebrovascular events and cervical irradiation first appeared in the mid-1970s.[109–111] In justifying radiation-induced carotid disease as a distinct clinical entity, Silverberg and colleagues[111] noted that these patients tended to be younger, have less coronary and peripheral vascular disease, and have lower serum lipid levels than nonirradiated patients with atherosclerotic carotid occlusive disease. Furthermore, they noted that the distribution of disease was unusual in that the arterial lesions were limited to the field of radiation.

Pathophysiology

Animal studies have led to the conclusion that arterial changes induced by radiation are in many ways indistinguishable from atherosclerosis. Lindsay and associates demonstrated that irradiation of the canine aorta was followed by the development of atherosclerotic lesions similar to those that occur naturally in older dogs.[112] Notably, the advanced atherosclerotic changes appeared to be localized to irradiated aortic segments.

Fonkalsrud and coworkers administered a total of 4000 roentgens to the femoral arteries of dogs over a 10-day period and observed two distinct phases of morphologic change.[113] In the acute phase, radiation injury appeared primarily to affect the endothelial cells while sparing the media and adventitia. Within 48 h, marked nuclear disruption and endothelial sloughing were noted, with deposition of platelets and fibrin. Gradual repopulation of the endothelial layer was apparent within three weeks, but was still incomplete at four months. After a few weeks, the media demonstrated fibrosis and decreased muscular cellularity with focal areas of necrosis and round cell infiltration. The adventitia showed focal hemorrhage and chronic inflammation during this later stage. Two to four months after radiation, progressive medial fibrosis, combined with endothelial thickening, resulted in moderate to marked narrowing of the vessel lumen. The authors suggested that the late changes in the media and adventitia of large arteries were caused by injury to the vasa vasorum. Furthermore, they postulated that radiation injury to the vasa vasorum with subsequent medial fibrosis may account for the increased incidence of rupture in large elastic arteries.

Animal studies have also suggested that diet and hypertension may affect arterial susceptibility to the degenerative changes induced by radiation. Gold noted only minimal changes in the intima and media of rats subjected to precordial radiation.[114] However, when rats given the same amount of radiation were fed a high fat and cholesterol diet, significant intimal proliferation, medial degeneration, and fibrosis were noted in the pulmonary and coronary arteries. Similarly, Asscher and associates found that irradiated mesenteric arteries in rats were more sensitive to hypertension-induced lesions than nonirradiated vessels.[115]

Thomas and Forbus have been credited with the first description of radiation injury to large vessels in humans.[107] They described autopsy findings from a 19-year-old man who had undergone two courses of radiation therapy for mediastinal lymphoma two and one-half years prior to death. Full-thickness changes consistent with atherosclerosis were found in the irradiated portion of the aortic arch with sparing of the nonirradiated aortic segments. Since that time, there have been numerous case reports and small series describing radiation injury to the carotid, vertebral, axillary, subclavian, coronary, splanchnic, iliac, and femoral arteries.[107,109,116–119]

Clinical Presentation

In their series of 20 patients with radiation-induced vascular lesions, McCready and colleagues noted two patterns of clinical presentation: luminal occlusion and arterial disruption.[117] Atypical stenoses or occlusions developed in six patients from seven to 24 years after irradiation. Three of these patients had disease of the extracranial carotid arteries presenting with cerebrovascular insufficiency, and three patients had iliofemoral disease presenting with severe lower extremity ischemia. Among the 11 patients with carotid disruptions, a typical sequence of events occurred. All had undergone resection of their primary tumor and radical neck dissection three to eight weeks following 5000 to 6500 rads of cervical irradiation. In addition, all of the patients with rupture had infection surrounding their carotid arteries, manifested either by disrupted skin flaps or an orocutaneous fistula. Rupture of the arteries occurred from 14 days to 16 weeks after the initial operation. In an earlier study, Marcial-Rojas and Castro reported a similar experience with six carotid artery ruptures in patients with head and neck carcinomas.[120] Arterial disruption was consistently preceded by necrosis of skin flaps in association with a salivary fistula.

Butler and coworkers described radiation-induced occlusive lesions as having three distinct pathologic patterns.[121] The first presents within the first five years following radiation and consists of mural thrombosis secondary to intimal damage. The second pattern occurs within 10 years and involves fibrotic occlusion of the vessel. The third can occur 20 or more years following irradiation and appears as periarterial fibrosis and accelerated atherosclerosis. Thus, the clinical presentation may be similar to atherosclerotic carotid artery occlusive disease with cervical bruits, amaurosis fugax, hemispheric TIA, or stroke. Angiographically, the lesions produced by cervical irradiation are indistinguishable from atherosclerosis with two possible exceptions: first, the lesions appear to be limited to the irradiated area; second, the disease occurs in locations atypical for atherosclerotic occlusive disease (Fig. 5-10).

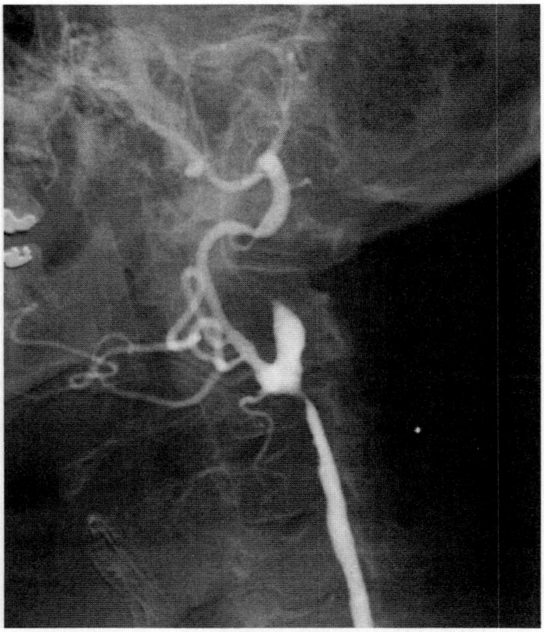

Figure 5-10. Carotid angiogram of a 56-year-old man who had undergone high-dose radiation therapy for salivary gland cancer. He presented with amaurosis fugax. There is severe, extensive narrowing of the distal common and internal carotid arteries with relative sparing of the carotid bulb. An endarterectomy of the common and external carotid arteries was performed with ligation of the internal carotid artery. (*Courtesy of Kaj H. Johansen, M.D., Ph.D.*)

Treatment

Silverberg and associates recommend that patients with radiation-induced carotid occlusive disease be approached as if the radiation were not a factor.[111] In their series of eight carotid endarterectomies performed in seven patients, there were no deaths and one postoperative carotid occlusion. Carotid rupture, which has been described following radiation and radical neck dissection, was not encountered. However, none of these patients had a previous history of neck infection or fistula formation, both of which have been associated with an increased risk of carotid rupture.[117,122,123] Also of note, patients who had radical neck surgery as part of their tumor treatment and patients whose carotid arteries were encased by tumor were excluded from the study.

Atkinson and colleagues in a more recent study concluded that carotid endarterectomy after cervical irradiation was technically more demanding but was feasible and produced good long-term results.[124] In a series of nine endarterectomies with an average follow-up of 49 months, one patient who underwent primary closure of the arteriotomy site developed transient hemispheric events postoperatively, and two patients suffered transient cranial nerve palsies. The authors acknowledged that not only was the arterial dissection more difficult owing to periarterial fibrosis, but the endarterectomy was complicated by adherence of the plaque to the vessel wall. Furthermore, they noted that following removal of the lesion, the arterial wall was often attenuated to the degree that segmental resection and reconstruction were required.

Patients presenting with carotid artery rupture predictably suffer a dismal prognosis. Among nine patients with carotid rupture in the series of McCready and coworkers, ligation of the vessel resulted in stroke or death in five.[117] Two patients in the latter study and two of six patients with carotid rupture reported by Marcial-Rojas and Castro[120] presented with a small bleed followed soon thereafter by exsanguinating hemorrhage. In the few patients who have such "herald bleeds," the authors recommend prompt surgical exploration and carotid ligation if no neurologic deficit is produced by carotid cross-clamping. Otherwise, extracranial-intracranial bypass with autogenous tissue is recommended, using the subclavian artery as the inflow site.

In asymptomatic patients who survive five years or more after cervical radiation therapy, Atkinson and associates[124] and Elerding and colleagues[125] have recommended serial monitoring for the development of carotid occlusive disease with duplex ultrasonography.

REFERENCES

1. Graham JM, Miller T, Stinnett DM: Spontaneous dissection of the common carotid artery. Case report and review of the literature. *J Vasc Surg* 7:811–813, 1988.
2. Jentzer A: Dissecting aneurysm of the left internal carotid artery. *Angiology* 5:232, 1954.
3. Bogousslavsky J, Despland PA, Regli F: Spontaneous carotid dissection with acute stroke. *Arch Neurol* 44:137–140, 1987.
4. Hart RG, Easton JD: Dissections of cervical and cerebral arteries. *Neurol Clin* 1:155–182, 1983.
5. Anson J, Crowell RM: Cervicocranial arterial dissection. *Neurosurgery* 29:89–96, 1991.
6. Meissner I, Mokri B: Vascular diseases of the cervical carotid artery. *Cardiovasc Clin* 22: 161–188, 1992.
7. Houser OW, Mokri B, Sundt TM Jr, et al: Spontaneous cervical cephalic arterial dissection and its residuum: angiographic spectrum. *Am J Neuroradiol* 5:27–34, 1984.
8. Zelenock GB, Kazmers A, Whitehouse WM Jr, et al: Extracranial internal carotid artery dissections: Noniatrogenic traumatic lesions. *Arch Surg* 117:425–432, 1982.
9. Lee NS, Jones HR Jr: Extracranial cerebrovascular disease. *Cardiol Clin* 9:523–534, 1991.
10. Trosch RM, Hasbani M, Brass LM: "Bottoms up" dissection (letter). *N Engl J Med* 320: 1564–1565, 1989.
11. Fisher CM, Ojemann RG, Roberson GH: Spontaneous dissection of cervico-cerebral arteries. *Can J Neurol Sci* 5:9–19, 1978.
12. Wiebers DO, Mokri B: Internal carotid artery dissection after childbirth. *Stroke* 16:956–959, 1988.
13. Jackson MA, Hughes RC, Ward SP, McInnes EG: "Headbanging" and carotid dissection. *Br Med J Clin Res Ed* 287:1262, 1983.
14. O'Connell BK, Towfighi J, Brennan RW, et al: Dissecting aneurysms of head and neck. *Neurology* 35:993–997, 1985.
15. Mokri B, Sundt TM Jr, Houser OW, Piepgras DG: Spontaneous dissection of the cervical internal carotid artery. *Ann Neurol* 19:126–138, 1986.
16. Anderson RM, Schecter MM: A case of spontaneous dissecting aneurysm of the internal carotid artery. *J Neurol Neurosurg Psychiat* 22:195, 1959.
17. Bostrom K, Liliequist B: Primary dissecting aneurysm of the extracranial part of the internal carotid and vertebral arteries. A report of three cases. *Neurology* 17:179–186, 1967.
18. Brice JG, Crompton MR: Spontaneous dissecting aneurysms of the cervical internal carotid artery. *Br Med J* 2:790, 1964.
19. Barnes WT, Jacoby GE: Aneurysm of the common carotid artery due to cystic medial

necrosis treated by excision and graft. *Ann Surg* 155:82–85, 1962.
20. Austin MG, Schaefer RF: Marfan's syndrome with unusual blood vessel manifestations: primary media necrosis dissection of right innominate, right carotid, and left carotid arteries. *Arch Pathol* 64:205–209, 1957.
21. Mokri B, Piepgras DG, Houser OW: Traumatic dissections of the extracranial internal carotid artery. *J Neurosurg* 68:189–197, 1988.
22. Gauthier G, Rohr J, Wildi E, Megret M: [Spontaneous dissecting aneurysm of the internal carotid artery. General review of 205 published cases with 10 personal cases]. *Schweiz Arch Neurol Psychiatr* 136:53–74, 1985.
23. Mokri B: Traumatic and spontaneous extracranial internal carotid artery dissections. *J Neurol* 237:356–361, 1990.
24. Mokri B, Sundt TM Jr., Houser OW: Spontaneous internal carotid dissection, hemicrania, and Horner's syndrome. *Arch Neurol* 36:677–680, 1979.
25. Friedman AH, Drake CG: Subarachnoid hemorrhage from intracranial dissecting aneurysm. *J Neurosurg* 60:325–334, 1984.
26. Grosman H, Fornasier VL, Bonder D, et al: Dissecting aneurysm of the cerebral arteries. Case report. *J Neurosurg* 53:693–697, 1980.
27. Yonas H, Agamanolis D, Takaoka Y, White RJ: Dissecting intracranial aneurysms. *Surg Neurol* 8:407–415, 1977.
28. Mokri B, Schievink WI, Olsen KD, Piepgras DG: Spontaneous dissection of the cervical internal carotid artery. Presentation with lower cranial nerve palsies. *Arch Otolaryngol Head Neck Surg* 118:431–435, 1992.
29. Petro GR, Witwer GA, Cacayorin ED, et al: Spontaneous dissection of the cervical internal carotid artery: correlation of arteriography, CT, and pathology. *Am J Roentgenol* 148:393–398, 1987.
30. Ojemann RG, Fisher CM, Rich JC: Spontaneous dissecting aneurysm of the internal carotid artery. *Stroke* 3:434–440, 1972.
31. Hart RG, Easton JD: Dissections. *Stroke* 16: 925–927, 1985.
32. Farrell MA, Gilbert JJ, Kaufmann JC: Fatal intracranial arterial dissection: Clinical pathological correlation. *J Neurol Neurosurg Psychiatry* 48:111–121, 1985.
33. West TE, Davies RJ, Kelly RE: Horner's syndrome and headache due to carotid artery disease. *Br Med J* 1:818–820, 1976.
34. Stanley JC: Pathology of carotid and vertebral arterial fibrodysplasia, in Ernst CB, Stanley JC (eds): *Current Therapy in Vascular Surgery,* 3d ed. Philadelphia, BC Decker, pp 4–8, 1991.
35. Leadbetter WF, Burkland CE: Hypertension in unilateral renal disease. *J Urol* 39:611–626, 1938.
36. Palumbinskas AJ, Ripley HR: Fibromuscular hyperplasia in extra-renal arteries. *Radiology* 82:451–455, 1964.
37. Corrin LS, Sandok BA, Houser OW: Cerebral ischemic events in patients with carotid artery fibromuscular dysplasia. *Arch Neurol* 38:616–618, 1981.
38. Mettinger KL, Ericson K: Fibromuscular dysplasia and the brain. I. Observations on angiographic, clinical and genetic characteristics. *Stroke* 13:46–52, 1982.
39. Phadke RV, Taori KB, Divekar VK, Bhutada VR: Fibromuscular dysplasia of common carotid artery. A case report. *Australas Radiol* 34:350–352, 1990.
40. Sandok BA: Fibromuscular dysplasia of the internal carotid artery. *Neurol Clin* 1:17–26, 1983.
41. Mettinger KL: Fibromuscular dysplasia and the brain. II. Current concept of the disease. *Stroke* 13:53–58, 1982.
42. Effeney DJ, Ehrenfeld WK, Stoney RJ, Wylie EJ: Fibromuscular dysplasia of the internal carotid artery. *World J Surg* 3:179–186, 1979.
43. Stanley JC, Fry WJ, Seeger JF, et al: Extracranial internal carotid and vertebral artery fibrodysplasia. *Arch Surg* 109:215–222, 1974.
44. Starr DS, Lawrie GM, Morris GC Jr: Fibromuscular disease of carotid arteries: Long term results of graduated internal dilatation. *Stroke* 12:196–199, 1981.
45. Stanley JC, Gewertz BL, Bove EL, et al: Arterial fibrodysplasia. Histopathologic character and current etiologic concepts. *Arch Surg* 110:561–566, 1975.
46. Effeney DJ, Krupski WC, Stoney RJ, Ehren-

feld WK: Fibromuscular dysplasia of the carotid artery. *Aust N Z J Surg* 53:527–531, 1983.
47. Stewart MT, Moritz MW, Smith RB3, et al: The natural history of carotid fibromuscular dysplasia. *J Vasc Surg* 3:305–310, 1986.
48. Joyce JW: Giant cell arteritis, in: Ernst CB, Stanley JC (eds): *Current Therapy in Vascular Surgery,* 2d ed. Philadelphia, BC Decker, pp 173–174, 1991.
49. Brown MM: Balloon angioplasty for cerebrovascular disease. *Neurol Res* 14:159–163, 1992.
50. Tsai FY, Matovich V, Hieshima G, et al: Percutaneous transluminal angioplasty of the carotid artery. *Am J Neuroradiol* 7:349–358, 1986.
51. Wilms GE, Smits J, Baert AL, De-Wolf L: Percutaneous transluminal angioplasty in fibromuscular dysplasia of the internal carotid artery: One year clinical and morphological follow-up. *Cardiovasc Intervent Radiol* 8:20–23, 1985.
52. Dublin AB, Baltaxe HA, Cobb CA: Percutaneous transluminal carotid angioplasty in fibromuscular dysplasia. Case report. *J Neurosurg* 59:162–165, 1983.
53. Jooma R, Bradshaw JR, Griffith HB: Intimal dissection following percutaneous transluminal carotid angioplasty for fibromuscular dysplasia. *Neuroradiology* 27:181–182, 1985.
54. Flandroy P, Lenelle J, Collignon J, Stevenaert A: Carotid cavernous fistula associated with Fogarty catheter angioplasty. *Am J Neuroradiol* 9:1242, 1988.
55. Bengtsson BA, Andersson R: Giant cell and Takayasu's arteritis. *Curr Opin Rheumatol* 3:15–22, 1991.
56. Nordborg E, Bengtsson BA: Epidemiology of biopsy-proven giant cell arteritis (GCA). *J Intern Med* 227:233–236, 1990.
57. Machado EB, Michet CJ, Ballard DJ, et al: Trends in incidence and clinical presentation of temporal arteritis in Olmsted County, Minnesota, 1950–1985. *Arthritis Rheum* 31:745–749, 1988.
58. Hunder GG: Giant cell (temporal) arteritis. *Rheum Dis Clin North Am* 16:399–409, 1990.
59. Fauchald P, Rygvold O, Oystese B: Temporal arteritis and polymyalgia rheumatica. Clinical and biopsy findings. *Ann Intern Med* 77:845–852, 1972.
60. Hall S, Persellin S, Lie JT, et al: The therapeutic impact of temporal artery biopsy. *Lancet* 2:1217–1220, 1983.
61. Hall S, Hunder GG: Is temporal artery biopsy prudent? *Mayo Clin Proc* 59:793–796, 1984.
62. Klein RG, Campbell RJ, Hunder GG, Carney JA: Skip lesions in temporal arteritis. *Mayo Clin Proc* 51:504–510, 1976.
63. Stanson AW, Klein RG, Hunder CG: Extracranial angiographic findings in giant cell (temporal) arteritis. *Am J Roentgenol* 127: 957–963, 1976.
64. Ehsan M, Lange RK, Waxman J: Overdiagnosis of temporal arteritis. *South Med J* 74: 1198–1200, 1981.
65. Allison MC, Gallagher PJ: Temporal artery biopsy and corticosteroid treatment. *Ann Rheum Dis* 43:416–417, 1984.
66. Andersson R, Malmvall BE, Bengtsson BA: Long-term survival in giant cell arteritis including temporal arteritis and polymyalgia rheumatica. A follow-up study of 90 patients treated with corticosteroids. *Acta Med Scand* 220:361–364, 1986.
67. Takayasu M: A case with peculiar changes of the central retinal vessels. *Acta Soc Ophth Japan* 12:554, 1908.
68. Di-Giacomo V: A case of Takayasu's disease occurred over two hundred years ago. *Angiology* 35:750–754, 1984.
69. Giordano JM, Leavitt RY, Hoffman G, Fauci AS: Experience with surgical treatment of Takayasu's disease. *Surgery* 109:252–258, 1991.
70. Hall S, Barr W, Lie JT, et al: Takayasu arteritis: A study of 32 North American patients. *Medicine (Baltimore)* 64:89–99, 1985.
71. Rose G, Sinclair-Smith CC: Takayasu's arteritis. A study of 16 autopsy cases. *Arch Pathol Lab Med* 104:231–237, 1980.
72. Vinijchaikul K: Primary arteritis of the aorta and its main branches (Takayasu's arteriopathy). A clinicopathologic autopsy study of eight cases. *Am J Med* 43:15–27, 1967.
73. Hall S, Buchbinder R: Takayasu's arteritis. *Rheum Dis Clin North Am* 16:411–422, 1990.

74. Liu YQ: Radiology of aortoarteritis. *Radiol Clin North Am* 23:671–688, 1985.
75. Ishikawa K: Natural history and classification of occlusive thromboartopathy (Takayasu's disease). *Circulation* 57:27–35, 1978.
76. Ishikawa K: Patterns of symptoms and prognosis in occlusive thromboaortopathy (Takayasu's disease). *J Am Coll Cardiol* 8:1041–1046, 1986.
77. Shelhamer JH, Volkman DJ, Parrillo JE, et al: Takayasu's arteritis and its therapy. *Ann Intern Med* 103:121–126, 1985.
78. Pajari R, Hekali P, Harjola PT: Treatment of Takayasu's arteritis: An analysis of 29 operated patients. *Thorac Cardiovasc Surg* 34: 176–181, 1986.
79. Kelly AB: Large pulsating vessels in the pharynx. *Glasgow Med J* 49:28–34, 1898.
80. Connolly JH: Large pulsating vessels in the right portion of the posterior pharyngeal wall, partly concealed behind the right tonsil in a boy aged five. *Proc R Soc Med (Laryngol Sect)* 7:25–26, 1913.
81. Fisher AGT: Sigmoid tortuosity of the internal carotid artery and its relation to tonsil and pharynx. *Lancet* 2:128–130, 1915.
82. Skillern PG: Anomalous internal carotid artery and its clinical significance in operations of the tonsils. *JAMA* 60:172–173, 1913.
83. Quattlebaum JK Jr., Upson ET, Neville RL: Stroke associated with elongation and kinking of the internal carotid artery. *Ann Surg* 150: 824–832, 1959.
84. Weibel J, Fields WS: Tortuosity, coiling and kinking of the internal carotid artery. I. Etiology and radiographic anatomy. *Neurology* 15: 7–11, 1965.
85. Metz H, Murray-Leslie RM, Bannister RG, et al: Kinking of the internal carotid artery in relation to cerebrovascular disease. *Lancet* 1: 424–426, 1961.
86. Kelly AB: Tortuosity of the internal carotid in relation to the pharynx. *J Laryngol* 40:15–23, 1925.
87. Mukherjee D, Inahara T: Management of the tortuous internal carotid artery. *Am J Surg* 149:651–655, 1985.
88. Poindexter JM Jr, Patel KR, Clauss RH: Management of kinked extracranial cerebral arteries. *J Vasc Surg* 6:127–133, 1987.
89. Desai B, Toole JF: Kinks, coils, and carotids: A review. *Stroke* 6:649–653, 1975.
90. Cioffi FA, Meduri M, Tomasello F, et al: Kinking and coiling of the internal carotid artery: Clinical-statistical observations and surgical perspectives. *J Neurosurg Sci* 19:15–22, 1975.
91. Collins PS, Orecchia P, Gomez E: A technique for correction of carotid kinks and coils following endarterectomy. *Ann Vasc Surg* 5: 116–120, 1991.
92. Vannix RS, Joergenson EJ, Carter R: Kinking of the internal carotid artery. Clinical significance and surgical management. *Am J Surg* 134:82–89, 1977.
93. Stanton PE Jr, McClusky DA Jr, Lamis PA: Hemodynamic assessment and surgical correction of kinking of the internal carotid artery. *Surgery* 84:793–802, 1978.
94. Smith BM, Starnes VA, Maggart MA: Operative management of the kinked carotid artery. *Surg Gynecol Obstet* 162:70–72, 1986.
95. Schechter DC: Cervical carotid aneurysms: Part I. *N Y State J Med* 79:892–901, 1979.
96. Zwolak RM, Whitehouse WM Jr, Knake JE, et al: Atherosclerotic extracranial carotid artery aneurysms. *J Vasc Surg* 1:415–422, 1984.
97. Ohyama T, Ohara S, Momma F: Aneurysm of the cervical internal carotid artery associated with Marfan's syndrome—case report. *Neurol Med Chir Tokyo* 32:965–968, 1992.
98. Welling RE, Taha A, Goel T, et al: Extracranial carotid artery aneurysms. *Surgery* 93: 319–323, 1983.
99. McCollum CH, Wheeler WG, Noon GP, DeBakey ME: Aneurysms of the extracranial carotid artery. Twenty-one years' experience. *Am J Surg* 137:196–200, 1979.
100. Ledgerwood AM, Lucas CE: Mycotic aneurysm of the carotid artery. *Arch Surg* 109:496–498, 1974.
101. Jebara VA, Acar C, Dervanian P, et al: Mycotic aneurysms of the carotid arteries—case report and review of the literature. *J Vasc Surg* 14:215–219, 1991.
102. Shipley AM, Winslow N, Walker WW: Aneu-

rysm in the cervical portion of the internal carotid artery: An analytical study of the cases recorded in the literature between August 1, 1925, and July 31, 1936; report of two new cases. *Ann Surg* 105:673, 1937.

103. Grossi RJ, Onofrey D, Tvetenstrand C, Blumenthal J: Mycotic carotid aneurysm. *J Vasc Surg* 6:81–83, 1987.
104. Krupski WC, Effeney DJ, Ehrenfeld WK, Stoney RJ: Aneurysms of the carotid arteries. *Aust N Z J Surg* 53:521–525, 1983.
105. Sundt TM Jr, Pearson BW, Piepgras DG, et al: Surgical management of aneurysms of the distal extracranial internal carotid artery. *J Neurosurg* 64:169–182, 1986.
106. Gassman A: Zur Histologie der Röntgenulcera. *Fortschr Geb Roentgenstr* 2:199–207, 1899.
107. Thomas E, Forbus WB: Irradiation injury to the aorta and the lung. *Arch Pathol* 67:256–263, 1959.
108. Cade S: *Malignant Disease and Its Treatment by Radium.* Baltimore: Williams & Wilkins, pp 161–248, 1940.
109. Levinson SA, Close MB, Ehrenfeld WK, Stoney RJ: Carotid artery occlusive disease following external cervical irradiation. *Arch Surg* 107:395–397, 1973.
110. Conomy JP, Kellermeyer RW: Delayed cerebrovascular consequences of therapeutic radiation. A clinicopathologic study of a stroke associated with radiation-related carotid arteriopathy. *Cancer* 36:1702–1708, 1975.
111. Silverberg GD, Brit RH, Goffinet DR: Radiation-induced carotid artery disease. *Cancer* 41:130–137, 1978.
112. Lindsay S, Kohn HI, Dakin RL, Jew J: Aortic arteriosclerosis in the dog after localized aortic x-irradiation. *Circ Res* 10:51–60, 1962.
113. Fonkalsrud EW, Sanchez M, Zerubavel R, Mahoney A: Serial changes in arterial structure following radiation therapy. *Surg Gynecol Obstet* 145:395–400, 1977.
114. Gold H: Production of arteriosclerosis in the rat: Effect of x-ray and a high-fat diet. *Arch Pathol* 71:268–273, 1961.
115. Asscher AW, Wilson C, Anson SG: Sensitisation of blood-vessels to hypertensive damage by x-radiation. *Lancet* 1:580–583, 1961.
116. Hayward RH: Arteriosclerosis induced by radiation. *Surg Clin North Am* 52:359–366, 1972.
117. McCready RA, Hyde GL, Bivins BA, et al: Radiation-induced arterial injuries. *Surgery* 93:306–312, 1983.
118. Savlov ED, Hahhas WA, May AG: Iliac and femoral arteriosclerosis following pelvic irradiation for carcinoma of the ovary. *Obstet Gynecol* 34:345–351, 1969.
119. Feher J: Myocardial infarction following irradiation. *Lancet* 2:643–644, 1965.
120. Marcial-Rojas RA, Castro JR: Irradiation injury to elastic arteries in the course of treatment for neoplastic disease. *Ann Otol* 71:945–958, 1962.
121. Butler MJ, Lane RH, Webster JH: Irradiation injury to large arteries. *Br J Surg* 67:341–343, 1980.
122. Huvos AG, Leaming RH, Moore OS: Clinicopathologic study of the resected carotid artery. Analysis of sixty-four cases. *Am J Surg* 126:570–574, 1973.
123. Fajardo LF, Lee A: Rupture of major vessels after radiation. *Cancer* 36:904–913, 1975.
124. Atkinson JL, Sundt TM Jr, Dale AJ, et al: Radiation-associated atheromatous disease of the cervical carotid artery: Report of seven cases and review of the literature. *Neurosurgery* 24:171–178, 1989.
125. Elerding SC, Fernandez RN, Grotta JC, et al: Carotid artery disease following external cervical irradiation. *Ann Surg* 194:609–615, 1981.

Part Two

Clinical Manifestations

6

Ischemia in the Carotid Artery Distribution

Phillip D. Swanson

TEMPORAL PATTERN

MAJOR ARTERIES ARISING FROM THE INTERNAL CAROTID
- Variability of Territories Supplied by the Major Arteries

SYMPTOMS AND SIGNS
- Visual loss
- Aphasia
- Hemiparesis
- Hemisensory Loss
- Perceptual Problems
- Disconnection Syndrome
- Hemianopia

FREQUENCY OF SYMPTOMS IN CAROTID ARTERY ISCHEMIA

With knowledge of the territories supplied by the internal carotid arteries and the location of the neurons responsible for definable neurologic functions, it should be relatively easy to predict which symptoms and signs will be found with ischemia in the carotid artery distribution. For the following reasons, however, such correlation is not always so straightforward: some symptoms can occur with ischemia at more than one location; territories supplied by the internal carotid artery and its branches can vary; and symptoms sometimes can be interpreted incorrectly by either the patient or the physician.

Ischemic events can be categorized in three ways: by temporal pattern; by location of the affected neurons and axons within the central nervous system; and by the presumed pathophysiology. The location of the pathology usually allows one to determine which arterial supply area is involved.

TEMPORAL PATTERN

Four terms are commonly used to characterize the temporal pattern of cerebrovascular events: transient ischemic attack (TIA); reversible ischemic neurologic deficit (RIND); stroke-in-evolution; and completed stroke. A TIA is defined as "transient (less than 24 h) hypofunction of the nervous system thought to be related to ischemia in the recognized distribution of the carotid or vertebral-basilar arterial system without residua from that attack (migraine or migraine equivalent excluded)."[1,2] The 24-h time limit for a TIA is arbitrary. In fact, most TIAs last less than 6 h, with the usual duration ranging from 8 to 14 min. A RIND resembles a TIA, but the neurologic signs persist beyond 24 h. An evolving stroke or "stroke-in-evolution" initially may resemble a TIA; however, neurologic signs fluctuate during the initial period of observation, with the outcome being a fixed neurologic deficit or completed stroke.

MAJOR ARTERIES ARISING FROM THE INTERNAL CAROTID

The first major branch of the internal carotid artery is the ophthalmic which gives rise to the central retinal artery (Chap. 2). Thus, unilateral visual loss is an important indicator of ischemia in the internal carotid distribution. The next major branch is the anterior choroidal artery, which supplies portions of the globus pallidus and posterior limb of the internal capsule. The internal carotid artery then branches into the middle and anterior cerebral arteries. The anterior cerebral artery usually supplies the medial surface of the ipsilateral cerebral hemisphere and the underlying corpus callosum. There is also a recurrent artery of Heubner that often arises from this vessel. It supplies part of the head of the caudate nucleus and anterior limb of the internal capsule. Ischemia in the anterior cerebral artery distribution may produce weakness more in the leg than the arm and sometimes a "disconnection syndrome" between the two cerebral hemispheres, as discussed later in this chapter.

The middle cerebral artery usually supplies the bulk of the convexity of the cerebral hemisphere. Through its penetrating lenticulostriate branches it also supplies part of the internal capsule, as well as the putamen and caudate nucleus. Patterns of infarction that occur with middle cerebral artery occlusions are shown in Fig. 6-1.

Variability of Territories Supplied by the Major Arteries

Van der Zwan and coworkers[3] have reexamined the territorial supply of the major cerebral arteries. Using 25 unfixed human brain specimens, they simultaneously injected each major artery under the same pressure with different colored mixtures of the polymer Araldite F. The territories of the anterior, middle, and posterior cerebral arteries were found to be highly variable in extent. Thus, on the medial surface of a cerebral hemisphere, the anterior cerebral artery in one case might supply the anterior 20 percent of the cortex, and in another two-thirds of that territory. These differences contribute to the variability in extent of infarction following occlusion of a major cerebral vessel (Figs. 6-2 and 6-3).

Another reason for the variability in the extent of infarction after vascular occlusion is the variation in collateral blood supply from other vessels (Chap. 2). In some people, occlusion of an internal carotid artery may lead to no hemispheric ischemia because of adequate collaterals from the anterior or posterior communicating arteries or from cortical collaterals. In others with poor collateral supply, infarction may ensue. The clinical outcome of internal carotid occlusion was reported by Nicholls and associates in 24 patients with carotid stenoses that progressed to complete

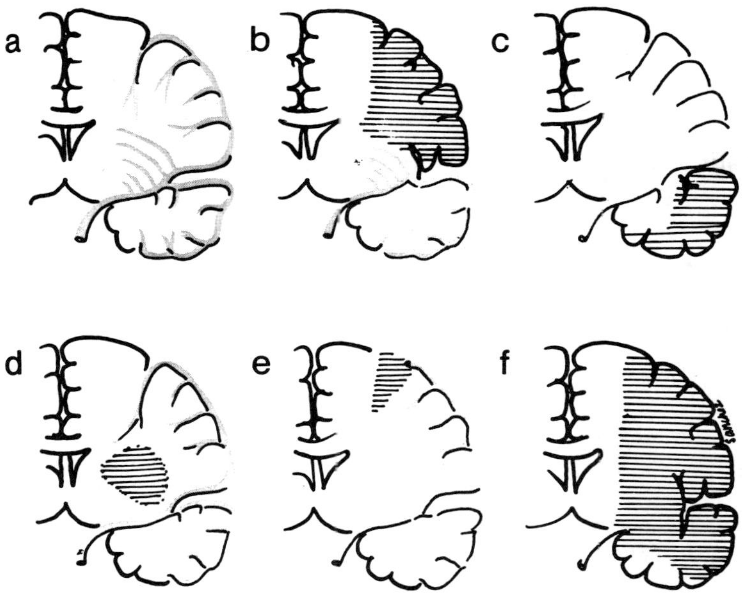

Figure 6-1. Typical patterns of infarction with middle cerebral artery (MCA) occlusion. *A.* Diagram of the MCA distribution in coronal section. *B.* Occlusion of the upper trunk of the MCA. *C.* Occlusion of the lower trunk of MCA. *D.* Infarct of the deep basal ganglia. *E.* Wedge infarct in the pial territory. *F.* Total MCA occlusion. *(From Caplan LR: Stroke: A Clinical Approach. 2d ed. Boston, Butterworth. Heinemann, 1993:215. Used with permission.)*

occlusion as documented by serial duplex scanning.[4] Progression to occlusion was associated with ipsilateral stroke in six (25 percent), ipsilateral TIA in four (16 percent), and nonhemispheric symptoms in one (5 percent). Thirteen patients remained asymptomatic. During a mean follow-up period of 39 months, the average annual rate of stroke and TIA were 10 and 13 percent, respectively, and the combined rate of stroke and TIA was 20 percent per year. Thus, progression of internal carotid stenosis to occlusion is associated with a relatively high risk for both immediate and late neurologic events.

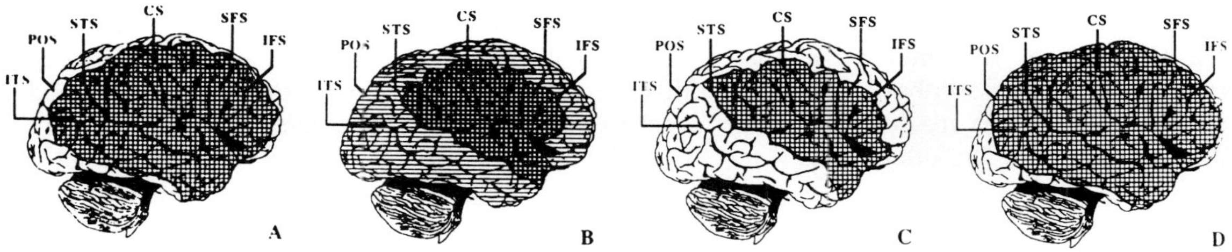

Figure 6-2. Cortical distribution of the middle cerebral artery (MCA). *A.* Most common distribution on the lateral surface of the hemisphere (crossed area). *B.* Area of variation on the lateral surface of the hemisphere (uncrossed horizontal lines). *C.* and *D.* Examples of the cortical MCA distribution in two individual cerebral hemispheres (crossed areas). CS = central sulcus; IFS = inferior frontal sulcus; ITS = inferior temporal sulcus; POS = parieto-occupital sulcus; SFS = superior frontal sulcus; STS = superior temporal sulcus. *(From van der Zwan et al.[3] Used with permission.)*

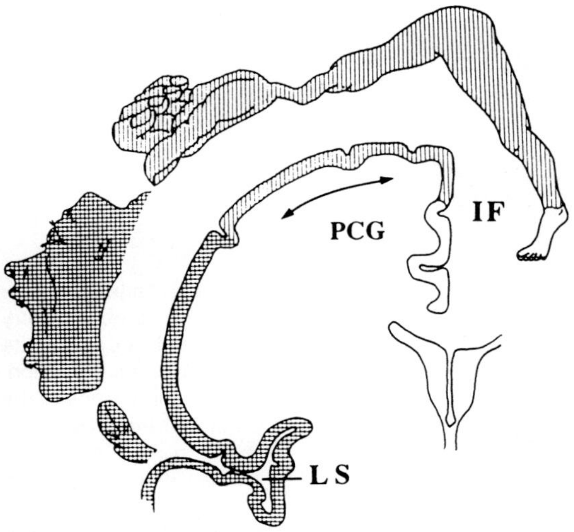

Figure 6-3. Diagram representing a composite of the minimum (horizontal lines) and maximum (vertical lines) areas supplied by the middle cerebral artery in the precentral gyrus reflected on the motor homunuculus. IF = interhemispheric fissure; LS = lateral sulcus; PCG = precentral gyrus. (*From van der Zwan et al.*[3] *Used with permission.)*

SYMPTOMS AND SIGNS

Visual Loss

Transient monocular blindness is called *amaurosis fugax*. If it can be stated unequivocally that the visual alteration was in one eye only and not in one or the other visual field, this symptom is a strong indicator of ischemia in the territory of the internal carotid artery rather than the vertebrobasilar system. In this situation, symptoms are due to either reduced flow or emboli to the ophthalmic artery. Occasionally fibrin-platelet or cholesterol emboli can be visualized during ophthalmoscopic examination. Cholesterol crystals or *Hollenhorst plaques* sometimes are visualized at the bifurcations of retinal arterioles. These have also been referred to as "bright plaques" and typically appear highly refractile in the light from the ophthalmoscope.

The visual manifestations of amaurosis fugax may vary. Wray classifies this symptom into four types based on the presumed pathophysiology (Table 6-1).[5] Amaurosis fugax due to reduced perfusion (Type II) typically comes on more slowly and lasts longer than that due to emboli or vasospasm. The visual impairment may be described as a curtain moving across the visual field from above, below, or the side; or it may involve loss of vision in the entire eye, with everything going black.[6] This contrasts with the visual phenomena of ocular migraine in which scintillations are characteristic.

Aphasia

The other symptom that most clearly points to the internal carotid distribution is aphasia. Aphasias are classified in different ways. Probably the most useful clinically is the Geschwind classification into *fluent* and *nonfluent* aphasias, which are distinguished by the volume of speech (Table 6-2).[7,8] Patients with nonfluent aphasias have slow, labored speech with hesitancy in initiating words, a tendency to leave out connective words, and poor articulation. Patients with fluent aphasias may have a naturally flowing spontaneous speech, but with little content and frequent word and syllable substitutions. There may be marked difficulty in naming. In practice, it often is difficult to fit an aphasia into one or the other category; however, it is important to recognize that a patient has aphasia and to describe the nature and severity of the problem. Bedside testing should, whenever possible, examine verbal and visual comprehension, output of spoken and written language, repetition of simple phrases, and naming of common objects. Most aphasic patients have a problem with language that is also evident in their handwriting.

Even in left-handed patients, language function usually is located in the left cerebral hemisphere in areas supplied by the middle cere-

Table 6-1 Types of Amaurosis Fugax[a]

	Type I	Type II	Type III	Type IV
Mechanism	Embolus Arteritis	Hypoperfusion	Vasospasm	Other
Onset	Abrupt	Less rapid	Abrupt	Abrupt
Duration	Seconds to minutes	Minutes to hours	Minutes	Variable
Visual Loss	All or partial	All or partial	Total or progressive visual field contraction	Partial
Pain	No	Rare	Often	No
Recovery	Complete	Complete	Usually complete	Complete
Unusual Features	Vision may black out completely	Sunlight-provoked	Vision loss may spare fixation	Alternating between eyes; multiple attacks

[a]After Wray.[5]

bral artery. Thus, the acute onset of aphasia usually signifies ischemia in the distribution of the left internal carotid artery.

Hemiparesis

Rapid onset of weakness on one body side is the most frequent symptom that suggests brain ischemia. It must be recognized, however, that hemiparesis can also occur with dysfunction below the level of the cerebral hemispheres. In the brain stem, motor fibers descend through the base of the pons. Therefore, a small ischemic lesion on one side of the pons can produce weakness of the opposite face, arm, and leg. Weakness of an arm and leg on the same body side also can occur with unilateral spinal cord lesions in the high cervical area, although in this situation the face would not be involved.

The hemiparesis that results from ischemia in the territory of the internal carotid artery may be accompanied by sensory loss, visual field loss, or aphasia. As discussed later, when hemiparesis is related to right brain dysfunction, it may be associated with such perceptual problems as denial of disability or inattention to the affected body side.

The pattern of weakness that occurs with hemispheric ischemia is extremely variable. Classically, in lesions of the cerebral convexity, weakness is worse in the face and arm than in the leg. However, information from the Stroke Data Bank suggests that an infarct at a given site in the motor cortex can produce quite different degrees and patterns of weakness.[9]

Hemisensory Loss

Hemisensory loss can result from ischemia in the territory of the middle cerebral artery with involvement of the sensory cortex or subcortical region underlying the postcentral gyrus. It should be remembered, however, that the

Table 6-2 Geschwind's Subtypes of Fluent Aphasia

Type of Aphasia	Comprehension	Repetition	Location of Lesion
Wernicke's	Impaired	Impaired	Posterior superior temporal
Conduction	Normal	Impaired	Suprasylvian-parietal
Anomic	Normal	Normal	Angular gyrus or lower temporal lobe
Isolation	Impaired	Normal	Surrounds intact speech areas

thalamus is primarily supplied by branches from the posterior cerebral arteries and is not typically in the territory supplied by the internal carotid arteries. A small infarct in the thalamus may produce numbness of the opposite side of the body in isolation or associated with hemiparesis if the internal capsule is involved.

The presence of perceptual problems indicates that the sensory loss is most likely cortical rather than thalamic. Another differentiating feature is the type of sensory loss that is found. With a cortical lesion, there may be intact pain and temperature sensation with prominent loss of tactile sensibility and stereognosis, whereas with a thalamic lesion pain and temperature sensations are likely to be impaired.

Perceptual Problems

Damage to the right cerebral hemisphere may be associated with alterations in the patient's perception of space and other, often bizarre symptoms, sometimes called the *right parietal syndrome*. Such patients may deny any disability, even when a severe hemiparesis is present. Patients may ignore the left side of their bodies and visual stimuli from the left side. When asked to draw a clock, they may crowd all the numbers into the right side of the circle.

Disconnection Syndrome

Damage to the corpus callosum from anterior cerebral artery occlusion can separate some functions of the two cerebral hemispheres. The resulting *disconnection syndrome* depends not only on involvement of cortical regions, but on the interruption of interhemispheral fiber tracts. In such cases, the language and perception areas of the left hemisphere are isolated from the right hemisphere. A recent patient with this problem complained of a "third hand." At times her hands would compete with each other for a cup of liquid. She had difficulty tapping her hands simultaneously and synchronizing the hands when propelling a wheelchair.

Hemianopia

Hemianopia or quadrantanopia without other symptoms or signs usually implicates the opposite occipital cortex, which is supplied by

Table 6-3 Symptoms Occurring in More Than 20 Percent of Cases with Transient Ischemic Attacks in the Carotid Artery Distribution

	Frequency (%)	
Symptoms	Left TIA	Right TIA
Weakness and sensory complaint, contralateral arm	67	70
Weakness, contralateral arm	56	50
Sensory complaint, contralateral arm	44	53
Dysphasia	45	
Weakness, contralateral leg	24	34
Ipsilateral loss of vision	20	27
Dysarthria	21	24
Sensory complaint, contralateral face		29
Sensory complaint, contralateral leg		28
Weakness, contralateral face	26	26

SOURCE: Futty DE, Conneally PM, Dyken ML, et al.[2]

the posterior cerebral artery. Unless this artery arises from the internal carotid through a large posterior communicating artery, a transient or permanent visual field deficit is not likely to result from ischemia in a carotid artery distribution. On the other hand, a hemianopia also can occur with ischemia to the part of the cerebral hemisphere containing the optic radiation fibers, which carry visual information from the lateral geniculate body to the occipital cortex. Thus, ischemia in the internal carotid artery distribution can affect the visual fields. Certainly, the presence of a hemianopia along with a hemisensory loss or hemiparesis excludes the brain stem as the site of pathology.

FREQUENCY OF SYMPTOMS IN CAROTID ARTERY ISCHEMIA

In the Cooperative Study of Hospital Frequency and Character of Transient Ischemic Attacks, a symptom analysis of patients thought to have a definite TIA in the territory of the internal carotid arteries showed that weakness and sensory complaints in the contralateral arm occurred in about 70 percent of cases, dysphasia in 45 percent of left hemispheric events, and ipsilateral loss of vision in 20–27 percent.[2] Dysarthria also occurred in about 20 percent of cases, as it did in vertebrobasilar TIA (Table 6-3).

REFERENCES

1. Dyken ML: Frequency and symptom analysis of transient ischemic attacks: A cooperative hospital study, in Scheinberg P (ed): *Cerebrovascular Diseases*. New York, Raven Press, pp 31–38, 1976.
2. Futty DE, Conneally PM, Dyken ML, Price TR, Haerer AF, Poskanzer DC, Swanson PD, Calanchini PR, Gotshall RA: Cooperative study of hospital frequency and character of transient ischemic attacks versus symptom analysis. *JAMA* 238:2386–2390, 1977.
3. van der Zwan A, Hillen B, Tullenken CAF, Dujovny M, Dragovic L: Variability of the territories of the major cerebral arteries. *J Neurosurg* 77: 927–940, 1992.
4. Nicholls SC, Bergelin R, Strandness DE: Neurologic sequelae of unilateral carotid artery occlusion: Immediate and late. *J Vasc Surg* 13: 175–176, 1991.
5. Wray SH: The management of acute visual failure. *J Neurol Neurosurg Psychiat* 56:234–240, 1993.
6. Burde RM: Amaurosis fugax. An overview. *J Clin Neuro-ophth* 9:185–189, 1989.
7. Geschwind N: Language and the brain. *Sci Am* 226:76–83, 1972.
8. Geschwind N: Aphasia. *N Engl J Med* 284:654–656, 1971.
9. Mohr JP, Foulkes MA, Polis AT, Hier DB, Kase CS, Price TR, Tatemichi TK, Wolf PA: Infarct topography and hemiparesis profiles with cerebral convexity infarction: the Stroke Data Bank. *J Neurol Neurosurg Psychiat* 56:344–351, 1993.

7

Ischemia in the Vertebrobasilar Distribution

Phillip D. Swanson

Diagnosing vertebrobasilar ischemia on clinical grounds alone is often difficult, especially in patients with transient ischemic attack (TIA) or early stroke. Several questions should be considered when assessing such a patient: Is a homonymous hemianopia due to a lesion in the occipital cortex (posterior cerebral artery) or in the optic radiation (middle cerebral artery)? Is weakness of a limb or limbs due to ischemia in the motor cortex or internal capsule (carotid artery distribution) or in the base of the pons (basilar artery)? Which specific artery is likely to supply the affected area in this patient and from which major vessel does that artery arise?

It must be remembered that the two vertebral arteries and the basilar artery that originates from them supply more than the brain stem. There is a "top of the basilar" syndrome, with symptoms resulting from ischemia to deep hemispheral structures, especially the thalamus, caused by reduced flow in the thalamo-perforating arteries. Furthermore, the two posterior cerebral arteries usually originate from the basilar artery, but in some cases one or both may fill primarily from the carotid arteries (Chap. 2). The posterior cerebral arteries supply important areas of the cerebral hemispheres, including the medial and inferior temporal lobes and the medial occipital lobes, which contain the visual cortex (Fig. 7-1). Symptoms and signs caused by ischemia to these areas are sometimes difficult to distinguish from those due to ischemia in areas supplied by the internal carotid system.

SYMPTOMS AND SIGNS OF VERTEBROBASILAR ISCHEMIA

In the Cooperative Study of Hospital Frequency and Character of Transient Ischemic Attacks, symptoms that occurred in more than 20 percent of cases with TIA in the vertebrobasilar distribution were ataxia (60 percent), dizziness or vertigo (43 percent), diplopia (39 percent), bilateral visual blurring (37 per-

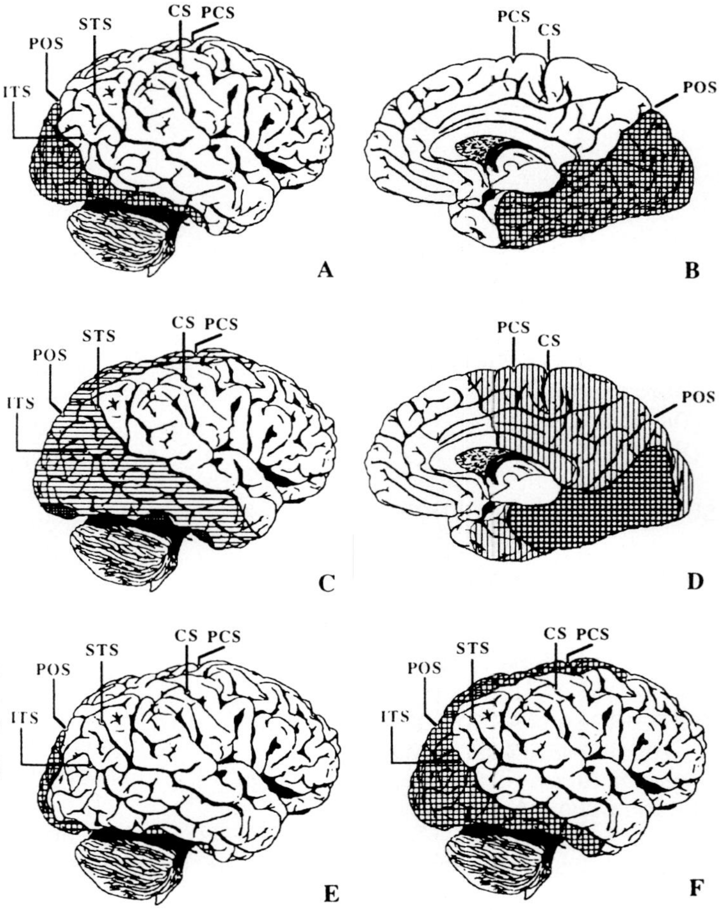

Figure 7-1. Cortical distribution of the posterior cerebral artery (PCA). CS = central sulcus; ITS = inferior temporal sulcus; PCS = precentral sulcus; POS = parieto-occipital sulcus; STS = superior temporal sulcus. *A*. Most common distribution on the lateral surface of the hemisphere (crossed area). *B*. Most common distribution on the medial surface of the hemisphere (crossed area). *C*. Area of variation on the lateral surface (uncrossed horizontal lines). *D*. Area of variation on the medial surface (uncrossed vertical lines); horizontal lines represent minimum areas and vertical lines represent maximum areas. *E* and *F*. Examples of the cortical PCA distribution in two individual cerebral hemispheres (crossed areas). (*From van der Zwan A, Hillen B, Tulleken CAF, Dujovny M, Dragovic L: Variability of the territories of the major cerebral arteries. J Neurosurg 77:927, 1992. Used with permission.*)

cent) and dysarthria (27 percent).[1] Bilateral limb weakness occurred in fewer than 10 percent of patients (Table 7-1).

Ataxia and Vertigo

Rapid onset of ataxia can be a symptom of posterior circulation ischemia. Ataxia is generally defined as incoordination of movement; it may be due to a lesion in the cerebellum or in the sensory pathways that control movement. The cerebellum is concerned with the regulation of muscular tone, the coordination of movement (particularly skilled voluntary movement), and the control of posture and gait. Dysfunction of the cerebellum or the vestibular system can result in difficulty with balance.

Vertigo is commonly associated with ataxia. True vertigo is characterized by the sensation that objects in the environment are spinning around or that the head and body are whirling. It is frequently accompanied by varying degrees of nausea, vomiting, pallor, and perspiration. Dizziness is a less distinct symptom typically described as a feeling of swaying or lightheadedness. Nystagmus should be searched for on neurological examination. Vertical nystagmus usually indicates brain stem pathology.

Diplopia

Since the nuclei of the third, fourth, and sixth cranial nerves are in brain stem structures supplied by branches of the basilar artery, one of the best indicators of brain stem dysfunction is the presence of diplopia or double vision. Diplopia can arise from involvement of an individual cranial nerve nucleus or from a lesion of the nerve itself. A cranial nerve paresis is more likely to signify damage within the brain stem rather than the peripheral portion of the nerve if there are associated findings that point to involvement of adjacent brain stem structures such as the cerebral peduncle or seventh cranial nerve.

Diplopia can also occur with small infarcts involving the medial longitudinal fasciculus (MLF), a pathway located in the dorsomedial brain stem containing fibers that coordinate the actions of the extraocular muscles. Damage to the ipsilateral MLF produces difficulty looking medially upon attempting horizontal gaze. This usually is associated with nystagmus of the contralateral (abducting) eye. In many cases such an *internuclear ophthalmoplegia* can be differentiated from a partial third nerve palsy by noting the patient's ability to turn the eye medially when attempting to converge.

Table 7-1 Symptoms Occurring in More Than 20 Percent of Cases with Transient Ischemic Attacks in the Vertebrobasilar Distribution

Symptom	Frequency (%)
Ataxia	60
Dizziness	43
Diplopia	39
Bilateral blurring of vision	37
Dysarthria	27

SOURCE: Futty DE, Conneally PM, Dyken ML, et al.[1]

Palatal Myoclonus

Rhythmic movements involving the soft palate, and often the pharynx and eyes, at frequencies from 40 to 200 per minute result from damage to dentato-olivary fibers in the brain stem. The most common cause is brain stem infarction.[2]

SUBCLAVIAN STEAL SYNDROME

The term "subclavian steal syndrome" was coined by Fisher[3] in an editorial that discussed a paper by Reivich and coauthors.[4] Two patients were shown to have reversed flow through the left vertebral artery associated with stenosis of the left subclavian artery proximal to the vertebral artery origin. Patient One had exercise-induced left postauricular headaches and had experienced four episodes of left arm weakness that were not exercise-induced. Patient Two had multiple episodes of visual blurring brought about by looking up or turning the head to the left, and one episode of aphasia and right hand weakness. However, this patient also had occlusion of the left internal carotid artery. Both patients had reduced blood pressures and pulses in the left arm. Patient One had a systolic bruit over the left subclavian artery. In these patients, the authors were able to demonstrate reversal of blood flow in the left vertebral arteries; they also showed similar effects in a dog model by occluding the subclavian artery on the left.

In 125 cases of subclavian steal syndrome reviewed by Patel and Toole, the most common symptoms were pain, numbness or fatigue of an arm, blurred vision or diplopia, vertigo or dizziness, and headaches.[5] Eleven of 68 patients reported that the symptoms were related to arm exercise. The most important physical findings were a diminished or absent radial pulse on the affected side, a supraclavicular bruit, and a difference in systolic blood pressure between the two arms ranging from 20 to 230 mmHg.

In spite of the underlying pathophysiology, it is rare to encounter a patient whose symptoms of ischemia are brought about by use of an upper extremity. Nevertheless, it is important for clinicians to be aware that retrograde vertebral flow can occur in this setting. The physical examination should include palpating for pulse differences, obtaining blood pressures from both arms, and careful listening for subclavian bruits. The surgical management of the subclavian steal syndrome is discussed in Chap. 29.

BRAIN STEM SYNDROMES

A variety of clinical syndromes can occur after brain stem infarction from occlusion of the vertebral or basilar arteries or their branches. These include the lateral medullary plate syndrome and several midbrain and pontine syndromes.

The Lateral Medullary Plate Syndrome

Infarction of a portion of the lateral medulla gives rise to a constellation of symptoms and signs that is readily recognizable upon neurological examination because of the ipsilateral loss of pain and temperature on the face and the contralateral loss of these sensory modalities on the body and limbs (Fig. 7-2). The usual symptoms include dizziness or vertigo,

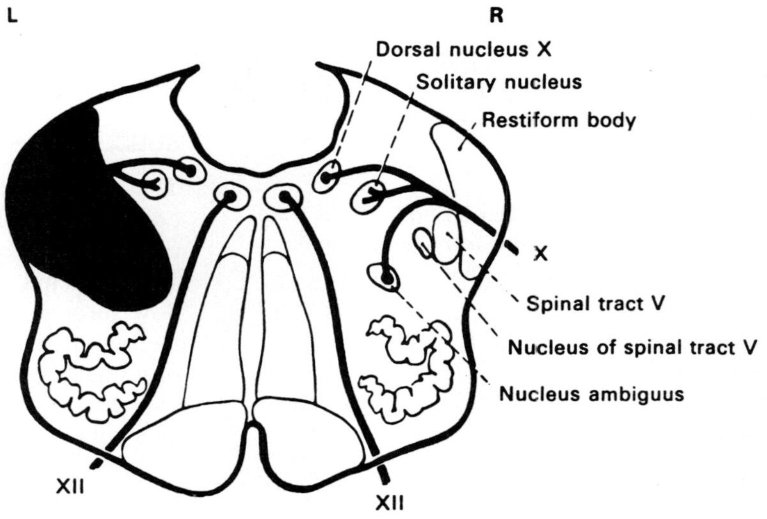

Figure 7-2. The medulla lesion which produces the lateral medullary plate syndrome. (*From Haymaker W: Bing's Local Diagnosis in Neurological Diseases. St. Louis, CV Mosby, 1969. Used with permission.*)

difficulty swallowing, and loss of balance. Infarction also may involve the ipsilateral cerebellum. This syndrome is sometimes the consequence of neck manipulation, either self-administered or secondary to chiropractic treatment, resulting in vertebral artery dissection and thrombosis.

Clinical case. A 71-year-old retired Army officer noticed difficulty standing after a morning bath. He felt dizzy and would fall to the left. He then developed a numb feeling on the left side of his lips, cheek, and throat. Within 30 min he was unable to walk. His voice seemed hoarse and he noted difficulty swallowing, although he could swallow small amounts down the right side of his throat. Neurological examination revealed clearly enunciated, but hoarse speech. There was mild pupil miosis and ptosis on the left. A corneal reflex could not be elicited on the left, and sensation to pinprick and temperature was impaired in the distribution of all three divisions of the left trigeminal nerve, including the left side of the tongue. The left side of the soft palate elevated less well than the right, and the gag reflex could not be elicited on the left. Over the body, sensations to pinprick and temperature were impaired on the right side up to the jaw, but other sensations were intact. The left hand was moderately clumsy, but was not weak. He was markedly ataxic when he attempted to walk.

Comment. This patient's signs and symptoms indicated damage to the left side of the lateral medulla, an area supplied by a branch of the vertebral artery, often the posterior inferior cerebellar artery. Autopsied cases of Wallenberg's syndrome or the lateral medullary plate syndrome are often found to have occlusion of the ipsilateral vertebral artery.

The Locked-in Syndrome

A large infarct in the brain stem at the level of the pons can produce a clinical state in which the patient has normal sleep-waking cycles but has no voluntary motor function of the limbs because of damage to the descending motor pathways. Often horizontal gaze is absent because the horizontal gaze pathways and both sixth cranial nerves are involved. However, the patient may be able to elevate or depress the eyes and eyelids, and thereby communicate with eye blinks or eye movements in the vertical plane. Infarctions in this area usually result from thrombosis of the basilar artery, occasionally as an extension of a vertebral artery occlusion.

Other Brain Stem Syndromes

Infarction can also occur in other areas of the brain stem. When there are typical signs, usually affecting an ipsilateral cranial nerve and a descending or ascending fiber tract which serves the contralateral body side, it will be apparent that the site of the infarct is in the brain stem (Figs. 7-3 and 7-4). However, when there is no cranial nerve involvement, as with a small infarct in the base of the pons, there may be no clear indication that the damage is in the brain stem.

A common diagnostic error is to misinterpret the presence of certain "cranial nerve" abnormalities found on neurological examination. Failure to demonstrate a gag reflex

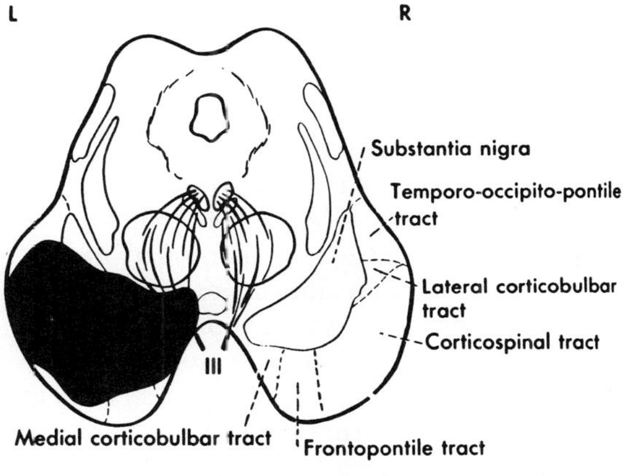

Figure 7-3. Midbrain lesion involving the cerebral peduncle and third nerve fibers. (*From Haymaker W: Bing's Local Diagnosis in Neurological Diseases. St. Louis, CV Mosby, 1969. Used with permission.*)

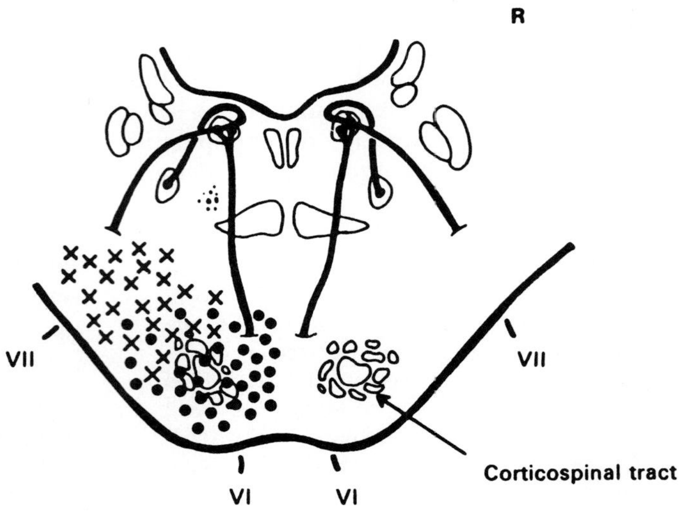

Figure 7-4. Caudal pons lesions involving the corticospinal tract, facial nerve (×), and 6th nerve fibers (●). (*From Haymaker W: Bing's Local Diagnosis in Neurological Diseases. St. Louis, CV Mosby, 1969. Used with permission.*)

should not lead to the conclusion that the reflex arc is interrupted in the brain stem. It is much more likely that the reflex is depressed because of dysfunction in descending "supranuclear" pathways. Similarly, equivocal corneal reflexes, asymmetry of the face, or slight deviation of the tongue can be mistakenly thought to indicate damage to the midbrain, pons, or medulla.

VERTEBROBASILAR SYNDROMES FROM HEMISPHERIC ISCHEMIA

It is sometimes forgotten that several important structures located in the cerebral hemispheres receive their blood supply from the vertebrobasilar system. These include the thalamus (supplied by "thalamo-perforating" branches), the hippocampal and occipital cortex, and often the posterior corpus callosum, all supplied by the posterior cerebral arteries. Although it is true that a posterior cerebral artery may originate from the ipsilateral internal carotid artery if there is a large posterior communicating branch, the posterior cerebral arteries receive their flow from the vertebrobasilar system in most individuals.

Hemiballismus

This term refers to involuntary twisting or rotating movements of the limbs on one side of the body, often involving the proximal limb muscles. When less violent they may resemble choreiform movements. The cause is usually a small infarction in or adjacent to the contralateral subthalamic nucleus which is usually supplied by a branch from a posterior cerebral artery. The movements usually lessen spontaneously in days or weeks.

Alexia without Agraphia

This rare syndrome can occur with infarction of the left occipital cortex and the posterior corpus callosum, both structures being supplied by the posterior cerebral artery.

Clinical case. A 58-year-old systems analyst with a known history of diabetes mellitus, hypertension, and heart disease was found by a friend to be difficult to arouse and seemed confused. When brought to the hospital he was able to respond to simple questions but had difficulty recognizing his friend. He could not see objects in the right visual field and could not move his eyes to the right. He had transient problems with naming and disorientation, which improved after a few days; however, he had profound difficulty reading. He would read letters of words instead of whole words, phrases, or sentences. He had good comprehension of spoken language and could spell words when asked, but had difficulty recognizing letters and numbers. He could write his name, could write words to dictation, and could formulate simple written sentences, such as "I write with a pen." However, when asked to read what he had written a few minutes before, he was unable to recognize the material. If he traced the letters with his finger, he could often recognize the letter and word. He also made some errors on naming objects in pictures. At the time of discharge five weeks after his stroke he could recognize single words three to five letters in length by writing the letters in the air, speaking the letters aloud, and putting them together to form a word.

The initial head CT scan was normal. A repeat CT scan showed infarction in the distribution of the left posterior cerebral artery. The infarct involved the left occipital cortex and the posterior portion of the corpus callosum.

Comment. Presumably this patient's brain received visual information only in the right cerebral hemisphere because of the left occipital infarction. He was then unable to transfer the information from the right hemisphere to the left because of damage to the posterior corpus callosum. By tracing the letter with his hand he was able to provide tactile information to the left hemisphere which could then be conveyed to appropriate language areas.

Visual Symptoms

It is not always easy for a patient with visual symptoms to recognize that the symptoms are related to a visual field rather than to the vision of one eye. For this reason, a TIA may be misinterpreted as being in a carotid artery territory rather than having a vertebrobasilar distribution. Therefore, it is important to ask if the patient was blind or nearly blind in one eye when the other eye was closed and to determine whether the visual symptom may have been on one side rather than in one eye. Occurrence of a *homonymous hemianopia* or *quadrantanopia* without other symptoms is likely to be due to ischemia in the territory of a posterior cerebral artery.

Rapid onset of blindness in both eyes is most likely to be due to ischemia in the territory of both posterior cerebral arteries. If the blindness persists, the patient may deny having visual loss (Anton's syndrome). In this situation the pupils will react to light, in contrast to the pupil unreactivity associated with ischemia in both optic nerves. Some patients with bilateral occipital infarction will spare a portion of the central visual field because of the presence of collateral supply from the anterior cerebral arteries.

Memory Loss and Transient Global Amnesia

Consolidation and retrieval of memory utilize neuronal systems in the hippocampal region of the temporal lobes and portions of the thalamus.[6,7] Damage to these structures on one side does not usually result in significant cognitive difficulty. Bilateral damage can bring about profound problems with memory, even when other cognitive functions such as speech and perception are unaffected. The basilar artery divides into the two posterior cerebral arteries that supply the thalamic and hippocampal regions on their way to the occipital cortex. The thalamic branches arise at the origin of the posterior cerebral arteries. The term "top of the basilar" syndrome has been used for the constellation of symptoms and signs that occurs with occlusion in this area, most commonly from embolism.

Clinical case. A 34-year-old woman became unresponsive during sleep. She showed decerebrate posturing, but over the next few days became more alert. On the eighth day of her illness she was conscious but withdrawn. By the end of the second week she was awake but apathetic. She was disoriented to time, place, and person. On formal psychological testing she could comprehend most paragraphs but could remember almost nothing of the content after several minutes. However, she was able to recall much information learned in the areas of vocabulary, general information, and basic arithmetic.

Six months after her illness began her IQ was 100, although the memory deficits persisted. She was totally unable to look up or down on command, but she was able to follow slowly moving objects, and Bell's phenomenon (reflex upward deviation of the eyes in response to forced closure of the eyelids) was present. Two and one-half years after the onset of her illness, the CT scan showed symmetrical zones of low absorption thought to be located in the dorsomedial region of the thalamus.

Comment. This patient has been reported in detail.[6] She probably had an infarction of the medial thalamus and adjacent periventricular gray matter around the third ventricle due to an embolus that obstructed the paramedian arteries arising from the basilar bifurcation. An isolated amnesic syndrome also can result from infarction in both medial temporal (hippocampal) regions due to occlusion of both posterior cerebral arteries.[7]

Transient global amnesia is the term given to episodes of confusion and amnesia that occur without loss of consciousness and last minutes to hours. These episodes typically occur in middle-aged and elderly persons, and the memory deficit involves events of the present and recent past. The underlying cause is often unclear, although a possible precipitating factor such as an emotional experience or minor head trauma may be apparent. Some cases appear to be related to seizures arising from a temporal lobe (complex partial seizures). Similar cases occurring during cerebral angiography or migraine episodes have been described. It seems likely that a TIA in the distribution of the basilar artery can cause a similar syndrome.

REFERENCES

1. Futty DE, Conneally PM, Dyken ML, et al: Cooperative study of hospital frequency and character of transient ischemic attacks: V. Symptom analysis. *JAMA* 238:2386–2390, 1977.
2. Swanson PD, Luttrell CN, Magladery JW: Myoclonus—a report of 67 cases and review of the literature. *Medicine* 41:339–356, 1962.
3. Fisher CM: A new vascular syndrome—the subclavian steal. *N Engl J Med* 265:913–914, 1961.
4. Reivich M, Holling E, Roberts B, Toole JF: Reversal of blood flow through the vertebral artery and its effect on cerebral circulation. *N Engl J Med* 265:878–885, 1961.
5. Patel A, Toole JF: Subclavian steal syndrome-reversal of cephalic blood flow. *Medicine* 44: 289–303, 1965.
6. Mills RP, Swanson PD: Vertical oculomotor apraxia and memory loss. *Ann Neurol* 4:249–153, 1978.
7. DeJong RN, Itabashi HH, Olson JR: Memory loss due to hippocampal lesions. *Arch Neurol* 20:339–348, 1969.

8

Epidemiology and Natural History of Adult Ischemic Cerebrovascular Disease

Anthony J. Orencia
José Biller

Cerebrovascular disease plays a major role in morbidity and mortality worldwide. Each year, approximately 500,000 people in the United States suffer a new or recurrent stroke, and 150,000 of them die. Based on U.S. 1992 estimates, cerebrovascular disease-related expenditures amount to at least 16.7 billion dollars.[1] Stroke is the third largest cause of death, after cardiovascular disease and cancer, in the United States alone. While it is recognized that stroke mortality primarily affects the elderly, stroke ranks third as a cause of death among individuals in the fifth and sixth decades of life.[2]

Stroke is also a major cause of chronic disability. The American Heart Association estimates that of stroke survivors: 31 percent require living assistance; 20 percent need help walking; 16 percent are institutionalized; 35 percent are between 35 and 65 years of age and unemployable; and 71 percent have some impaired vocational capacity years after the stroke.[3]

This chapter reviews the observational epidemiology of adult ischemic cerebrovascular disease, including its distribution, magnitude, and risk factors. Emphasis is placed on ischemic stroke risk factors. The epidemiology of transient ischemic attacks (TIAs) is covered as a risk factor for ischemic stroke. A separate section reviews the observational epidemiology of extracranial atherosclerotic carotid artery disease. While clinical series and reviews document intracranial carotid and vertebrobasilar artery occlusive disease, substantive epidemiologic data are limited. Although there may be some overlap with other chapters in this book, the major focus here is on disease frequency and distribution, risk and prognostic factors in the general population, and the probabilities of disease occurrence, recurrence, survival, or mortality.

THE FREQUENCY AND MAGNITUDE OF STROKE

Stroke Prevalence and Short-Term and Long-Term Survival

Prevalence is the expression of the interrelationships among incidence, survivorship, mortality, and disease recovery. Based on the U.S. National Health Interview Survey, the proportion of strokes occurring at any given time in the white population is 720 per 100,000. The corresponding prevalence of stroke in the U.S. nonwhite population is 910 per 100,000.[4]

Improvements in observed survival after first episodes of cerebral infarction in Rochester, Minnesota, suggest possible modifications in stroke management.[5] An improvement in long-term survival following a first cerebral infarction was seen in a higher proportion of individuals in the 1970 to 1974 period compared with the earliest period of the study, 1945 to 1949. The improvement in short-term (30-day) survival following a cerebral infarction was modest. The 3-week ischemic stroke case fatality for men and women of Tilburg, Netherlands was higher than the Rochester, Minnesota, population for comparable calendar periods.[6,7]

The relative survival following a first stroke is highest for strokes occurring at home. The 30-day survival for patients who had a first stroke in the home was 80 percent. Thirty-day survival estimates for patients whose first strokes occurred in a nursing home or hospital were 54 and 61 percent, respectively.[7] Hospitalized individuals whose first stroke occurred at home had a lower five-year observed survival than those who were not hospitalized, an indication that those with the most severe strokes were more likely to be hospitalized. Potential cardiac sources of emboli were detected in more than 40 percent of strokes occurring in a nursing home and in over 50 percent of strokes occurring in a hospital.[7]

Stroke Mortality

International comparisons of stroke mortality rates show that the rate of decline from 1970 through 1985 was greater among women. The African continent was not represented in this mortality comparison study involving 27 countries.[8] Although U.S. stroke mortality rates have gradually declined, the greatest decrease was evident around 1968 and 1973 for the black and white populations, respectively. The annual rate of stroke mortality decline has slowed remarkably since 1979, while the mortality rates for coronary heart disease and for all causes have leveled off.[9]

Analyses of aggregate risk studies on the U.S. decline in stroke mortality suggest that

Table 8-1 Age-adjusted Mortality Rates per 100,000 from Cerebrovascular Disease by Race and Calendar Period, U.S. New Mexico Men, 1958–1987

	Calendar period					
Race	1958–1962	1963–1967	1968–1972	1973–1977	1978–1982	1983–1987
Hispanic	82.9	75.8	82.5	65.5	48.9	45.8
Native American	52.2	54.2	70.1	58.3	39.8	31.3
Non-Hispanic white	95.0	78.8	94.6	77.5	54.7	36.1
US white	121.6	108.7	105.5	90.4	66.6	52.5

SOURCE: From Kattapong and Becker.[15] Reproduced by permission.

pharmacologic therapy for high blood pressure caused at most a small drop.[10–11] Reduction in blood pressure levels, cigarette smoking, coronary heart disease mortality, and improved treatment of cardiorespiratory complications of stroke may have contributed to this decline.[10] Longitudinal trends in Minneapolis-St. Paul, Minnesota showed a substantial stroke mortality decline of more than 50 percent from 1960 through 1990, attributed to both primary and secondary disease prevention. The average level of cardiovascular disease risk factors including systolic blood pressure, diastolic blood pressure, current cigarette smoking, and average serum total cholesterol also fell.[12]

The increasing emphasis on studies concerning distribution and risk factor differences for stroke in minority populations is appropriate, since approximately one-quarter of the U.S. population will consist of "minorities" by the year 2000.[13] Further understanding of cerebrovascular disease in groups other than the white population also provides insight regarding probable migratory, environmental, or genetic influences. Recently analyzed New Mexico vital statistics data collected from 1958 through 1987 showed that Native Americans had the lowest cerebrovascular disease mortality rates, followed by Hispanics, during a 25-year span.[13] (Tables 8-1–8-2). The 1983 U.S. data showed a remarkable difference in stroke mortality rates between African-Americans and whites. The former are approximately three and one-half to four times more likely to die of stroke in the age group 35 to 54, and they have approximately a twofold to threefold increase in mortality rates in the age group 55 to 74.[14–15]

Stroke Incidence

Stroke incidence has been documented worldwide.[16–31] However, worldwide comparisons of stroke rates are limited by nonuniform methods of case identification and diagnostic

Table 8-2 Age-adjusted Mortality Rates per 100,000 from Cerebrovascular Disease by Race and Calendar Period, U.S. New Mexico Women, 1958–1987

	Calendar period					
Race	1958–1962	1963–1967	1968–1972	1973–1977	1978–1982	1983–1987
Hispanic	74.6	62.7	76.5	66.9	43.8	43.1
Native American	36.5	32.8	55.7	43.9	34.6	19.3
Non-Hispanic white	69.9	60.2	76.1	70.7	48.3	39.3
US white	108.7	95.7	80.8	78.1	60.8	78.1

SOURCE: From Kattapong and Becker[15] Reproduced by permission.

criteria.[32] With the 1976 U.S. population as the standard for age and gender distributions, standardized incidence rate ratios for first stroke in 37 regions varied slightly, except for rates from China and Japan, which showed the highest ratios (Fig. 8-1).[32] Age-adjusted ischemic stroke rates present an interesting geographic divergence in secular trends among the Shibata, Akita, and Hisayama Japanese populations for men and women age 40 through 79. The average annual cerebral infarction incidence rate was highest among the men and women of Hisayama.[22,24,30] Ischemic stroke rates from the Ni-Hon-San study were compared for 45- to 69-year-old Japanese men and 45- to 68-year-old Japanese-American men living in Hawaii. Age-specific rates for ischemic strokes in Japan were three to five and one-half times higher than the rates in Hawaii.[28]

The average annual incidence rate of stroke among Rochester, Minnesota residents declined from 213 to 115 per 100,000 population between the 1950 to 1954 and 1975 to 1979 periods for all age groups.[33] The increase in stroke incidence rates during the 1980 to 1984 period coincided with the general use of cranial computerized tomography (CT), which appeared to increase the detection of milder strokes. Ischemic stroke rates declined from 183 to 102 per 100,000 between 1945 to 1954 and 1975 to 1984, respectively. The decline in incidence occurred earlier in women than in men (Fig. 8-2). A Rochester, Minnesota study among pregnant women for the period 1955

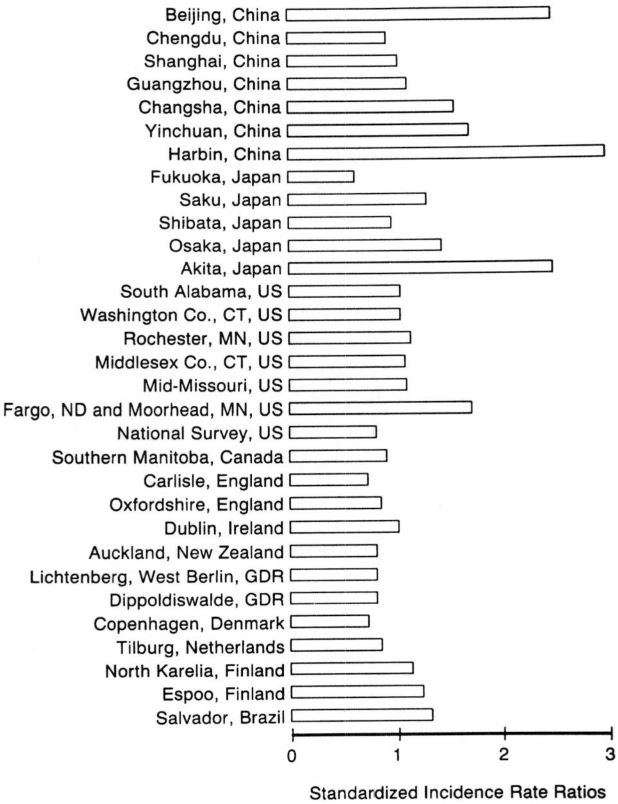

Figure 8-1. Age-standardized incidence rate ratios for a first stroke in selected communities. Age standardization is based on the 1976 U.S. population.

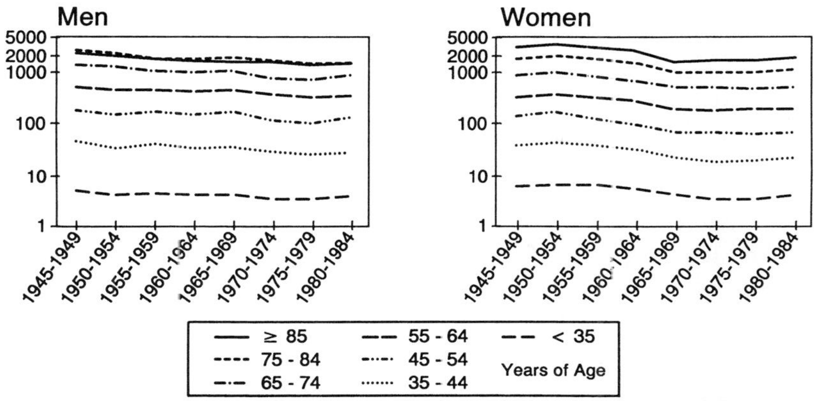

Figure 8-2. Poisson regression model predicted age group-specific incidence rates of first stroke in Rochester, Minnesota. x-axis: calendar years; y-axis: average annual incidence rate per 100,000 population.

to 1979 suggested that the observed 5.1 per 100,000 cerebral infarctions during pregnancy was lower than in previous reports.[21] The decline in stroke incidence for both men and women was observed not only in Rochester, Minnesota, but also in North Karelia, Finland, and Hisayama, Japan.[22,33–34] For reasons that could not be explained satisfactorily, stroke incidence increased among the women of Soderhamn, Sweden, from 262 to 362 per 100,000 in the 1975 to 1978 and 1983 to 1986 periods, respectively.[31]

The reasons for the decline in stroke incidence have been the subject of a lively debate.[33,35–39] Ebrahim identified four probable reasons for the observed decline: (1) effective treatment of high blood pressure; (2) reduced exposure to risk factors associated with high blood pressure; (3) reduced exposure to other risk factors for stroke; and (4) the competing risk of ischemic heart disease and mortality that seems to keep prone individuals from developing a stroke.[38]

Methodologic concerns affecting reported trends in stroke incidence could be influenced, in part, by the case ascertainment process used, degree of error reduction in the diagnostic coding system for national surveillance data, and the study sample selected. A record linkage system shows that approximately 14 percent of persons with stroke are not hospitalized.[7] This proportion may be an underestimation in study projects that lack comprehensive accounting for first stroke cases in a community. Inadequate ascertainment may lead to misguided conclusions regarding time trends or the impact of risk factor levels on stroke outcomes.

THE NATURAL HISTORY OF EXTRACRANIAL CAROTID ATHEROSCLEROTIC DISEASE

A considerable body of evidence has focused on the descriptive and analytic epidemiology of atherosclerotic carotid artery disease.[40–53] Although epidemiologic information on vertebrobasilar and intracranial carotid artery disease is emerging, discussion here is limited to the more extensive understanding of extracranial carotid atherosclerotic disease.

Distribution and Occurrence of Carotid Artery Disease in the Community

Asymptomatic carotid bruits discovered during routine physical examination may be a marker for carotid atherosclerotic disease and stroke. The prevalence of localized, asymptomatic carotid bruits in a randomly sampled white population has been found to increase with age from 1 to 3 percent in persons 45 years and older, and from 4 to 7 percent in persons 65 years and older.[46,54–55] Asymptomatic carotid bruits are more common among women than men in population-based studies.[46,54–55] Diffuse or localized carotid bruits, irrespective of lateralization, are 85 percent predictive of moderate to severe atherosclerosis of the extracranial carotid artery.[41]

Asymptomatic carotid atherosclerotic lesions in men and women age 39 years and younger are uncommon.[56] The highly varied estimates for the prevalence of a significant asymptomatic carotid stenosis depend partly on the diagnostic modality used (Table 8-3), constitutional or demographic factors, and history of concurrent disease. The prevalence of extracranial carotid artery atherosclerosis in Eastern Finnish men, assessed with high-resolution B-mode ultrasonography, showed a proportional increase over age 40 years: 14.1 percent at 42 years; 32.0 percent at 48 years; 67.7 percent at 54 years; and 81.9 percent at 60 years. Although complicated by methodologic and equipment differences in the diagnosis of carotid artery disease, the overall prevalence among Eastern Finnish men (49 percent) was higher than the reports from Friuli-Venezia Giulia in Italy, Northern France, and the Netherlands.[52,56] The severity of carotid disease was found to increase with age among men and women over 65 years living in retirement homes in Seattle, Washington. The internal, external, or common carotid arteries were stenotic in 31.4 percent of these patients who underwent Doppler examination.[57]

Risk Factors for Extracranial Carotid Artery Atherosclerotic Disease

Cigarette smoking, advanced age, male gender, diabetes mellitus, obesity, high systolic blood pressure, and serum lipids and lipoproteins are positive independent predictors of significant extracranial carotid artery atherosclerosis.[42–45] Serum uric acid levels appear to have an inverse relationship.[42] Duration of cig-

Table 8-3 Proportion of Significant Asymptomatic Carotid Stenosis as Determined by Ultrasound Examination

Principal author	Source of study subjects	Age (years)	Method	Number screened	Percentage (%) with stenosis ≥50%
Hennerici	Referral to vascular laboratory	Mean and error: men = 58.1 ± 7.1 women = 56.2 ± 6.8	Doppler	1370	5.9
Colgan	Hospital-sponsored health fairs	24–91	Duplex	348	3.7
		≥50		280	4.3
Fowl	Noninvasive vascular laboratory, VA Medical Center	≥50	Duplex		
	(a) without peripheral vascular disease			153	6.5
	(b) with peripheral vascular disease			116	12.9
Ricci	Stratified sample from health districts in Perugia, Italy	≥50	Doppler	320	5.0

SOURCE: Modified from Adams et al.[53] With permission.

arette smoking is a powerful predictor of extracranial carotid artery atherosclerosis.[42,44–45] The risk of severe carotid atherosclerosis for a person who has smoked for 40 years is three and one-half times higher than that of an individual who has never smoked. Clearly, cessation of smoking has a major impact on lessening the cumulative effects of smoking.[44]

Low-density lipoprotein-cholesterol increases the risk of carotid artery atherosclerosis (based on arteriographic assessment) by 6 percent for every 10 mg/dl increase in serum levels. Serum cholesterol, triglycerides, high-density lipoprotein-cholesterol, and apolipoprotein A-I are not related independently to severe extracranial carotid artery atherosclerosis.[45] On the basis of B-mode ultrasound evaluations, and after multivariable adjustment for other risk factors, high-density lipoprotein-cholesterol and low-density lipoprotein-cholesterol predict linearly the extent of extracranial carotid atherosclerosis.[43,52] Despite limitations in methodology across various studies, this trend toward a direct relationship between low-density lipoproteins and the extent or severity of carotid atherosclerotic disease is clear.[40]

Cross-sectional data from the Lausanne Stroke Registry showed that light to moderate alcohol consumption was inversely related to internal carotid artery stenosis.[51] Follow-up studies are needed to assess internal carotid artery morphology among individuals who may or may not consume alcohol regularly. An ancillary study to the Systolic Hypertension in the Elderly Program found that isolated systolic hypertension was associated strongly with carotid stenosis and atherosclerosis. This relationship was independent of smoking, diastolic blood pressure, alcohol use, heart rate, or concentration of apolipoprotein-B levels.[50]

The inconsistency of risk factor findings in studies of extracranial carotid atherosclerosis may be explained, in part, by: (1) differences in measurement techniques used, such as carotid arteriography, B-mode ultrasonography, or Doppler analysis; (2) differences in defining severity of stenosis, such as wall thickness measurement rather than disturbed flow patterns;[42] and (3) biases related to the selection of a study population from patients with a range of cerebrovascular problems referred for carotid arteriography. Pooled risk factor analyses for assessing the impact of serum lipids and lipoproteins on carotid artherosclerosis are not possible because of the methods used for serum lipid analysis, interstudy variations in lipoprotein fractions analyzed, the arterial segment examined, the study population, control selection in case-control studies, and the techniques used for evaluating carotid disease.[40] Difficulties also arise in making generalizations based on risk factor studies that use arteriography because subjects are chosen on the basis of specific clinical indications during an atherosclerotic disease work-up. The inclusion of minimal to severe carotid disease, however, may support the validity of these investigations.[58]

Risk of Neurologic Events

Risk estimates for asymptomatic carotid bruit or stenosis are pertinent to developing management plans for the secondary prevention of strokes. Comparisons between studies on the stroke risk of patients with asymptomatic carotid bruits or stenoses may not be possible owing to the different types of evaluations performed and the characteristics of the study populations.

Patients with asymptomatic carotid bruits from an outpatient referral practice were followed by questionnaire for five years or until they died. Evaluations were based on standardized auscultation of the heart, neck, and orbits, and retinal arterial pressure measurements. The annual stroke risk, given survival, was 1.5 percent at one year, or 7.5 percent at five years. Among patients with asymptomatic diffuse or localized carotid bruits, the annual ischemic stroke risk, given survival, was approximately three times higher than for patients without bruits. The risk of future ischemic strokes was predicted independently by a history of myocardial infarction (MI), recent MI, presence of peripheral vascular disease, or a history of congestive heart failure (CHF).[59]

Clinical series-based reports estimate that approximately 3 to 6 percent of patients who have ≥50 percent asymptomatic carotid stenosis develop a subsequent stroke (Table 8-4). Patients with asymptomatic, hemodynamically significant internal carotid artery lesions examined by ocular pneumoplethysmography were approximately two times more likely to suffer an ischemic stroke than those with normal ocular pneumoplethysmography, or seven times more likely than an age- and gender-matched population.[49] The annual stroke risk, given survival, at three years was 0.5 percent in the general population, 1.5 percent in persons with normal ocular pneumoplethysmography, and 3.4 percent among patients with abnormal ocular pneumoplethysmography.

The annual risk of a TIA progressing to a stroke in patients with atherosclerotic cerebrovascular disease is probably in the range of 3 or 4 percent per year. The recurrent stroke risk for patients with atherosclerotic carotid disease who have had strokes probably varies from 7 to 10 percent per year (Table 8-5). Whether the entry event is a TIA or a stroke, some overlap seems to exist in the annual stroke risk estimates. Caution should be exercised in interpreting pooled or aggregate data from different clinical samples and study protocols or meta-analytic statistical summary estimates.[60]

RISK FACTORS FOR FIRST ISCHEMIC STROKE

Recent excellent reviews have explored the risk factors for ischemic stroke in detail.[61–63]

Table 8-4 Proportion with Subsequent Stroke in Patients with Significant (≥50 Percent) Asymptomatic Carotid Artery Stenosis Who Have Not Undergone Carotid Endarterectomy

Principal author	Method	Follow-up (mo)	Patients N	% with strokes	% with ipsilateral strokes
Humphries	Angiogram	32	168	2.4	—
Kartchner	OPG[a]	24	389	6.2	—
Johnson	Angiogram	24	22	0	0
Durward	Angiogram	NA[b]	73	12.3	2.7
Guitierrez	OPG	NA	19	15.8	—
Ford	Doppler ultrasound/ angiogram	48	36	2.8	2.8
Chambers	Doppler ultrasound	23	113	5.3	—
O'Halleran	Duplex ultrasound	46	121	11.6	—
Moll	OPG	NA	274	3.3	—
Hennerici	Doppler ultrasound	32	235	3.0	—
Donaldson	Duplex ultrasound	24	69	2.9	—
Meissner	OPG	35	292	5.5	4.4
AbuRhama	Duplex ultrasound	32	72	2.8	—

[a]OPG = oculoplethysmography
[b]NA = information not included in the article
SOURCE: Modified from Adams et al.[53] With permission.

Table 8-5 Annual Vascular Event Risk for Individuals with Various Features of Atherothrombotic Cerebrovascular Disease

Population	Principal author	Subgroups	Duration of study, years	Number of patients	Annual stroke risk[a]	Standard error in stroke risk
TIA	Hurwitz		5.37	212	4.33	0.65
	Muuronen		7.80	314	0.63	0.16
	Haerer		1.00	299	14.78	2.31
	Friedman		2.28	44	8.80	3.12
	Candelise	Aspirin	0.94	63	3.43	2.43
		Sulfinpyrazone	0.94	61	3.55	2.51
	Whisnant		2.00	198	12.57	1.90
TIA plus stroke	Fields	Aspirin	2.00	88	6.03	1.91
		Placebo	2.00	90	8.45	2.26
	Sorenson	Aspirin	2.08	107	8.86	2.15
		Placebo	2.08	102	5.49	1.66
	Harrison		4.10	188	3.04	0.65
	CCSG[b]	Aspirin	2.17	290	6.11	1.02
		Placebo	2.17	139	7.16	1.60
	ACCSG[b]	Aspirin	2.08	442	7.01	0.91
		Dipyridamole/aspirin	2.08	448	6.05	0.83
	UK-TIA Study group	Placebo	4.00	814	3.95	0.36
		Low-dose aspirin	4.00	806	3.35	0.33
		High-dose aspirin	4.00	815	3.27	0.33
	Hass	Ticlopidine	3.28	1529	3.64	0.28
		Aspirin	3.25	1540	4.56	0.31
	NASCET Collaborators[b]	Medical group	2.00	331	16.15	1.70
	Bousser	Placebo	3.00	204	5.49	0.99
		Aspirin	3.00	198	2.99	0.73
		Dipyridamole/aspirin	3.00	202	3.11	0.73
	ESPSG[b]	Dipyridamole/aspirin	2.00	1250	4.78	0.45
		Placebo	2.00	1250	7.96	0.59
	EC/IC Bypass Study group[b]		4.65	714	7.28	0.51
		Carotid occlusion	4.65	147	9.16	1.29
		Asymptomatic	4.65	276	6.50	0.77
Stroke	Britton	Aspirin	2.00	253	6.76	1.20
		Placebo	2.00	252	6.79	1.20
	Sacco		5.00	222	7.97	0.94
	Gent	Placebo	1.67	220	9.09	1.64
		Suloctidil	1.67	213	9.51	1.68
	Matsumoto		1.00	575	10.44	1.38
	Gent	Placebo	2.00	523	10.27	1.04
		Ticlopidine	2.00	525	8.27	0.93

[a]Annual event risk given as percent per year

[b]Abbreviations: CCSG = Canadian Cooperative Study Group; ACCSG = American-Canadian Cooperative Study Group; NASCET Collaborators = North American Symptomatic Carotid Endarterectomy Trial Collaborators; ESPSG = European Stroke Prevention Study Group; EC/IC Bypass Study Group = Extracranial/intracranial Bypass Study Group.

SOURCE: From Wilterdink and Easton.[60] Reprinted with permission.

The following sections discuss both the well-documented and controversial risk factors for an initial stroke. A tabular summary provides an overview of the independent risk factors for ischemic stroke from selected population-based studies (Table 8-6).

Risk Factors That Are Nonmodifiable

Age, Race, and Gender Since the descriptive epidemiology of age, race, and gender as stroke risk factors was covered earlier in this chapter, a synopsis is presented here. The risk of stroke at least doubles each de-

Table 8-6 Multivariable Risk Factor Model for Ischemic Stroke

Principal author	Davis, 1987[78]	Harmsen, 1990[72]	Wolf, 1988[158]	Wolf, 1988[158]	Boysen, 1988[18]
	Rochester, MN, US	Göteborg, Sweden	I. Framingham, MA, US (men)	II. Framingham, MA, US (women)	Copenhagen, Denmark
Advancing age	1.6 per 10 years[a]	Not tested[b]	(+)[c]	(+)	(+)
Male gender	2.0	(men only)	Not applicable	Not applicable	(+)
Hypertension	4.0	2.5 diastolic	3.1	2.1	(+) (systolic)
Hypertensive heart disease	2.2	Not tested	Not tested	Not tested	Not tested
Coronary heart disease	2.2	Not significant[d]	Not tested	Not tested	(+)
Atrial fibrillation	Not significant	11.5	Not tested	Not tested	(+)
Congestive heart failure	1.7	Not tested	Not tested	Not tested	Not tested
Smoking	Not tested	1.8	1.6	1.9	(+)
Alcohol	Not tested	Not significant	Not tested	Not tested	Not significant
Physical activity	Not tested	Not significant	Not tested	Not tested	Not tested
Cholesterol	Not tested	Not significant	(+)	Not tested	(+)
Body mass index/ relative weight	Not tested	Not significant	(+)	Not tested	Not significant
Diabetes mellitus/ glucose intolerance	1.7	Not significant	2.6	2.0	(+)
Arterial peripheral vascular disease	Not significant	Not tested	Not tested	Not tested	Not tested
Family history of stroke	Not tested	Not significant	Not tested	Not tested	Not significant
Transient ischemic attack	3.9	3.5	Not tested	Not tested	Not tested
Regression model	Time-dependent proportional hazards	Logistic	Baseline proportional hazards	Baseline proportional hazards	Baseline proportional hazards

[a]Relative risk (its corresponding 95% confidence interval does not contain 1.0).
[b]Variable was not tested in the specific model.
[c](+) Significant risk factor adjusted in the model but results are not presented. For the Copenhagen, Denmark Heart Study, results for all the variables adjusted simultaneously are not available.
[d]Not significant when incorporated as a variable in the risk factor model.

cade after the 35 to 44 year age group up to the 75 to 84 year age group. The greatest increase in stroke risk occurs between 35 and 54 years.[64] African-Americans have disproportionately higher stroke rates than other ethnic or racial groups.[14,64] Men and women have approximately a 1:1 age-adjusted stroke risk ratio.[33]

Circadian and Seasonal Factors The circadian variation of ischemic strokes peaking between 10:00 A.M. and 12:00 noon[65–67] has led to the hypothesis that diurnal changes in platelet function and fibrinolysis may be relevant to stroke.[69] A relationship between seasonal climatic variation and ischemic stroke occurrence has been postulated.[70] An increase in referral for cerebral infarctions was observed during the warmer months in Iowa.[71] The mean ambient temperature negatively correlated with the incidence of cerebral infarction in Hisayama, Japan.[70] Further study of the significance of seasonal temperature fluctuations in relationship to stroke risk factors may uncover patterns accounting for an increase in ischemic stroke incidence. For instance, seasonality has been correlated with a higher risk of cerebral infarction in 40 to 64-year-old individuals who are nonhypertensive and individuals with serum cholesterol below 160 mg/dl.[70] Further studies, however, are needed to determine whether these apparent associations are spurious or real.

Family History Few familial studies have investigated the influence of genetic and environmental factors on ischemic stroke occurrence.[18,72–77] A fivefold increase in stroke prevalence among monozygotic compared to dizygotic male twin pairs suggests a genetic predisposition to stroke. The proband concordance rates for monozygotic and dizygotic pairs are 17.7 and 3.6 percent, respectively.[76] The 1913 Swedish birth cohort study demonstrated a threefold increase in the incidence of stroke in men whose mothers died of stroke compared with men without such a maternal history. Blood pressure seemed not to affect the results.[73] Family history of stroke was not related independently to stroke among men and women from Copenhagen, Denmark, or men from Göteborg, Sweden.[18,72] A sibling history of stroke or TIA among original cohort members of the Framingham Study was not associated with cerebral ischemia. Parental history of coronary heart disease, however, was strongly associated with stroke or TIA among the Framingham offspring study members.[77]

Family history also seems to play a role in stroke mortality among the upper middle-class Caucasian population in Rancho Bernardo, Southern California. Women with a family history of stroke had a twofold greater risk of stroke mortality than those without such a history. This finding was independent of age, systolic blood pressure, plasma cholesterol, cigarette smoking, obesity, and fasting plasma glucose. Family history of stroke in men did not predict stroke mortality.[74]

Risk Factors That Can Be Modified, Controlled, or Treated

Transient Ischemic Attack The independent risk of a subsequent stroke is at least three times greater for individuals with a history of TIA than for those who have not experienced a TIA.[72,78] The median time from a TIA to a first ischemic stroke varies depending on the methods used to study the problem. If a TIA developed during the follow-up period, the median time to stroke was approximately 2.4 months (0.2 year); if TIAs present at the baseline evaluation were included, and events that developed during the study period were ignored, the median time to stroke was approximately 7.5 years.[78] In Rochester, Minnesota the incidence of stroke following TIA was approximately 10 percent in the first six months after onset, with an average of 6 percent per year thereafter.[79]

Diabetes Mellitus Diabetes is a definite risk factor for stroke. After controlling for other stroke risk factors, diabetes increases the risk of thromboembolic stroke by approximately twofold to threefold relative to persons without diabetes.[80–83] Diabetes increases the overall propensity toward large vessel complications such as coronary heart disease, ischemic stroke, and peripheral vascular disease.[84] Diabetes may predispose an individual to cerebral ischemia via acceleration of atherosclerosis or by local effects on the cerebral microcirculation.[85]

In the Honolulu Heart Program, men with glucosuria, in the absence of a diabetic history, also were at increased risk for stroke. Glucosuria increased the risk of a thromboembolic stroke by approximately 2.5-fold. This finding was independent of age, body mass, hypertensive status, serum cholesterol level, and cigarette smoking.[82]

Lipid and Lipoprotein Abnormalities The relationship between serum cholesterol, triglycerides, or apolipoproteins and ischemic stroke or stroke mortality remains unsettled. A 12-year study of women, age 38 to 60 in Göteborg, Sweden showed an 8.7-fold greater risk of stroke for serum triglyceride values of 2.2 mmol/liter or greater relative to lower values.[86] Serum cholesterol did not predict strokes after adjustment for systolic blood pressure, smoking, obesity, and serum triglycerides. Serum triglyceride levels independently predicted subsequent strokes. None of the women who had strokes were on lipid-lowering agents.[86]

While the association of intracranial hemorrhage and cholesterol appears to be inverse, there is a positive association between serum cholesterol and nonhemorrhagic stroke mortality after controlling for age, race, blood pressure, and cigarette smoking in men 35 to 57 years of age. Serum cholesterol levels of 5.16 to 6.18 mmol/liter (200 to 239 mg/dl) or more doubled the risk of nonhemorrhagic stroke deaths. This association probably reflects accelerated atherosclerosis due to elevated levels of low-density lipoprotein-cholesterol.[87]

In a case-control study of Chinese individuals living in Hong Kong who had acute strokes, a serum high-density lipoprotein-cholesterol concentration greater than 1.59 mmol/liter and serum apolipoprotein A-I concentration of 130 mg/dl or higher were independent predictors of stroke risk reduction. Lipoprotein (a) concentrations greater than 29.2 mg/dl predicted all strokes.[88] Combining all stroke types may obscure the true association between ischemic strokes and serum lipoproteins. Furthermore, serum lipoprotein abnormalities may occur during the acute phase of stroke.[88–90] For individuals without lipid measurements before stroke, comparing values obtained within 48 h after admission to control values may incorrectly identify lipoprotein fractions as potential risk factors.[90] Additional studies of lipoprotein fractions may yield clues to the pathogenesis of ischemic strokes.

Arterial Hypertension The age-adjusted risk of stroke for men or women with definite hypertension is threefold greater than for persons without hypertension. Men or women with borderline hypertension have a 50 percent greater risk of stroke than do normotensive individuals.[62] Improved control of hypertension was coincident with the decline in stroke incidence for the population of Rochester, Minnesota (Fig. 8-3).[91]

Arterial hypertension is the most crucial risk factor where active therapeutic management of both diastolic and systolic blood pressures can dramatically reduce stroke morbidity and mortality. Through reduction in diastolic blood pressure levels, reduction in stroke rates favored the stepped care instead of the community-treated referred care group of black or white men and women participating in the Hypertension, Detection and Follow-up Program.[92] Clinical trial results from the Systolic Hypertension in the Elderly Program also demonstrated the benefits of stroke prevention by antihypertensive drug treatment in older persons with isolated systolic hypertension.[93–94]

However, efforts to control hypertension as a risk factor for stroke should not start only after hypertension develops. A key strategy for stroke prevention is the primary prevention of hypertension. Such evidence comes from dietary[95–96] and lifestyle studies of stroke risk factors. Blood pressure varies according to sodium intake, but variations in blood pressure for a particular sodium intake become greater as a function of both advancing age and higher blood pressure levels.[95] Urinary sodium excretion was associated positively with stroke mortality in men participating in the INTERSALT Study.[97] An estimated 26 percent reduction in stroke incidence

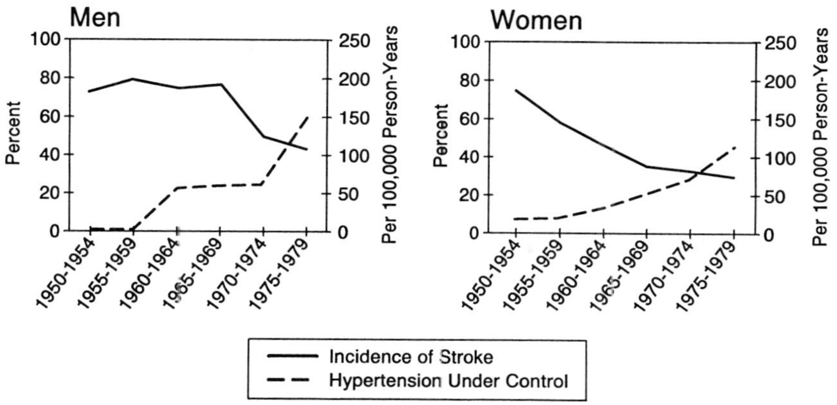

Figure 8-3. Average annual incidence for stroke in Rochester, Minnesota, and percentage of persons with hypertension under control (diastolic blood pressure <95 mmHg). Rates adjusted for age to the 1950 U.S. white population.

can be achieved with a reduction in salt intake.[98]

Cardiac Disease Cardiac diseases constitute the largest set of risk factors for ischemic stroke. The Cerebral Embolism Task Force reported the following facts: (1) one in six ischemic strokes is due to cardiogenic embolism; (2) nonrheumatic atrial fibrillation is the most frequent substrate for cerebral embolism; and (3) other major sources of cardiogenic strokes include coronary heart disease (25 percent), rheumatic mitral stenosis (10 percent), and prosthetic cardiac valves (10 percent).[99] The reader is referred to other excellent sources for additional review of the cardioembolic sources of ischemic stroke.[99–101] The treatment of cardiogenic embolism is discussed in Chap. 15.

Coronary heart disease almost triples the risk of a stroke, and cardiac failure quintuples the risk.[102] For patients with MI, the probability of stroke is increased significantly up to two months after the cardiac event. This increased risk is more pronounced in patients with Q wave than non-Q wave MIs. The cumulative probability of an MI or sudden unexpected death after a first diagnosis of cerebral infarction is not elevated significantly until five years after the cerebral infarction.[103]

Atrial fibrillation is clearly a significant contributor to stroke in both men and women.[104–110] As reported by the Framingham and Whitehall cohort studies, nonrheumatic atrial fibrillation is approximately five to seven times more likely to predispose an individual to stroke than the absence of this condition, after adjusting for age.[108,110] Within four deciles starting with the 50 to 59 year age group, atrial fibrillation, independent of hypertension, coronary heart disease, and CHF, retained a three- to fivefold greater risk of stroke.[111] Persons with mitral stenosis, CHF, previous stroke, or prosthetic mitral valves carried the highest risk of stroke.[112] As a long-recognized risk factor for stroke, atrial fibrillation has been the subject of several clinical trials in evaluating stroke prevention.[113–115] Antithrombotic prophylaxis with aspirin and warfarin is effective in preventing ischemic strokes among patients with nonrheumatic atrial fibrillation.[116]

Early studies reported conflicting results on the risk of an ischemic stroke among patients with mitral valve prolapse.[117–120] The reported four- to sevenfold increase in the risk of stroke among young to middle-aged adults with a history of mitral valve prolapse is probably exaggerated.[117–118] A cohort study of patients with echocardiographically confirmed mitral valve prolapse prospectively followed up for stroke showed a modest risk of stroke relative to those without prolapse (AJ Orencia, unpublished data).

Sinus node dysfunction is a cardiac rhythm abnormality difficult to assess as a risk factor for stroke. The confounding factors that may alter the magnitude of the association between sinus node dysfunction and ischemic stroke need further assessment.[121–122] Despite research into pacemaker types and their probable benefits in prolonging survival, studies on pacemakers and their influence on stroke or stroke mortality are yet to be addressed systematically.[123–125]

While atherothrombotic or small artery diseases comprise 80 percent of all cerebral infarctions, 15 to 20 percent of cerebral infarct cases have cardioembolic causes.[101] The list of putative cardiac risk factors for ischemic stroke continues to grow. For example, cardiac conditions such as the "shaggy aorta" syndrome or stroke due to paradoxical embolism have been recognized.[126–128]

Hematologic or Hemostatic Disorders Primary hematologic disorders may be associated with ischemic strokes. Severe strokes tend to have more extensive hemorrheologic abnormalities.[129] Since fibrinogen levels are closely correlated with such other stroke risk factors as smoking, hypertension, diabetes, obesity, and hematocrit, it is necessary to present multivariable risk factor-adjusted results to avoid misinterpretation. The risk of stroke increases with increasing fibrinogen levels in men.[130] These results in men are corroborated by a study from Göteborg, Sweden. After taking into account systolic blood pressure, smoking, and serum cholesterol, fibrinogen retained its direct relationship with stroke; factors II, VII, X, VIII-C, plasminogen, and fibrinolytic activities were not significant predictors.[131]

A study of rural inhabitants in Hisayama, Japan found low hematocrit levels (less than 30 percent) to be an independent risk factor for cerebral infarction in women but not in men. The pathogenesis of cerebral infarction due to low hematocrit values probably relates to hypooxygenation of the tissues.[132] The long-term atherogenic effect of high hematocrit levels on cerebral infarction has been suggested by various studies, including Framingham.[62] There is also evidence suggesting that changes in hemostatic function increase the risk of stroke in patients with nonvalvular atrial fibrillation.[133]

A heterogeneous family of antibodies directed against phospholipids, such as anticardiolipin antibodies and the lupus anticoagulant, may contribute to cerebral ischemia in young adults.[134–135] The consistency and temporality of the association between antiphospholipid antibodies and ischemic stroke need further verification.

The feasibility of conducting nested case-control studies in clinical neuroepidemiology is supported by the increasing number of blood samples stored over long periods in cohorts of healthy men and women. With a priori issues addressed to minimize measurement and selection bias, nested case-control studies are powerful designs that could assist in addressing questions about the hematologic factors for ischemic stroke.

Cigarette Smoking Cigarette smoking is an unequivocal, independent risk factor for ischemic stroke in men and women of all ages.[136–141] Whether the measurement of exposure is by pack-years, carbon monoxide-years, or nicotine-years, the cumulative lifetime exposure to cigarette smoking is associated directly with cerebrovascular disease.[141]

Inferences drawn from longitudinal studies, such as the Honolulu Heart Program and the Nurses' Health Study, implicate cigarette smoking as an independent risk factor for stroke. Individuals who smoked cigarettes had a twofold to threefold greater risk of developing an ischemic stroke when compared to nonsmokers.[136–137] Evidence also exists that passive smoking increases the risk of an ischemic stroke independently of other risk factors. The risk approximately doubled for the spouse of a smoker compared with that of the spouse of a nonsmoker.[140]

Smoking cessation may reduce the progression of atherosclerotic carotid artery disease or the direct complications of an ischemic stroke.[44,140] However, more than five years may be required before a reduction in stroke risk is observed after smoking cessation.[141] The hazards of smoking also should be viewed in conjunction with its effects on hemorrhagic strokes, lung cancer, coronary heart disease, and other disorders.

Alcohol Consumption Although several mechanisms have been proposed to explain how alcohol increases the risk for ischemic strokes, the epidemiologic evidence is not strongly convincing.[142–146] The physiologic role of alcohol as a stroke risk factor may relate to hypertension, local disturbances in cerebral autoregulatory mechanisms, the influence of smoking as a cofactor in atherogenesis among drinkers, hemostatic problems (abnormal platelet reactivity, thromboxane formation, decreased fibrinolytic activity), cardiac tachyarrhythmias during drinking sprees, or deterioration of an underlying cardiomyopathic condition.[147–148]

Early studies that lacked control for stroke-confounding factors suggested that both occasional and regular ethanol intoxication increased the risk of cerebral infarction in middle-aged women and young men.[149–150] This apparent relationship between alcohol ingestion and ischemic stroke may be due to the confounding effect of smoking.[144–146] The Nurses' Health Study reported that moderate alcohol consumption among middle-aged women did not increase their risk for ischemic stroke.[151] Neither acute alcohol ingestion nor weekly alcohol consumption independently elevated the risk of cerebral infarction in middle-aged and elderly men and women.[146]

While findings of a modestly increased risk for stroke associated with alcohol consumption have been consistent with previous studies,[142] it should be noted that alcohol has disparate relations to other diseases.[152] Reliance on properly designed longitudinal or nested case-control studies[144–151] may resolve the conflicting results that have stemmed from the choice of a control group in previously reported case-control designs.

Oral Contraceptive Use Owing to the combined reporting of stroke outcomes, it is difficult to distinguish the magnitude of either the thrombotic or hemorrhagic stroke risk attributable to oral contraceptives. Current oral contraceptive use is believed to be linked with platelet reactivity and fibrin deposition.[153] Results of studies on the relationship between oral contraceptive use and ischemic stroke, or between oral contraceptive use and stroke mortality, have been equivocal.[18,151,154–155] An earlier review concluded strongly that oral contraceptive use increases the risk of ischemic strokes.[156] In contrast, stratifying the duration of past oral contraceptive use failed to show an association with strokes in the Nurses' Health Study.[151] Postmenopausal hormone treatment also had no significant effect on stroke for participants in the Copenhagen City Heart Study.[18]

Residents of a California retirement community who received estrogen replacement were approximately half as likely to die of stroke when compared with women who did not receive such treatment. This finding was unaffected by the presence of hypertension, smoking, alcohol, exercise, or obesity.[157] Conclusions from the longtitudinal Women's Health Initiative Study, which is in progress, may clarify the role of postmenopausal hormone replacement therapy in ischemic stroke.

Obesity With the exception of the Copenhagen Heart Study,[18] obesity, measured in terms of relative weight or body mass index, consistently predicted subsequent strokes.[18,62,158–159] Its association with stroke could be explained, in part, by the presence of hypertension and diabetes.[159] Relative weight more than 30 percent above average was an independent contributor to a subsequent atherothrombotic brain infarction.[62,158]

Physical Inactivity and Disability Despite adequate documentation that physical inactivity is a risk factor for coronary heart disease, data on stroke outcomes have been sparse. Few studies exist on physical inactivity and disability in the elderly as risk factors for stroke. Physical inactivity-correlated factors in the pathogenesis of stroke may involve an increase in blood pressure and weight, uncontrolled blood sugar levels, increases in low-density lipoprotein-cholesterol levels, and cardiovascular deconditioning.[160]

A Roscow-Breslau one-point increment in the worsening of patient physical functioning increased stroke incidence by 50 percent, as compared with elderly subjects who performed activities independently. This finding from the Yale Health and Aging Project was independent of age, hypertension, angina, diabetes, and gender.[161] Decreased physical activity at work, independent of age, serum cholesterol, diastolic blood pressure, body mass index, and tobacco consumption was related to a 60 percent increased risk of stroke compared with those who had normal to elevated levels of physical activity at work. Neither the Finnish men or women who had low physical activity in their leisure times were at increased risk of stroke.[162] In a British study of men aged 40 to 59 years who were followed-up for 9.5 years, there was a dose-response trend for an increasing risk of stroke or heart disease as physical activity level decreased.[163] The small number of strokes precluded the authors from presenting their data separately for strokes and heart attacks, especially in assessing the protective effect of sporting (vigorous) activity.

The predominant bias affecting studies of physical activity and disease concerns the process of self-selection for recruitment into the study. For example, individuals who reported no sports activities may have undiagnosed or subclinical diseases, and persons who reported vigorous activities may have adopted additional health-promoting behaviors.[164]

RISK FACTORS FOR RECURRENT ISCHEMIC STROKES

An understanding of the risk factors for stroke recurrence is important in the prevention of recurrent stroke and stroke-related complications, as well as in stroke rehabilitation. Limited information exists on the natural history of recurrent ischemic strokes. While stroke incidence declined in Rochester, Minnesota, stroke recurrence did not change during the period from 1950 through 1979. The cumulative risk of stroke recurrence, given survival to one, five, and 10 years, was 5.7, 19.3, and 28.8 percent, respectively. The risk of stroke recurrence was similar for men and women. The majority of strokes were cerebral infarctions: 92 percent at first occurrence and 88 percent at recurrence. Blood pressure level prior to the first stroke or hypertension management did not have any apparent effect on stroke recurrence throughout the follow-up period.[165]

Stroke recurrence after a first stroke or TIA in the Söderhamn, Sweden community was approximately 10 percent per year.[166] Recurrence risk from another population-based cohort study in Umea, Sweden was also much higher than the Rochester, Minnesota figures. The risk of a recurrent stroke, given survival to one and five years, was 14 and 37 percent, respectively.[167]

For ischemic stroke subtypes, the risk of early recurrence is highest for atherothrombotic infarction (7.9 percent) and lowest for lacunar infarction (2.2 percent). Both cardioembolic infarction and infarction of undetermined cause have intermediate risks. In the Stroke Data Bank study, early recurrence was defined as a stroke within 30 days after the index stroke that clearly resulted in a new deficit involving a different anatomic or vascular territory or a different stroke subtype than the index cerebrovascular event.[168]

The following factors from the Stroke Data Bank were investigated to ascertain their influence on early stroke recurrence: age, race, gender, handedness, initial neurologic syndrome, cerebral site, systolic and diastolic blood pressures, blood sugar concentration, history of hypertension, MI, valvular heart disease, atrial fibrillation, other arrhythmias, angina, CHF, diabetes mellitus, previous stroke or TIAs, stroke severity, and cranial CT findings. Multivariable analysis of risk factors identified history of hypertension and blood sugar concentration at admission as significant predictors of early recurrence. In the absence of hypertension and hyperglycemia, the baseline risk of recurrence was 0.8 percent. The risk increased to 4.9 percent in the presence of hypertension and a blood sugar concentration of 200 mg/dl, and to 8.6 percent in the presence of hypertension and a blood sugar concentration of 300 mg/dl. Age, gender, handedness, valvular heart disease, and CHF were not associated with an early recurrence of stroke.[168]

Based on a median follow-up of 13 months in the Stroke Data Bank ischemic stroke recurrence study, a history of diabetes mellitus, diastolic hypertension (100 mmHg or greater), and a prior stroke were significant risk factors for increased stroke recurrence. Patients with an unknown ischemic infarct subtype had a lower risk of stroke recurrence than patients with such subtypes as embolism, atherosclerosis, or lacunae. Age, gender, race, history of hypertension, atrial fibrillation, TIAs, or stroke location were not associated with an increased risk of stroke recurrence.[169] The conclusions or generalizations from this study may hold true for other hospital-based patient populations with similar characteristics.

Hypertension, TIA, MI, other heart disease, diabetes mellitus, age, and male gender were multivariable factors predicting recurrent strokes in the Lehigh Valley study.[170] In contrast, a Swedish study of stroke recurrence found that advancing age and a history of cardiac failure were the only variables associated with an increased risk of recurrent stroke.[167] Middle-aged adults with coronary artery disease had a threefold greater risk for recurrent TIA or stroke than those without this condition.[171]

Recent attention has focused on antiphospholipid antibodies in recurrent thromboembolism.[171–172] Prothrombotic states in patients with atherosclerosis and other structural lesions who experience recurrent ischemia continue to be investigated.[173]

Policy guidelines regarding the value of medical or surgical[174] interventions in reducing the morbidity and mortality of recurrent stroke may be established in the near future. The design and implementation of a comprehensive medical rehabilitation plan should also be at the center of a recurrent stroke prevention program.[175]

FUTURE DIRECTION AND PERSPECTIVE

Cerebrovascular disease will continue to be the dominant cause of neurologic morbidity and mortality. As well-established risk factors for stroke are controlled, new and emerging risk factors will become more important. Advances in the epidemiology of cerebrovascular disease and continued refinement of neuroimaging techniques will improve disease classification and diagnostic accuracy.

Much work in cerebrovascular disease epidemiology remains to be done in vulnerable populations. Investigators cannot assume that the risk factors for an initial or recurrent stroke or predictors for atherosclerotic carotid disease documented in white populations will be present to the same extent in other racial or ethnic groups. The genetics of cerebrovascular disease is unique and probably separate from the genetics of coronary artery disease. Future studies may identify genetic markers in subgroups of families at risk for stroke.

Additional improvements in health care and technologic advances should promote longevity. However, it is unlikely that concern over cerebrovascular diseases will decrease for the growing elderly population. In view of the substandard care for cerebrovascular disease in the developing world, epidemiologic studies will continue to identify risk factors and disease clusters that could be the focus of preventive efforts by national and international health organizations.

Primary stroke prevention is a key factor that should be started in the young. Educational efforts should focus on modifiable risk factors for cerebrovascular disease that may contribute to further reductions in incidence and disability.

REFERENCES

1. American Heart Association: *Heart and Stroke Facts*. Dallas, 1992.
2. American Heart Association: *Facts about Stroke*. Dallas, 1992.
3. American Heart Association: *Heart and Stroke Facts*. Dallas, 1993.
4. Department of Health and Human Services Task Force: *Department of Health and Human Services Task Force on Black and Minority Health, 1984–1985: National Health Interview Survey,* 1972.
5. Garraway WM, Whisnant JP, Drury I: The changing pattern of survival following stroke. *Stroke* 58:520–523, 1983.
6. Herman B, Leyten ACM, Van Luijk JH, et al: Epidemiology of stroke in Tilburg, The Netherlands. The population-based stroke incidence register: 2. Incidence, initial clinical picture and medical care, and three-week case fatality. *Stroke* 13:629–634, 1982.
7. Feng EJ, Orencia AJ, Whisnant JP: Outcome and pathogenesis of stroke is conditioned by place of stroke occurrence. *J Stroke Cerebrovasc Dis* 3:3–8, 1993.
8. Bonita R, Stewart A, Beaglehole R: International trends in stroke mortality: 1970–1985. *Stroke* 21:989–992, 1990.
9. Cooper R, Sempos C, Hsieh SC, Kovar MG: Slowdown in the decline of stroke mortality in the United States, 1979–1986. *Stroke* 21:1274–1279, 1990.
10. Jacobs DR, McGovern PG, Blackburn H: The US decline in stroke mortality: What does ecological analysis tell us? *Am J Public Health* 82:1596–1599, 1992.
11. Casper M, Wing S, Strogatz D, et al: Antihypertensive treatment and US trends in stroke mortality, 1962 to 1980. *Am J Public Health* 82:1600–1606, 1992.
12. McGovern PG, Burke GL, Sprafka JM, et al: Trends in mortality, morbidity, and risk factor levels for stroke from 1960 through 1990: The Minnesota heart survey. *JAMA* 268:753–759, 1992.
13. American Heart Association: Cardiovascular diseases and stroke in African-Americans and other racial minorities in the United States: A statement for health professionals. *Circulation* 83:1462–1480, 1991.
14. Gillum RF: Stroke in blacks. *Stroke* 19:1–9, 1988.
15. Kattapong VJ, Becker TM: Ethnic differences in mortality from cerebrovascular disease among New Mexico's Hispanics, Native Americans, and Non-Hispanic whites, 1958 through 1987. *Ethnicity Dis* 3:75–82, 1993.
16. Ahmed OI, Orchard TJ, Sharma R, et al: De-

clining mortality from stroke in Allegheny County, Pennsylvania: Trends in case fatality and severity of disease, 1971–1980. *Stroke* 19:181–184, 1988.
17. Alfredsson L, von Arbin M, De Faire U: Mortality from the incidence of stroke in Stockholm. *Br Med J* 292:1299–1303, 1986.
18. Boysen G, Nyboe J, Appleyard M, et al: Stroke incidence and risk factors for stroke in Copenhagen, Denmark. *Stroke* 19:1345–1353, 1988.
19. Malmgren R, Bamford J, Warlow C, Sandercock P: Geographical and secular trends in stroke incidence. *Lancet* 1:1196–1200, 1987.
20. Giroud M, Beuriat P, Vion P, et al: Stroke in a French prospective population study. *Neuroepidemiology* 8:97–104, 1989.
21. Wiebers DO, Whisnant JP: The incidence of stroke among pregnant women in Rochester, MN 1955 through 1979. *JAMA* 254:3055–3057, 1985.
22. Ueda K, Omae T, Hirota Y, et al: Decreasing trend in incidence and mortality from stroke in Hisayama residents, Japan. *Stroke* 12:154–160, 1981.
23. Gillum RF, Gomez-Marin O, Kottke TE, et al: Acute stroke in a metropolitan area, 1970 and 1980: The Minnesota Heart Survey. *J Chron Dis* 38:891–898, 1985.
24. Tanaka H, Ueda Y, Date C, et al: Incidence of stroke in Shibata, Japan: 1976–1978. *Stroke* 12:460–466, 1981.
25. Ashok PP, Radhakrishnan K, Sridhadran R, El-Mangoush M: Incidence and pattern of cerebrovascular disease in Benghazi, Libya. *J Neurol Neurosurg Psychiatry* 49:519–523, 1986.
26. Li SC, Schoenberg BS, Wang CC, et al: Cerebrovascular disease in the People's Republic of China. *Neurology* 35:1708–1717, 1985.
27. Oxfordshire Community Stroke Project: Incidence of stroke in Oxfordshire: First year's experience of a community stroke register. *Br Med J* 287:713–717, 1983.
28. Takeya Y, Popper JS, Shimizu Y, et al: Epidemiologic studies of coronary heart disease and stroke in Japanese men living in Japan, Hawaii and California: Incidence of stroke in Japan and Hawaii. *Stroke* 15:15–23, 1984.
29. Haberman S: Sex differences in the incidence of cerebrovascular disease. *J Epidemiol Commun Health* 35:45–50, 1981.
30. Suzuki K, Kutsuzawa T, Takita K, et al: Clinico-epidemiologic study of stroke in Akita, Japan. *Stroke* 18:402–406, 1987.
31. Terent A: Increasing incidence of stroke among Swedish women. *Stroke* 19:598–603, 1988.
32. Alter M, Zhang ZX, Sobel E, et al: Standardized incidence ratios of stroke: A worldwide review. *Neuroepidemiology* 5:148–158, 1986.
33. Broderick JP, Phillips SJ, Whisnant JP, et al: Incidence rates of stroke in the eighties: The end of the decline in stroke? *Stroke* 20:577–582, 1989.
34. Salonen JT, Puska P, Mustaniemi H: Changes in morbidity and mortality during comprehensive community program to control cardiovascular diseases during 1972–1977 in North Karelia. *Br Med J* 2:178–183, 1979.
35. Garraway WM, Whisnant JP, Furlan AJ, et al: The declining incidence of stroke. *N Engl J Med* 300:440–452, 1979.
36. Garraway WM, Whisnant JP, Drury I: The continuing decline in the incidence of stroke. *Mayo Clin Proc* 58:520–523, 1983.
37. Whisnant JP: The decline of stroke. *Stroke* 15:160–168, 1984.
38. Ebrahim S: *Clinical Epidemiology of Stroke*. Oxford, Oxford University Press, 1990.
39. Hachinski V: Decreased incidence and mortality of stroke. *Stroke* 15:376–378, 1984.
40. Tell GS, Crouse JR, Furberg CD: Relation between blood lipids, lipoproteins and cerebrovascular atherosclerosis: A review. *Stroke* 19:423–430, 1988.
41. Ingall TJ, Homer D, Whisnant JP, et al: Predictive value of carotid bruit for carotid arteriosclerosis. *Arch Neurol* 46:418–422, 1989.
42. Crouse JR, Toole JF, McKinney WM, et al: Risk factors for extracranial carotid artery atherosclerosis. *Stroke* 18:990–996, 1987.
43. Rubens J, Espeland MA, Ryu J, et al: Individual variation in susceptibility to extracranial carotid atherosclerosis. *Arteriosclerosis* 8:389–397, 1988.
44. Whisnant JP, Homer D, Ingall TJ, et al: Duration of cigarette smoking is the strongest

predictor of severe extracranial carotid artery atherosclerosis. *Stroke* 21:707–714, 1990.

45. Homer D, Ingall TJ, Baker HL Jr, et al: Serum lipids and lipoproteins are less powerful predictors of extracranial carotid artery atherosclerosis than are cigarette smoking and hypertension. *Mayo Clin Proc* 66:259–267, 1991.
46. Sandok BA, Whisnant JP, Furlan AJ, Mickell JL: Carotid artery bruits prevalence survey and differential diagnosis. *Mayo Clin Proc* 57:227–230, 1982.
47. Dempsey RJ, Moore RW: Amount of smoking independently predicts carotid artery atherosclerosis severity. *Stroke* 23:693–696, 1992.
48. Norris JW, D'Alton JG: Outcome of patients with asymptomatic carotid bruits, in Reivich M, Hurtig HI (eds): *Cerebrovascular Diseases*. New York, Raven, pp 63–76, 1983.
49. Meissner I, Wiebers DO, Whisnant JP, O'Fallon WM: The natural history of asymptomatic carotid artery occlusive lesions. *JAMA* 258: 2704–2707, 1987.
50. Sutton-Tyrrell K, Alcorn HG, Wolfson SK Jr, et al: Predictors of carotid stenosis in older adults with and without isolated systolic hypertension. *Stroke* 24:355–361, 1993.
51. Bogousslavsky J, Melle GV, Despland PA, Regli F: Alcohol consumption and carotid atherosclerosis in the Lausanne Stroke Registry. *Stroke* 21:715–720, 1990.
52. Salonen R, Seppanen K, Rauramaa R, Salonen JT: Prevalence of carotid atherosclerosis and serum cholesterol levels in Eastern Finland. *Arteriosclerosis* 8:788–792, 1988.
53. Adams HP Jr, Kappelle LJ, Birgitte HB: Asymptomatic carotid artery stenosis: Evaluation and treatment, in Adams HP Jr (ed): *Handbook of Cerebrovascular Diseases*. New York, Marcel Dekker, pp 13–34, 1993.
54. Heyman A, Wilkinson WE, Heyden S, et al: Risk of stroke in asymptomatic persons with cervical arterial bruits. *N Engl J Med* 302: 838–841, 1980.
55. Wolf PA, Kannel WB, Sorlie P, McNamara P: Asymptomatic carotid bruit and risk of stroke: The Framingham study. *JAMA* 245:1442–1445, 1981.
56. Prati P, Vanuzzo D, Casaroli M, et al: Prevalence and determinants of carotid atherosclerosis in a general population. *Stroke* 23:1705–1711, 1992.
57. Pujia A, Rubba P, Spencer MP: Prevalence of extracranial carotid artery disease detectable by echo-Doppler in an elderly population. *Stroke* 23:818–822, 1992.
58. Tell GS: Cigarette smoking, lipids, lipoproteins, and extracranial carotid artery atherosclerosis (editorial). *Mayo Clin Proc* 66:327–331, 1991.
59. Wiebers DO, Whisnant JP, Sandok BA, O'Fallon WM: Prospective comparison of a cohort with asymptomatic carotid bruit and a population-based cohort without carotid bruit. *Stroke* 21:984–988, 1990.
60. Wilterdink JL, Easton JD: Vascular event rates in patients with atherosclerotic cerebrovascular disease. *Arch Neurol* 49:857–863, 1992.
61. Ueda K, Omae T: Risk factors for stroke and transient ischemic attack, in Whisnant JP (ed): *Stroke: Populations, Cohorts, and Clinical Trials*. Oxford, Butterworth-Heinemann, pp 80–110, 1993.
62. Wolf PA, Cobb JL, D'Agostino RB: Epidemiology of stroke, in Barnett HJM, Mohr JP, Stein BM, Yatsu FM (eds): *Stroke: Pathophysiology, Diagnosis and Management*. New York, Churchill Livingstone, pp 3–27, 1992.
63. Davis PH, Hachinski V: Stroke: Epidemiology of cerebrovascular disease, in Anderson DW, Schoenberg DG (eds): *Neuroepidemiology: A Tribute to Bruce Schoenberg*. Boca Raton, CRC Press, pp 28–53, 1991.
64. Kurtzke JF: Epidemiology of cerebrovascular disease, in McDowell F, Caplan LF (eds): *Cerebrovascular Survey Report for the National Institute of Neurological and Communicative Disorders and Stroke*. Rochester, MN, Whiting Press, 1985.
65. Marler JR, Price TR, Clark GL, et al: Morning increase in onset of ischemic stroke. *Stroke* 20:473–476, 1989.
66. Tsementzis SA, Gill JS, Hitchcock ER, et al: Diurnal variation of an activity during the onset of stroke. *Neurosurgery* 17:901–904, 1985.

67. Marsh III E, Biller J, Adams HP Jr, et al: Circadian variation in onset of acute ischemic stroke. *Arch Neurol* 47:1179–1180, 1990.
68. Argentino C, Toni D, Rasura M, et al: Circadian variation in the frequency of ischemic stroke. *Stroke* 21:387–389, 1990.
69. Andreotti F, Davies GJ, Hackett DR, et al: Major circadian fluctuations in fibrinolytic factors and possible relevance to time of onset of myocardial infarction, sudden cardiac death and stroke. *Am J Cardiol* 62:635–636, 1988.
70. Shinkawa A, Ueda K, Hasuo Y, et al: Seasonal variation in stroke incidence in Hisayama, Japan. *Stroke* 21:1262–1267, 1990.
71. Biller J, Jones MP, Bruno A, et al: Seasonal variation of stroke. Does it exist? *Neuroepidemiology* 7:89–98, 1988.
72. Harmsen P, Rosengren A, Tsipogianni A, Wilhelmsen L: Risk factors for stroke in middle-aged men in Göteborg, Sweden. *Stroke* 21: 223–229, 1990.
73. Welin L, Svardsudd K, Wilhelmsen L, et al: Analysis of risk factors for stroke in a cohort of men born in 1913. *N Engl J Med* 317:521–526, 1987.
74. Khaw KT, Barrett-Connor E: Family history of stroke as an independent predictor of ischemic heart disease in men and stroke in women. *Am J Epidemiol* 123:59–66, 1986.
75. Diaz JF, Hachinski VC, Pederson LL, Donald A: Aggregation of multiple risk factors for stroke in siblings of patients with brain infarction and transient ischemic attacks. *Stroke* 17:1239–1242, 1986.
76. Brass LM, Isaacsohn JL, Merikangas KR, Robinette CD: A study of twins and stroke. *Stroke* 23:221–223, 1992.
77. Kiely DK, Wolf PA, Cupples A, et al: Familial aggregation of stroke: The Framingham Study. *Stroke* 24:1366–1371, 1993.
78. Davis PH, Dambrosia JM, Schoenberg BS, et al: Risk factors for ischemic stroke: A prospective study in Rochester, Minnesota. *Ann Neurol* 22:319–327, 1987.
79. Whisnant JP: The role of the neurologist in the decline of stroke. *Ann Neurol* 14:1–7, 1983.
80. Brand FN, Abbott RD, Kannel WB: Diabetes, intermittent claudication, and risk of cardiovascular events: The Framingham study. *Diabetes* 38:504–509, 1989.
81. Barrett-Connor E, Khaw KT: Diabetes mellitus: An independent risk factor for stroke. *Am J Epidemiol* 128:116–123, 1988.
82. Abbott RD, Donahue RP, MacMahon SW, et al: Diabetes and the risk of stroke. *JAMA* 257:949–952, 1987.
83. Manson JE, Colditz GA, Stampfer MJ, et al: A prospective study of maturity-onset diabetes mellitus and risk of coronary heart disease and stroke in women. *Arch Intern Med* 151: 1141–1147, 1991.
84. Schumacher MA, Smith KR: Diabetes in Utah among adults: Interaction between diabetes and other risk factors for microvascular and macrovascular complications. *Am J Public Health* 78:1195–1201, 1988.
85. Hallenbeck JM, Dutka AJ, Kochanek PM, et al: Stroke risk factors prepare rat brain stem tissues for modified local Shwartzman reaction. *Stroke* 19:863–869, 1988.
86. Lapidus L, Bengtsson C, Lindquist L, et al: Triglycerides—Main lipid risk factor for cardiovascular disease in women? *Acta Med Scand* 217:481–489, 1985.
87. Iso H, Jacobs DR Jr, Wentworth D, MRFIT Research Group: Serum cholesterol levels and six-year mortality from stroke in 350,977 men screened for the multiple risk factor intervention trial. *N Engl J Med* 320:904–910, 1989.
88. Woo J, Lau E, Lam CWK, et al: Hypertension, lipoprotein(a), and apolipoprotein A-I as risk factors for stroke in the Chinese. *Stroke* 22:203–208, 1991.
89. Jurgens G, Koltringer P: Lipoprotein (a) in ischemic cerebrovascular disease: A new approach to the assessment of risk for stroke. *Neurology* 37:513–515, 1987.
90. Woo J, Lam CWK, Kay R, et al: Acute and long-term changes in serum lipids after acute stroke. *Stroke* 21:1407–1411, 1990.
91. Garraway WM, Whisnant JP: The changing pattern of hypertension and the declining incidence of stroke. *JAMA* 258:214–217, 1987.
92. Hypertension Detection and Follow-up Program Cooperative Group: Five-year findings of the hypertension detection and follow-up

program III. Reduction in stroke incidence among persons with high blood pressure. *JAMA* 247:633–638, 1982.
93. SHEP Cooperative Research Group: Prevention of stroke by antihypertensive drug treatment in older persons with isolated systolic hypertension: final results of the Systolic Hypertension in the Elderly Program (SHEP). *JAMA* 265:3255–3264, 1991.
94. Perry HM, Smith WM, McDonald RH, et al: Morbidity and mortality in the Systolic Hypertension in the Elderly Program (SHEP) Pilot Study. *Stroke* 20:4–13, 1989.
95. Law MR, Frost CD, Wald NJ: I. By how much does dietary salt reduction lower blood pressure? I-Analysis of observational data among population. *Br Med J* 302:811–815, 1991.
96. Frost CD, Law MR, Wald NJ: II. Analysis of observational data within populations. *Br Med J* 302:815–818, 1991.
97. Xie JX, Sasaki S, Joossens JV, Kesteloot H: The relationship between urinary cations obtained from the INTERSALT study and cerebrovascular mortality. *J Hum Hypertens* 6:17–21, 1992.
98. Law MR, Frost CD, Wald NJ: III. Analysis of data from trials of salt reduction. *Br Med J* 302:819–824, 1991.
99. Cerebral Embolism Task Force: Cardiogenic brain embolism. *Arch Neurol* 43:71–84, 1986.
100. Sherman DG, Dyken ML, Fisher M, Harrison MJG, Hart RG: Cerebral embolism. *Chest* 89(suppl):82S–98S, 1986.
101. Sherman DG, Dyken ML, Fisher M, et al: Antithrombotic therapy for cerebrovascular disorders. *Chest* 102(suppl):529S–537S, 1992.
102. Kannel WB, Wolf PA, Verter J: Manifestations of coronary disease predisposing to stroke. *JAMA* 250:2942–2946, 1983.
103. Dexter DD Jr, Whisnant JP, Connolly DC, O'Fallon WM: The association of stroke and coronary heart disease: A population study. *Mayo Clin Proc* 62:1077–1083, 1987.
104. Wolf PA, Abbott RD, Kannel WB: Atrial fibrillation: A major contributor to stroke in the elderly: The Framingham Study. *Arch Intern Med* 147:1561–1564, 1987.
105. Petersen P, Godtfredsen J: Risk factors for stroke in chronic atrial fibrillation. *European Heart J* 9:291–294, 1988.
106. Kopecky SL, Gersh BJ, McGoon MD, et al: The natural history of lone atrial fibrillation. A population-based study over three decades. *N Engl J Med* 317:669–674, 1987.
107. Moulton AW, Singer DE, Haas JS: Risk factors for stroke in patients with nonrheumatic atrial fibrillation: A case-control study. *Am J Med* 91:156–161, 1991.
108. Flegel KM, Shipley MJ, Rose G: Risk of stroke in nonrheumatic atrial fibrillation. *Lancet* 1:526–529, 1987.
109. Brand FN, Abbott RD, Kannel WB, Wolf PA: Characteristics and prognosis of lone atrial fibrillation: 30-year follow-up in the Framingham Study. *JAMA* 254:3449–3453, 1985.
110. Wolf PA, Dawber TR, Thomas HE Jr, Kannel WB: Epidemiologic assessment of chronic atrial fibrillation and risk of stroke: The Framingham Study. *Neurology* 28:973–977, 1978.
111. Wolf PA, Abbott RD, Kannel WB: Atrial fibrillation as an independent risk factor for stroke: The Framingham Study. *Stroke* 22:983–988, 1991.
112. Halperin JL, Hart RG: Atrial fibrillation and stroke: New ideas, persisting dilemmas. *Stroke* 19:937–941, 1988.
113. Petersen P, Boysen G, Godtfredsen J, et al: Placebo controlled, randomized trial of warfarin and aspirin for prevention of thromboembolic complications in chronic atrial fibrillation: The Copenhagen AFASAK study. *Lancet* 1:175–179, 1989.
114. The Stroke Prevention in Atrial Fibrillation Investigators: Design of a multicenter randomized trial for the stroke prevention in atrial fibrillation study. *Stroke* 21:538–545, 1990.
115. The Boston Area Anticoagulation Trial for Atrial Fibrillation Investigators: The effect of low-dose warfarin on the risk of stroke in patients with nonrheumatic atrial fibrillation. *N Engl J Med* 323:1505–1511, 1990.
116. Stroke Prevention in Atrial Fibrillation Investigators: Stroke prevention in atrial fibrillation study: Final results. *Circulation* 84:527–539, 1991.
117. Barnett HJM, Boughner DR, Taylor DW, et

al: Further evidence relating mitral valve prolapse to cerebral ischemic events. *N Engl J Med* 302:139–144, 1980.
118. Scharf RE, Hennerici M, Bluschke V, et al: Cerebral ischemia in young patients: Is it associated with mitral valve prolapse and abnormal platelet activity in vivo? *Stroke* 13:454–458, 1982.
119. Egeblad H, Sorensen PS: Prevalence of mitral valve prolapse in younger patients with cerebral ischemic attacks: A blinded controlled study. *Acta Med Scand* 216:385–391, 1984.
120. Kelley RE, Pina I, Lee SC: Cerebral ischemia and mitral valve prolapse: Case-control study associated factors. *Stroke* 19:443–446, 1988.
121. Fairfax AJ, Lambert CD, Leatham A: Systemic embolism in chronic sinoatrial disorder. *N Engl J Med* 295:190–192, 1976.
122. Bathen J, Sparr S, Rokseth R: Embolism in sinoatrial disease. *Acta Med Scand* 203:7–11, 1978.
123. Jelic V, Belkic K, Djordjevic M, Kocovic D: Survival in 1,431 pacemaker patients: Prognostic factors and comparison with the general population. *Pace* 15:141–147, 1992.
124. Stangl K, Seitz K, Wirtzfeld A, et al: Differences between atrial single chamber pacing (AAI) and ventricular single chamber pacing (VVI) with respect to prognosis and antiarrhythmic effect in patients with sick sinus syndrome. *Pace* 13:2080–2085, 1990.
125. Rosenqvist M, Brandt J, Schuller H: Long-term pacing in sinus node disease: Effects of stimulation mode on cardiovascular morbidity and mortality. *Am Heart J* 116:16–22, 1988.
126. Kazmier FJ: Shaggy aorta syndrome and disseminated atheromatous embolization, in Bergan JJ, Yao JST (eds): *Aortic Surgery*. Philadelphia, WB Saunders, pp 189–194, 1989.
127. Jones HR Jr, Caplan LR, Come PC, et al: Cerebral emboli of paradoxical origin. *Ann Neurol* 13:314–319, 1983.
128. Lechat PH, Mas JL, Lascault G, et al: Prevalence of patent foramen ovale in patients with stroke. *N Engl J Med* 318:1148–1152, 1988.
129. Fisher M, Meiselman HJ: Hemorrheological factors in cerebral ischemia. *Stroke* 22:1164–1169, 1991.
130. Kannel WB, Wolf PA, Castelli WP, D'Agostino RB: Fibrinogen and risk of cardiovascular disease. *JAMA* 258:1183–1186, 1987.
131. Wilhelmsen L, Svardsudd K, Korsan-Bengtsen K, et al: Fibrinogen as a risk factor for stroke and myocardial infarction. *N Engl J Med* 311:501–505, 1984.
132. Kiyohara Y, Ueda K, Hasuo Y, et al: Hematocrit as a risk factor of cerebral infarction: Long-term prospective population survey in a Japanese rural community. *Stroke* 17:687–692, 1986.
133. Gustafsson C, Blomback M, Britton M, Hamsten A, Svensson J: Coagulation factors and the increased risk of stroke in nonvalvular atrial fibrillation. *Stroke* 21:47–51, 1990.
134. Kushner M, Simonian N: Lupus anticoagulants, anticardiolipin antibodies, and cerebral ischemia. *Stroke* 20:225–229, 1989.
135. Kittner SJ, Gorelick PB: Antiphospholipid antibodies and stroke: An epidemiological perspective. *Stroke* 23(suppl I):I19–I22, 1992.
136. Colditz GA, Bonita R, Stampfer MJ, et al: Cigarette smoking and risk of stroke in middle-aged women. *N Engl J Med* 318:937–941, 1988.
137. Abbott RD, Yin Y, Reed DM, Yano K: Risk of stroke in male cigarette smokers. *N Engl J Med* 315:717–720, 1986.
138. Bonita R, Scragg R, Stewart A, et al: Cigarette smoking and risk of premature stroke in men and women. *Br Med J* 293:6–8, 1986.
139. Shinton R, Beevers G: Meta-analysis of relation between cigarette smoking and stroke. *Br Med J* 298:789–794, 1989.
140. Donnan GA, McNeil JJ, Adena MA, et al: Smoking as a risk factor for cerebral ischemia. *Lancet* 1:643–647, 1989.
141. Molgaard CA, Bartok A, Peddecord KM, Rothrock J: The association between cerebrovascular disease and smoking: A case-control study. *Neuroepidemiology* 5:88–94, 1986.
142. Ben-Shlomo Y, Markowe H, Shipley M, Parot G: Stroke risk for alcohol consumption using different control groups. *Stroke* 23:1093–1098, 1992.
143. Gill JS, Zezulka AV, Shipley MJ, et al: Stroke and alcohol consumption. *N Engl J Med* 315:1041–1046, 1986.

144. Ellekjaer EF, Wyller TB, Sverre JM, Holmen J: Lifestyle factors and risk of cerebral infarction. *Stroke* 23:829–834, 1992.
145. Gorelick PB, Rodin MB, Langenberg P, et al: Is acute alcohol ingestion a risk factor for ischemic stroke? Results of a controlled study in middle-aged and elderly stroke patients at three urban medical centers. *Stroke* 18:359–364, 1987.
146. Gorelick PB, Rodin MB, Langenberg P, et al: Weekly alcohol consumption, cigarette smoking, and the risk of ischemic stroke: Results of a case-control study at three urban medical centers in Chicago, Illinois. *Neurology* 39: 339–343, 1989.
147. Gorelick PB: Alcohol and stroke. *Stroke* 18: 267–271, 1987.
148. Hillbom ME: What supports the role of alcohol as risk factor for stroke? *Acta Med Scand* 717(suppl):93–106, 1987.
149. Hillbom ME, Kaste M: Ethanol intoxication. A risk factor for ischemic brain infarction. *Stroke* 14:694–699, 1983.
150. Taylor JR, Combs-Orme T: Alcohol and strokes in young adults. *Am J Psychiatry* 142:116-118, 1985.
151. Stampfer MJ, Willett WC, Colditz GA, et al: A prospective study of past use of oral contraceptive agents and risk of cardiovascular diseases. *N Engl J Med* 319:1313–1317, 1988.
152. Klatsky AL, Armstrong MA, Friedman GD: Risk of cardiovascular mortality in alcohol drinkers, ex-drinkers and nondrinkers. *Am J Cardiol* 66:1237–1242, 1990.
153. Stadel BV: Medical progress oral contraceptives and cardiovascular disease (second of two parts). *N Engl J Med* 305:672–677, 1981.
154. Royal College of General Practitioners' Oral Contraception Study: Further analyses of mortality in oral contraceptive users. *Lancet* 1:541–546, 1981.
155. Collaborative Group for the Study of Stroke in Young Women: Oral contraceptives and stroke in young women. *JAMA* 231:718–722, 1975.
156. Longstreth WT Jr, Swanson PD: Oral contraceptives and stroke. *Stroke* 15:747–750, 1984.
157. Paganini-Hill A, Ross RK, Henderson BE: Postmenopausal estrogen treatment and stroke: A prospective study. *Br Med J* 297:519–522, 1988.
158. Wolf PA, D'Agostino RB, Kannel WB, et al: Cigarette smoking as a risk factor for stroke. *JAMA* 259:1025–1029, 1988.
159. Folsom AR, Prineas RJ, Kaye SA, Munger RG: Incidence of hypertension and stroke in relation to body fat distribution and other risk factors in older women. *Stroke* 21:701–706, 1990.
160. Bouchard C, Shephard RJ, Stephens T, et al: *Exercise, Fitness, and Health: A Consensus of Current Knowledge*. Champaign, IL, Human Kinetics Books, 1990.
161. Colantonio A, Kasl SV, Ostfeld AM: Level of function predicts first stroke in the elderly. *Stroke* 23:1355–1357, 1992.
162. Salonen JT, Puska P, Tuomilehto J: Physical activity and risk of myocardial infarction, cerebral stroke and death. *Am J Epidemiol* 115: 526–537, 1982.
163. Wannamethee G, Shaper AG: Physical activity and stroke in British middle-aged men. *Br Med J* 304:597–601, 1992.
164. Curfman GD: The health benefits of exercise: A critical reappraisal. *N Engl J Med* 328:574–576, 1993.
165. Meissner I, Whisnant JP, Garraway WM: Hypertension management and stroke recurrence in a community (Rochester, Minnesota, 1950–1979). *Stroke* 19:459–463, 1988.
166. Terent A: Survival after stroke and transient ischemic attacks during the 1970s and 1980s. *Stroke* 20:1320–1326, 1989.
167. Vittanen M, Eriksson S, Asplund K: Risk of recurrent stroke, myocardial infarction and epilepsy during long-term follow-up after stroke. *Eur Neurol* 28:227–231, 1988.
168. Sacco RL, Foulkes MA, Mohr JP, et al: Determinants of early recurrence of cerebral infarction: The stroke data bank. *Stroke* 20:983–989, 1989.
169. Hier DB, Foulkes MA, Swiontoniowski M, et al: Stroke recurrence within 2 years after ischemic infarction. *Stroke* 22:155–161, 1991.
170. Sobel E, Alter M, Davanipour Z, et al: Stroke in the Lehigh Valley: Combined risk factors for recurrent stroke. *Neurology* 39:669–672, 1989.

171. Levine ST, Brey RL, Joseph CLM, Havstad S, on behalf of the Antiphospholipid Antibodies in Stroke Study Group: Risk of recurrent thromboembolic events in patients with focal cerebral ischemia and antiphospholipid antibodies. *Stroke* 23(suppl I):I-29–I-32, 1992.
172. The Antiphospholipid Antibodies in Stroke Study Group: Clinical and laboratory findings in patients with antiphospholipid antibodies and cerebral ischemia. *Stroke* 21:1268–1273, 1990.
173. Brey RL, Hart RG, Sherman DG, Tegeler CH: Antiphospholipid antibodies and cerebral ischemia in young people. *Neurology* 40: 1190–1196, 1990.
174. Rubin JR, Goldstone J, McIntyre KE Jr, et al: The value of carotid endarterectomy in reducing the morbidity and mortality of recurrent stroke. *J Vasc Surg* 4:443–449, 1986.
175. Goldberg G, Berger GG: Secondary prevention in stroke: A primary rehabilitation. *Arch Phys Med Rehabil* 69:32–40, 1988.

9

Clinical Evaluation of the Patient with Cerebrovascular Disease

Phillip D. Swanson

Patients with cerebrovascular disease seek medical attention in several different clinical situations: (1) as outpatients in a clinic or emergency room for transient symptoms of cerebral dysfunction; and (2) in the emergency room following rapid onset of neurologic symptoms. Presenting symptoms that suggest a rapidly progressing cerebral disorder include unilateral weakness, unilateral sensory changes, headache, loss of consciousness, loss of language abilities, and alterations of vision.

It is convenient to distinguish the assessment of a patient with transient symptoms from that of a patient with an evolving or completed stroke whose symptoms are not evanescent. However, as pointed out by Caplan, "none of the time courses is specific for any single pathology or pathophysiology."[1] In other words, some patients who fit the definition of a transient ischemic attack (TIA) will have had a small infarction with only fleeting symptoms.

The evaluation of patients with suspected stroke or TIA must be broad enough to cover a variety of possible etiologies. Although the focus of this book is on cerebral ischemia, "cerebrovascular disease" includes both hemorrhagic and ischemic conditions. Furthermore, stroke can be caused by occlusion of cerebral veins or venous sinuses rather than cerebral arteries.

TRANSIENT ISCHEMIC ATTACKS

Most definitions of a TIA use a 24-h cut-off point for the duration of symptoms and signs beyond which the diagnosis changes to a reversible ischemic neurologic deficit (RIND), stroke-in-evolution, or completed stroke (Chap. 6). However, the typical duration of a TIA is much shorter than 24 h, most often in the range of 8 to 14 min.[2,3] To be considered as a TIA, the episode must be consistent with an ischemic event in the territory supplied by a cerebral artery. Therefore, in the absence of further defining symptoms, dizziness, faintness, and loss of consciousness usually exclude the diagnosis of TIA.

Conditions that can mimic TIA include presyncope, hyperventilation, partial seizures, vertiginous attacks due to labyrinthine disease, and migraine episodes (Table 9-1). Episodes of presyncope usually occur when the patient is in the upright position, and the predominant symptom is lightheadedness. Localized limb weakness, clear diplopia, or unilateral visual symptoms should not be present, but dimming of vision may be mentioned by the patient. Hyperventilation episodes are often accompanied by a sense of breathlessness and tingling of the lips and fingers. Partial motor seizures are usually associated with symptoms such as face or limb jerking and are rarely mistaken for a TIA. However, partial seizures can occur without motor involvement. Partial sensory seizures can be manifested by numbness or discomfort in the affected limb. Partial seizures with interruption of speech can easily be mistaken for a TIA, as illustrated by the following case.

Clinical case. A 59-year-old engineer passed out while jogging. His memory was impaired for several hours. He was briefly hospitalized, and a CT scan showed a small lacune in the left putamen; an EEG was normal. A month later he had the first of several episodes of difficulty speaking. These lasted 10 to 60 min and occurred once or twice per week. They were diagnosed as TIAs in the distribution of the left internal carotid artery. After the two most recent episodes his speech did not return to normal. He had difficulty understanding both written words and speech. He also had some difficulty spelling. Spontaneous speech was halting, with word-finding errors and occasional word substitutions. Four months after the initial episode of loss of consciousness, MRI examination demonstrated an enhancing mass in the left temporal lobe with surrounding edema. The mass was shown at biopsy to be a glioblastoma multiforme.

Comment. The above case illustrates that TIA-like symptoms can occur in patients with underlying structural disease. This patient's symptoms changed with time, and eventually it became clear that his aphasic symptoms

Table 9-1 Features of Conditions Producing TIA-Like Symptoms

Condition	Features
Presyncope	Lightheadedness, upright position
Hyperventilation	Breathlessness, finger and lip tingling
Partial seizures	Aura, stereotyped episodes, altered awareness, sensory or motor "march"
Episodic or positional vertigo	Spinning sensation, nystagmus during attack, vertigo on lying down
Migraine	Evolving symptoms, longer duration, visual scintillations, history going back months to years

were progressing. Because of the possibility of nonvascular causes, an imaging study usually is indicated in patients with TIA-like symptoms. It is noteworthy, however, that in this clinical case the initial CT scan did not show a mass lesion.

Vertigo can occur during a posterior circulation TIA (Chap. 7), but when it occurs in isolation it is more likely due to labyrinthine conditions such as benign positional vertigo or Meniere's disease. Migraine is often but not always associated with headache. The terms *migraine accompaniment* or *migraine aura without headache* have been applied to episodes of cerebral dysfunction attributed to cerebral ischemia during a migraine attack.[4,5] These episodes usually last somewhat longer (15 to 24 min) than typical TIAs, and the symptoms often evolve during this interval. Visual symptoms are frequent and usually include such "positive" features as flashing lights, haloes, or jagged lines (fortification spectra). Patients with migraine auras often say that they have had similar episodes months or years before. They also may have had migraine headaches in the past.

Diagnostic Approach to the Patient with TIA

Transient ischemic attacks are usually divided into "carotid" and "vertebrobasilar" according to the most likely arterial system producing the symptoms (Chaps. 6 and 7). The clinical features of the episodes give the most important clues for reaching the correct diagnosis. Critical to how far one goes with the diagnostic evaluation is whether the patient is likely to be a candidate for carotid endarterectomy. Thus, it is less likely that a patient with vertebrobasilar symptoms will be subjected to angiography than will a patient with TIAs in the territory of the internal carotid artery.

The physical examination may be helpful in directing further diagnostic studies. In suspected cases of hyperventilation syndrome, observing the patient during 1 to 3 min of voluntary hyperventilation can be diagnostic. It is important to assess for postural hypotension, hypertension, unequal arm blood pressures, carotid or supraclavicular bruits, evidence of retinal emboli, cardiac murmurs or arrhythmias, and persistent neurologic signs. However, the chance of a physician's examining a patient during a TIA is less than 10 percent.[6]

Diagnostic testing should be more comprehensive in young individuals, in whom atherosclerotic disease is less likely to be the cause of symptoms. Laboratory tests should include: a CBC with platelet count to detect blood dyscrasias such as idiopathic thrombocythemia or polycythemia vera; lupus anticoagulant and coagulation factors, including protein S and protein C that may indicate a hypercoagulable state; and antinuclear antibodies (ANA), erythrocyte sedimentation rate (ESR), complement, and other autoantibodies to search for evidence of collagen vascular diseases. Blood chemistries should include serum glucose, cholesterol, lipoproteins, and triglycerides to look for factors that predispose to atherosclerosis. An elevated ESR in an elderly individual should raise the level of suspicion for temporal arteritis. A CT or MRI study of the brain is valuable to rule out such causes of transient ischemic symptoms as an arteriovenous malformation or an unsuspected brain tumor.

The cardiac assessment begins with an electrocardiogram. Echocardiography should be considered to evaluate for the presence of mitral valve prolapse, nonbacterial thrombotic endocarditis, or a patent foramen ovale. Transesophageal or contrast echocardiography will increase the likelihood of detecting a patent foramen ovale or proximal aortic atheromata that might be a source of cerebral emboli. Transesophageal echocardiography is most likely to be helpful in young patients without clinical evidence of heart disease.[7]

It is now routine in patients with suspected

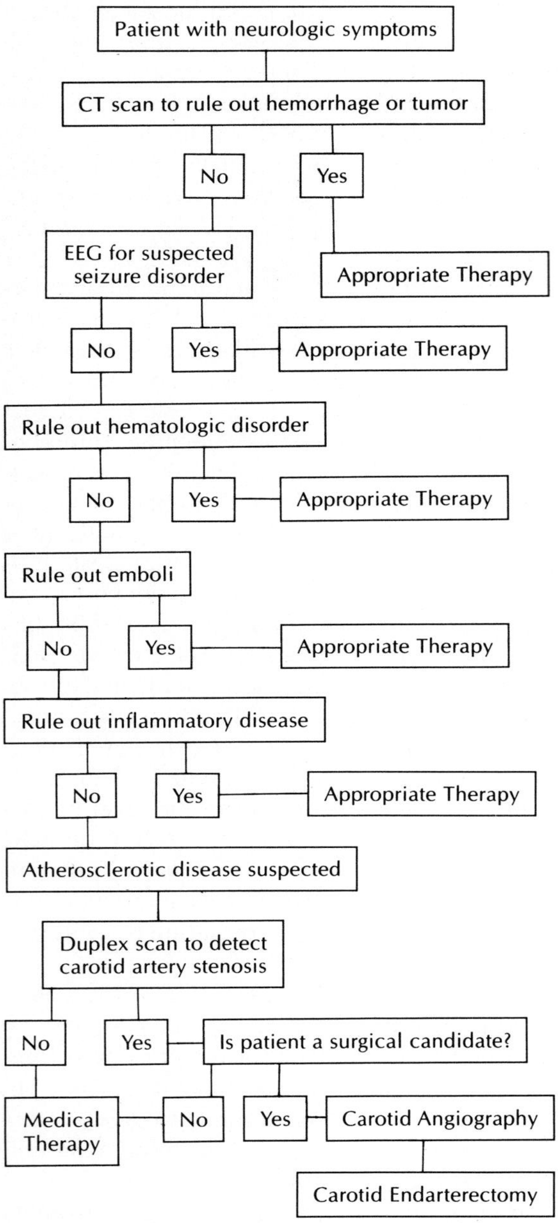

Figure 9-1. Algorithm for the diagnostic evaluation of a patient with neurologic symptoms.

TIA to perform a duplex scan to evaluate the extracranial carotid arteries (Chap. 11). Transcranial Doppler is becoming more widely used to assess for the presence of intracranial arterial stenosis or emboli (Chap. 12).

Electroencephalography (EEG) is no longer routinely done. However, it can be extremely useful in selected cases to rule out the possibility of partial seizures manifested by episodes of sensory loss or aphasia. In some patients who have frequent episodes suspected to be partial seizures accompanied by aphasia, admission to a unit equipped with closed circuit television and EEG monitoring equipment may be needed to record one or more episodes.[8]

Cerebral angiography should be considered in patients with TIA if it is believed that the results of the study will make a difference in managing the patient. If noninvasive studies suggest extracranial arterial stenosis amenable to surgery, or if treatment might be modified by visualization of the intracranial vessels as in patients with granulomatous angiitis, then angiography is indicated. Continued advances in imaging of the extracranial and intracranial cerebral vessels by duplex scanning and magnetic resonance angiography are likely to reduce the necessity for performing contrast angiography in TIA patients (Chap. 21).

A suggested general algorithm for the diagnostic evaluation of patients with neurologic symptoms is given in Fig. 9-1.

EVOLVING OR COMPLETED STROKE

The symptoms and signs of stroke occur rapidly, evolving within minutes to hours. They indicate dysfunction in localized anatomic areas within the cerebral hemispheres or brain stem that can be understood as resulting from occlusion or rupture of blood vessels. Brain tumors, degenerative diseases, and multiple sclerosis are conditions whose time courses usually differ from those of stroke syndromes. The differential diagnosis of suspected stroke is depicted in Fig. 9-2.[9–11]

Hemorrhage

The diagnosis of intracranial hemorrhage must be made rapidly. Intracranial hemorrhages can be classified as follows:

(1) Subarachnoid hemorrhage secondary to ruptured berry aneurysm
(2) Intracerebral hemorrhage
  (A) Primary, associated with hypertension
  (B) Rupture of an arteriovenous malformation
  (C) Lobar, associated with congophilic (amyloid) angiopathy

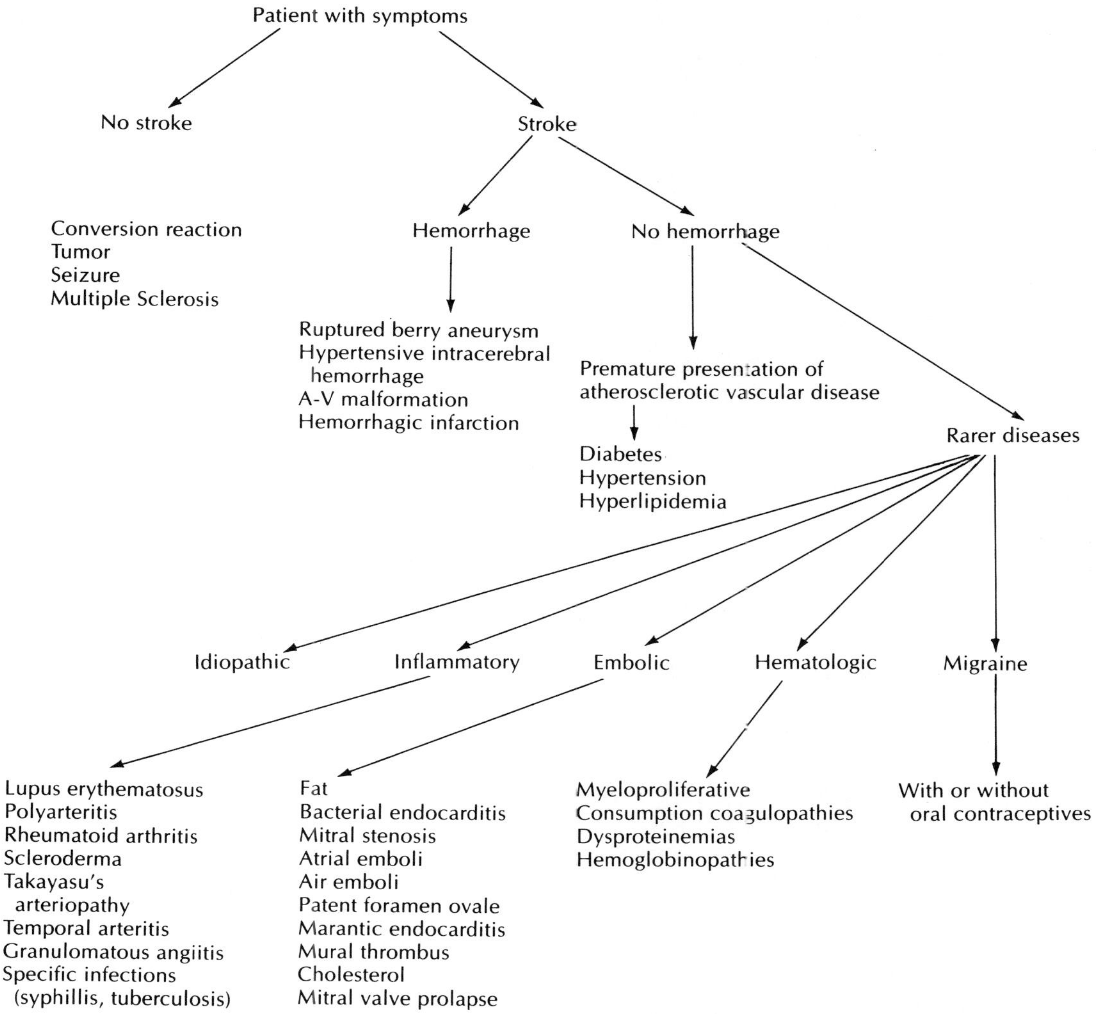

Figure 9-2. The differential diagnosis of stroke.

(D) Lobar, associated with intravenous drug abuse
(E) Contusions from head trauma
(F) Hemorrhagic infarction from cerebral embolus or cerebral vein thrombosis
(G) Hemorrhage into a brain tumor

A ruptured berry aneurysm usually presents without warning, and the clinical picture evolves rapidly. In some patients, premonitory leaking from the aneurysm will have occurred a day or more before the major event, producing headache, transitory unilateral weakness and numbness, or speech disturbances. Since the bleeding is directly into the subarachnoid space, the predominant symptom will almost always be severe headache and neck stiffness. Other symptoms and signs that suggest a ruptured aneurysm include altered level of consciousness and subhyaloid hemorrhages in the retina related to the rapid rise in intracranial pressure. The retinal hemorrhages can be quite large and confluent. If the aneurysm is located on the internal carotid artery at the junction with the posterior communicating artery, it is common to find an ipsilateral third cranial nerve palsy (ptosis, dilated pupil that is poorly reactive, and externally rotated eyeball with inability to look medially, up, or down). Since the fourth cranial nerve is intact, the superior oblique muscle will intort the eye when the patient tries to look down. There may also be signs of cerebral ischemia due to spasm of the middle cerebral, anterior cerebral, or basilar arteries.

Intracerebral hemorrhage associated with leaking from a perforating artery or from an arteriovenous malformation is also typically associated with a severe headache. Neurologic signs appear rapidly and are determined by the location of bleeding. With an intracerebral hemorrhage from perforating arteries off the middle cerebral artery, hemiplegia is likely. With an intracerebellar hemorrhage, ataxia and vertigo may occur initially, followed by loss of consciousness. Hemorrhage into the pons will be associated with quadriplegia, inability to move the eyes horizontally, and coma.

Thrombosis can occur in cortical or deeper veins or in cerebral venous sinuses. The infarcts that result are typically hemorrhagic. Venous thrombosis may occur in the postpartum period or in other clinical situations associated with dehydration or fever. Venous or sinus thromboses may be septic or nonseptic. Seizures, often of the partial type, are a frequent associated finding in patients with cortical vein thrombosis. These patients may also have focal neurologic findings resulting from damage to underlying cerebral tissue. Increased intracranial pressure may accompany thrombosis of the superior sagittal or lateral venous sinuses. Cavernous sinus thrombosis is often associated with proptosis, retinal hemorrhages, and ophthalmoplegias.

Ischemic Stroke

Ischemic strokes can be due to thrombotic or embolic occlusions of the cerebral vessels. Specific causes of ischemic strokes are listed below:

Thrombotic (nonembolic) stroke

(1) Associated with atherosclerosis
(2) Associated with hematologic abnormalities
  (A) Polycythemia vera
  (B) Essential thrombocythemia
  (C) Consumption coagulopathies
  (D) Dysproteinemias (cryoglobulinemia)
  (E) Hemoglobinopathies (sickle cell disease)
  (F) Lupus anticoagulant
(3) Inflammatory
  (A) Specific infections (meningovascular syphilis, tuberculous or fungal meningitis)
  (B) Collagen vascular diseases
    (a) Systemic lupus erythematosus
    (b) Periarteritis nodosa
  (C) Granulomatous angiitis

  - **(D)** Associated with amphetamine or cocaine use
- **(4)** Infarct associated with migraine
- **(5)** Miscellaneous
  - **(A)** Fibromuscular dysplasia
  - **(B)** Dissecting aneurysm of ascending aorta or of large arteries (carotid or vertebral)
  - **(C)** Moya-moya arteriopathy
  - **(D)** Trauma (vertebral occlusion associated with neck manipulation)

Embolic Stroke

- **(1)** Bacterial endocarditis
- **(2)** Rheumatic heart disease
- **(3)** Atrial fibrillation with other heart disease
- **(4)** Left ventricular mural thrombus with acute MI, ventricular aneurysm, or dilated cardiomyopathy
- **(5)** Atrial myxoma
- **(6)** Marantic (nonbacterial thrombotic) endocarditis associated with malignancy
- **(7)** Libman-Sacks endocarditis associated with SLE
- **(8)** Paradoxical embolus associated with patent foramen ovale or septal defect
- **(9)** Air or fat emboli
- **(10)** Mitral valve prolapse
- **(11)** Artery-artery emboli
- **(12)** Embolus associated with angiography or cardiac surgery

Lacunar infarcts are usually due to occlusion of small perforating arterioles in individuals with chronic hypertension or diabetes mellitus. Clinical presentations that are associated with lacunar infarction include pure motor hemiparesis, pure hemisensory syndrome, dysarthria-clumsy hand syndrome, and ataxic hemiparesis syndrome.

Diagnostic Approach to the Patient with Acute Stroke

A careful history should be taken from the patient and, if possible, a family member to assess the circumstances surrounding the onset of symptoms. Sudden onset of neurologic symptoms during sleep is common with ischemic stroke. If symptoms began during exertion, acute hemorrhage or paradoxical embolism should be suspected. Have similar symptoms occurred previously, suggesting TIA episodes? Is headache a prominent symptom? Are there other underlying conditions such as hypertension, cardiac disease, or diabetes mellitus? Is the patient taking anticoagulants?

The physical examination will assist in determining the likely cause of the event. Of particular importance is the presence or absence of nuchal rigidity, the level of blood pressure, and the presence of cardiac arrhythmias or murmurs. Elevated body temperature should suggest the possibility of bacterial endocarditis. It is important to differentiate between hemorrhagic and ischemic stroke early in the diagnostic process. Further diagnostic and therapeutic interventions will be quite different in each category.

Lumbar puncture is rarely necessary with acute stroke patients, unless there is a suspicion that the stroke is associated with an infectious process such as meningovascular syphilis. Assessment of cardiac function is important in patients with ischemic stroke to look for a potential source of emboli. Electrocardiography is done routinely, and echocardiography is recommended in young individuals or in others where cardiac disease is strongly suspected.[12,13] A CT scan without contrast is the most important initial study to differentiate between ischemia and hemorrhage. When a subarachnoid hemorrhage is suspected, the CT scan can be carried out with infusion of a double dose of contrast material, which frequently will demonstrate the presence of an arterial aneurysm. If aneurysm clipping would be indicated, cerebral angiography is done to locate the lesion and demonstrate its size, shape, and the presence or absence of an aneurysmal neck. Transcranial Doppler ultrasonography is useful for demonstrating spasm of large arteries.

If no hemorrhage is demonstrated on CT scan, the patient is assumed to have an ischemic event. The initial CT scan may show little change with an early infarct, but after a few days a repeat CT scan with contrast or an MRI study may be carried out to better delineate the location and extent of an ischemic infarct (Chap. 13). In cases where a patent foramen ovale associated with paradoxical embolism is suspected, transesophageal echocardiography should be obtained. Additional diagnostic tests to be considered in patients with acute ischemic stroke are similar to those for patients being evaluated for TIA. These include: a CBC, platelet count, lupus anticoagulant, and coagulation factors; serum glucose, cholesterol, lipoproteins, and triglycerides; and an ESR, ANA, and rheumatoid factor. A toxicology screen should be obtained if drug abuse is suspected and blood cultures carried out if endocarditis seems likely.

Duplex scanning of the neck vessels is recommended for most patients with ischemic stroke, since it is noninvasive and gives important information about the status of the carotid and vertebral arteries (Chap. 11). Cerebral angiography is recommended if the stroke is minor and if noninvasive studies suggest an extracranial arterial stenosis amenable to surgery, or when there is a suspicion of arterial dissection, fibromuscular dysplasia, or cerebral angiitis. Meningeal biopsy may be indicated in rare instances of strongly suspected cerebral angiitis.

MEDICAL MANAGEMENT OF THE ACUTE STROKE PATIENT

Most patients with acute ischemic events are not considered candidates for vascular surgical procedures such as carotid endarterectomy because of the inherent danger of restoring blood flow to an infarcted area. Nonsurgical approaches to the acute stroke patient include: (1) drugs and other therapies designed to minimize ischemic damage; (2) thrombolytic agents to dissolve acute thrombi; (3) anticoagulants to prevent thrombus propagation in patients whose stroke is incomplete and to prevent recurrence in patients whose ischemic events are embolic; and (4) rehabilitation techniques.

It must be acknowledged that there is little evidence at the present time that the size of an infarct can be changed significantly by medical measures. Medical management of most stroke patients is directed principally toward preventing complications while the patient is in the acute phase of illness. Prevention of contractures, deep vein thrombosis, and decubiti are important goals best achieved by early involvement of physical therapy.

The rationale for the use of anticoagulation and other antithrombotic measures to prevent stroke is discussed in Chap. 15. Here it may be stated that the only clearly established situation in which anticoagulants should be used is when the patient has had an embolic stroke and is at risk for recurrent emboli. Such patients include those with rheumatic heart disease, those with artificial heart valves, and patients with mural thrombi after MI. Nevertheless, it is common practice for physicians to administer anticoagulants to patients whose neurologic symptoms fluctuate (so called "stroke-in-evolution") and to patients with rather mild "incomplete" ischemic events. Unfortunately, data are not available that substantiate the efficacy of such treatment.

REFERENCES

1. Caplan LR: Stroke. *A Clinical Approach,* 2d ed. Boston, Butterworth-Heinemann, 1993.
2. Dyken ML: Frequency and symptom analysis of transient ischemic attacks: A cooperative hospital study, in Scheinberg P (ed.) *Cerebrovascular Diseases*. New York, Raven Press, pp 31–38, 1976.
3. Dyken ML, Conneally PM, Haerer AF, et al: Cooperative study of hospital frequency and character of transient ischemic attacks. I.

Background, organization, and clinical survey. *JAMA* 237:882–886, 1977.
4. Fisher CM: Late-life migraine accompaniments as a cause of unexplained transient ischemic attacks. *Can J Neurol Sci* 7:9–17, 1980.
5. Dennis M, Warlow C: Migraine aura without headache: Transient ischemic attack or not? *J Neurol Neurosurg Psychiat* 55:437–440, 1992.
6. Price TR, Gotshall RA, Poskanzer DC, et al: Cooperative study of hospital frequency and character of transient ischemic attacks. VI. Patients examined during an attack. *JAMA* 238: 2512–2515, 1977.
7. DeRook FA, Comess KA, Albers GW, Popp RL: Transesophageal echocardiography in the evaluation of stroke. *Ann Intern Med* 117:922–932, 1992.
8. Pierelli F, Chatrian GE, Erdly WW, Swanson PD: Long-term EEG video-audio monitoring: Detection of partial epileptic seizures and psychogenic episodes by twenty-four hour EEG record review. *Epilepsia* 30:513–523, 1989.
9. Levine J, Swanson PD: Nonatherosclerotic causes of stroke. *Ann Intern Med* 70:807–816, 1969.
10. Hart RG, Miller VT: Cerebral infarction in young adults: a practical approach. *Stroke* 14: 110–114, 1983.
11. Swanson PD, Strandness DE Jr: Diagnosis of ischemic stroke. *Univ Wash Med* 7:23–20, 1980.
12. Come PC, Riley MF, Bivas NK: Role of echocardiography and arrhythmia monitoring in the evaluation of patients with suspected systemic embolism. *Ann Neurol* 12:527–531, 1983.
13. Greenland P, Knopman DS, Mikell FL, et al: Echocardiography in diagnostic assessment of stroke. *Ann Intern Med* 95:51–53, 1981.

Part Three

Diagnostic Evaluation

10

Indirect Noninvasive Tests for Cerebrovascular Disease

R. Eugene Zierler

In 1927 Moniz first described a technique for performing cerebral arteriography in a living patient.[1] Over the ensuing years, contrast arteriography has remained the standard diagnostic investigation for cerebrovascular disease. However, owing to its invasive nature, arteriography is not readily applicable in many clinical situations, such as screening asymptomatic patients and performing serial follow-up studies. In addition, arteriography is a strictly anatomic investigation that gives no direct information about the physiologic significance of the observed lesions.

During the past two decades, the risk and limitations of arteriography have stimulated the development of numerous noninvasive methods for the evaluation of cerebrovascular disease.[2] These newer tests are characterized by minimal risk, absence of patient discomfort, and relatively low cost. An ideal noninvasive test could differentiate between normal and diseased arteries, classify a wide range of lesions, detect disease progression over time, identify the structural features of atherosclerotic plaque, and assess the collateral circulation associated with carotid disease. Although no single method has all these capabilities, many of these goals can be achieved with currently available techniques.

Noninvasive tests for extracranial carotid

Table 10-1 Noninvasive Tests for Extracranial Carotid Artery Disease

Indirect tests
Periorbital Doppler examination
Supraorbital photoplethysmography
Posterior orbital study
Oculoplethysmography (OPG)
Pulse delay OPG
Pressure OPG (OPG-Gee)
Direct tests
Ultrasonic arteriography
B-mode imaging
Duplex scanning
B-mode imaging
Pulsed Doppler flow detection
Spectral waveform analysis
Color-flow imaging

artery disease can be considered as either indirect or direct (Table 10-1). The first tests to be applied clinically were indirect tests, such as the periorbital Doppler examination.[3] Of all the noninvasive methods described, only a few are still in widespread clinical use. Although indirect tests may be of value in selected patients, the direct approach of duplex scanning is clearly the current technique of choice for routine diagnosis (Chap. 11).

In spite of the diminished clinical role of indirect noninvasive tests, their underlying principles are still highly relevant to the study of cerebrovascular disease. The purpose of this chapter is to provide a brief review of the features of the major indirect tests. Further details on the performance and interpretation of these tests can be found in the References.

PHYSIOLOGIC BASIS FOR INDIRECT TESTING

Indirect tests rely on pressure or flow changes in the distal branches of the internal and external carotid arteries to diagnose lesions at the carotid bifurcation. Thus, these methods require the presence of a "hemodynamically significant" lesion. However, because pressure and flow are not significantly reduced in the carotid system until the arterial diameter is narrowed by 50 percent or more, indirect tests can detect only severely stenotic or occlusive lesions.[4] Consequently, as indicated in Fig. 10-1, these tests cannot distinguish between normal and minimally diseased arteries or differentiate high-grade stenosis from occlusion. Furthermore, since the results are typically reported as either "positive" or "negative," indirect tests are of limited value in classifying lesion severity and monitoring disease progression. These limitations are largely overcome by the use of direct methods, particularly duplex scanning (Fig. 10-1).

As discussed in Chap. 2, the ophthalmic artery is a branch of the supraclinoid segment of the internal carotid artery. The ophthalmic ar-

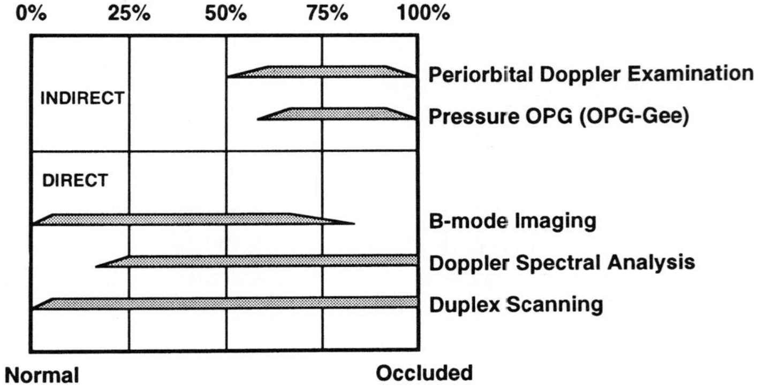

Figure 10-1. Approximate range of internal carotid artery diameter reduction detected by various indirect and direct tests. (*Adapted from Bandyk.*[2])

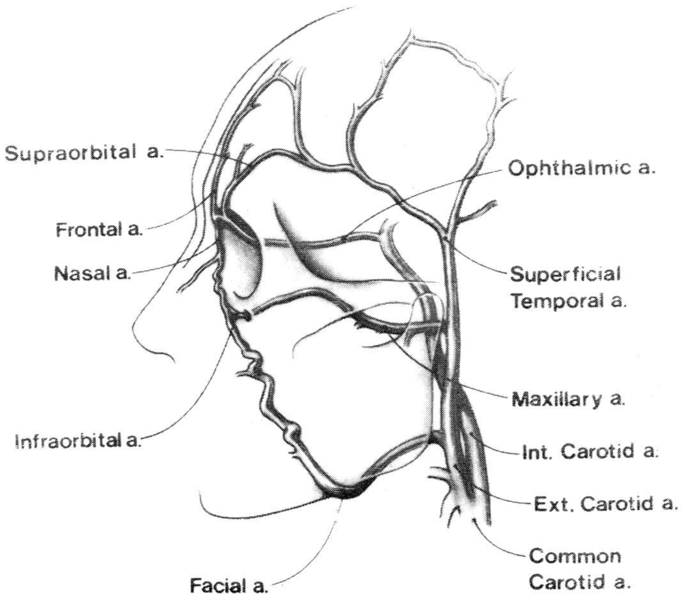

Figure 10-2. Branches of the internal and external carotid arteries showing the potential collateral routes through the periorbital circulation. [*From Lynch TG, Hobson RW: Noninvasive cerebrovascular diagnostic techniques, in Wilson SE (ed): Vascular Surgery Principles and Practice. New York, McGraw-Hill, 1987, chap 10, p 108, used with permission.*]

tery gives off the central retinal artery and a variable number of smaller branches that supply the area around the eye. Several of these branches eventually exit from the orbit and form anastomoses with the facial and superficial temporal branches of the external carotid artery. Thus, the periorbital circulation is an important collateral route between the internal and external carotid territories (Fig. 10-2). The major periorbital branches are the frontal, supraorbital, and nasal arteries (Fig. 10-3).

In general, indirect tests identify either directional flow changes in the periorbital arteries or alterations in the ocular pulse or blood pressure. Indirect tests include the periorbital Doppler examination,[5,6] supraorbital photoplethysmography,[7] the posterior orbital study,[8,9] pulse delay oculoplethysmography,[10,11] and pressure oculoplethysmography[12,13] (Table 10-1). The periorbital Doppler examination and oculoplethysmography have been the most widely used of the indirect tests and will be discussed further.

PERIORBITAL DOPPLER EXAMINATION

In the periorbital Doppler examination, a direction-sensing Doppler system is used to determine the presence and direction of flow in the branches of the ophthalmic artery that supply the periorbital area of the face. Because the arteries of interest are located just beneath the skin, a relatively high frequency

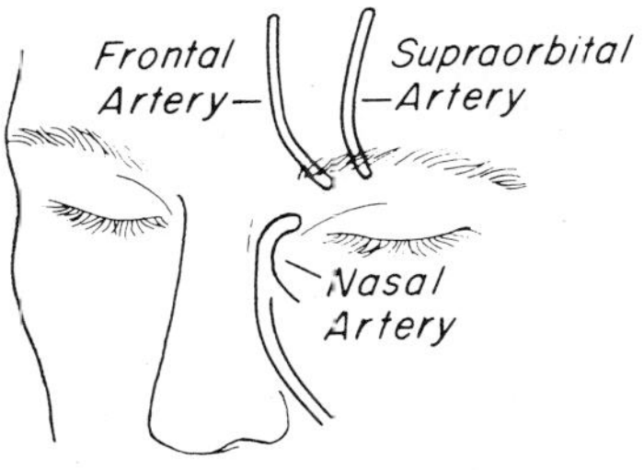

Figure 10-3. Approximate locations of the major periorbital arteries. [*From Zwiebel WJ: Doppler cerebrovascular techniques, in Zwiebel WJ (ed): Introduction to Vascular Ultrasonography, 2d ed. Orlando, Grune and Stratton, 1986, chap 6, p 110, used with permission.*]

Doppler transducer (5 to 10 MHz) can be used. The flow signals are located by moving the transducer carefully over the orbital rim in the characteristic location of the periorbital arteries (Fig. 10-3). The superior branches (frontal and supraorbital) are usually the most reliable for Doppler evaluation. It is important to point the transducer into the orbit for accurate identification of flow direction and changes in flow direction. In addition, the transducer must be held steady throughout the examination to avoid artifactual changes in signal strength, particularly during compression of the external carotid branches.

As shown in Fig. 10-4*A*, blood flow in the periorbital arteries normally proceeds from the inside to the outside of the orbit or toward the face. A severe stenosis or occlusion of the internal carotid that reduces the perfusion pressure in the ophthalmic artery can result in several characteristic changes in the normal periorbital flow pattern. When the branches of the external carotid artery serve as a major source of collateral flow to the ipsilateral cerebral circulation, reversed flow is noted in the periorbital arteries, and flow is directed from the face into the orbit (Fig. 10-4*B*).

Specific sources of collateral flow can be identified by a series of external carotid compression maneuvers.[6] The usual compression points are the facial artery along the lower border of the mandible and the superficial temporal artery in front of the ear directly above the temporomandibular joint (Fig. 10-4*B*). When the internal carotid artery is widely patent, compression of an external carotid branch usually produces an augmentation of the Doppler flow signal in the periorbital vessels. This change is the result of compensatory flow to the face from the internal carotid circulation. A less common normal response to compression maneuvers is no change in periorbital flow. When a hemodynamically significant lesion is present in the internal carotid circulation and the external carotid branches are functioning as collaterals, the periorbital flow signals will cease or diminish with compression. In some cases, there will be a complete change in flow direction in response to compression. These normal and abnormal changes in the periorbital flow pattern are summarized in Table 10-2.

Sources of collateral flow originating from the contralateral carotid system can be identified by noting the periorbital flow response to compression of each common carotid ar-

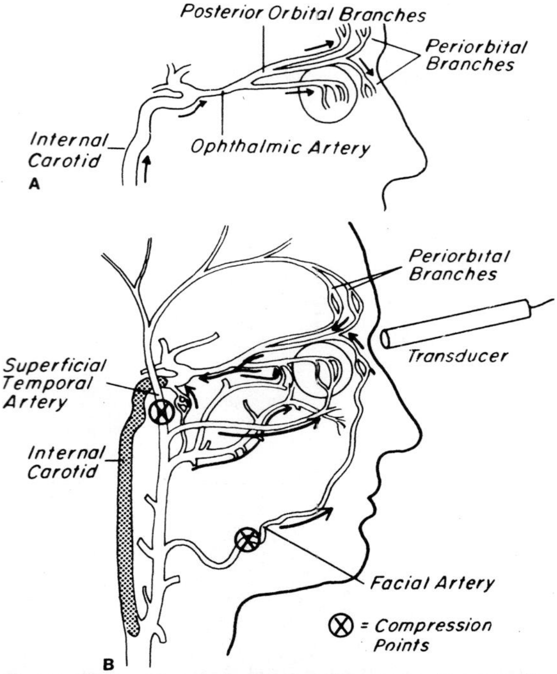

Figure 10-4. Flow in the periorbital arteries is normally directed toward the face or from the inside to the outside of the orbit (*A*). When a hemodynamically significant lesion is present in the internal carotid artery, collateral flow from the external carotid branches may result in reversed flow in the periorbital arteries (*B*). Digital compression points for assessing the collateral contributions of various external carotid branches are marked with an X. (*From Zwiebel WJ: Doppler cerebrovascular techniques, in Zwiebel WJ (ed): Introduction to Vascular Ultrasonography, 2d ed. Orlando, Grune and Stratton, 1986, chap 6, p 109, used with permission.*)

Table 10-2 Periorbital Doppler Examination Normal and Abnormal Changes in Periorbital Arterial Flow

Normal
Flow directed out of the orbit (toward the face)
Augmentation of flow with external carotid compression
No change in flow with external carotid compression
Abnormal
Flow reversal (into the orbit)
Cessation of flow with external carotid compression
Diminished flow with external carotid compression
Reversal of flow with external carotid compression (flow into the orbit changes to flow out of the orbit)

tery and the contralateral external carotid branches.[14] Collateral flow to the internal carotid territory from the vertebrobasilar system cannot be detected by the periorbital Doppler examination.

The principal advantage of the periorbital Doppler test is that it requires inexpensive equipment and can be performed relatively rapidly. However, this test requires considerable skill on the part of the examiner, and the reported accuracy has been quite variable. Although an abnormal (positive) test is a good indicator of a hemodynamically significant internal carotid lesion, false-negative results are

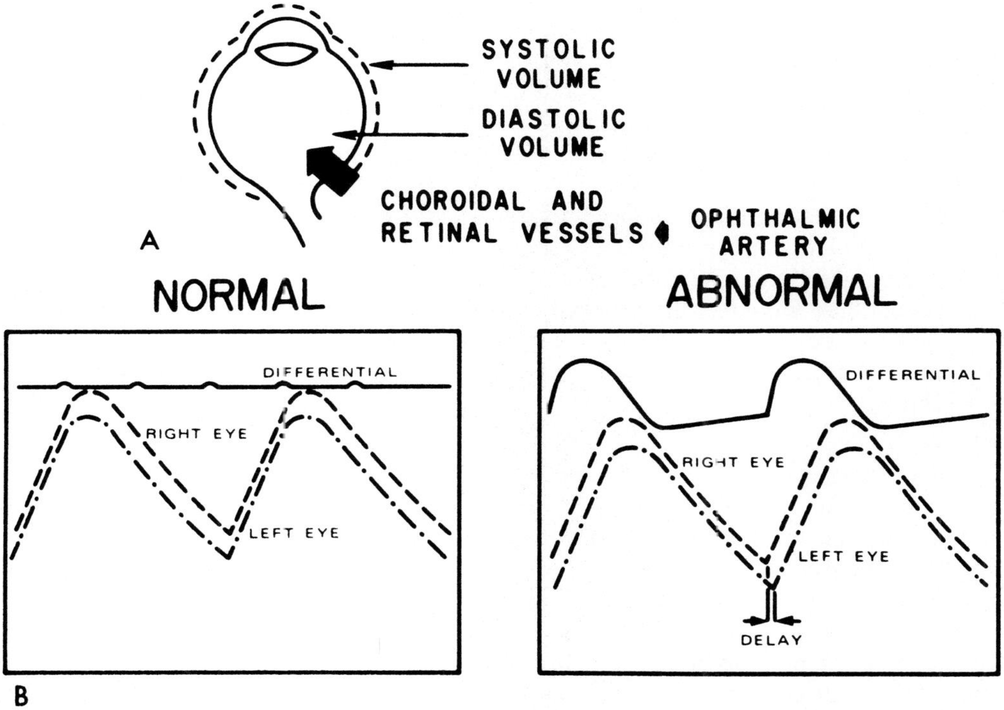

Figure 10-5. Pulse delay or fluid-filled OPG. The ocular pulse originates in the choroidal and retinal vessels that are supplied by the ophthalmic artery (*A*). Waveforms represent the left and right ocular pulsations, and the differential tracing indicates the difference between the pulse arrival times in the two eyes (*B*). The abnormal tracing shows a significant delay between the ocular pulse arrival times. (*From Bernstein EF: Additional noninvasive techniques for cerebrovascular diagnosis, in Zwiebel WJ (ed): Introduction to Vascular Ultrasonography, 2d ed. Orlando, Grune and Stratton, 1986, chap 10, p 248, used with permission.*)

frequently associated with ipsilateral common or external carotid stenoses and efficient collateral pathways. In a review of 102 carotid arteries evaluated by both the periorbital Doppler test and arteriography, the false-positive rate was only 3 percent, but the false-negative rate was 22 percent.[15] Thus, this test is most reliable when it shows abnormalities. Furthermore, it appears that the sensitivity of the periorbital Doppler examination increases with the severity of internal carotid disease and is highest for internal carotid occlusion.[16] While overall accuracy rates exceeding 90 percent have been reported,[6,17,18] a number of studies have been unable to duplicate such favorable results.[19,20]

OCULOPLETHYSMOGRAPHY (OPG)

When a hemodynamically significant lesion is present in the carotid system, flow through the collateral pathways may result in a delay of the ocular pulse or a reduction in the ocular perfusion pressure. The indirect noninvasive tests that rely on detecting these changes are referred to as oculoplethysmography. Because these methods require direct application of devices to the eyes, they are generally contraindicated in the presence of conjunctivitis, glaucoma, recent ocular trauma, or a history of retinal detachment.

Pulse Delay OPG

Kartchner and McRae described an indirect test based on detecting the difference in pulse arrival times between the two eyes.[11] Ocular pulsations were sensed through saline-filled tubes connected to small plastic cups applied to the anesthetized corneas and held in place by a negative pressure of 40 to 50 mmHg. External carotid pulsations were detected by photoplethysmograph transducers clipped on each ear. The external carotid pulsations were used to detect external carotid lesions and as a reference baseline to help identify bilateral internal carotid disease. Pulse waveforms from the eyes and ears were compared electronically and any delay noted (Fig. 10-5).

One advantage of the pulse delay OPG method over the periorbital Doppler examination is that the former is less dependent on examiner skill. However, clinical experience with this type of OPG has produced inconsistent results. Although Kartchner and coworkers[10] initially reported an overall accuracy of 90 percent, a subsequent study by Blackshear and coworkers noted a false-positive rate of 19 percent, a false-negative rate of 48 percent, and an overall accuracy of 68 percent using the same instrument and diagnostic criteria.[21] Adjunctive use of carotid phonoangiography with the pulse delay OPG did not appear to improve the results. The reasons for these differences in accuracy probably include such physiologic factors as arterial wall properties, intracranial atheroscle-

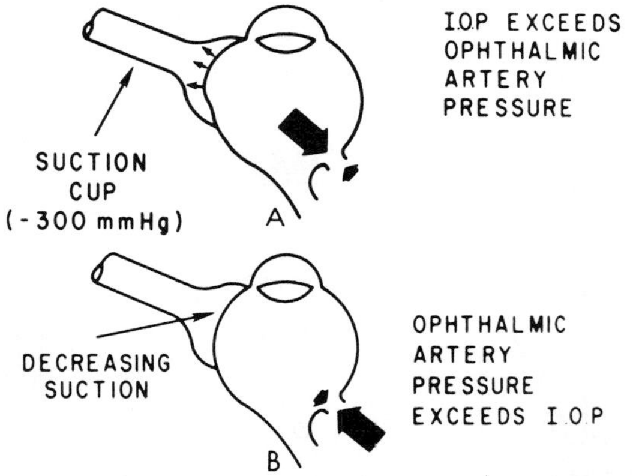

Figure 10-6. Pressure or air-filled OPG (OPG-Gee). A suction cup is placed on the eye lateral to the cornea and the negative pressure gradually increased to obliterate the ocular pulsation (*A*). As the pressure in the system is restored, the pressure at which ocular pulsations return is noted and correlated with the ophthalmic artery pressure (*B*). I.O.P. = intraocular pressure (*From Bernstein EF: Additional noninvasive techniques for cerebrovascular diagnosis, in Zwiebel WJ (ed): Introduction to Vascular Ultrasonography, 2d ed. Orlando, Grune and Stratton, 1986, chap 10, p 249, used with permission.*)

rotic lesions, collateral flow patterns, and bilateral carotid disease. Since most of these factors are impossible to control, this method is now considered unsuitable for routine diagnosis of cerebrovascular disease.

Pressure OPG (Oculopneumoplethysmography)

The air-filled OPG system developed by Gee (OPG-Gee) has been the most widely used of the oculoplethysmographic methods.[13] This instrument measures ophthalmic artery pressure (OAP) through small suction cups placed on the sclera lateral to each cornea. As suction is applied to the cups, the intraocular pressure increases and flow in the ophthalmic artery eventually ceases. In clinical practice, the ocular pulsations are temporarily obliterated by applying a negative pressure of 300 or 500 mmHg to the suction cups. The higher negative pressure is necessary to obliterate ocular pulsations in some hypertensive patients. As the pressure in the system is gradually restored, the pressure at which the ocular pulsations reappear is noted (Fig. 10-6). There is a close correlation between the OAP as measured by the air-filled OPG and operative

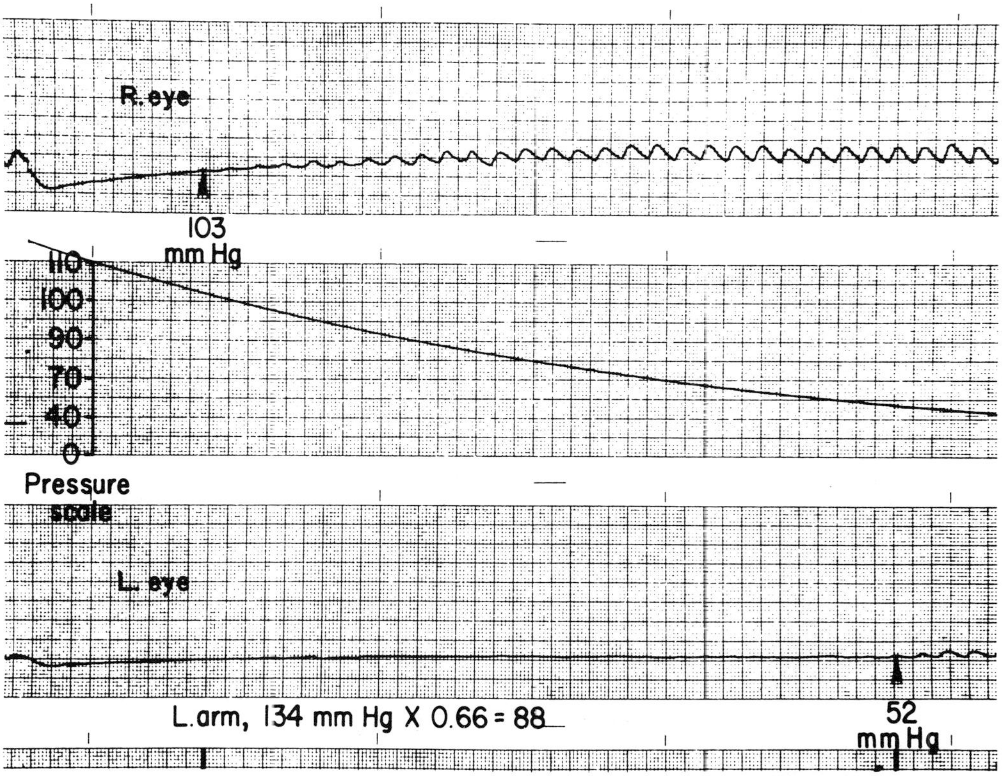

Figure 10-7. Air-filled OPG study (OPG-Gee) indicating a hemodynamically significant lesion involving the left common or internal carotid artery. The OAP for each side is determined by referring to the center scale which displays the pressure in the OPG system. The left OAP is 52 mmHg, giving an OAP/BSP ratio of less than 0.66. (*From Lynch TG, Hobson RW: Noninvasive cerebrovascular diagnostic techniques, in Wilson SE (ed): Vascular Surgery Principles and Practice. New York, McGraw-Hill, 1987, chap 10, p 116, used with permission.*)

measurement of internal carotid artery stump pressure.[13] The cerebral collateral circulation can also be evaluated by performing this test with common carotid artery compressions.

Although various criteria have been proposed for interpreting the air-filled OPG test, they are all based on either the difference between the pressures in the two eyes or the relationship between the OAP and the brachial artery systolic pressure.[22] One commonly applied set of criteria consists of a difference in OAP of 5 mmHg or more between the two eyes or a ratio of OAP to brachial artery systolic pressure (OAP/BSP ratio) of 0.66 or less.[23] Figures 10-7 and 10-8 show examples of air-filled OPG studies.

In spite of some controversy over the degree of stenosis required to produce a positive air-filled OPG test, the reported accuracy for detecting severe carotid lesions has generally been quite high. If a stenosis of 65 to 75 percent diameter reduction is considered significant, the overall accuracy is in the range of 94 to 98 percent.[12,22,23] In addition, the false-negative rate with the air-filled OPG has been consistently lower than that of the periorbital

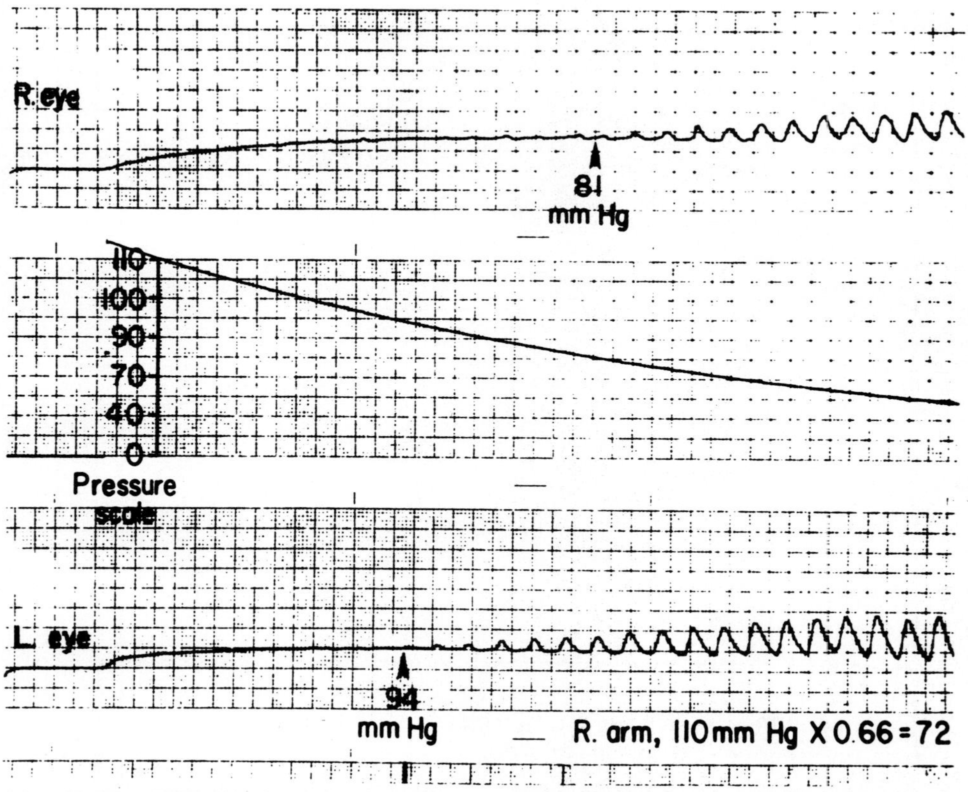

Figure 10-8. Air-filled OPG study (OPG-Gee) suggesting a hemodynamically significant stenosis in the right carotid system. Both OAP/BSP ratios are greater than 0.66, but the right OAP is 13 mmHg less than the left OAP. (*From Lynch TG, Hobson RW: Noninvasive cerebrovascular diagnostic techniques, in Wilson SE (ed): Vascular Surgery Principles and Practice. New York, McGraw-Hill, 1987, chap 10, p 116, used with permission.*)

Doppler examination, and it is superior to the other indirect tests in identifying bilateral carotid disease.[12]

Although this test may be reliable for detecting hemodynamically significant carotid stenoses, like the other indirect tests it does not indicate the exact location of lesions and does not distinguish between severe stenosis and occlusion. The ability of air-filled OPG to assess the potential collateral circulation to the cerebral hemispheres has been useful in the management of patients requiring carotid resection for head and neck tumors,[24] and carotid interruption for treatment of aneurysmal disease.[25] Finally, characteristic changes in the normal ocular pulse wave that correlate with increased intracranial pressure have been observed in head-injured patients.[26]

CLINICAL APPLICATIONS

Because of limitations discussed earlier in this chapter, indirect tests are no longer of value in the routine clinical diagnosis of cerebrovascular disease. However, they occasionally may be helpful when it is necessary to evaluate the collateral circulation to the brain. Indirect tests may indicate the presence of intracranial arterial disease when the duplex scan shows a normal carotid bifurcation. In this situation, an abnormal result suggests a more distal pressure or flow reducing lesion in the carotid system. A transcranial Doppler examination (Chap. 12) also may be useful in this setting.

In the report of the Ad Hoc Committee of the Western Vascular Society on vascular laboratory utilization and payment,[27] the only indirect testing method listed as "acceptable equipment for studies" is ocular pneumoplethysmography (OPG-Gee). The report also emphasizes that this test has limitations and should not be used as the only screening method for extracranial carotid artery disease. The testing methods listed as "no longer acceptable for reimbursement" are the periorbital Doppler examination, OPG-Kartchner (pulse delay OPG), and carotid bruit analysis. Although the era of indirect testing for carotid artery disease has clearly passed, these methods represent an important stage in the development of physiologic testing for vascular disease.

REFERENCES

1. Moniz E: L'encephalographie arteriel, son importance dans la localisation des tumeurs cerebrales. *Rev Neurol* 2:72, 1927.
2. Bandyk DF, Thiele BL: Noninvasive assessment of carotid artery disease. *West J Med* 139:486, 1983.
3. Strandness DE Jr: Historical aspects, in *Duplex Scanning in Vascular Disorders*. New York, Raven, chap 1, pp 1–24, 1990.
4. May AG et al: Critical arterial stenosis. *Surgery* 54:250, 1963.
5. Brockenbrough EC: Periorbital Doppler velocity evaluation of carotid obstruction, in Bernstein EF (ed): *Noninvasive Diagnostic Techniques in Vascular Disease*. St. Louis, CV Mosby, chap 23, pp 231–238, 1982.
6. Barnes RW et al: The Doppler cerebrovascular examination: Improved results with refinements in technique. *Stroke* 8:468, 1977.
7. Barnes RW et al: Supraorbital photoplethysmography: Simple, accurate screening for carotid occlusive disease. *J Surg Res* 22:319, 1977.
8. Spencer MP: Technique of Doppler examination, in Spencer MP, Reid JM (eds): *Cerebrovascular Evaluation with Doppler Ultrasound*. The Hague, Martinus Nijoff, pp 77–80, 1981.
9. Maroon JC et al: Ophthalmosonometry: An ultrasonic method for assessing carotid blood flow. *J Neurosurg* 30:328, 1969.
10. Kartchner MM et al: Oculoplethysmography: An adjunct to arteriography in the diagnosis of extracranial carotid occlusive disease. *Am J Surg* 132:728, 1976.
11. Kartchner MM et al: Noninvasive detection and evaluation of carotid occlusive disease. *Arch Surg* 106:528, 1973.

12. Gee W: Carotid physiology with ocular pneumoplethysmography. *Stroke* 13:666, 1982.
13. Gee W et al: Measurement of collateral hemispheric blood pressure by ocular pneumoplethysmography. *Am J Surg* 130:121, 1975.
14. Bone GE, Barnes RW: Limitations of the Doppler cerebrovascular examination in hemispheric cerebral ischemia. *Surgery* 79:577, 1976.
15. Lye CR et al: The accuracy of the supraorbital Doppler examination in the diagnosis of hemodynamically significant carotid disease. *Surgery* 79:42, 1976.
16. Lynch TG et al: Evaluation of cerebrovascular Doppler examination and oculopneumoplethysmography in a clinical perspective. *Stroke* 12:325, 1981.
17. Bone GE, Barnes RW: Clinical implications of the Doppler cerebrovascular examination: A correlation with angiography. *Stroke* 7:271, 1976.
18. Barnes RW et al: Doppler ultrasound and supraorbital photoplethysmography for noninvasive screening of carotid occlusive disease. *Am J Surg* 134:183, 1977.
19. Gross et al: Comparison of noninvasive diagnostic techniques in carotid artery occlusive disease. *Surgery* 82:271, 1977.
20. Archie JP et al: Improved accuracy of cerebral vascular noninvasive testing using combined methods. *Surg Gynecol Obstet* 151:791, 1980.
21. Blackshear WM et al: A prospective evaluation of oculoplethysmography and carotid phonoangiography. *Surg Gynecol Obstet* 148:201, 1979.
22. Eikelboom B et al: Criteria for interpretation of oculopneumoplethysmography (Gee). *Arch Surg* 118:1169, 1983.
23. McDonald PT et al: Ocular pneumoplethysmography: Detection of carotid occlusive disease. *Ann Surg* 189:44, 1979.
24. Nolph MB et al: Ophthalmoplethysmography in head and neck surgery. *Arch Otolaryngol* 105:492, 1979.
25. Oiler DW et al: Treatment for high extracranial internal carotid artery aneurysm. *Ann Surg* 42:311, 1976.
26. Gee W et al: Ocular pneumoplethysmography in head-injured patients. *J Neurosurg* 59:46, 1983.
27. Strandness DE Jr et al: Vascular laboratory utilization and payment: Report of the Ad Hoc Committee of the Western Vascular Society. *J Vasc Surg* 16:163, 1992.

11

Duplex Scanning and Color-Flow Imaging

R. Eugene Zierler

In contrast to the indirect noninvasive tests discussed in Chap. 10, the direct tests for extracranial cerebrovascular disease are based on an evaluation of anatomic or hemodynamic features in the vessels of interest. Thus, while the indirect tests are reported as either "positive" or "negative," direct tests can be used to classify the severity of stenosis at the carotid bifurcation and to distinguish between high-grade stenosis and occlusion. Furthermore, the well-established association between extracranial carotid artery disease and cerebrovascular symptoms provides a strong rationale for direct testing.

Several methods that do not incorporate some type of imaging system can be considered as direct tests, including qualitative carotid phonoangiography, quantitative phonoangiography, and the continuous wave Doppler scan.[1] However, early experience with these techniques indicated that they are generally no more useful than the indirect tests, and they are not widely used. While other approaches, such as ocular pneumoplethysmography and transcranial Doppler, may play a limited clinical role, duplex scanning has emerged as the preferred noninvasive test for carotid artery disease.[2]

THE DUPLEX CONCEPT

Continuous Wave and Pulsed Doppler

The Doppler effect is the change in frequency of a wave that is produced by relative motion between the wave source and the point of observation. Although the most common examples of the Doppler effect involve sound waves, this shift in frequency is not limited to sound but occurs with all propagated waves, including light waves. When the sound source and observer move toward each other, the Doppler frequency shift is positive and the frequency is increased; a decrease in frequency results when the sound source and observer move away from each other. For vascular applications of Doppler ultrasound, the red blood cells are the principal moving sound reflectors, and the relationship between the frequency of the reflected and transmitted sound waves is defined by the equation:

$$\Delta f = \frac{2fV \cos\theta}{C}$$

where Δf is the Doppler shifted frequency, f is the frequency of the transmitted ultrasound, V is the velocity of the blood cells, θ is the angle between the incident ultrasound beam and the direction of blood cell motion (Fig. 11-1), and C is the speed of sound in tissue (approximately 154,000 cm/sec). The constant 2 in this equation accounts for the round-trip path traveled by the sound waves from the source to the reflectors and back to the source. It is necessary to use the cosine of θ to account for the component of the velocity vector along the axis of the ultrasound beam.[3] For the special

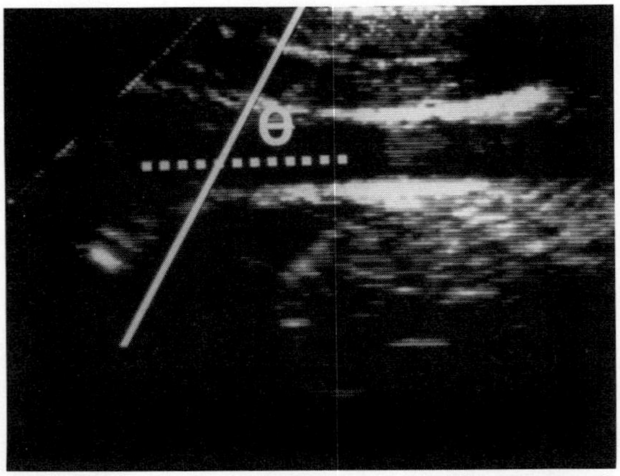

Figure 11-1. B-mode image from a duplex scanner illustrating the Doppler angle θ between the incident ultrasound beam and the direction of blood flow. Flow is assumed to be parallel to the vessel wall.

case in which the axis of the ultrasound beam and the direction of blood flow are the same, $\theta = 0$ and $\cos\theta = 1$; however, in most clinical applications the transducer is positioned to create an angle of 30 to 60° between the ultrasound beam and the vessel wall. When $\theta = 90°$, $\cos\theta = 0$ and there is, theoretically, no Doppler shift. Therefore, beam angles approaching 90° should be avoided when using Doppler techniques for blood flow detection (Fig. 11-2). If the angle θ is held constant, and f and C are also assumed to be constant, the Doppler shifted frequency is directly proportional to the blood cell velocity. For ultrasound frequencies in the megahertz (MHz) range and physiologic blood cell velocities, the Doppler frequency shift is typically in the audible kilohertz (kHz) range.

In 1959 Satomura published the first report describing the use of ultrasound and the Doppler effect to derive information on the velocity of blood flow through intact skin.[4] These early observations led a group of physiologists and clinicians at the University of Washington to develop ultrasound techniques for "nondestructive" testing of cardiovascular function.[5]

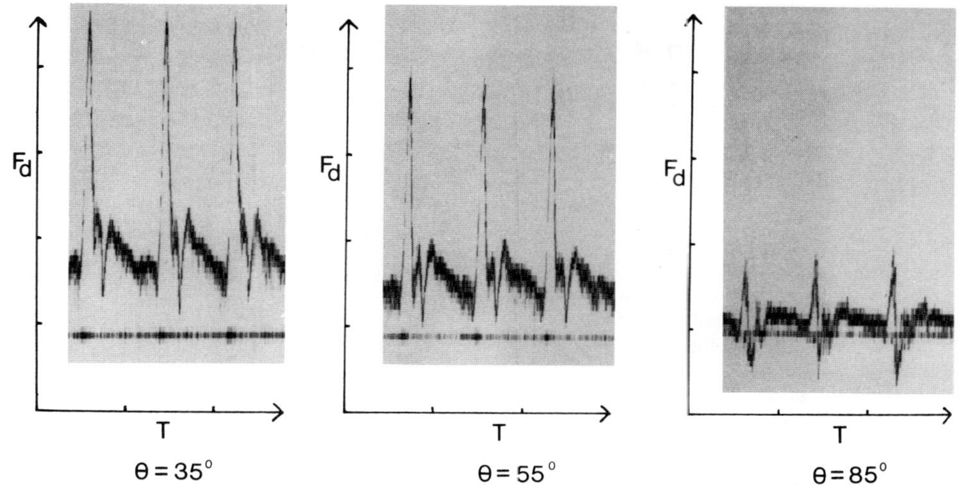

Figure 11-2. Effect of variation in the Doppler angle θ on common carotid artery spectral waveforms. The Doppler shifted frequencies increase for smaller angles and decrease as the angle approaches 90°. F_d, Doppler shifted frequency; *T*, time. [*From Zierler RE, Roederer GO, Strandness DE Jr: The use of frequency spectral analysis in carotid artery surgery, in Bergan JJ, Yao JST (eds): Cerebrovascular Insufficiency. Orlando, Grune & Stratton, 1983, chap 10, p 142, used with permission.*]

The application of Doppler ultrasound to the evaluation of the arterial system was described by Strandness and coworkers in 1966.[6]

The first commercially available Doppler instrument consisted of a probe containing the transducer elements combined with a loudspeaker that provided an audible output of the Doppler shifted frequency signal.[7] While the audible characteristics of the Doppler signal could be interpreted as normal or abnormal, the information provided was quite subjective and of limited clinical value. Thus, more objective and quantitative methods for analysis of Doppler signals were needed. These early instruments were continuous wave Doppler systems in which separate transmitting and receiving transducers operated continuously to detect flow. Although some continuous wave instruments can differentiate between flow toward and away from the transducers, they lack any ability to identify flow at a specific site in tissue. Consequently, the continuous wave Doppler signal actually represents a combination of signals obtained from flow at various points along the path of the ultrasound beam (Fig. 11-3). Interpretation of continuous wave Doppler signals can be difficult when vessels are superimposed within the ultrasound beam or when complex flow disturbances are present within a single vessel. These disadvantages have been overcome by the development of pulsed Doppler systems and more sophisticated techniques for Doppler signal analysis.

In a pulsed Doppler system a single ultrasound transducer alternates between transmitting and receiving functions. A short burst or pulse of ultrasound is transmitted into the tis-

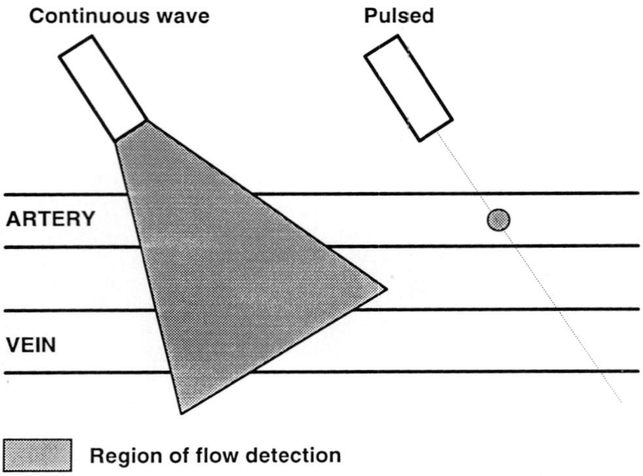

Figure 11-3. Continuous wave and pulsed Doppler systems. In a continuous wave system, the region of flow detection extends as far as the ultrasound beam penetrates and includes any vessels in the path of the beam. A pulsed Doppler detects flow only in a small region of tissue called the "sample volume," which can be positioned at any point along the ultrasound beam.

sue and, after waiting for the return of the reflected signal from a specific depth, the receiver is activated. The speed of sound in tissue determines the time required for a round trip to a particular depth. This provides the ability to sample flow at discrete sites in tissue. The region of flow detection is called the "sample volume" and can be positioned electronically at any point along the ultrasound beam (Fig. 11-3). To be certain that flow is sampled from only one depth, the reflected signal from each ultrasound pulse must be received before transmission of the next pulse. This limits the rate at which ultrasound pulses can be transmitted. The maximum pulse repetition frequency or PRF is defined as:

$$\text{PRF (maximum)} = \frac{C}{2d}$$

where C is the constant speed of sound in tissue and d is the distance between the transducer and the site of flow detection. Like directional continuous wave Doppler systems, a pulsed Doppler can distinguish between flow toward and away from the transducer.

Ultrasound Imaging

A pulsed Doppler system with multiple sample volumes or "range gates" was the basis for an early vascular imaging system described by Hokanson and coworkers in 1971.[8] This method, which was called "ultrasonic arteriography," used a directional 5-MHz pulsed Doppler mounted on a position-sensing mechanical arm. The pulsed Doppler had six range gates that could be placed at various depths in tissue; whenever flow was detected by one or more range gates, a spot was stored on an oscilloscope screen. In this way, a two-dimensional flow image of the carotid bifurcation could be created by moving the Doppler transducer slowly over the neck (Fig. 11-4). Although it was hoped that ultrasonic arteriography might provide diagnostic information comparable to that obtained by contrast arteriography, the quality of the flow images was relatively poor. In addition, ultrasonic arteriography gave no direct information on arterial wall anatomy and did not allow the examiner to control the incident angle of the pulsed Doppler beam. However, this approach did permit selective sampling of flow in the

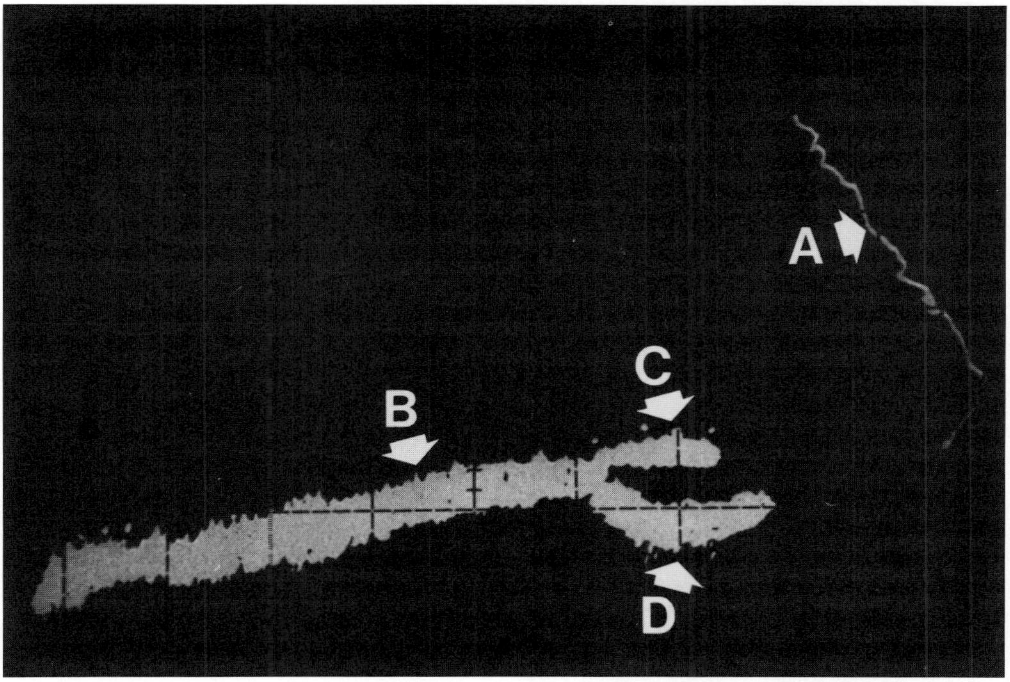

Figure 11-4. Ultrasonic arteriographic image of a normal carotid bifurcation. *A* indicates the lower border of the mandible; *B*, common carotid artery; *C*, external carotid artery; *D*, internal carotid artery. [*From Zierler RE, Strandness DE Jr: Noninvasive dynamic and real-time assessment of extracranial cerebrovasculature, in Wood JH (ed): Cerebral Blood Flow: Physiologic and Clinical Aspects. New York, McGraw-Hill, 1987, chap 19, p 315, used with permission.*]

branches of the carotid bifurcation and suggested that analysis of flow velocity patterns could be valuable in the detection of arterial disease.

At the same time that Doppler techniques were first being applied to the clinical evaluation of arterial problems, ultrasound methods for visualizing tissues were also being developed.[7] The initial investigations concerned the effects of atherosclerotic plaques on the transmission of ultrasound through arterial walls.[9] These studies showed that the major component of the arterial wall that influenced the transmission of ultrasound was calcium, and even microscopic calcium deposits produced significant attenuation of the ultrasound beam. A prototype real-time scanning system was designed and built at the University of Washington that contained three ultrasound transducers mounted on a rapidly rotating wheel. The images generated by this system were crude by modern standards, but they clearly demonstrated that real-time imaging of the carotid bifurcation was feasible. An image from one of the first patients evaluated is shown in Fig. 11-5. This is a longitudinal view of the carotid bifurcation with the common, internal, and external branches all visualized and apparently patent. However, when an arteriogram was done, the internal carotid artery was

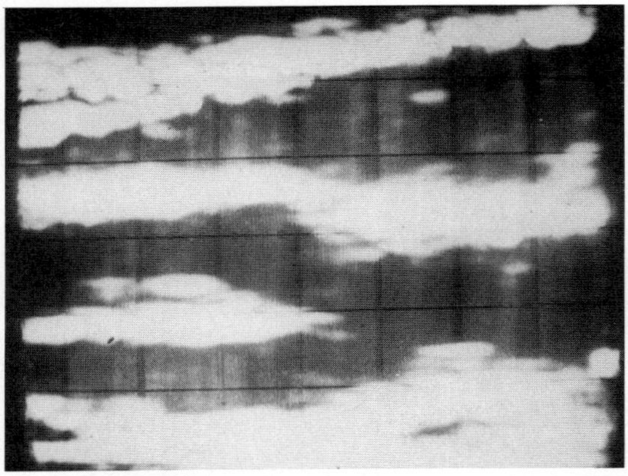

Figure 11-5. Real-time ultrasound image of a carotid bifurcation obtained with the prototype scanning system. The carotid bifurcation is seen in longitudinal view, with the common carotid on the right, the internal carotid on the bottom left, and the external carotid on the top left. The internal jugular vein is seen above the carotid bifurcation. The internal carotid artery was found to be occluded by arteriography. (*From Strandness,*[7] *used with permission.*)

found to be occluded. This experience indicated that the thrombus and plaque occluding the vessel had acoustic properties similar to those of blood and therefore could not be identified by the image alone. Since the problem appeared to be one of determining whether an artery was patent or occluded, a logical solution was the addition of a Doppler system to detect flow in the imaged vessels. It was this single case that stimulated the development of the duplex concept—the combination of real-time ultrasound imaging and pulsed Doppler flow detection.[7,10]

A block diagram of the first duplex scanning system is shown in Fig. 11-6. The scanhead for this system (Fig. 11-7) contained separate B-mode and Doppler transducers coupled to the skin through a water-filled boot. The transducers were aligned to allow detection of blood flow in the plane of the B-mode image, and the position of the Doppler beam and the

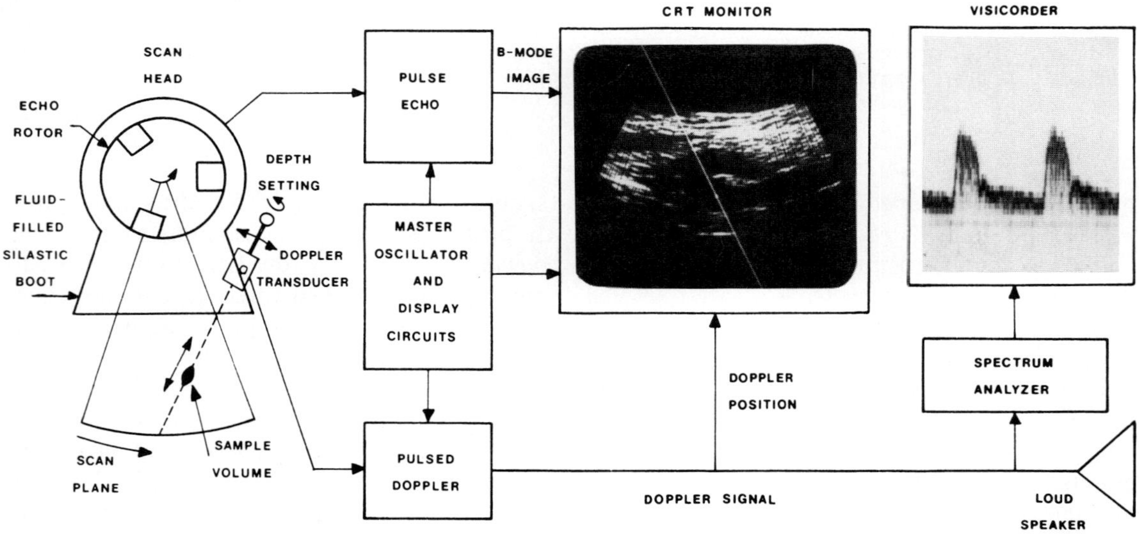

Figure 11-6. Diagram of the first duplex scanning system. The pulse echo (B-mode) transducers were mounted on a rotating wheel, and the separate Doppler transducer was attached to the side of the scanhead. Position of the pulsed Doppler sample volume was indicated by a cursor superimposed on the B-mode image. The Doppler signal was displayed through both a loudspeaker and a spectrum analyzer.

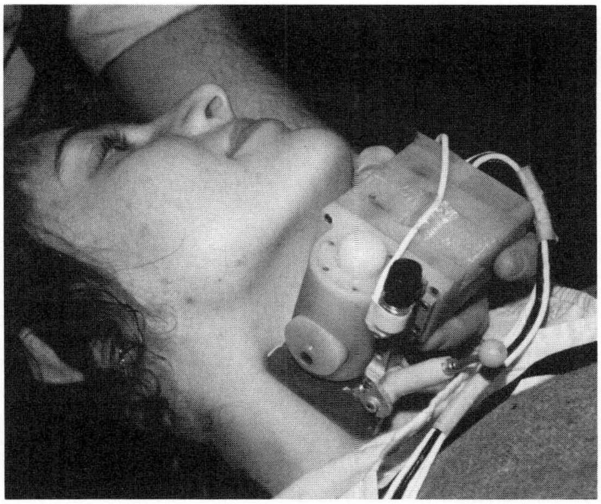

Figure 11-7. Scanhead of the first duplex scanning system. The pulsed Doppler transducer was attached to the short arm mounted on the water-filled boot.

single pulsed Doppler sample volume were indicated by a line and a dot superimposed on the B-mode image. This transducer was quite large, making it difficult to evaluate the internal carotid artery high in the neck. Another problem with this scanhead was keeping the B-mode and Doppler transducers mechanically aligned in the same plane. These problems eventually were solved by designing scanheads that used the same transducers for both the B-mode and Doppler functions.

During the early experience with this duplex scanning system for the evaluation of carotid artery disease it became apparent that certain blood flow patterns were associated with specific arteries. For example, the external carotid, which supplies a high-resistance vascular bed, shows a triphasic flow pattern with a brief reverse flow component in late systole or early diastole and low end-diastolic flow velocities (Fig. 11-8). Since the brain is normally a low-resistance organ, the internal carotid flow pattern has forward flow throughout the cardiac cycle and high end-diastolic

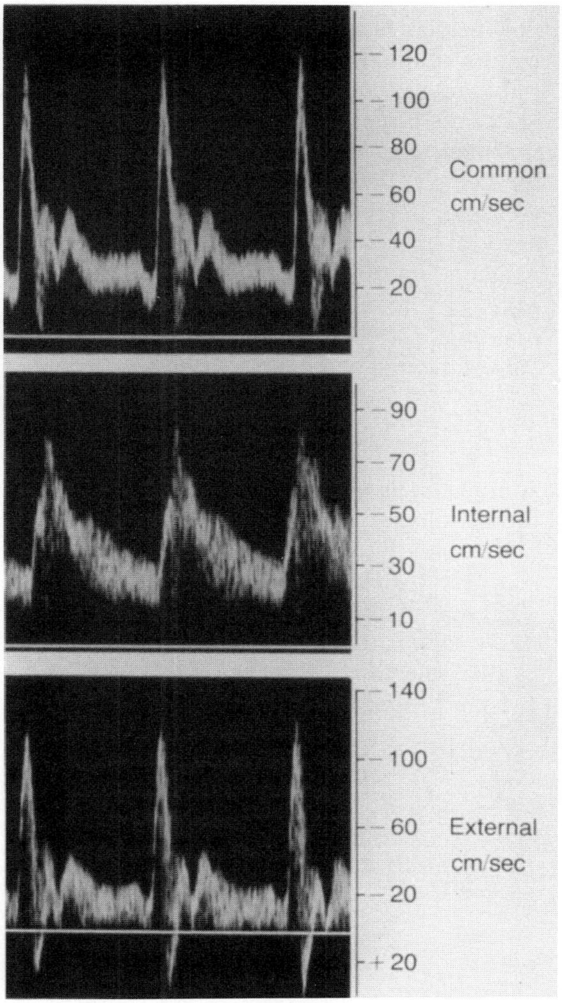

Figure 11-8. Normal carotid bifurcation spectral waveforms. The internal carotid (*center*) shows a typical low resistance flow pattern with forward flow throughout the cardiac cycle and high end-diastolic velocities. The external carotid (*bottom*) has a triphasic, high resistance flow pattern with a reverse flow component. The common carotid flow pattern (*top*) contains features of both the internal and external carotid flow patterns.

flow velocities (Fig. 11-8). Accurate characterization of the flow patterns produced by arterial lesions required the development of sophisticated methods for analysis of pulsed Doppler signals. The first techniques used for Doppler signal processing were the zero-crossing detector and off-line sonographic spectral analysis; however, these were unsatisfactory for routine clinical applications and gave way to spectral analysis based on the real-time fast Fourier transform method and color-flow imaging.[7]

B-MODE IMAGING

B-mode imaging alone has been used to assess the histologic and surface features of carotid bifurcation lesions with varying degrees of success.[11–13] Although the sonographic appearance of a plaque may correlate qualitatively with its histologic composition, the clinical relevance of this information is controversial.[14] Lipid is generally the least echogenic component of an atherosclerotic plaque, but as the collagen content of a plaque increases relative to its lipid content, echogenicity also increases. Predominantly fibrous plaques produce a homogeneous B-mode image, but focal deposits of thrombus or lipid can result in a more heterogeneous appearance. As noted previously, the presence of calcium in the arterial wall leads to marked attenuation of ultrasound. Consequently, calcified atherosclerotic plaque is extremely echogenic and results in bright echoes with acoustic shadows (Fig. 11-9). The B-mode characteristic of plaque that appears to correlate most closely with clinical outcome is heterogeneity, a feature that has been attributed to intraplaque hemorrhage.[15] This particular feature has been observed more frequently in symptomatic than in asymptomatic patients.[16]

Since ulcerated plaque at the carotid bifurcation is commonly regarded as a source of cerebral emboli, there has been considerable interest in the sonographic evaluation of plaque

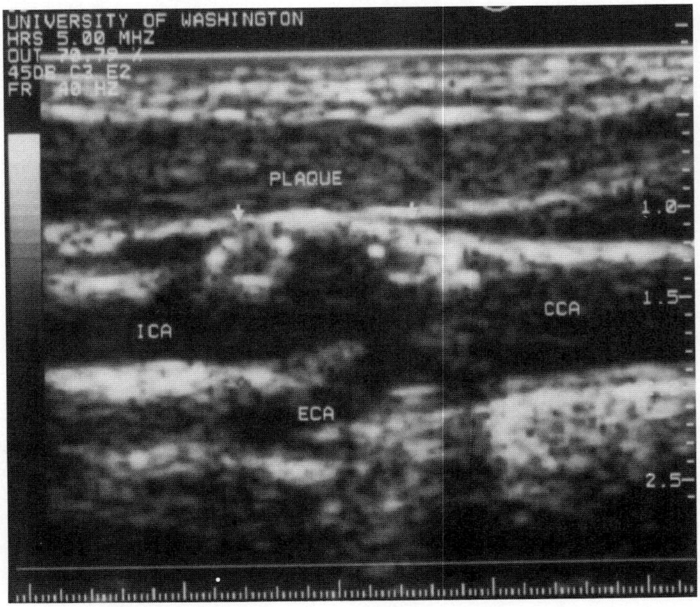

Figure 11-9. B-mode image of a diseased carotid bifurcation. A calcified atherosclerotic plaque is present along the near wall of the carotid bulb, indicated by the arrows, with acoustic shadowing in the distal common carotid artery (*CCA*). *ICA,* internal carotid artery; *ECA,* external carotid artery.

surface characteristics. Although some favorable results have been reported, the overall reliability of B-mode imaging for the detection of ulcerated atherosclerotic plaque generally has been poor.[13,16,17] Experience with B-mode imaging for the classification of carotid artery disease has shown that interpretation of the image is most accurate for lesions of minimal to moderate severity and least accurate for high-grade stenoses or occlusions.[12] It is often difficult to estimate the size of the arterial lumen from a B-mode image because the acoustic properties of noncalcified plaque, thrombus, and flowing blood are similar. In addition, acoustic shadows from calcified plaques may prevent complete visualization of the arterial wall and lumen. These limitations are largely overcome by the addition of pulsed Doppler information and classification of disease severity based on the degree of flow disturbance produced by a particular lesion.

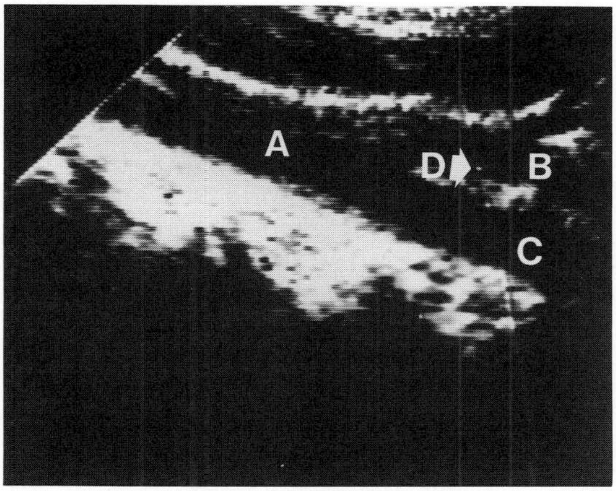

Figure 11-10. Standard duplex scan image of a left carotid bifurcation. *A*, common carotid artery; *B*, external carotid artery; *C*, internal carotid artery. A white line indicates the position of the Doppler beam, and the sample volume is represented by a dot *D*. [*From Zierler RE, Strandness DE Jr: Noninvasive dynamic and real-time assessment of extracranial cerebrovasculature, in Wood JH (ed): Cerebral Blood Flow: Physiologic and Clinical Aspects. New York, McGraw-Hill, 1987, chap 19, p 316, used with permission.*]

SPECTRAL WAVEFORM ANALYSIS

In standard carotid duplex scanning, the B-mode image is used to locate the arteries and facilitate placement of the pulsed Doppler sample volume at the site of interest (Fig. 11-10). The severity of disease is then determined by spectral analysis of the Doppler signal. Pulsed Doppler signals are best suited for this approach because they permit evaluation of flow patterns at discrete sites within the arterial lumen. Spectral waveform analysis is a signal processing technique that displays the complete frequency and amplitude content of the Doppler signal. As indicated by the Doppler equation, the Doppler shifted frequency is directly proportional to blood cell velocity. The amplitude of the signal depends on the number of blood cells moving through the Doppler sample volume. As the number of blood cells producing the Doppler frequency shift increases, the signal amplitude becomes stronger. Spectral information usually is presented graphically, with frequency or velocity on the vertical axis, time on the horizontal axis, and amplitude indicated by shades of gray. Although several methods have been developed for performing real-time spectral analysis, the digital fast Fourier transform is most commonly used in duplex scanning.

As shown in Figure 11-11, the flow pattern in a normal artery is uniform or laminar, and a spectral waveform taken with the pulsed Doppler sample volume in the center of the lumen shows a relatively narrow band of frequencies. Stenoses and other arterial wall abnormalities disrupt this normal pattern and produce flow disturbances that are apparent in the Doppler spectral waveform as a wider range of frequencies and amplitudes (Fig.

11-11). This increase in the width of the frequency band is referred to as "spectral broadening." An abnormal increase in the peak systolic frequency is associated with severe stenoses that produce high velocity jets. End-diastolic frequency is also increased in very severe stenoses. The spectral waveform criteria given in Table 11-1 and illustrated in Fig. 11-12 have been developed for classifying the severity of internal carotid disease. These criteria have been validated by a series of comparisons with independently interpreted contrast arteriograms; they can distinguish between normal and diseased internal carotid arteries with a specificity of 84 percent and a sensitivity of 99 percent.[18–20] The accuracy for detecting 50 to 99 percent diameter stenosis or occlusion is 93 percent.[20]

It is important to recognize that changes in both Doppler shifted frequency and spectral width can result from artifacts or errors in examination technique. For example, as shown in Fig. 11-13, if the pulsed Doppler sample volume is placed near the arterial wall instead of

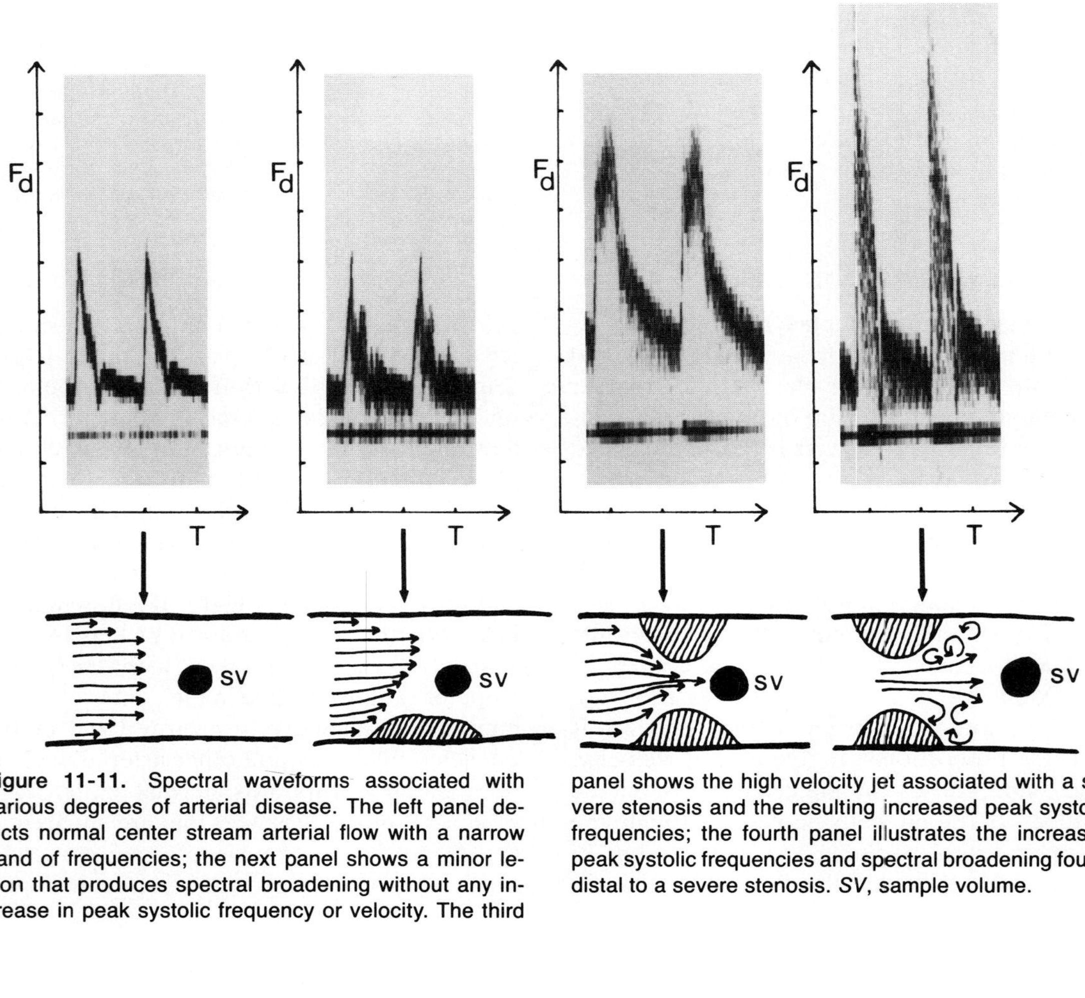

Figure 11-11. Spectral waveforms associated with various degrees of arterial disease. The left panel depicts normal center stream arterial flow with a narrow band of frequencies; the next panel shows a minor lesion that produces spectral broadening without any increase in peak systolic frequency or velocity. The third panel shows the high velocity jet associated with a severe stenosis and the resulting increased peak systolic frequencies; the fourth panel illustrates the increased peak systolic frequencies and spectral broadening found distal to a severe stenosis. *SV*, sample volume.

Table 11-1 Criteria for Classification of Internal Carotid Artery Disease by Duplex Scanning with Spectral Waveform Analysis of Pulsed Doppler Signals

	Arteriographic diameter reduction[a]	Peak systolic frequency[b] or velocity[c]	End-diastolic frequency or velocity	Spectral waveform characteristics
A	0% (normal)	<4 kHz <125 cm/s		Minimal or no spectral broadening; boundary layer separation present in the carotid bulb
B	1–15%	<4 kHz <125 cm/s		Spectral broadening during deceleration phase of systole only
C	16–49%	<4 kHz <125 cm/s		Spectral broadening throughout systole
D	50–79%	≥4 kHz ≥125 cm/s	<4.5 kHz <140 cm/s	Marked spectral broadening
D+	80–99%	≥4 kHz ≥125 cm/s	≥4.5 kHz ≥140 cm/s	Marked spectral broadening
E	100% (occlusion)			No flow signal in the internal carotid artery; decreased diastolic flow in the ipsilateral common carotid artery

[a]Diameter reduction is based on arteriographic measurements of stenosis using methods that compared the residual internal carotid artery lumen diameter to the estimated diameter of the carotid bulb.

[b]Frequency criteria are based on a pulsed Doppler with a 5 MHz transmitting frequency, a sample volume that is small relative to the internal carotid artery, and a 60-degree Doppler angle.

[c]Velocity criteria are based on the angle-adjusted velocity using a Doppler angle of 60 degrees or less.

in the center of the flow stream, spectral broadening will be produced by the velocity gradients normally present at that site. If this situation is not recognized, the severity of disease may be overestimated. Similarly, a sample volume that is large in relation to the vessel being examined will detect velocity gradients near the arterial wall even when it is correctly positioned in the center stream. Therefore, in most clinical applications, a small sample volume size provides the most reliable information.[21]

The angle θ between the incident Doppler ultrasound beam and the vessel wall (Fig. 11-1) can be adjusted during a duplex scan using the B-mode image and the superimposed Doppler cursor (Fig. 11-10). Most duplex scanning instruments allow this angle to be set manually and use the cosine of θ to calculate a blood flow velocity based on the Doppler equation. However, the assumption that blood flow is parallel to the vessel wall may be incorrect, particularly when atherosclerotic lesions are present. Variations in this angle between measurements, or use of angles approaching 90°, can produce significant errors in the calculation of velocity using the Doppler equation.[22] Therefore, whether the Doppler scale is set to units of frequency or velocity, a constant angle should be maintained throughout the examination, preferably 60° or less.

An adequate PRF is also required for accurate display of Doppler shifted frequencies by a pulsed Doppler system. With higher PRF values, more ultrasound pulses are available to sample flow, and a better representation of the Doppler signal is obtained. The highest frequency that can be displayed is equal to one-half of the PRF and is called the "Nyquist limit."[3] For example, if a pulsed Doppler has a PRF of 10kHz, the highest Doppler shift that can be correctly displayed is 5 kHz. When the

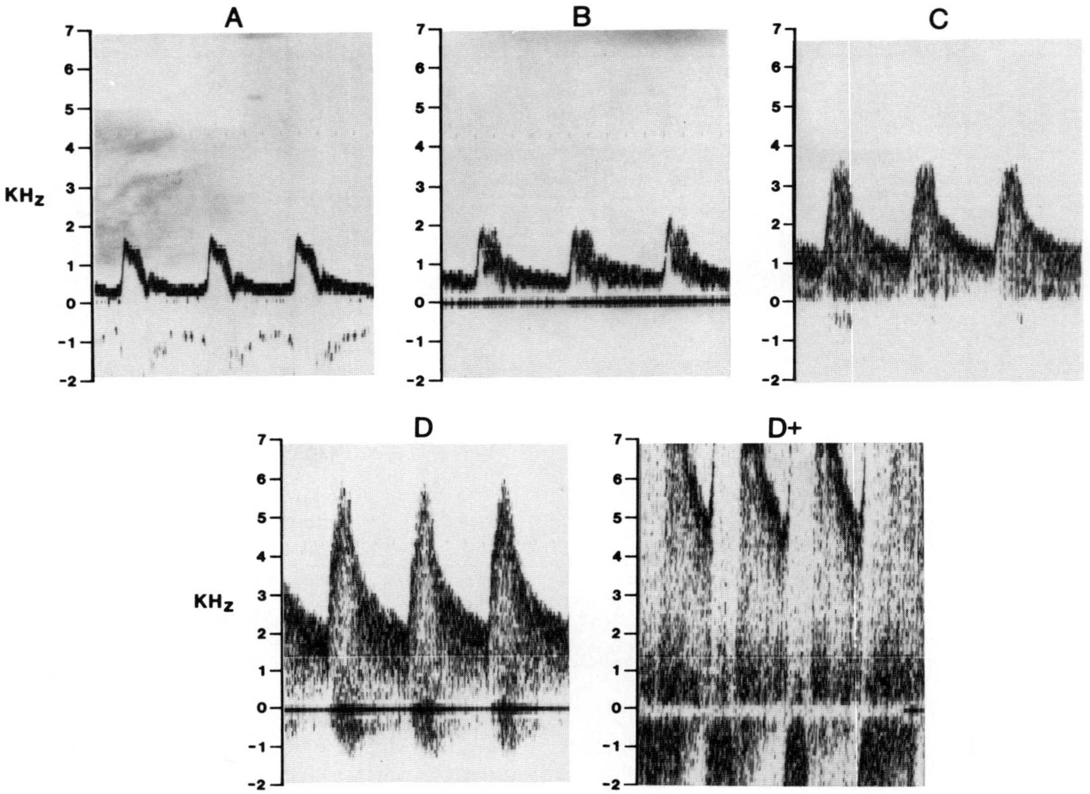

Figure 11-12. Examples of internal carotid spectral waveforms classified according to the criteria given in Table 11-1. *A*, Normal; *B*, 1 to 15 percent diameter reduction; *C*, 16 to 49 percent diameter reduction; *D*, 50 to 79 percent diameter reduction; and *D*$^+$, 80 to 99 percent diameter reduction. [*From Zierler RE, Strandness DE Jr: Noninvasive dynamic and real-time assessment of extracranial cerebrovasculature, in Wood JH (ed): Cerebral Blood Flow: Physiologic and Clinical Aspects. New York, McGraw-Hill, 1987, chap 19, p 317, used with permission.*]

Nyquist limit is exceeded, the phenomenon of aliasing is observed. Aliasing is most likely to occur when blood flow velocity is increased, as in a high velocity jet associated with a severe stenosis. The low PRF values that must be used to detect flow in deep vessels also tend to produce aliasing. A spectral waveform with aliasing is "cut off" at the Nyquist limit, and the missing portion of the waveform appears as flow in the opposite direction (Fig. 11-14). It should be emphasized that aliasing does not represent actual flow but is an artifact of the pulsed Doppler sampling process.

COLOR-FLOW DOPPLER IMAGING

Real-time color-flow imaging is an alternative to spectral waveform analysis for displaying the pulsed Doppler information obtained by duplex scanning.[23] In contrast to spectral analysis, which evaluates the entire frequency and amplitude content of the signal at a selected

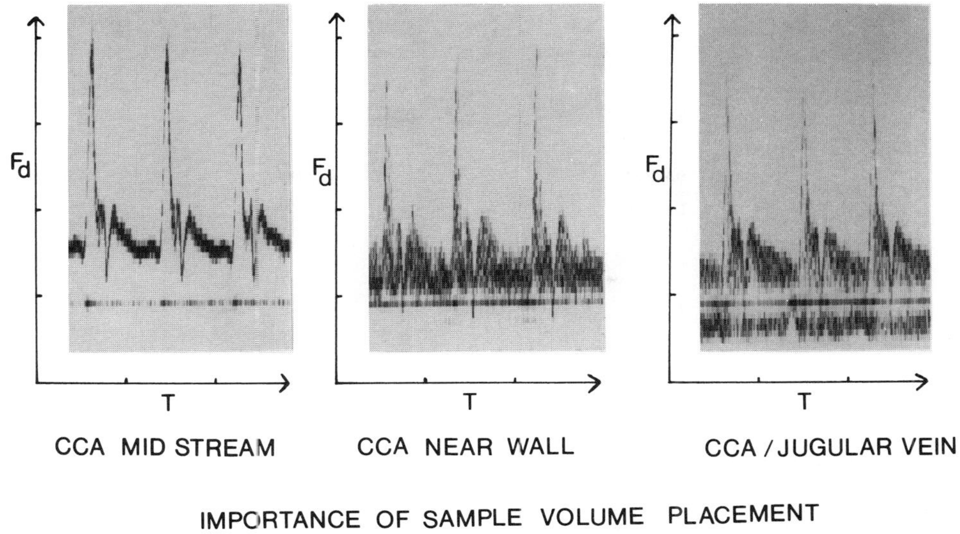

Figure 11-13. Effect of sample volume placement on spectral waveforms taken from the common carotid artery (*CCA*). Pulsed Doppler sample volume was placed in the middle of the flow stream, near the vessel wall, and between the arterial lumen and the adjacent internal jugular vein. F_d, Doppler shifted frequency; *T*, time. [*From Zierler RE, Roederer GO, Strandness DE Jr: The use of frequency spectral analysis in carotid artery surgery, in Bergan JJ, Yao JST (eds): Cerebrovascular Insufficiency. Orlando, Grune & Stratton, 1983, chap 10, p 141, used with permission.*]

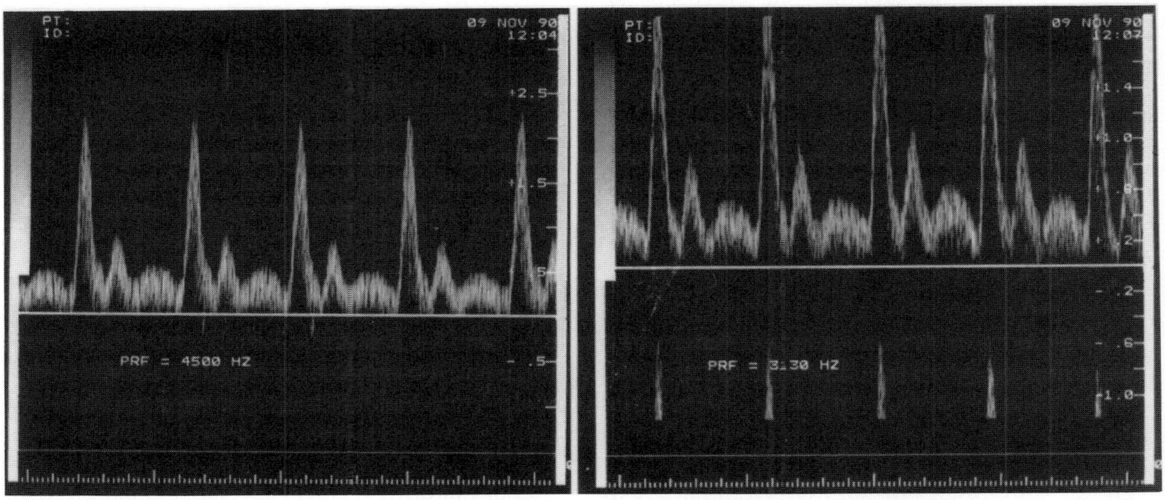

Figure 11-14. Aliasing in spectral waveforms. Waveform on the left is taken with a PRF of 4500 Hz and does not show aliasing. Waveform on the right is taken from the same vessel with a PRF of 3130 Hz and aliasing is present. The peaks of the aliased waveforms are "cut off" and appear below the zero-flow baseline. [*From Zierler RE, Zierler BK: Duplex sonography of lower extremity arteries, in Zwiebel WJ (ed): Introduction to Vascular Ultrasonography, 3d ed. Philadelphia, WB Saunders Company, 1992, chap 16, p 240, used with permission.*]

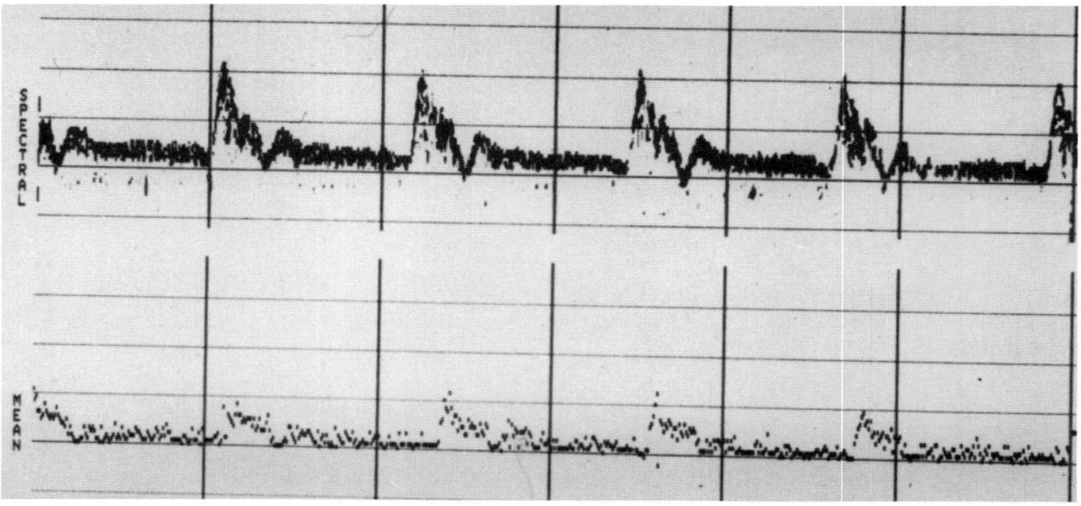

Figure 11-15. Spectral waveforms from a common carotid artery. The upper waveform contains the complete spectra with all the frequency and amplitude information. The lower waveform displays only the mean spectral frequencies. Note that the peak systolic frequencies of the mean waveform are much lower than those of the complete spectral waveform.

sample site, color-flow imaging provides a single estimate of the Doppler shifted frequency or flow velocity for each site within the B-mode image. Thus, spectral waveforms actually contain more information on flow patterns at each individual site than color-flow images. The main advantage of the color-flow display is that it presents simultaneous flow information on the entire image, even though the amount of data for each sample site is reduced.

Spectral waveforms contain a range of frequencies and amplitudes, allowing determination of flow direction and spectral parameters such as mean, mode, peak, and bandwidth. The color assignments for the color-flow image are based on flow direction and a single mean or average frequency estimate for each site in the B-mode image plane. Consequently, the peak Doppler frequency shifts or velocities shown by spectral waveforms generally are higher than the frequencies or velocities indicated by color-flow imaging (Fig. 11-15).

Because color-flow imaging is based on pulsed Doppler ultrasound, it is subject to the same physical limitations as spectral waveform analysis of pulsed Doppler signals. For example, since the Doppler frequency shift depends on the angle θ in the Doppler equation, color assignments in the color-flow image will be accurate only if this angle is properly adjusted and remains constant along the length of a vessel. Unfortunately, blood vessels are seldom straight, so different colors may represent either true velocity changes or variations in the frequency shift resulting from changes in the Doppler angle. This potential source of error always should be considered when interpreting color-flow images (Fig. 11-16). Aliasing is a pulsed Doppler artifact that occurs in both spectral waveform analysis and color-flow imaging. As mentioned previously, an aliased spectral waveform shows an abrupt loss of the waveform peak, with the missing portion appearing below the baseline as flow in the reverse direction (Fig. 11-14). When aliasing is present in a color-flow image, high ve-

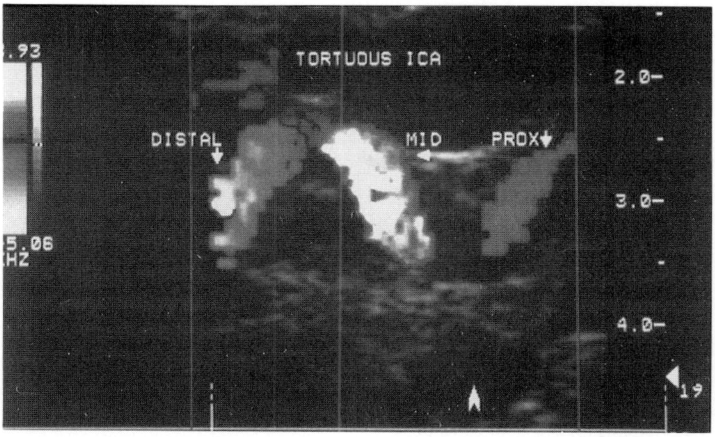

Figure 11-16. Color-flow image of a tortuous internal carotid artery (*ICA*). Changes in color from shades of red to shades of blue result from different angles between the flow stream and the ultrasound scan lines. No color appears when the angle approaches 90° and the Doppler shift is very small. (See Color Plate 1.)

locity jets are assigned colors that indicate flow in the direction opposite to arterial flow (Fig. 11-17). Theoretically, aliasing should be more common with color-flow imaging than with spectral waveform analysis, since relatively low PRF values are required to generate color-flow images.

In a color-flow image, shades of two or more distinct colors, usually red and blue, indicate the direction of flow relative to the ultrasound scan lines. A color bar near the image illustrates the particular color scale being used. The display is generally set up by the examiner to show flow in the arterial direction as red and flow in the venous direction as blue (Fig. 11-18). Variations in the Doppler shifted frequency or flow velocity are then indicated by changes in color, with lighter shades typically representing higher flow velocities. The specific features of color-flow images vary considerably among the commercially available duplex scanning instruments; however, a

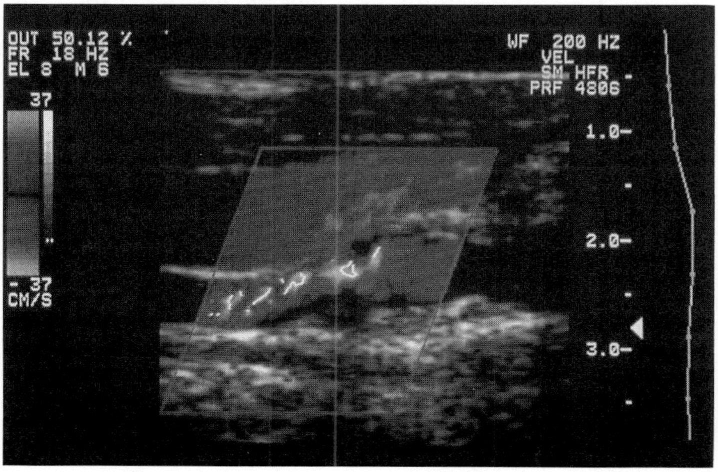

Figure 11-17. Aliasing in a color-flow image. The colors in this image represent blood flowing through a stenotic carotid artery lesion. Flow in the arterial direction is indicated by shades of red and yellow, while flow in the venous direction is indicated by shades of blue. However, the blue areas in the arterial lumen where the flow velocities are highest represent aliasing of the color-flow image and not true reversed flow. This is analogous to aliasing in spectral waveforms. (See Color Plate 2.)

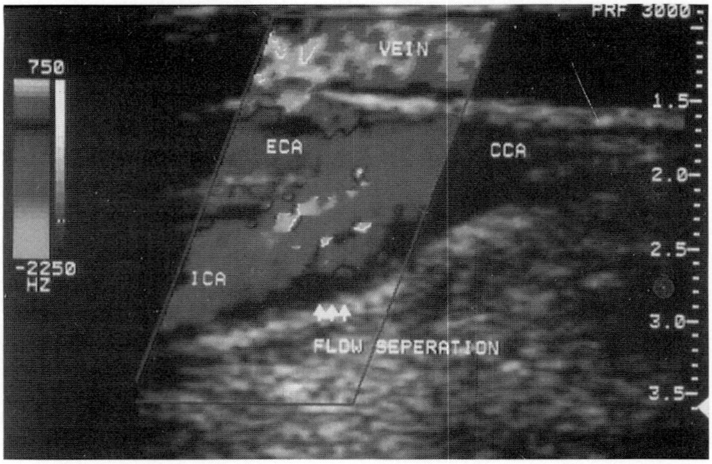

Figure 11-18. Color-flow image of a normal carotid bifurcation. As shown by the color bar to the left of the image, flow in the arterial direction is indicated by shades red and yellow; flow in the venous direction is indicated by shades of blue. *CCA*, common carotid artery; *ECA*, external carotid artery; *ICA*, internal carotid artery; and *VEIN*, internal jugular vein. An area of flow separation is present along the posterior or outer wall of the carotid bulb. (See Color Plate 3.)

single sample volume pulsed Doppler and spectrum analyzer are always available for a detailed evaluation of flow patterns at selected arterial sites.

A complete color-flow image includes the color-coded Doppler information superimposed on the real-time B-mode image. Because of the extremely large amount of Doppler and B-mode information needed to produce color-flow images, they are acquired at relatively slow frame rates. Consequently, some of the rapid variations in flow velocity that occur during the cardiac cycle may not be accurately displayed. For example, if it takes approximately 33 msec to generate each frame of a color image (30 frames per sec), flow transients with time constants near 20 msec, such as those occurring at the onset of systole, will not be reliably detected. This can result in temporal and spatial distortion in the color-flow image.

INSTRUMENTATION AND EXAMINATION TECHNIQUE

The attenuation of ultrasound as it travels through tissue is directly proportional to the transmitting frequency. Therefore, lower frequencies can penetrate to greater depths than higher frequencies. Stated another way, lower ultrasound frequencies are required for obtaining image and Doppler information from deeply located structures such as those in the abdomen. Since the blood vessels in the neck are relatively superficial, ultrasound transmitting frequency is generally not a major consideration in carotid duplex scanning. Transducers with frequencies in the range of 5 to 10 MHz give optimal results.

One of the principal limitations of the standard approach to carotid duplex scanning is the small region of the arterial lumen that can be evaluated at any one time. To obtain complete information on flow patterns throughout the B-mode image, the single pulsed Doppler sample volume must be moved serially to various sites. Even with extreme diligence on the part of the examiner, flow disturbances that are confined to a small section of the vessel may be overlooked. Furthermore, it is more difficult to appreciate the complex three-dimensional features of flow in the carotid bifurcation with the single sample volume technique than it is with color-flow imaging.

The basic examination technique is the same for both color-flow imaging and standard duplex scanning. First, the common carotid artery is imaged low in the neck and then followed distally. The common carotid bifurcation usually is at the level of the upper border of the thyroid cartilage, and the internal and external carotid arteries can be distinguished by their typical location, with the internal carotid posterolaterally and the external carotid anteromedially. The carotid sinus or bulb may be seen as a dilatation of the arterial lumen at the origin of the internal carotid artery (Fig. 11-19). Once the internal carotid artery is identified, it should be followed as far distally as possible; however, there is usually no need to follow the external carotid beyond its proximal portion. Flow patterns are most easily visualized when the arteries are scanned in longitudinal section. Occasionally, transverse scans are useful for showing unusual anatomic relationships between the various carotid branches.

As the carotid branches are visualized on the B-mode image, pulsed Doppler signals are obtained at frequent intervals along the vessels. This is necessary because the flow disturbances produced by arterial lesions are propagated only for a short distance downstream. Particular care is taken to completely assess the flow pattern in the carotid bulb or proximal internal carotid artery. Abnormal flow disturbances such as high velocity jets and poststenotic turbulence are noted. The color-flow image can be useful for locating the vessels, particularly when kinks, coils, or other anatomic variants are present. Although the color-flow image also may be helpful for identifying flow disturbances, some high velocity jets may not be apparent on the color-flow image because the colors are based on a mean Doppler frequency estimate rather than the true peak systolic frequency.

There are no formal criteria for classifying the severity of vertebral artery disease by duplex scanning. However, the cervical and in-

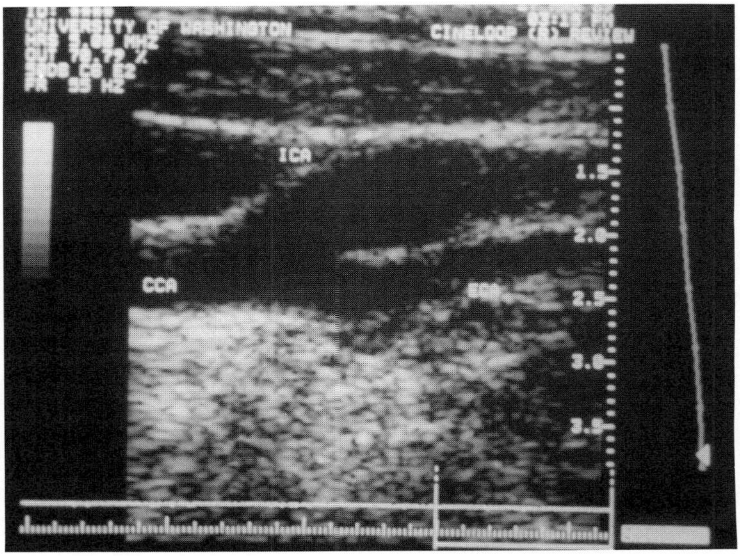

Figure 11-19. B-mode image of a normal carotid bifurcation. The carotid bulb is seen as a dilatation of the proximal internal carotid artery (*ICA*). *CCA*, common carotid artery; *ECA*, external carotid artery.

tervertebral portions of the vertebral artery can be examined by both standard duplex scanning and color-flow imaging. When this is clinically indicated, the presence and direction of flow in the vertebral arteries are noted.

NORMAL AND ABNORMAL CAROTID FLOW PATTERNS

As shown in Figure 11-8, the normal internal carotid artery has a low resistance flow pattern with forward flow throughout the cardiac cycle. This pattern is similar to other arteries, such as the renal and celiac axis, which also supply low resistance organs.[24,25] In contrast, the external carotid displays the triphasic flow pattern typical of peripheral arteries that supply a high-resistance vascular bed.[26] The flow pattern in the common carotid combines features of both the internal and external carotid arteries.

The peak systolic flow velocity in the common carotid artery normally is higher in the center stream than near the vessel wall. This can be demonstrated by serial sampling of the flow pattern across the lumen with a pulsed Doppler as shown in Fig. 11-20. Higher flow velocities also may be apparent on the color-flow image by a predominance of lighter shades in the center of the lumen, particularly during systole.[27,28]

The carotid bulb occupies a variable portion of the distal common and proximal internal carotid arteries (Fig. 11-19). The unique diverg-

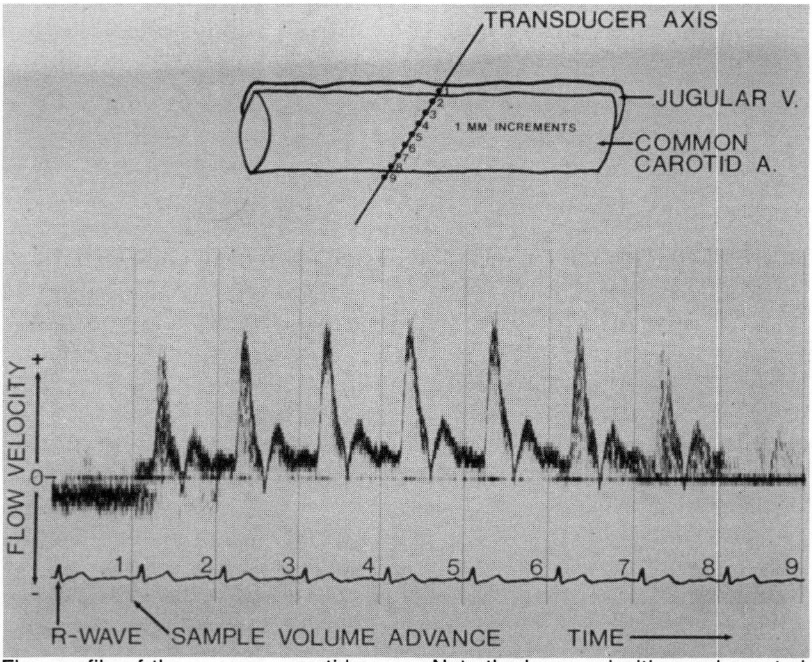

Figure 11-20. Flow profile of the common carotid artery demonstrated by serial sampling with a small sample volume pulsed Doppler. One cardiac cycle has been obtained for each 1-mm increment of lumen diameter. Note the lower velocities and spectral broadening near the vessel wall. Peak velocities are highest in the center of the flow stream.

ing and converging geometry of the bulb can create local pressure gradients that affect the flow pattern in the boundary layer—that layer of blood immediately adjacent to the arterial wall. When flow within the boundary layer stops or reverses direction, a localized flow pattern called "boundary layer separation" or "flow separation" results. A region of boundary layer separation is normally present along the posterior or outer wall of the bulb on the side opposite the flow divider. This region is characterized by low flow velocity with alternating forward and reverse components. Continuous forward flow is present in the bulb along the flow divider, and a more laminar flow pattern is reestablished in the internal carotid artery distal to the bulb. The features of boundary layer separation in normal carotid bifurcations have been demonstrated by model studies and clinical pulsed Doppler examinations.[27,29–33] The characteristic spectral waveforms of boundary layer separation in the carotid bulb are illustrated in Fig. 11-21 and 11-22. Figure 11-18 shows the typical appearance of boundary layer separation in a color-flow image. Since flow in the region of boundary layer separation is mainly in the reverse direction, the area usually appears as an oval-shaped blue area that fluctuates in size during the cardiac cycle. A smaller area of flow separation occasionally is found near the origin of the external carotid artery. Recognizing flow separation in the carotid bulb is important, since these normal flow patterns may be mistaken for the flow disturbances associated with arterial disease. The presence of flow separation in the carotid bulb with normal flow patterns proximal and distal to that site is highly predictive of normal carotid bifurcation anatomy.[34] Mild to moderate lesions of the carotid bifurcation that "fill in" the carotid bulb are characterized by absence of flow separation.

A significant stenosis in the proximal common carotid artery will cause the flow pattern in the more distal common carotid to be damped, with reduced peak systolic velocities. Asymmetry in the common carotid artery

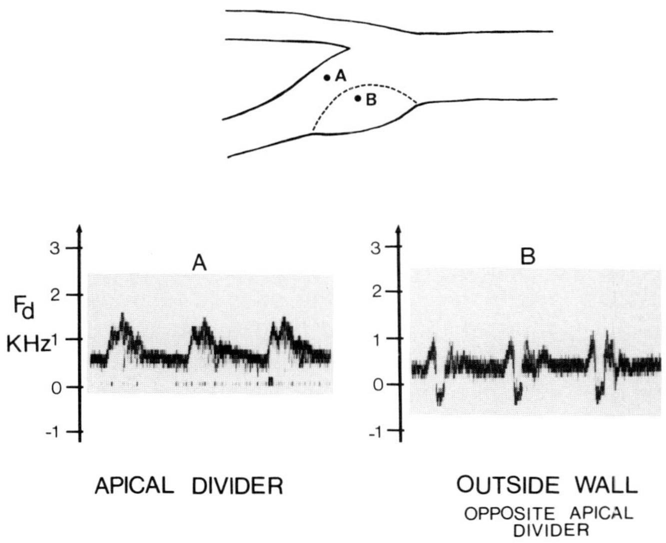

Figure 11-21. Spectral waveforms from a normal carotid bulb. There is forward flow throughout the cardiac cycle near the apical divider (*A*), while the flow pattern along the outer wall of the bulb (*B*) contains both forward (positive) and reverse (negative) velocity components. The latter pattern is typical of an area of boundary layer separation.

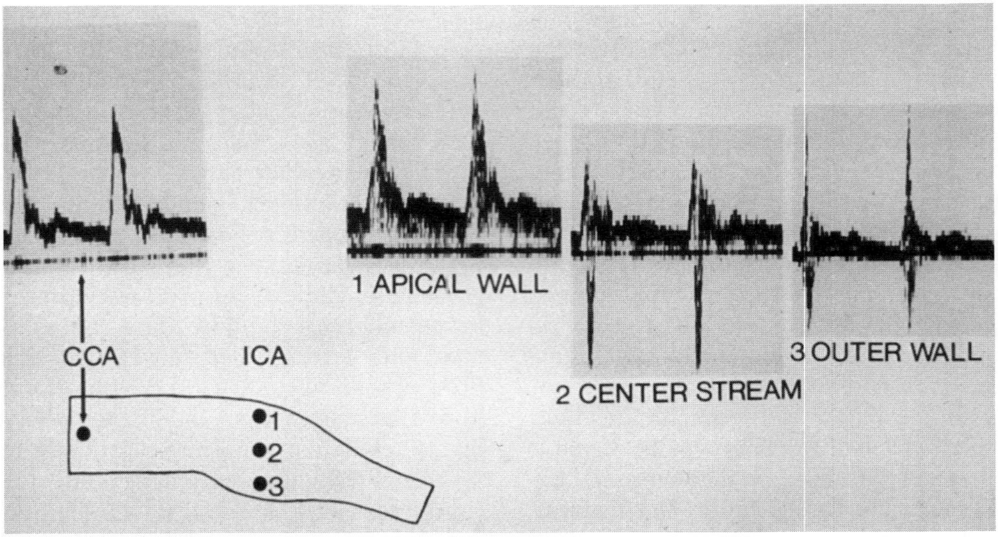

Figure 11-22. Spectral waveforms illustrating boundary layer separation in the carotid bulb. The flow pattern in the common carotid artery (*CCA*) shows forward flow throughout the cardiac cycle. A similar flow pattern is seen in the internal carotid artery (*ICA*) at site *1* (Apical Wall). Sites *2* (Center Stream) and *3* (Outer Wall) indicate the area of boundary layer separation with lower flow velocities and both forward and reverse flow components.

waveforms will be evident if the proximal common carotid disease is unilateral. Even when it is not possible to position the pulsed Doppler sample volume at the exact location of the high velocity jet, the presence of a proximal stenosis may be indicated by spectral broadening in the waveform obtained from the distal common carotid. However, these findings may not be present with stenoses that reduce the common carotid artery diameter by less than 50 percent.

Stenoses that narrow the carotid artery diameter by 50 percent or more are associated with high velocity jets and characteristic changes in the center stream flow pattern. Spectral waveform criteria for classification of internal carotid artery stenoses are described in Table 11-1 and illustrated in Fig. 11-12. The color-flow image of a severe internal carotid stenosis is shown in Fig. 11-23. While flow proximal to the stenosis appears relatively normal, a high-velocity stenotic jet is seen as a slight narrowing in the flow stream with aliasing of the color-flow image. The mixed color pattern in the poststenotic segment represents turbulent flow immediately distal to the stenosis and is analogous to the broadening of poststenotic spectral waveforms (Figs. 11-11 and 11-12). Another example of poststenotic turbulence in a color-flow image is shown in Fig. 11-24.

The color-flow image has been particularly useful for identifying unusual anatomic features of the carotid bifurcation, such as tortuosity or kinking, which can be difficult to recognize with standard duplex scanning techniques (Figs. 11-16 and 11-24). Color-flow imaging also is valuable for documenting internal carotid occlusion. With standard duplex scanning, internal carotid occlusion is indicated by

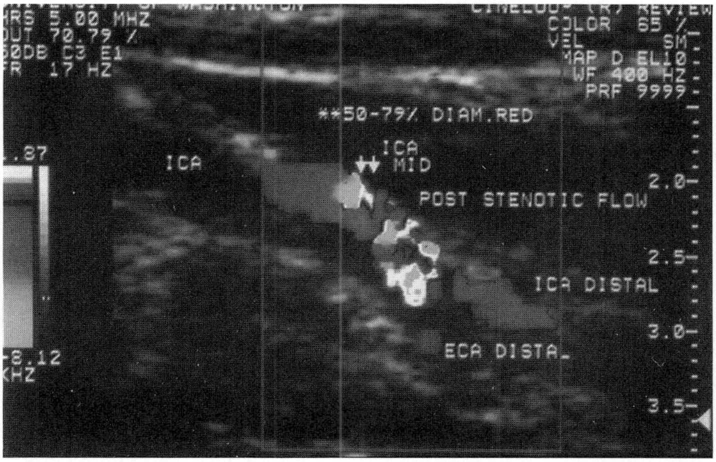

Figure 11-23. Color-flow image of a severe internal carotid artery (*ICA*) stenosis. The color-flow image shows normal flow in the prestenotic segment, a high velocity jet with aliasing, and poststenotic turbulence. (See Color Plate 4.)

the absence of a pulsed Doppler flow signal in that vessel, decreased diastolic flow velocity in the ipsilateral common carotid artery, and the presence of flow in the external carotid artery (Fig. 11-25). In this situation, the flow pattern in the common carotid artery on the side of the occlusion resembles that found in the external carotid. The site of occlusion in the proximal internal carotid often can be visualized on the color-flow image (Fig. 11-26).

When there is unilateral internal carotid occlusion, flow velocities in the contralateral carotid bifurcation may be increased owing to compensatory collateral flow, resulting in overestimation of stenosis severity in the patent internal carotid artery.[35,36] To avoid this problem, a minor modification of the standard duplex criteria has been proposed that increases the frequency or velocity thresholds between stenosis categories.[35] In the presence

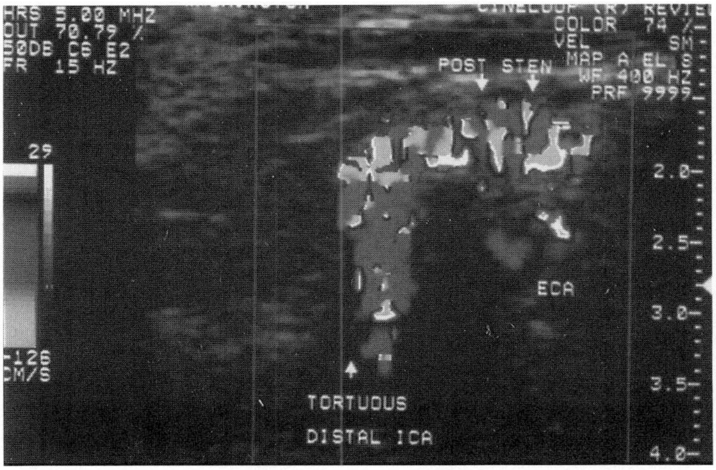

Figure 11-24. Color-flow image of a tortuous internal carotid artery (*ICA*) with the mixed color pattern characteristic of poststenotic turbulence. *ECA*, external carotid artery. (See Color Plate 5.)

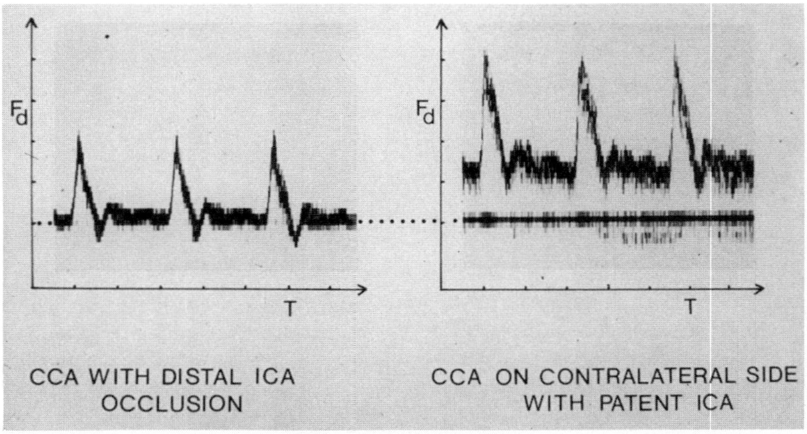

Figure 11-25. Spectral waveform features of the common carotid artery (*CCA*) with internal carotid artery (*ICA*) occlusion. Spectral waveform on the left is ipsilateral to the occlusion and shows a typical high resistance pattern similar to an external carotid, with a reversed flow phase and low diastolic flow velocity. Spectral waveform on the right is from the contralateral side with a patent ICA and shows a characteristic low resistance flow pattern.

of contralateral internal carotid occlusion, increased peak systolic frequencies up to 4.5 kHz, particularly with minimal spectral broadening, should be considered consistent with a 16 to 49 percent diameter reducing stenosis, and the end-diastolic frequency required for an 80 to 99 percent stenosis should be increased from 4.5 to 5.0 kHz.

CLINICAL APPLICATIONS

Duplex scanning was first developed for assessing the carotid bifurcation, and it continues to be regarded as the preferred noninvasive method for evaluating the extracranial carotid artery. However, advances in technology have also expanded the capabilities of du-

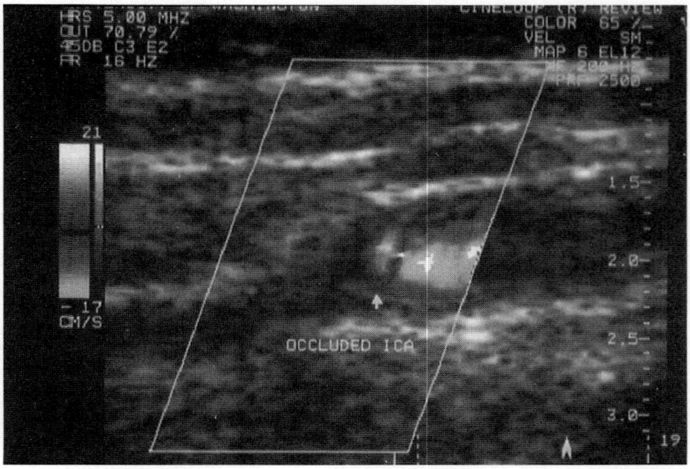

Figure 11-26. Occluded internal carotid artery (*ICA*.) Occlusion is indicated by failure to visualize flow distal to the bifurcation. The small blue area represents transient reversal of flow at the site of occlusion. (See Color Plate 6.)

Color Plates

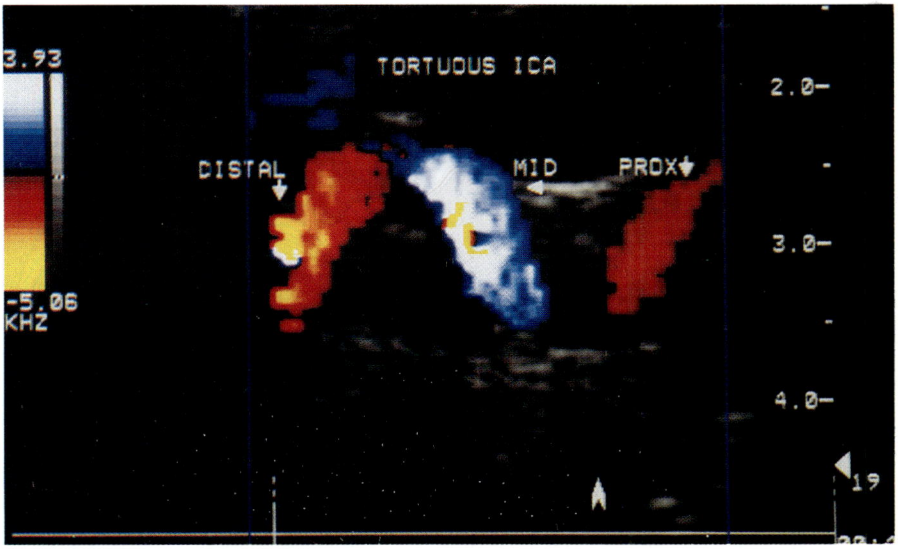

Plate 1. Color-flow image of a tortuous internal carotid artery (***ICA).*** Changes in color from shades of red to shades of blue result from different angles between the flow stream and the ultrasound scan lines. No color appears when the angle approaches 90° and the Doppler shift is very small.

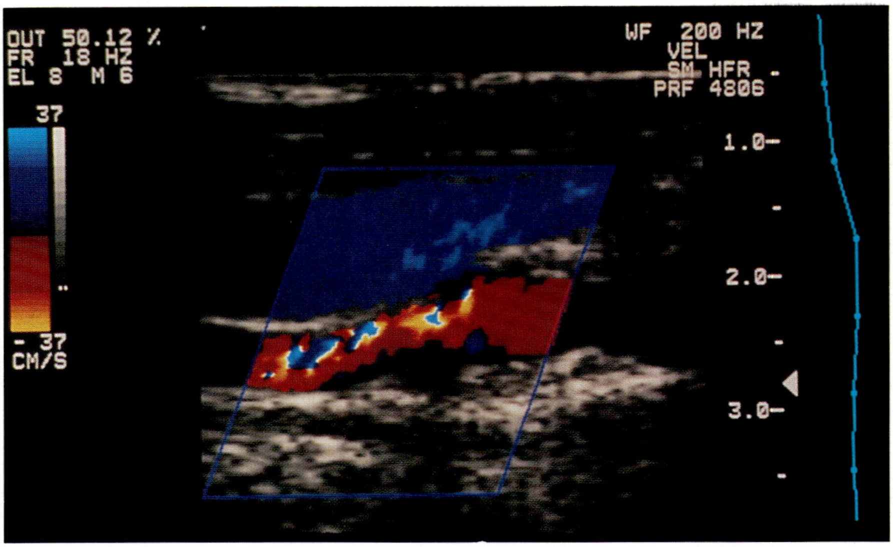

Plate 2. Aliasing in a color-flow image. The colors in this image represent blood flowing through a stenotic carotid artery lesion. Flow in the arterial direction is indicated by shades of red and yellow, while flow in the venous direction is indicated by shades of blue. However, the blue areas in the arterial lumen where the flow velocities are highest represent aliasing of the color-flow image and not true reversed flow. This is analagous to aliasing in spectral waveforms.

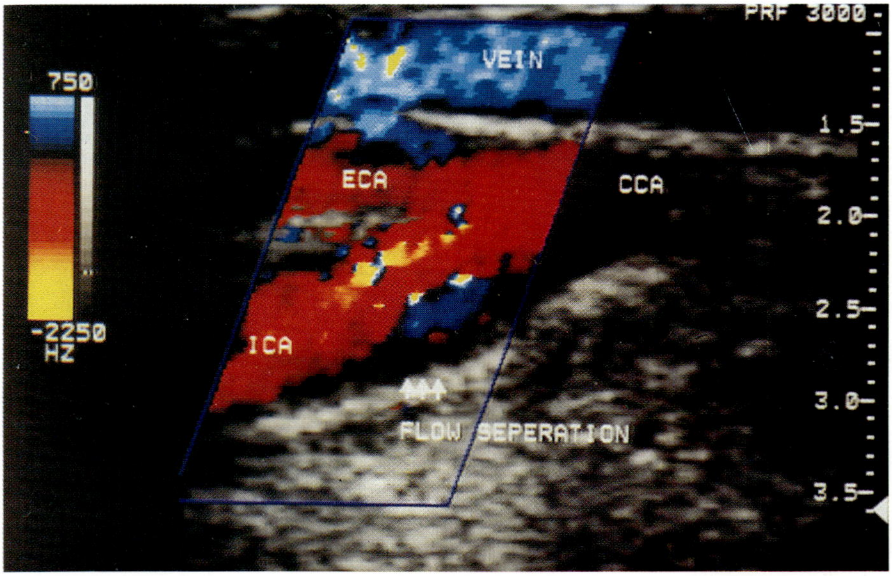

Plate 3. Color-flow image of a normal carotid bifurcation. As shown by the color bar to the left of the image, flow in the arterial direction is indicated by shades of red and yellow, while flow in the venous direction is indicated by shades of blue. ***CCA***, common carotid artery; ***ECA***, external carotid artery; ***ICA***, internal carotid artery; and ***VEIN***, internal jugular vein. An area of flow separation is present along the posterior or outer wall of the carotid bulb.

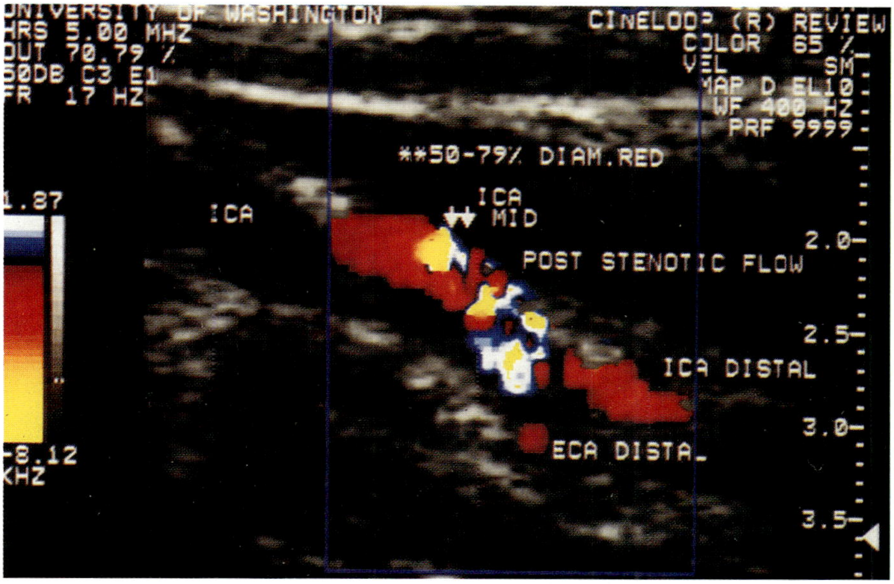

Plate 4. Color-flow image of a severe internal carotid artery (***ICA)*** stenosis. The color-flow image shows normal flow in the prestenotic segment, a high velocity jet with aliasing, and post-stenotic turbulence.

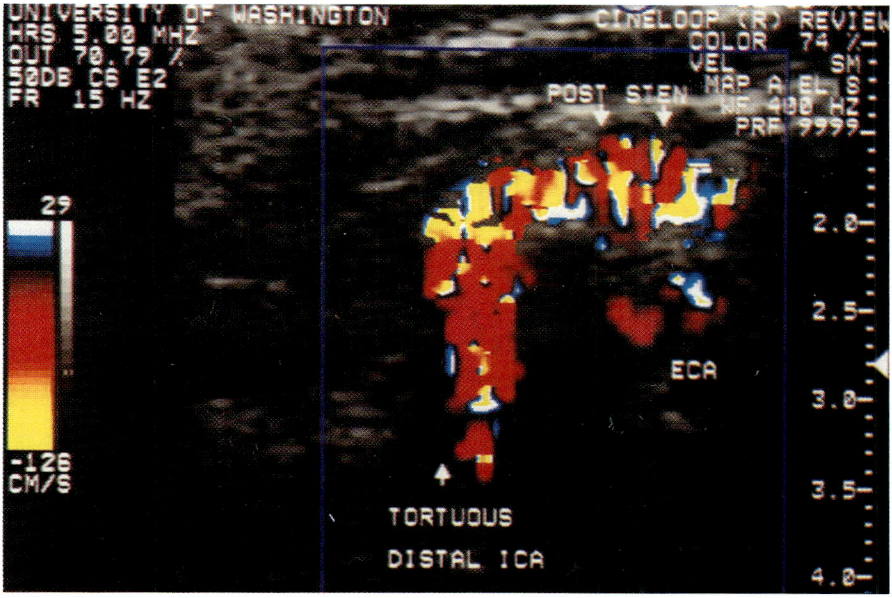

Plate 5. Color-flow image of a tortuous internal carotid artery (***ICA)*** with the mixed color pattern characteristic of poststenotic turbulence. ***ECA***, external carotid artery.

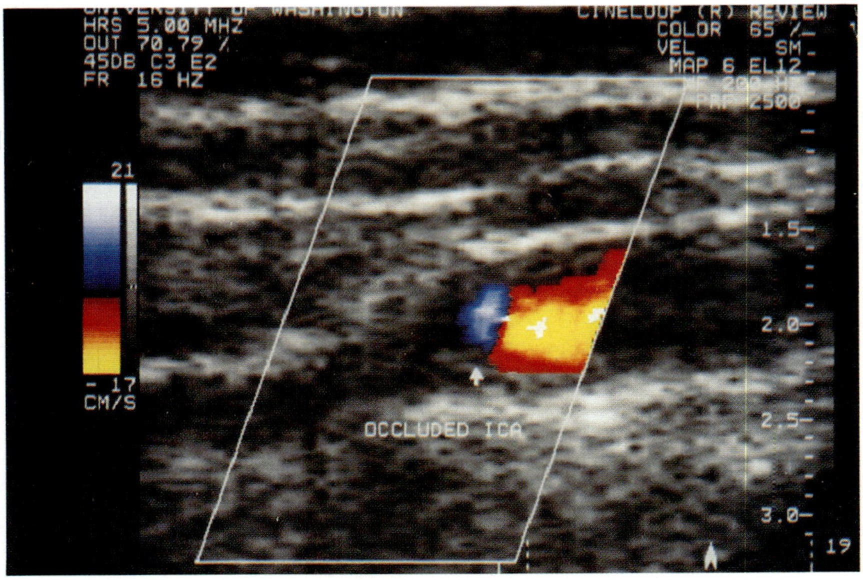

Plate 6. Occluded internal carotid artery (***ICA***). Occlusion is indicated by failure to visualize flow distal to the bifurcation. The small blue area represents transient reversal of flow at the site of occlusion.

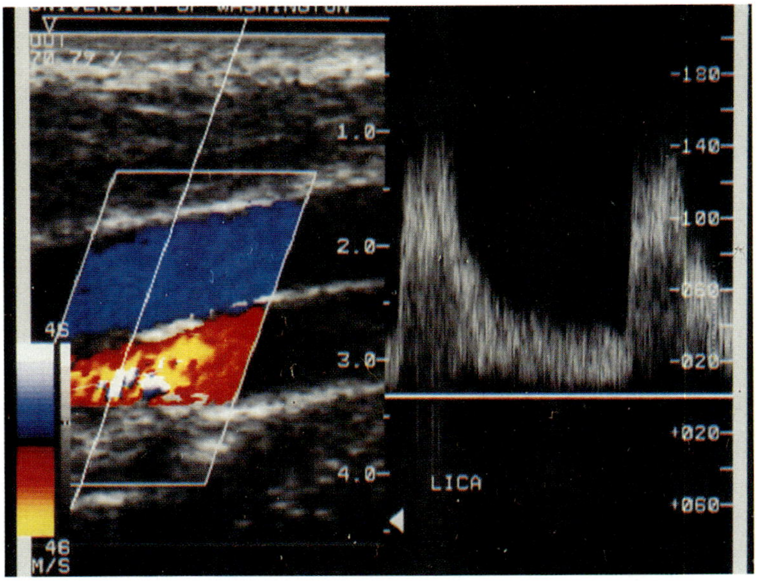

Plate 7. Color-flow image of an internal carotid stenosis and the corresponding pulsed Doppler spectral waveform. A significant flow disturbance is evident on the color-flow image, and the spectral waveform indicates a 50 to 79 percent diameter stenosis.

plex scanning to include detection of vascular disease in the abdomen and extremities.[24–26,37] The primary goal in the initial diagnostic evaluation of carotid artery disease is the identification of patients who are at risk for stroke. Once this is accomplished, decisions can be made regarding the need for arteriography and the potential benefits of carotid endarterectomy. Specific indications for carotid duplex scanning are as follows: (1) an asymptomatic carotid bruit; (2) hemispheric cerebral or ocular transient ischemic attacks (TIAs); (3) prior stroke with good neurologic recovery; (4) screening prior to major cardiac or peripheral vascular surgery; and (5) follow-up after carotid endarterectomy.[2]

The finding of a bruit in the neck is one of the most common indications for a noninvasive carotid evaluation. Among 100 patients with 165 asymptomatic neck bruits, duplex scanning showed a normal internal carotid in 12 (7 percent), less than 50 percent diameter reduction in 83 (50 percent), stenosis of 50 percent or greater diameter reduction in 61 (37 percent), and internal carotid occlusion in 9 (6 percent).[38] Thus, although the majority of neck bruits are associated with extracranial carotid artery disease, a relatively smaller proportion are related to severe internal carotid stenoses.

Therapeutic decisions for patients with asymptomatic carotid artery disease must take into account not only the severity of stenosis, but also the expected clinical outcome. In a serial follow-up study of 167 patients with asymptomatic neck bruits, duplex scanning showed progression of disease in 60 percent of the internal carotid arteries.[39] The mean annual rate of progression to greater than 50 percent diameter stenosis was 8 percent, and the mean annual rate for development of ipsilateral neurologic symptoms (TIA or stroke) was 4 percent. There was a strong correlation between the presence of an 80 to 99 percent internal carotid stenosis by duplex scanning and the occurrence of neurologic symptoms or internal carotid occlusion. Patients with 80 to 99 percent stenoses had a 46 percent incidence of one or more of these events, while those with less severe stenoses had only a 1.5 percent incidence. These data indicate that an asymptomatic 80 to 99 percent internal carotid stenosis identifies a group of patients who are at high risk for TIA, stroke, or internal carotid occlusion.

The purpose of carotid artery screening in patients with hemispheric neurologic symptoms is to identify lesions that could reduce hemispheric blood flow or be the source of cerebral emboli. As discussed in Chap. 16, the North American Symptomatic Carotid Endarterectomy Trial (NASCET) concluded that surgery was highly beneficial for patients with recent hemispheric TIAs or mild strokes and 70 to 99 percent stenosis of the ipsilateral internal carotid artery.[40] Although the specific NASCET guidelines require a 70 to 99 percent stenosis by arteriography, many of the lesions in the 50 to 79 percent stenosis category by duplex scanning (Table 11-1) will fall into this group. Thus, the finding of a 50 to 79 percent carotid lesion in a symptomatic patient should be considered an indication for further evaluation. A modification of the carotid duplex criteria has been proposed that is based on the ratio of the peak systolic velocities in the internal and common carotid arteries (ICA/CCA ratio). An ICA/CCA ratio of 4.0 or greater has a 91 percent sensitivity and 87 percent specificity for identifying a 70 to 99 percent diameter stenosis as defined in the NASCET.[41]

The role of screening for carotid artery disease prior to cardiac or other major surgical procedures has been difficult to define. Studies reviewing this issue have not shown a consistent relationship between perioperative neurologic events and the presence of asymptomatic carotid stenoses.[42] Consequently, routine prophylactic carotid endarterectomy cannot be recommended. Occasionally the duplex scan shows a normal or minimally diseased internal carotid artery in a patient with hemispheric neurologic symptoms. Follow-up of these patients generally supports a nonoperative approach, since the incidence of subsequent neurologic events is extremely low, and a noncarotid cause for symptoms may exist.[43] Other clinical applications of carotid duplex scanning include intraoperative assessment (Chap. 25), detection of recurrent stenosis after carotid endarterectomy (Chap. 27), and carotid surgery without arteriography (Chap. 21).

Some variability is unavoidable in the performance and interpretation of any diagnostic test. The greatest variability in carotid duplex scanning has been noted for the normal to moderate stenosis categories designated as A, B, and C in Table 11-1 and Fig. 11-12. Much better agreement has been observed for classification of lesions greater than 50 percent diameter reducing.[44] Similarly, the results of carotid arteriography are subject to the most variability when the arteries are normal or minimally diseased.[45] In general, the agreement between duplex scanning and arteriography is equivalent to the agreement between two radiologists interpreting the same arteriograms.

Color-flow imaging offers several potential advantages over the standard approach to duplex scanning. By visualizing areas of flow within a B-mode image, the branches of the carotid bifurcation are more easily identified. The color-flow image also expedites recognition of localized flow disturbances and should shorten the time required to perform an examination. However, since there are currently no definitive color criteria for classification of stenosis severity, spectral waveforms must still be used to determine the extent of carotid disease (Fig. 11-27). Color-flow imaging can facilitate spectral waveform analysis by allowing optimal positioning of the pulsed Doppler sample volume at sites of disease.

The value of color-flow imaging for the assessment of carotid artery disease was evaluated by a study conducted in two vascular laboratories—one with a color-flow imaging instrument and the other with a standard duplex scanner.[46] A total of 307 internal carotid arteries were evaluated by color-flow imaging

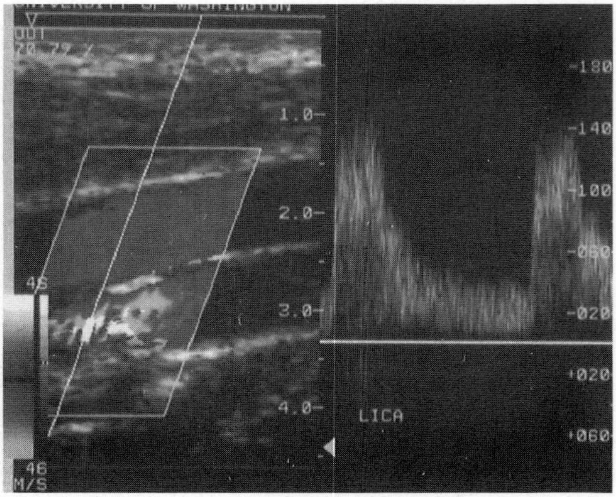

Figure 11-27. Color-flow image of an internal carotid stenosis and the corresponding pulsed Doppler spectral waveform. A significant flow disturbance is evident on the color-flow image, and the spectral waveform indicates a 50 to 79 percent diameter stenosis. (See Color Plate 7.)

and arteriography, while 206 internal carotid arteries had a standard duplex scan and arteriography. Perfect agreement between the duplex scan result and the arteriogram was achieved in 87 percent of the color-flow examinations and in 80 percent of the standard duplex scans. In addition, significantly fewer arteries were over-classified by one disease category when color-flow imaging was used. Although this study supported the overall accuracy of both duplex techniques, there was a strong trend toward improved diagnostic results with color-flow imaging. This difference was attributed to more precise placement of the pulsed Doppler sample volume when the color-flow image was used as a guide. It should be emphasized, however, that the accuracy of standard carotid duplex scanning is already quite favorable, and the additional value of color-flow imaging in routine carotid testing may be relatively small. Color-flow imaging is most likely to be helpful in selected patients who have atypical arterial anatomy or suspected internal carotid occlusion.

REFERENCES

1. Bandyk DF, Thiele BL: Noninvasive assessment of carotid artery disease. *West J Med* 139:486, 1983.
2. Strandness DE Jr, Andros G, Baker JD, Bernstein EF: Vascular laboratory utilization and payment: report of the Ad Hoc Committee of the Western Vascular Society. *J Vasc Surg* 216:163, 1992.
3. Beach KW, Phillips DJ: Doppler instrumentation for evaluation of arterial and venous disease. *Clin Diag Ultrasound* 13:5, 1984.
4. Satomura S: Study of flow patterns in peripheral arteries by ultrasonics. *J Acoust Soc Jpn* 15:151, 1959.
5. Rushmer RF, Baker DW, Stegall HF: Transcutaneous Doppler flow as a nondestructive technique. *J Appl Physiol* 2:554, 1966.
6. Strandness DE Jr, McCutcheon EP, Rushmer RF: Application of a transcutaneous Doppler flowmeter in evaluation of occlusive arterial disease. *Surg Gynecol Obstet* 122:1039, 1966.
7. Strandness DE Jr: *Duplex Scanning in Vascular Disorders*. New York, Raven, 1990.
8. Mozersky DJ, Hokanson DE, Baker DS, Strandness DE Jr: Ultrasonic arteriography. *Arch Surg* 103:663, 1971.
9. Hartley CJ, Strandness DE Jr: The effects of artherosclerosis on the transmission of ultrasound. *J Surg Res* 9:575, 1969.
10. Barber FE, Baker DW, Nation AWC, et al: Ultrasonic duplex echo-Doppler scanner. *IEEE Trans Biomed Eng* 21:109, 1974.
11. Comerota AJ, Cranley JJ, Katz AK, et al: Real-time B-mode carotid imaging: A three-year multicenter experience. *J Vasc Surg* 1:84, 1984.
12. Hennerici M, Reifschneider G, Trockel U, Aulich A: Detection of early atherosclerotic lesions by duplex scanning of the carotid artery. *J Clin Ultrasound* 12:455, 1984.
13. O'Donnell TF, Erdoes L, Mackay WC, et al: Correlation of B-mode ultrasound imaging and arteriography with pathologic findings at carotid endarterectomy. *Arch Surg* 120:443, 1985.
14. Reilly LM: Importance of carotid plaque morphology, in Bernstein EF (ed): *Vascular Diagnosis,* 4th ed. St. Louis, Mosby–Year Book, 1993, chap 35, pp 333–340.
15. Reilly LM, Lusby RJ, Hughes L, et al: Carotid plaque histology using real-time ultrasonography—Clinical and therapeutic implications. *Am J Surg* 146:188, 1983.
16. Lusby RJ, Ferell LD, Ehrenfeld WK, et al: Carotid plaque hemorrhage: Its role in production of cerebral ischemia. *Arch Surg* 117:1479, 1981.
17. O'Leary DH, Holen J, Ricotta JJ: Carotid bifurcation disease—Prediction of ulceration with B-mode US. *Radiology* 162:523, 1987.
18. Fell G, Phillips DJ, Chikos PM, et al: Ultrasonic duplex scanning for disease of the carotid artery. *Circulation* 64:1191, 1981.
19. Langlois YE, Roederer GO, Chan AW, et al: Evaluating carotid artery disease—The concordance between pulsed Doppler/spectrum analysis and angiography. *Ultrasound Med Bio* 9:51, 1983.

20. Roederer GO, Langlois YE, Chan AW, et al: Ultrasonic duplex scanning of extracranial carotid arteries: Improved accuracy using new features from the common carotid artery. *J Cardiovasc Ultrasonography* 1:373, 1982.
21. Knox RA, Phillips DJ, Breslau PJ, et al: Empirical findings relating sample volume size to diagnostic accuracy in pulsed Doppler cerebrovascular studies. *J Clin Ultrasound* 10:227, 1982.
22. Phillips DJ, Beach KW, Primozich J, Strandness DE Jr: Should results of ultrasound Doppler studies be reported in units of frequency or velocity? *Ultrasound Med Biol* 15:205, 1989.
23. Kremkau FW: Principles and pitfalls of real-time color flow imaging, in Bernstein EF (ed): *Vascular Diagnosis,* 4th ed. St. Louis, Mosby–Year Book, 1993, chap 12, pp 90–105.
24. Jager K, Bollinger A, Valli C, Ammann R: Measurement of mesenteric blood flow by duplex scanning. *J Vasc Surg* 3:462, 1986.
25. Hoffmann U, Edwards JM, Carter S, et al: Role of duplex scanning for the detection of atherosclerotic renal artery disease. *Kidney Int* 39:1232, 1991.
26. Zierler RE: Duplex and color-flow imaging of the lower extremity arterial circulation. *Semin Ultrasound CT MR* 11:168, 1990.
27. Zierler RE, Phillips DJ, Beach KW, et al: Noninvasive assessment of normal carotid bifurcation hemodynamics with color-flow ultrasound imaging. *Ultrasound Med Biol* 13:471, 1987.
28. Zierler RE, Primozich JF, Phillips, DJ, Strandness DE Jr: Color-flow ultrasound imaging of the normal and diseased carotid bifurcation. *Dynamic Cardiovasc Imaging* 1:34, 1987.
29. Ku DN, Giddens DP: Pulsatile flow in a model carotid bifurcation. *Arteriosclerosis* 3:31, 1983.
30. Ku DN, Phillips DJ, Giddens DP, et al: Hemodynamics of the normal human carotid bifurcation: in vitro and in vivo studies. *Ultrasound Med Biol* 11:13, 1985.
31. LoGerfo FW, Nowak MD, Quist WC: Structural details of boundary layer separation in a model human carotid bifurcation under steady and pulsatile flow conditions. *J Vasc Surg* 2:263, 1985.
32. Phillips DJ, Greene FM, Langlois YE, et al: Flow velocity patterns in the carotid bifurcations of young, presumed normal subjects. *Ultrasound Med Biol* 9:39, 1983.
33. Bharadvaj BK, Mabon RF, Giddens DP: Steady flow in a model of the human carotid bifurcation. Part I. Flow visualization. *J Biomechanics* 15:349, 1982.
34. Nicholls SC, Phillips DJ, Primozich JF, et al: Diagnostic significance of flow separation in the carotid bulb. *Stroke* 20:175, 1989.
35. Fujitani RM, Mills JL, Wang LM, Taylor SM: The effect of unilateral carotid arterial occlusion upon contralateral duplex study: Criteria for accurate interpretation. *J Vasc Surg* 16:459, 1992.
36. Spadone DP, Barkmeier LD, Hodgson KJ, et al: Contralateral internal carotid artery stenosis or occlusion: Pitfall of correct ipsilateral classification—A study performed with color-flow imaging. *J Vasc Surg* 11:642, 1990.
37. Zierler RE: The role of the vascular laboratory in clinical decision-making. *Semin Roentgenol* 27:63, 1992.
38. Fell G, Breslau P, Knox RA, et al: Importance of noninvasive ultrasonic Doppler testing in the evaluation of patients with asymptomatic carotid bruits. *Am Heart J* 102:221, 1981.
39. Roederer GO, Langlois YE, Jager KA, et al: The natural history of carotid arterial disease in asymptomatic patients with cervical bruits. *Stroke* 15:605, 1984.
40. North American Symptomatic Carotid Endarterectomy Trial Collaborators: Beneficial effect of carotid endarterectomy in symptomatic patients with high-grade stenosis. *N Engl J Med* 325:445, 1991.
41. Moneta GL, Edwards JM, Chitwood RW, et al: Correlation of North American Symptomatic Carotid Endarterectomy Trial (NASCET) angiographic definition of 70% to 90% internal carotid artery stenosis with duplex scanning. *J Vasc Surg* 17:152, 1993.
42. Barnes RW, Marszalek PB: Asymptomatic carotid disease in the cardiovascular surgical patient: Is prophylactic endarterectomy necessary? *Stroke* 12:497, 1981.
43. Zierler RE, Kohler TR, Strandness DE Jr: Duplex scanning of normal or minimally diseased

carotid arteries: Correlation with arteriography and clinical outcome. *J Vasc Surg* 12:447, 1990.
44. Kohler T, Langlois Y, Roederer GO, et al: Sources of variability in carotid duplex examination: A prospective study. *Ultrasound Med Biol* 4:571, 1985.
45. Chikos PM, Fisher LD, Hirsh JA, et al: Observer variability in evaluating extracranial carotid artery stenosis. *Stroke* 14:885, 1983.
46. Londrey GL, Spadone DP, Hodgson KJ: Does color-flow imaging improve the accuracy of duplex carotid evaluation? *J Vasc Surg* 13:659, 1991.

12

Transcranial Doppler in Extracranial Cerebrovascular Disease

David W. Newell

PRINCIPLES AND DEVELOPMENT OF TRANSCRANIAL DOPPLER

Transcranial Doppler (TCD) has expanded the capabilities of Doppler ultrasound to include examination of the intracranial circulation.[1] The use of ultrasound to measure blood flow velocity is based on the Doppler principle. As discussed in Chap. 11, the Doppler principle describes the frequency shift of a wave when the source of the wave and the receiver of the wave are moving with respect to each other. To measure the velocity of flowing blood, one can use the frequency shifts of an ultrasound beam reflected from flowing blood. These shifts are directly proportional to the blood flow velocity.

Satomura and Kaneko first described this application of ultrasound.[2,3] One of their goals was actually to record blood flow velocities from the intracranial vessels. However, they concluded that the skull would be too much of a barrier to useful recordings; therefore, they concentrated their attention on the extracranial circulation. Further developments in this field have led to the many applications and the widespread use of Doppler ultrasound in the cardiovascular system.

The first transcranial Doppler recordings were made by Dr. Rune Aaslid in 1981 using a 2 MHz pulsed Doppler manufactured by Vingmed.[4] Subsequently, the transcranial Doppler methodology was developed at the Department of Neurosurgery in Berne, Switzerland. The initial application of this technology concentrated on the diagnosis of cerebral vasospasm caused by subarachnoid hemorrhage. Subsequent refinements in this technology were made possible by small portable microprocessor–controlled equipment (TC264, Eden Medical Electronics, Uberlingen, Germany). This instrumentation consisted of a 2 MHz pulsed range-gated Doppler with analog and digital output of the velocity waveform.

Pulsed Doppler is essential for TCD purposes, since a small sample volume is required to locate the different arteries in the basal human cerebral circulation in and around the circle of Willis. The low frequency used for the Doppler system is required for maximum penetration through the natural cranial windows. Initial identification of the individual intracranial vessels was accomplished by knowledge of the anatomy and flow characteristics of the intracranial circulation and was performed using a freehand technique.[1,5] Subsequently, additional techniques have been described for improved vessel identification.

The applications of TCD have expanded greatly. In addition to its widely accepted use in detecting cerebral vasospasm,[6] other applications continue to develop. Detection of intracranial stenosis from a variety of pathologic conditions has been described,[7] as well as the assessment of intracranial hemodynamics, which can be affected by many disease processes.[8] Monitoring of intracranial blood flow velocity also can be performed, and this can be used to study cerebral blood flow changes during autoregulatory responses,[9] CO_2 changes[8] in response to some medications, and brain activation.[10] Monitoring of the intracranial velocity changes during vessel clamping and other surgical procedures is also being used for research and clinical purposes. Further development of time-sequenced Dopplers allows monitoring of more than one vessel simultaneously.[4] Multichannel Doppler enables comparisons between cerebral hemispheres during vessel clamping, cerebral activation, autoregulation, and CO_2 reactivity.

During the last several years, the ability to detect intracranial microemboli has been recognized and further refined. It is now possible to detect cerebral arterial emboli caused by entry into the circulation during open heart surgery, peripheral vascular surgery, and catheter procedures. The microemboli that occur during surgical procedures are largely due to air bubbles, but also may arise from intravascular formed elements.[11,12] In addition, intracranial emboli composed of formed elements have been detected in many asymptomatic patients with intravascular pathology and have been observed in patients experiencing transient ischemic attacks (TIAs).[11,13] The development of automated detection and quantitation devices for intracranial microemboli is now underway. The two major capabilities of TCD that are useful in patients with extracranial cerebrovascular disease are the ability to detect intracranial emboli and the ability to determine the intracranial hemodynamic effects of proximal vascular lesions.

EXAMINATION TECHNIQUES

The initial transcranial Doppler recordings were made through the temporal window or the thin portion of the squamous part of the temporal bone.[1] It has been observed in most humans that in the temporal region of the skull, the inner and outer tables can be either fused or closely approximated, which allows the transmission of ultrasound (Fig. 12-1). The thicker portions of the cranium have a middle layer of cancellous bone, or diploe, which contains bone spicules that have a tendency to scatter ultrasound in many directions. Most of the skull is composed of this type of bone and therefore is less suitable for ultrasound penetration.

Three acoustical windows for TCD examination have been described: the transtemporal window; the transorbital window; and the transforamenal window (Fig. 12-2). The transtemporal window is located directly superior to the zygomatic arch. In this location, there may be several areas in the temporal squama where ultrasound can penetrate, and therefore several temporal windows which can be used for examination. Grolimund found that probably less than 35 percent of the original ultrasonic power is transmitted through the temporal bone during TCD examination.[14] Through amplification techniques and enhancement of signal-to-noise ratio, smaller fractions of the original ultrasonic intensity can be used to record useful spectral signals. Approximately 90 percent of

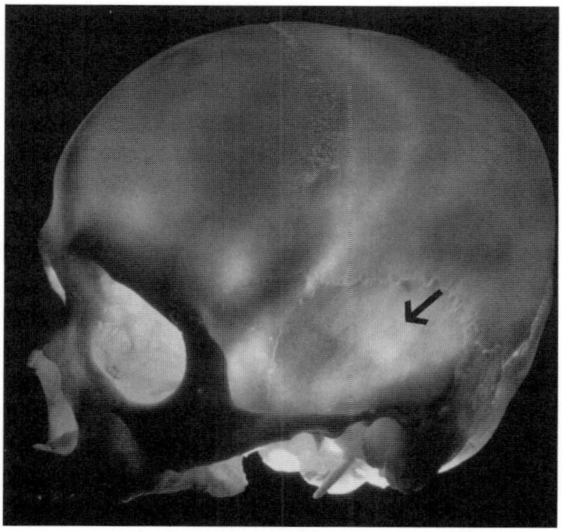

Figure 12-1. Transillumination of the human skull illustrating thin portions of the temporal bone (*arrow*) where ultrasound penetration using transcranial Doppler is possible. The inner and outer table of the skull are often fused in this region. This feature allows the penetration of low frequency ultrasound.

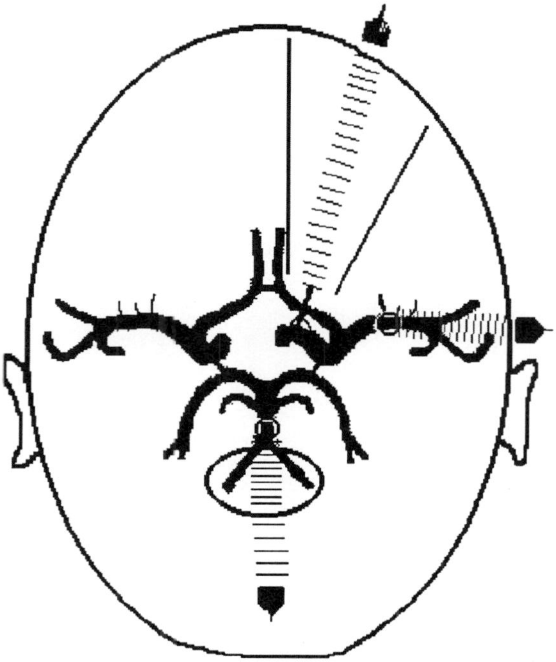

Figure 12-2. The three windows for transcranial Doppler examination of the basal cerebral vessels. Anteriorly, the transorbital window is used to examine the carotid siphon as well as the ophthalmic artery. On the lateral portion of the skull is the transtemporal window used to examine the middle cerebral artery, proximal anterior cerebral artery, distal internal carotid artery, and proximal posterior cerebral artery. The third window is the transforamenal window, which can be used to examine the posterior circulation vessels. The two vertebral arteries and basilar artery are easily examined using this window. The posterior inferior cerebellar arteries can also usually be examined.

subjects can be examined through the temporal window.[5] However, hyperostosis of the temporal bone may make it impossible to perform a complete examination of some individuals. Elderly females are particularly prone to having poor temporal windows. The temporal window can be used to examine the middle cerebral artery (MCA), proximal anterior cerebral artery (ACA), terminal internal carotid artery (ICA), proximal posterior cerebral artery (PCA), anterior communicating artery, and occasionally the posterior communicating artery (Fig. 12-3).

The most accurate determination of flow velocity is accomplished when an artery is parallel to the direction of the ultrasound beam. Generally, as arteries become more perpendicular to the ultrasound beam, they can no longer be examined adequately. Therefore, the standard TCD examination usually is limited to the basal cerebral arteries. It is not typically possible to examine the MCA branches as they become vertically oriented in the Sylvian fissure. Other arterial segments which are normally beyond the range of TCD are the ACA distal to the anterior communicating artery as it becomes vertically oriented in the interhemispheric fissure, and the PCA as it curves laterally around the brain stem and becomes oriented perpendicular to the ultrasound beam from the temporal window. The transorbital route can be used to examine the ophthalmic artery, the carotid siphon, and occasionally the ACAs. The transforamenal window utilizes the natural cranial opening through the foramen magnum. It can be used to examine both vertebral arteries (VA) as well as the basilar artery (BA). Branches from the vertebral arteries, particularly the posterior inferior cerebellar artery (PICA), also can be examined through these windows.

Vessel identification is accomplished through

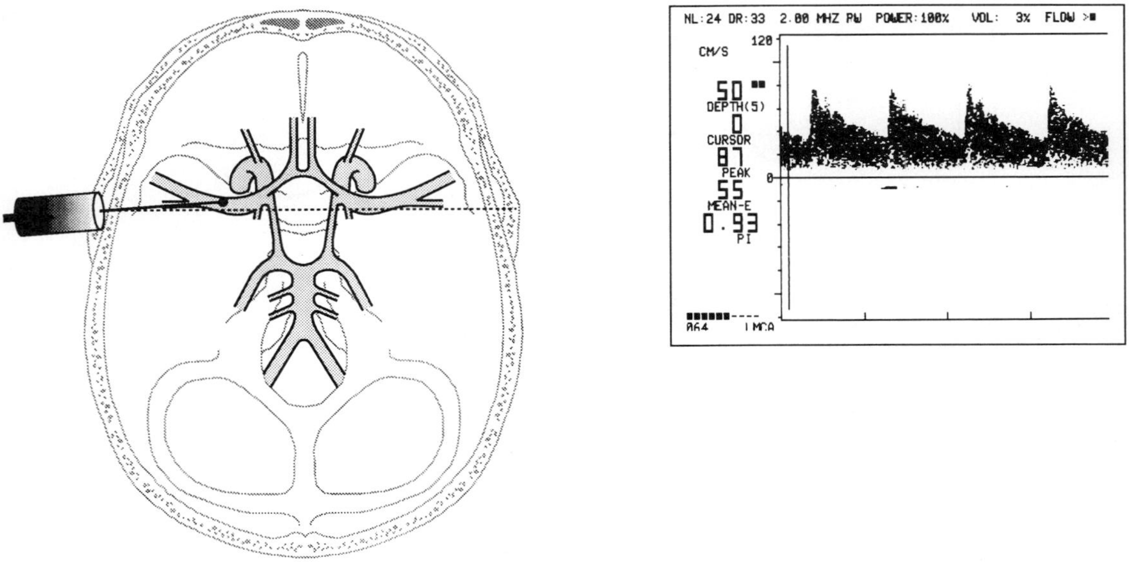

Figure 12-3. Recordings from the middle cerebral artery through the transtemporal window. Note that the spectral tracing is that of a low resistance vascular bed, which is typical of the intracranial circulation. Normally, the middle cerebral trunk is found at a depth of 55 mm from the scalp at the temporal window.

several techniques. The original and most widely used method for vessel identification involves the freehand technique, which utilizes six criteria to identify the intracranial vessels.[5] These are:

1. The cranial window used
2. The depth of the sample volume
3. The direction of flow in relation to the transducer
4. The spatial relationship of the vessel under examination to the internal carotid artery bifurcation
5. The relative flow velocity
6. The response to compression and oscillation maneuvers

Successful use of the freehand technique requires an ultrasonographer who is extremely familiar with the normal and abnormal intracranial vascular anatomy and who has performed multiple examinations on normal and abnormal subjects. Further technical developments in TCD equipment have led to the use of other modalities to facilitate vessel identification, such as vessel mapping and color-flow TCD.

The transcranial mapping technique was developed by Aaslid in cooperation with Eden Medical Electronics.[15] The principle behind transcranial vessel mapping is a computer-generated display produced by mapping the movement of the Doppler sample volume at different locations along the basal cerebral arteries. The computer saves a record of the placement of the sample volume as a three-dimensional plot with color-coded dots. With the aid of a vessel map, the branch points can be identified and the intracranial vessel anatomy can be reconstructed. Spectral waveforms saved from each of the dots may then be evaluated. In this way, one may record and provide positive documentation for the location of each waveform.

A more recent development for vessel identification is called transcranial color-coded real-time ultrasonography (TCCU).[16] This technology provides a B-mode image with a two-dimensional color-coded image of the basal cerebral arteries. Positive vessel identification is achieved using TCCU by enabling the sonographer to scan the basal vessels and obtain a real-time color-coded map of the vascular anatomy (Fig. 12-4). This technique also provides visualization of such intracranial landmarks as the sphenoid wing and the petrous ridge. Landmarks are useful reference points to locate the various intracranial vessels. Certain intracranial mass lesions can be identified at the same time and their effects on the normal vasculature can be evaluated.

The TCCU method involves scanning the intracranial basal vessels through the same three windows used in freehand examinations. The color-coded blood flow maps are then used to direct the sample volume to specific intracranial vessels. The color-coded map is renewed every two seconds during the scanning phase. Once a vessel is chosen for examination, the probe is held in the same position where optimal vessel visualization is achieved. Then the Doppler mode is selected and the sample volume is placed on the previously obtained color-flow map to record from each intracranial vessel. The TCCU technique is useful in providing documentation of the site at which recordings are obtained. It is also helpful in cases of difficult vessel identification or when vascular anomalies are present.[16–18] The equipment used for color-flow is currently more cumbersome than that commonly used for the freehand technique.

INTRACRANIAL STENOSIS

Intracranial arterial stenosis may be caused by a variety of pathologic processes. The devel-

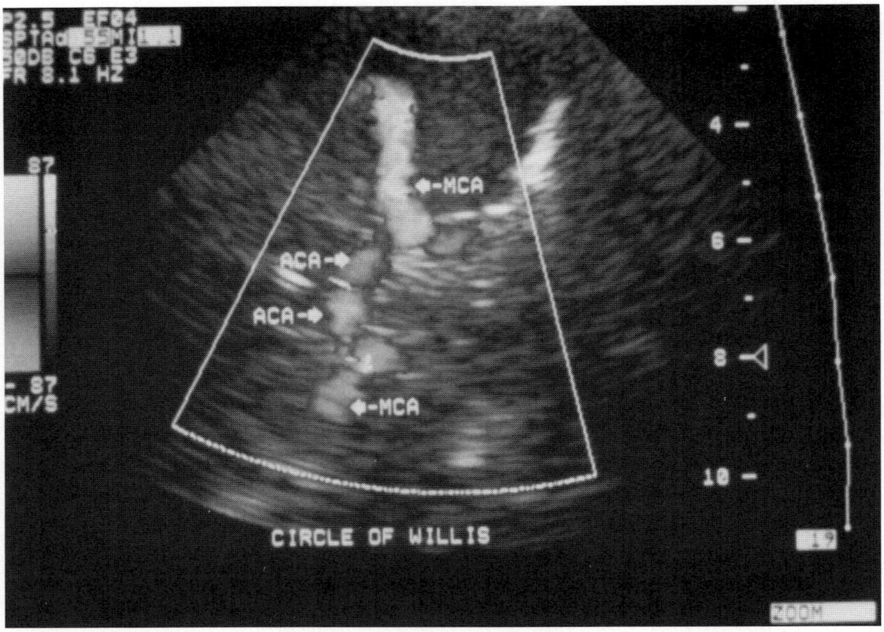

Figure 12-4. This is a sector scan from a color-flow Doppler instrument. This black and white illustration shows the major components of the circle of Willis. When the scan is obtained, the examiner can place the Doppler sample volume on preidentified vessels to record the blood flow velocity. This method provides the examiner with increased confidence for correct vessel identification.

opment of TCD ultrasonography has extended the capability of Doppler ultrasound to diagnose this condition reliably.[19–24] Reversible intracranial vessel narrowing is commonly caused by vasospasm following subarachnoid hemorrhage[6] and also can be seen in certain forms of vasculitis.[25] The most common cause of fixed intracranial stenosis in patients presenting with symptoms related to cerebrovascular disease is atherosclerosis involving the basal intracranial vessels.[22,26] Other conditions that can cause intracranial arterial stenosis include moyamoya disease, intracranial arterial dissection, sickle cell disease,[27] and arterial to arterial emboli undergoing various stages of recanalization.

Atherosclerotic disease of the intracranial vessels has received much less attention than lesions of the extracranial cerebral vessels. Probably one reason for this is that a noninvasive method was not available prior to the development of TCD to diagnose and follow the natural history of these lesions. Despite the fact that intracranial arterial stenosis due to atherosclerosis is less common than extracranial stenosis in western populations, the stroke rate from intracranial lesions can be significant. Bogousslavsky and coworkers[28] have analyzed the natural history of patients with MCA stenosis or occlusion entered into the extracranial–intracranial bypass study group. During a follow-up period of 42 months, recurrent cerebrovascular events (TIA and stroke) were experienced by 11.7 percent of the patients per year. The study found that atherosclerotic disease of the MCA was more common in Asian patients than in their Caucasian counterparts. A recent autopsy study comparing the severity of intracranial to extracranial atherosclerosis in Hong Kong Chinese also found that atherosclerosis of the intracranial cerebral vessels was more severe than that of the extracranial cerebral vessels in this population.[29]

The criteria for diagnosis of intracranial stenosis using TCD has been the subject of recent studies. The MCA, in addition to being commonly involved in intracranial atherosclerosis, is also the best suited for TCD examination. This is because it usually is parallel to the ultrasound beam and is considered an end artery in most cases. Leptomeningeal collateral vessels can be present; however, the collateral capacity of these vessels in humans is highly variable. Since increased velocities can be due either to stenosis or increased flow from collateral sources, four criteria have been established for making a positive identification of MCA stenosis.[7]

Criterion 1: Blood flow velocity increased to levels above those found in normal subjects.

Criterion 2: Localized increase in velocity at particular segments of the MCA.

Criterion 3: Side to side differences exceeding those encountered in normal subjects.

Criterion 4: Sonographic sounds of disturbed flow.

These criteria can also be applied to the other vessels commonly involved with intracranial atherosclerosis, namely, the distal ICA, and the other basal cerebral vessels (ACA, PCA, VA, BA). However, these arteries may be more likely than the MCA to have moderate increases in velocity when conducting increased collateral flow.

The differential diagnosis of intracranial stenosis includes vasospasm, feeding arteries to arteriovenous malformations, collateral circulation in the circle of Willis due to arterial occlusions, and carotid cavernous fistulas. Other less common occurrences include aneurysms, which can produce turbulence, and intracranial dissections, which may produce an intimal injury and stenosis.

Analysis of the accuracy of TCD for the diagnosis of intracranial stenosis has been reviewed by several authors.[19–21,23,24] Spencer and Whisler[24] compared carotid siphon stenosis assessed by angiography and TCD. In a group of 33 carotid siphons visualized angiographically, 11 demonstrated stenosis ranging from 30 to 75 percent. Comparison examinations using TCD revealed a sensitivity of 73 percent and specificity of 95 percent. Ley-Pozzo and Ringelstein[20] compared intra-arterial digital subtraction angiography to TCD in detecting occlusive disease of the carotid siphon and MCA. Sixteen of 17 cases of carotid siphon stenosis were correctly identified. Another study comparing TCD with angiography in a population of 196 patients reported the correct identification of stenosis using TCD in 16 of 21 cases documented angiographically.[21]

INTRACRANIAL HEMODYNAMICS

Using TCD to evaluate intracranial hemodynamics has added much new information concerning the control of the cerebral circulation. In addition to being able to evaluate intracranial stenoses by observing focal accelerations in the blood flow velocity, TCD can be used to measure relative changes in blood flow in the basal intracranial vessels. The use of TCD for this purpose is based on the principle that changes in velocity will be proportional to changes in flow through a vessel if the vessel diameter is constant. When using TCD to evaluate blood flow changes, a constant insonation angle (angle between the ultrasound beam and the vessel) is insured by the use of a fixed monitoring probe. Changes in blood flow velocity through the MCA can be used to assess relative changes in blood flow in that artery due to changes in CO_2 concentration or moderate changes in arterial blood pressure. Using these principles, the functional capacity of the distal regulating vessels in the cerebral circulation can be assessed.

The maintenance of adequate cerebral blood flow depends on sufficient cerebral perfusion pressure through the inflow vessels. Sufficient cerebral perfusion is dependent on the blood pressure, the anatomy of the extracranial and intracranial vasculature, and compensatory mechanisms when the vasculature or blood pressure becomes compromised. Under normal circumstances the human cerebral circulation contains two paired inflow arterial networks, the carotid and vertebral systems. At the base of the brain a normally configured circle of Willis will function as a manifold to normalize the perfusion pressure to the distal vessels if one or more extracranial vessels becomes occluded or hemodynamically compromised due to stenosis.

The collateral capacity of the circle of Willis normally allows nearly complete compensation "side-to-side" in cases of carotid occlusion.[30,31] The major pathways that compensate for a carotid occlusion are (1) crossover through the anterior communicating artery with reversed flow in the proximal anterior cerebral artery (A_1) ipsilateral to the occlusion; (2) reversed flow (forward flow) in the posterior communicating artery ipsilateral to the occlusion; and (3) reversed flow in the ipsilateral ophthalmic artery. The major pathways that normally compensate for hemodynamically significant posterior circulation occlusions are the posterior communicating arteries, which provide "front-to-back" collateral flow. The posterior communicating arteries also can provide "back-to-front" collateral flow in cases of bilateral carotid occlusion or severe stenosis. However, major differences in the functional capacity of the circle of Willis are found in the general population. It has been estimated that less than 50 percent of individuals possess an anatomically normal circle.[32] Figure 12-5 illustrates the normal configuration of the circle of Willis and common variants seen.

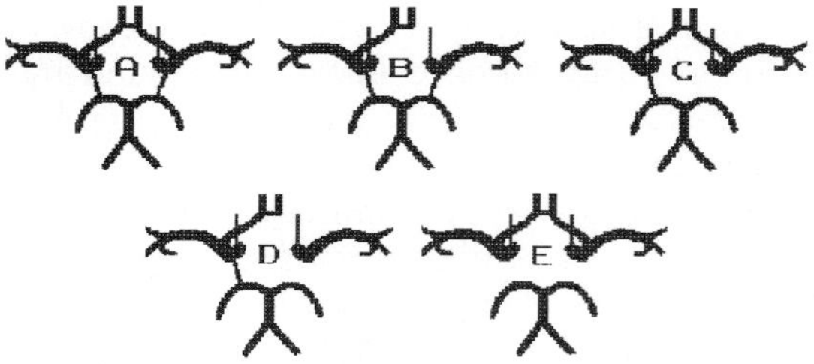

Figure 12-5. The common variations seen in the circle of Willis. *A.* Normal circle which can provide adequate collateral circulation to the distal cerebral vasculature with extracranial arterial occlusions. *B.* Functional impairment of the anterior crossover pathway due to an absent or atretic proximal anterior cerebral artery (*A1*). *C.* Functional impairment of anterior and posterior communication on one side due to an absent or atretic posterior communicating artery. *D.* Isolated carotid artery due to an inadequate anterior crossover pathway as well as inadequate posterior to anterior communication. The middle cerebral artery territory in this configuration is highly dependent on the flow through the ipsilateral internal carotid artery as well as the retrograde pathway through the ophthalmic artery. *E.* Absence of anterior to posterior communication due to bilateral agenesis or atresia of the posterior communicating arteries.

The effect of extracranial occlusive disease on intracranial hemodynamics and cerebral blood flow (CBF) is largely dependent on two factors: (1) the extent of the extracranial occlusive disease; and (2) the intracranial vascular anatomy and functional capacity of each individual patient. When the cerebral perfusion pressure is compromised owing to an acute extracranial arterial occlusion or a drop in blood pressure in the presence of extracranial occlusive disease, the collateral capacity of the circle of Willis will determine the distribution of perfusion to the intracranial vessels. Cerebral autoregulation then serves to dilate the distal regulatory vessels. This will effectively lower cerebrovascular resistance in an attempt to maintain cerebral blood flow. When this mechanism can no longer compensate and CBF begins to fall, increased extraction of oxygen from the blood by the brain can serve as an additional mechanism to maintain cerebral metabolism. When all these mechanisms are exhausted, cerebral ischemic symptoms or stroke on a hemodynamic basis can ensue.

TESTING OF VASOMOTOR RESERVE

The evaluation of vasomotor reserve in the cerebral circulation has served as an indirect method to evaluate the compensatory state of cerebral autoregulation. Normally, cerebral autoregulation preserves cerebral blood flow at a constant level between a mean arterial pressure of 50 to 150 mmHg.[33,34] This is accomplished by varying the resistance of the distal cerebral vasculature by vasoconstriction and vasodilation. As the blood pressure or cerebral perfusion pressure (CPP = systemic blood pressure − intracranial pressure) decreases, vasodilation of the distal regulating vessels lowers cerebrovascular resistance, maintaining constant CBF.

The distal cerebral vessels normally are very sensitive to the blood CO_2 concentration. They constrict in response to decreased CO_2 concentration (hyperventilation) and dilate in response to increased CO_2 concentration (CO_2 inhalation). When CPP decreases as a result of proximal arterial stenosis or occlusion, and the distal regulatory vessels become maximally dilated, they lose their responsiveness to CO_2. Diamox has also been used to effect distal cerebral vasodilation and probably works by a similar pH-dependent mechanism.[35] Lack of responsiveness to CO_2 or to Diamox can be used to indicate reduced CPP in the middle cerebral arteries due to the effects of proximal occlusive disease.

Several methods have been used to evaluate CO_2 reactivity.[133] Xenon has been used to measure CBF changes directly in response to CO_2 changes. Single photon emission tomography (SPECT) has been used for measuring regional differences in increased CBF induced by CO_2.[35] The use of TCD to measure vasoreactivity is based on its ability to measure relative changes in blood flow through the inflow vessels (MCAs) in response to changes in CO_2 concentration or to Diamox. The diameter of the MCA remains relatively constant during changes in CO_2 concentration.[36,37] Therefore, changes in velocity from baseline level correlate closely to relative changes in blood flow through that artery.[35,38] An important distinction between TCD and indicator methods is that TCD measures these responses in the MCA perfusion territory. This territory may become smaller in occlusive disease if the leptomeningeal collateral vessels provide increased perfusion to the cerebral hemisphere from the ACA and PCA.

The total percentage change in velocity between baseline and CO_2 inhalation and baseline and hyperventilation has been termed "vasomotor reactivity."[8] Ringelstein and coworkers,[8,31] have established normal values in a group of volunteers (age 20 to 75 years) for vasomotor reactivity in the MCA distribution. An average maximum increase in velocity of 52.5 percent with CO_2 inhalation and a decrease of 35.3 percent with hyperventilation was found, yielding an average vasomotor reactivity (VMR) of 87.8 percent. Figure 12-6 illustrates CO_2 reactivity testing using simultaneous bilateral monitoring of both MCAs. In a group of patients with carotid occlusions, VMR was significantly reduced in the ipsilateral MCA in 40 cases of unilateral occlusion. In 15 cases with bilateral occlusions, VMR was severely reduced on both sides. All patients with low-flow infarctions on CT ($n=5$), chronic ischemic ophthalmopathy ($n=2$), or repeated hypostatic TIAs ($n=2$) had VMR measurements of less than 38 percent.[8] The VMR present in patients with carotid occlusions is highly dependent on the configuration of the circle of Willis. In a group of 64 patients with carotid occlusions, Ringelstein

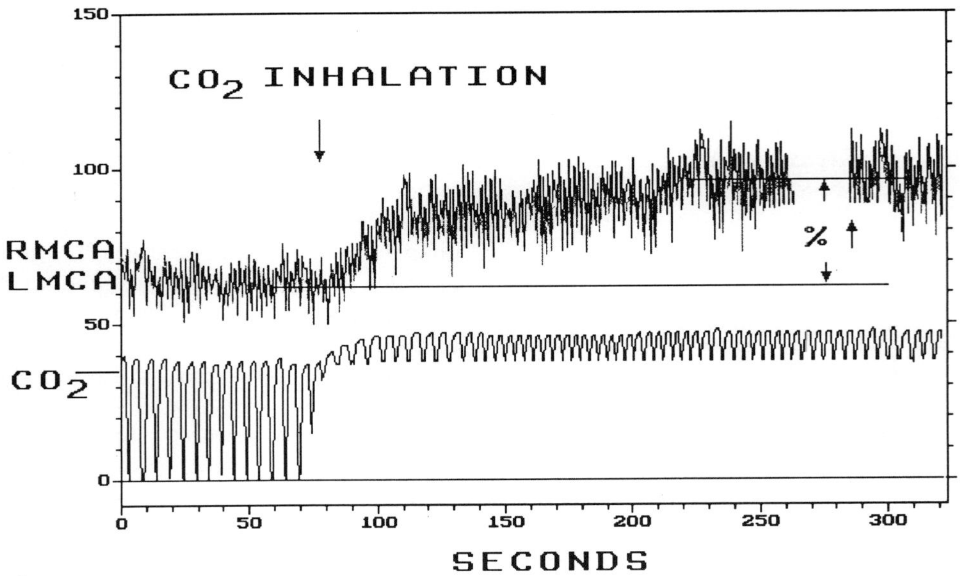

A

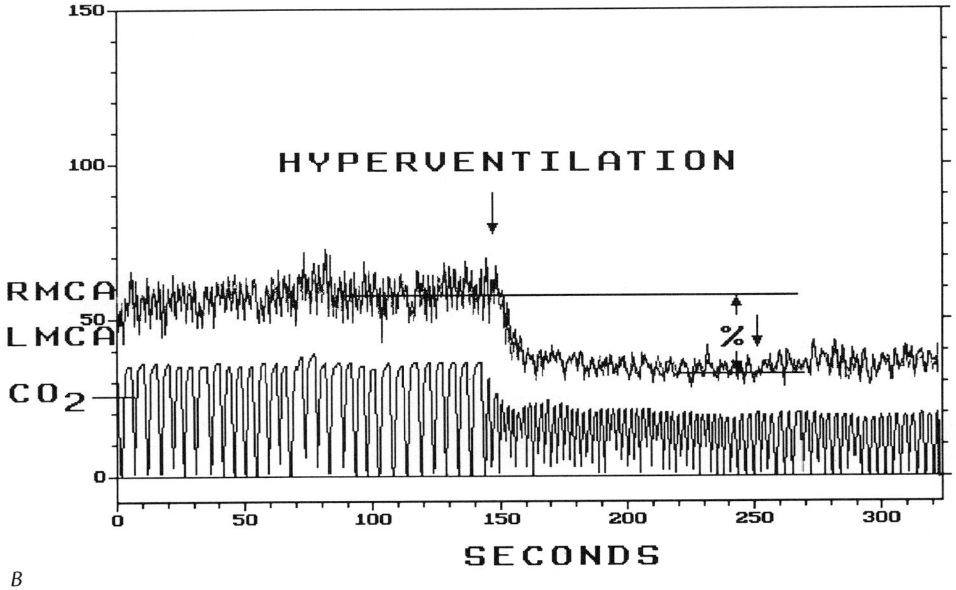

B

Figure 12-6. Blood flow velocity tracings illustrating normal and abnormal CO_2 reactivity. Continuous recordings are made from the middle cerebral arteries bilaterally and the patient is instructed to inhale 6 percent CO_2. Following this, the patient is instructed to hyperventilate. The percentage increase of flow velocity with CO_2 inhalation (*A*) and percentage decrease with hyperventilation (*B*) are used to indicate the cerebrovascular vasomotor reactivity. As the perfusion pressure to the cerebral circulation is decreased by extracranial or intracranial occlusive disease, the cerebral vasomotor reactivity becomes reduced. *C* and *D* indicate exhausted vasomotor reactivity on the left side with intact vasomotor reactivity on the right in a patient with an intracranial carotid occlusion. *LMCA* = left middle cerebral artery; *RMCA* = right middle cerebral artery.

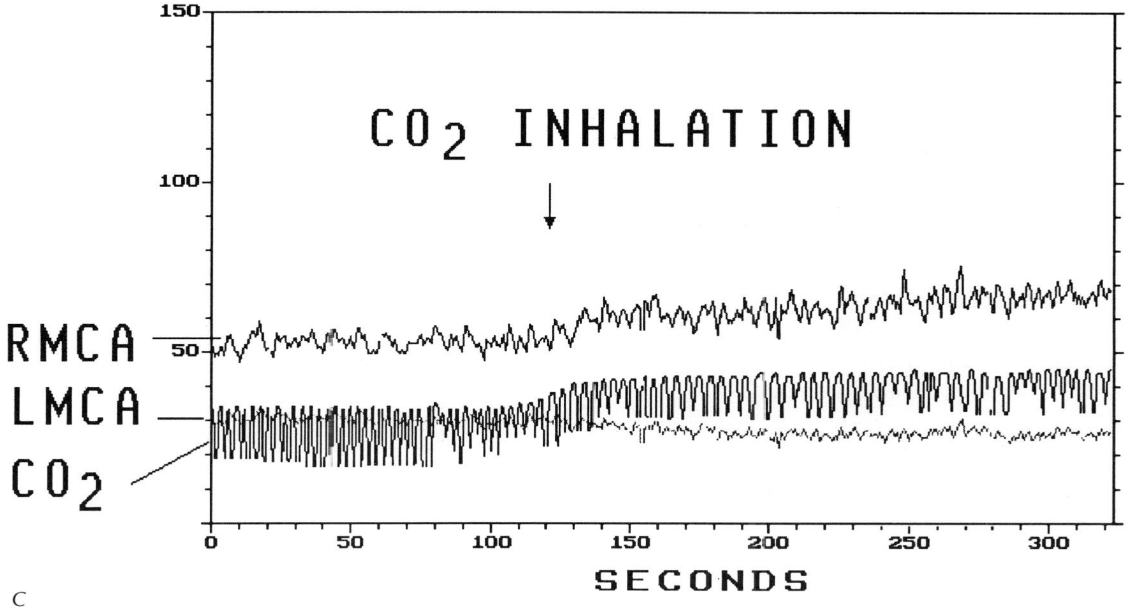

C

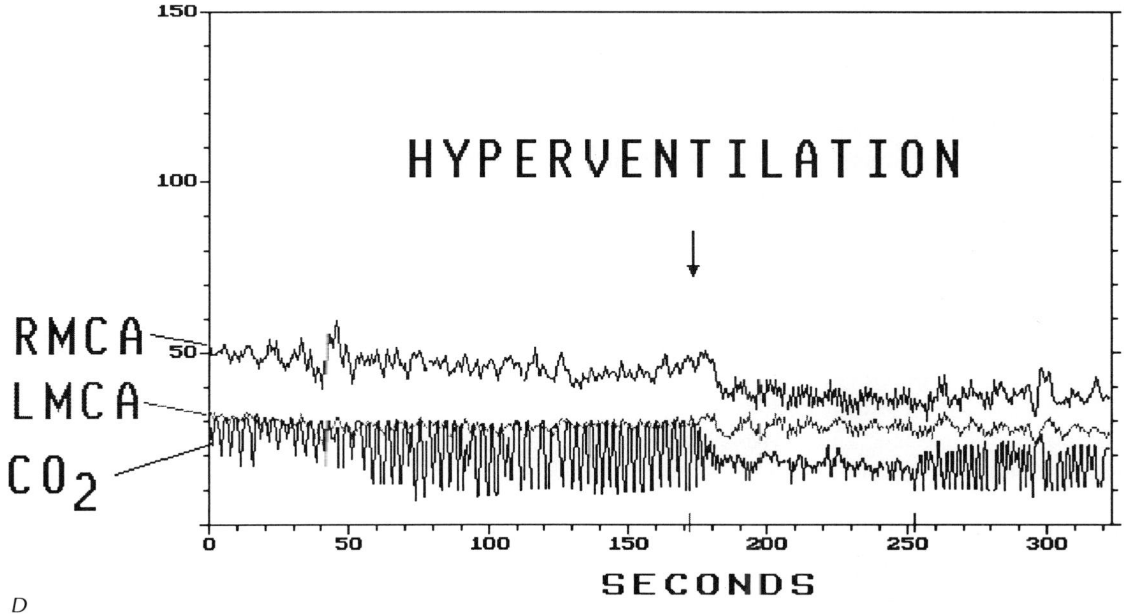

D

Figure 12-6. (*Continued*)

and coworkers[8] found a significantly reduced VMR in those with inadequate collateral vessels in the circle of Willis as compared to the subgroup with a normal circle.

Testing of VMR using TCD can provide valuable physiologic information about individual patients with extracranial occlusive disease or combinations of intracranial and extracranial occlusive disease. This information may be very helpful in establishing effective therapy, especially in patients who have recurrent transient ischemic events or repeated strokes. A carotid occlusion may have a benign natural history in patients who can maintain an adequate hemodynamic reserve through an intact circle of Willis. Other patients with the same lesion may have no hemodynamic reserve owing to inadequate collaterals and may be prone to repeated TIAs or strokes on a hemodynamic basis.

Kleiser and Widder[39] recently reported the results of a study of the natural history of patients with unilateral carotid occlusions who had VMR testing. In a group of 86 patients with unilateral carotid occlusion, 11 patients had exhausted VMR. This subgroup had a high ipsilateral stroke rate (17 percent per year over three years) compared with an ipsilateral stroke rate of 3 percent per year for the entire group (which is comparable to previously published series). Therefore, it appears possible by VMR testing to identify patients with poor hemodynamic reserve who have a high stroke risk and who may benefit from medical or surgical therapy to improve cerebral perfusion.

CEREBRAL AUTOREGULATION

Cerebral autoregulation refers to the ability of the brain to maintain constant cerebral blood flow despite changes in cerebral perfusion pressure. Lassen documented this phenomenon in humans by measuring CBF at different blood pressures and established that CBF was relatively constant in the normal physiologic range of blood pressures.[33] Below a mean arterial pressure of 50 mmHg CBF begins to fall with further reductions in pressure. The methodology for determining cerebral autoregulation in the past was cumbersome and invasive, requiring radioisotopes for CBF measurement and vasoactive medication to change the blood pressure. It is primarily because of the impracticality of autoregulation measurements and the ease of CO_2 reactivity measurements that CO_2 reactivity has been more thoroughly investigated in cerebrovascular disease.

Transcranial Doppler can now be used to noninvasively determine autoregulation in the MCA perfusion territories. Aaslid and coworkers[4] have introduced a method in which blood pressure and MCA velocity are monitored noninvasively and the relative change in flow through the MCA in response to a rapid step change in arterial blood pressure is observed.[9] Large thigh cuffs are inflated to suprasystolic pressures and rapidly released to produce a transient drop in blood pressure. Initial reluctance to accept this methodology was based on criticisms[40] subsequently shown to be completely incorrect.[41,42] Recent com-

Figure 12-7. Autoregulation can be assessed with TCD by using the middle cerebral artery velocity as an index of relative change in blood flow in response to a transient drop in blood pressure. *A.* Unfiltered tracing of the arterial blood pressure and right and left middle cerebral artery velocity spectral outline tracings in a patient with no vasomotor reserve on the left side and normal vasomotor reserve on the right assessed by CO_2 reactivity. The results of the autoregulation testing indicate impairment in autoregulation on the left and intact autoregulation on the right. *B.* Filtered tracings of the same recording showing the rapid return of the right middle cerebral velocity to the baseline level 10 seconds after the blood pressure drop and no similar return of the middle cerebral velocity on the left side where the blood flow is pressure passive. *LMCA* = left middle cerebral artery; *RMCA* = right middle cerebral artery; *ABP* = arterial blood pressure.

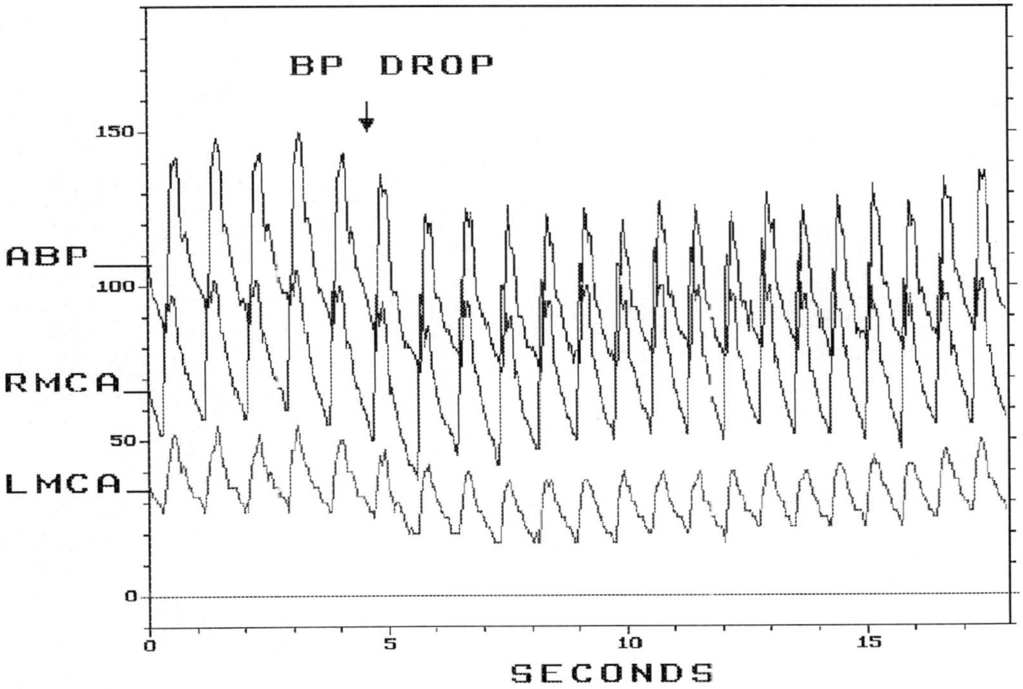

BP DROP
ABP
RMCA
LMCA
150
100
50
0
0
5
10
15
SECONDS

A

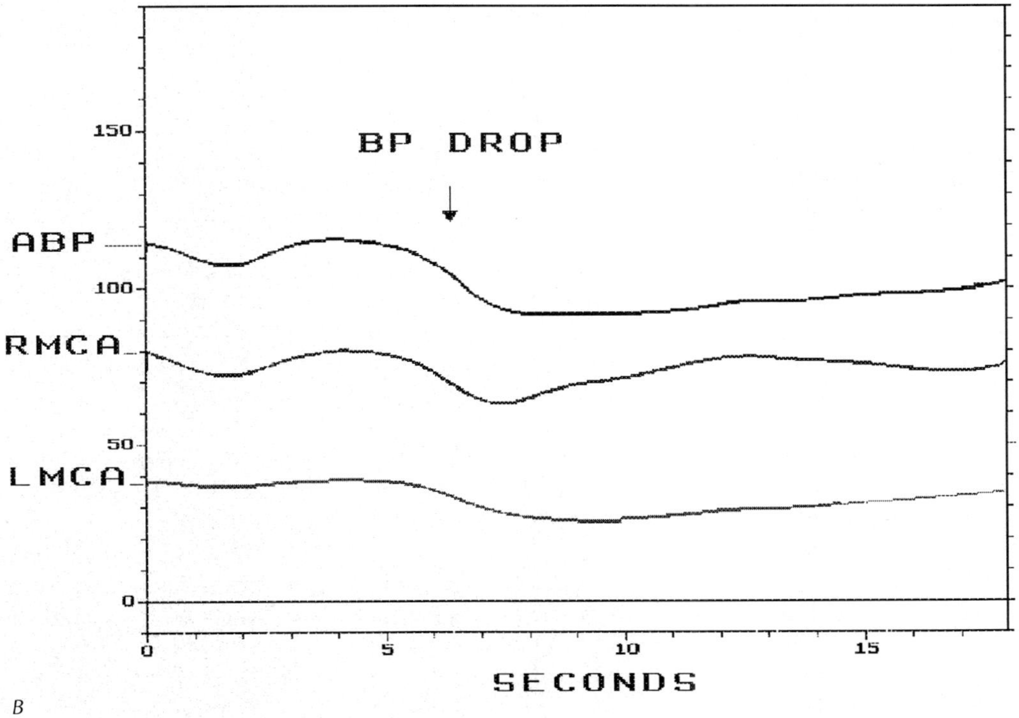

BP DROP
ABP
RMCA
LMCA
150
100
50
0
0
5
10
15
SECONDS

B

parisons between MCA velocity and internal carotid artery flow have confirmed the validity of this method.[42]

Preliminary clinical testing in patients with cerebrovascular occlusive disease indicates that cerebral autoregulation is absent in patients with severely impaired CO_2 reactivity (Fig. 12-7). Noninvasive testing of cerebral autoregulation using TCD may prove useful in the complete hemodynamic evaluation of patients with cerebrovascular occlusive disease.

INTRACRANIAL EMBOLI

Considerable interest has developed in the ability of TCD to detect intracranial microemboli passing through the basal cerebral vessels. Doppler ultrasound was first used to detect intravascular microemboli in the large vessels of animals exposed to decompression from hyperbaric air.[43] The first examination was performed using 5 MHz continuous wave ultrasound to produce audible, and later visual display signals. Ultrasound was utilized clinically to detect audible intravascular air microemboli during cardiac surgery[44] and during neurosurgical procedures.[45] Subsequent development of spectral analysis has allowed identification of embolic signatures in the spectral tracings (Fig. 12-8).

The ability of TCD to detect intra-arterial microemboli was first recognized by monitoring the MCA velocity during carotid endarterectomy (CEA) and open heart surgery.[46–49] Microemboli composed of air were identified following crossclamp release during CEA and heart operations. However, similar embolic signals were recognized during arterial dissection for CEA before the artery was entered. These microemboli also have been seen in patients with atrial fibrillation and prosthetic heart valves and are now recognized to be composed of formed elements.[11] In vivo animal experiments have confirmed the ability of Doppler ultrasound to detect microparticles

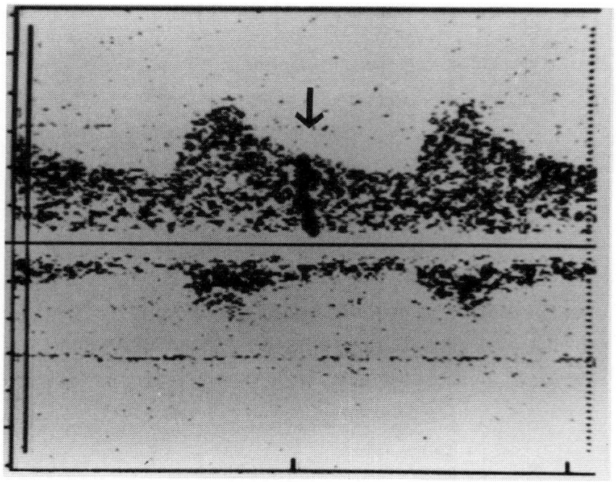

Figure 12-8. Spectral analysis tracing of intracranial arterial microembolus. The intermittent high frequency sound heard on the audio monitor is reflected in the spectral tracing as a discrete high-density signal (*arrow*).

composed of fat, platelet-rich thrombi, clotted blood, atheromatous materials, and air.[50,51]

Clinical evaluations of intracranial as well as extracranial microemboli detection have recently been described. Intracranial microemboli have been detected in patients with atrial fibrillation,[52] prosthetic heart valves,[53] carotid stenosis,[13] fibromuscular dysplasia, arterial dissection, intracranial stenosis,[54] and during such invasive procedures as angiography,[55,56] cerebrovascular and heart surgery.[46,49] Monitoring for intracranial air microemboli after venous injection also has been useful in identifying patients with cardiac and pulmonary defects causing right-to-left circulation shunts.[57]

Most microemboli do not cause overt symptoms. However, multiple microemboli have been associated with impaired neuropsychologic function following open heart surgery.[58] The clinical utility of intracranial emboli monitoring has not yet been fully established. It may serve a useful role in identifying patients at high risk for a poor outcome following stroke,[59] identifying the site of active embolization in the arterial system in patients with TIAs,[54] and distinguishing embolic versus hemodynamic causes of stroke and TIAs.[13]

CLINICAL UTILITY OF TCD IN OCCLUSIVE DISEASE

As with any new diagnostic tool that provides information about a particular disease process not previously obtainable, the clinical utility of TCD needs to be established. Part of this process involves the collection of data on new elements of pathophysiology revealed by this technique. It also requires categorizing patients, based on pathophysiology, into new subgroups that may have a different natural history. Studies using this approach are beginning to emerge.[8,39,59] The ability of TCD to disclose new information about patients with occlusive cerebrovascular disease can enable rational treatments and strategies for management. Several cases illustrating these principles follow.

Case 1 A 65-year-old male with a history of cerebrovascular disease complained of feeling faint upon turning his head to the right. TCD examination of the proximal PCAs revealed normal velocities in a neutral position; however, upon head turning, symptoms were elicited and a marked diminution in the velocity tracings was seen. Upon return to a neutral position, the velocity in both PCAs was increased above the baseline (hyperemia), indicating the occurrence of ischemia (Fig. 12-9). Cerebral angiography revealed an inadequate anterior-to-posterior communication through the circle of Willis (Fig. 12-5*E*) and an occluded left vertebral artery. The right vertebral artery became compressed on head turning owing to cervical spondylosis.

Case 2 A 35-year-old female presented to the hospital in status epilepticus. Work-up revealed an acute right frontal infarction on MRI. Carotid duplex examination was normal. TCD examination revealed normal velocities in the intracranial vessels; however, frequent emboli were seen in the right MCA. Cerebral angiography demonstrated fibromuscular dysplasia in the high right cervical ICA beyond the range of carotid duplex. The patient was placed on aspirin and had no further symptoms. Emboli monitoring two weeks later, showed no emboli.

Case 3 A middle-aged male presented with persistent TIAs following carotid endarterectomy. A CEA had been performed at another institution for TIAs in the hemisphere ipsilateral to a carotid stenosis identified by duplex scanning alone. Postoperatively, the patient continued to have TIAs, and TCD examination revealed emboli in the MCA ipsilateral to the surgery. No emboli were found in the ICA distal to the endarterectomy site. Cerebral angiography revealed resolution of the carotid stenosis and demonstrated an ipsilateral carotid siphon stenosis, presumed to be the source of the emboli. The patient was placed on anticoagulation therapy and the symptoms resolved.

Case 4 A 53-year-old male was referred with TIAs related to the right hemisphere that were unresponsive to aspirin therapy. A 90 percent stenosis of the right supraclinoid ICA was found, and he was considered for angioplasty. TCD studies revealed normal vasomotor reactivity in both hemispheres with good left-to-right collateral crossover. Emboli were detected in the right MCA. The patient was placed on anticoagulation and had one more TIA, followed by resolution of his symptoms. He was able to avoid angioplasty since he was well compensated hemodynamically above the lesion.

Case 5 A 30-year-old female had a stroke with onset of aphasia; then her symptoms resolved over one month. She then began having TIAs consisting of right hand numbness and clumsiness four to five times per week for several months, despite aspirin, Persantin, and Ticlopidine therapy. TCD examination revealed a low velocity in the left MCA with no emboli detected. Testing of VMR and autoregulation revealed absent VMR in the left MCA and normal VMR in the right MCA. Autoregulation was similarly absent in the left MCA and normal on the right. MRI showed a small infarct in a watershed zone between the left MCA and ACA distributions. The patient went on to have an extra-

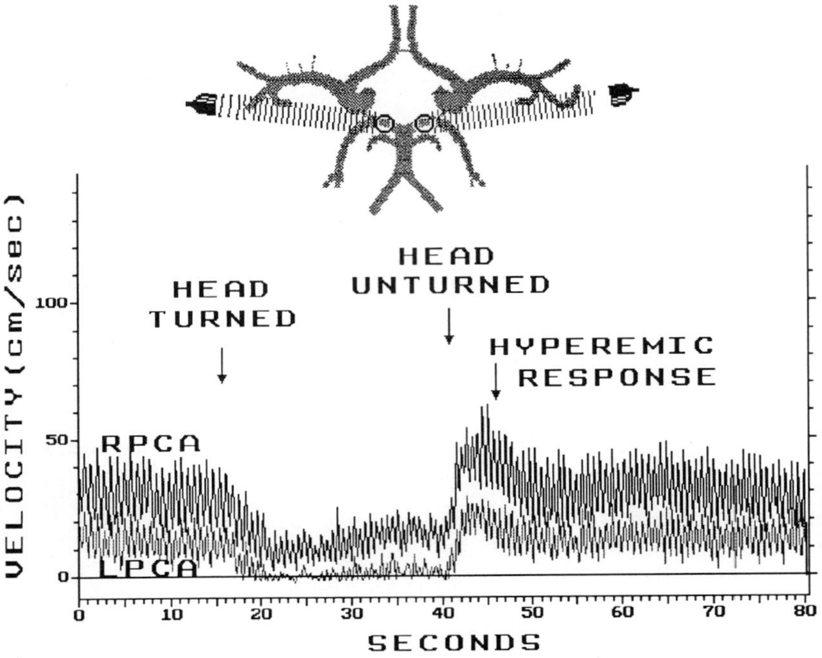
HEAD
TURNED
HEAD
UNTURNED
HYPEREMIC
RESPONSE
RPCA
LPCA
VELOCITY (cm/sec)
100
50
0
0
10
20
30
40
50
60
70
80
SECONDS

A

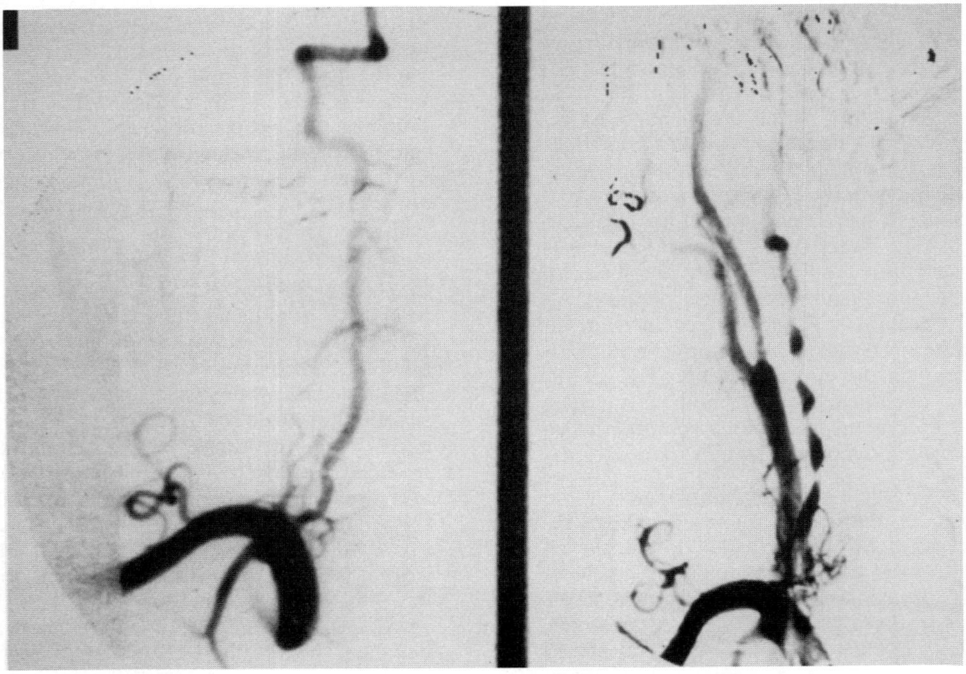

B

cranial to intracranial bypass procedure for presumed hemodynamic TIAs.

Case 6 A 69-year-old male was well until he had a stroke manifesting as a left hemiparesis and dysarthria. He recovered completely but had a subsequent TIA. An angiogram revealed a right internal carotid artery occlusion with retrograde flow through the ophthalmic artery and minimal forward flow through a small right posterior communicating artery. There was no filling of the right MCA from the left carotid system. His circle of Willis resembled that seen in Fig. 12-5*D*. VMR testing revealed severely reduced VMR on the right. He subsequently had a gastrointestinal bleed with hypotension and developed a new stroke manifested as a severe left hemiparesis. He has made a partial recovery. His CT scan is illustrated in Fig. 12-10. He is now being considered for a revascularization procedure.

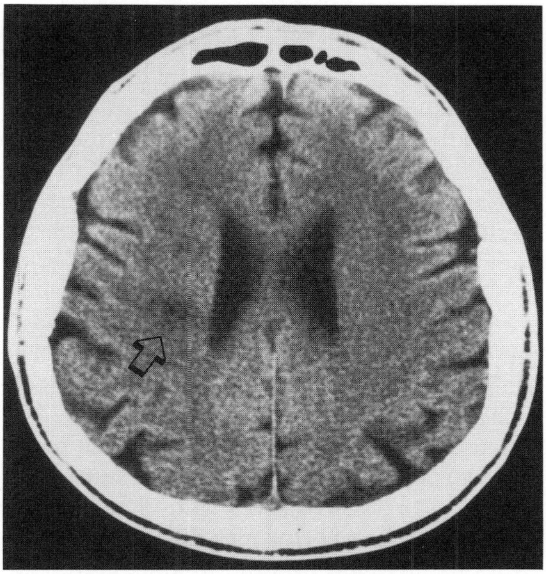

Figure 12-10. This is a typical low flow infarct (*arrow*) seen in the right hemisphere of a patient with severely impaired hemodynamic reserve on VMR testing (Case 6) and inadequate collateral pathways through the circle of Willis.

MONITORING DURING CAROTID ENDARTERECTOMY

Transcranial Doppler has been used to continuously monitor the blood flow velocity in the MCA trunk during carotid endarterectomy.[59–63] This can be accomplished using a head band or other probe fixation device to attach the probe to the temporal window ipsilateral to the endarterectomy site. Important technical considerations are to be sure that the MCA is the artery being monitored and to devise a system of probe fixation that will not be disturbed during the operative procedure. One drawback of this type of monitoring is that it cannot be used in a small percentage of patients because of temporal hyperostosis. In one recent series, temporal hyperostosis prevented adequate monitoring in 13 percent of 150 carotid endarterectomies.[60]

Intraoperative TCD monitoring can provide information that may be used to avoid surgical complications. Four aspects of TCD monitoring can be of value during carotid endarterectomy: (1) the ability to detect emboli; (2) detection of hypoperfusion during cross-clamping; (3) detection of postoperative thrombosis; and (4) detection of postoperative hyperperfusion. The detection of emboli during endarterectomy was first recognized when loud high frequency signals were heard on the audio output and high density spectral signals were seen

Figure 12-9. *A.* This tracing demonstrates monitoring of both posterior cerebral arteries in a patient with symptoms of cerebrovascular insufficiency on head turning. The velocity tracings diminished markedly with head turning and increased upon return to a neutral position, indicating proximal obstruction. Subsequent cerebral angiography revealed occlusion of the left vertebral artery, compression of the right vertebral artery due to cervical spondylosis, and absent anterior to posterior collateral pathways as seen in Fig. 12-5E. *B.* Angiogram showing vertebral artery in neutral position (left) and with head turned (right). LPCA = left posterior cerebral artery; RPCA = right posterior cerebral artery.

on TCD during cross clamp release. It was assumed that most of these signals represented air entrained in the arterial circulation and had no particular clinical significance. It has subsequently been recognized that formed element emboli were passing into the MCA during dissection of the carotid artery before the circulation was entered. Sporadic emboli are commonly seen after closure of the arteriotomy. However, large numbers of emboli increasing in frequency after the completion of the endarterectomy may alert the surgeon to the possibility of an intimal flap or other technical problems.

The assessment of adequate cerebral perfusion during carotid cross clamping has been a subject of extensive investigation and debate among surgeons performing CEA. Past investigations have led to a more complete understanding of cerebral physiology during carotid cross clamping, and several facts have become clear. The threshold for cerebral infarction depends on both the severity and the duration of cerebral ischemia. Therefore, if the cross clamp time is brief enough, even those patients with severe hypoperfusion may not sustain infarction, whereas patients with prolonged moderate hypoperfusion may sustain permanent infarction. Most patients do not sustain severe hypoperfusion during carotid cross clamping because they are protected by intact collateral pathways from the posterior circulation and from the contralateral carotid circulation. Schneider et al. evaluated these collateral pathways in 50 patients prior to undergoing CEA.[61] During cross-clamping, significantly higher MCA velocities and stump pressures were maintained in those patients who had intact collateral pathways, compared with patients with impaired or absent collateral pathways. There were also fewer ischemic changes on electroencephalography (EEG) in the group with intact collateral pathways.

The goal of the surgeon performing CEA is to avoid cerebral hypoperfusion during cross clamping and also to avoid other complications that can occur during shunt placement. A reasonable strategy utilized by many surgeons is to shunt selectively by only shunting those patients who have hypoperfusion during cross clamping. TCD can be used to monitor the changes in MCA velocity that occur during carotid cross clamping to identify those patients with hypoperfusion. The most useful method for doing this has been to calculate the percentage drop in MCA velocity from a stable baseline preceding the cross clamp maneuver.

Halsey et al. compared regional CBF, TCD, and EEG during CEA.[62] There was a high degree of variability between the changes in blood flow velocity on TCD and changes in CBF. It was concluded that TCD may be a better indicator of flow in the basal vessels supplying the deeper areas of the brain while CBF may be a better indicator of cortical perfusion. Spencer et al. compared MCA velocity changes to carotid stump pressures in response to cross clamping.[63] An exponential curve was established between the two measurements, with the velocity reaching zero at a stump pressure of 15 mmHg. After allowing 10 to 15 seconds following clamping for an autoregulatory adjustment, the percentage decrease in MCA velocity from the baseline was calculated. It was found that an MCA velocity value of 40 percent of the baseline corresponded to a stump pressure of approximately 25 mmHg. In this study, all hypoperfusion-related complications occurred when the MCA velocity fell below 40 percent of the baseline figure.

Halsey has reported the results of a multicenter study using TCD monitoring during CEA.[64] In this large group of patients, shunts were used routinely in some and selectively in others. If the MCA velocity during cross-clamping fell below 15 percent of the baseline value, there was a significantly higher stroke rate in patients who were not shunted. If the velocity in the MCA remained above 40 percent of the baseline, there was a higher stroke rate in patients who were shunted. The difference in stroke rate between shunted and nonshunted patients was not significantly different if the MCA velocity dropped between 16 and 40 percent of baseline. Each individual surgeon must determine how they will use the information gained from monitoring for hypoperfusion using TCD. However, intraoperative monitoring with TCD may give useful information regarding the level of residual perfusion through the MCA, which can aid the surgeon in the decision making process.

Monitoring of the MCA velocity during CEA may allow the early detection of two other potential complications: postoperative carotid thrombosis and postoperative hyperperfusion. To gain the maximum information from TCD monitoring, the monitoring should continue during the early postoperative period or longer if these complications are suspected. A sudden decrease in MCA velocity in the postoperative period to those levels seen during cross clamping can provide an early warning of postoperative carotid occlusion. Postoperative hyperperfusion is a dangerous complication which is associated with headaches and cerebral edema ipsilateral to the endarterectomy, and may result in intracerebral hemorrhage (Chap. 26).[60,65,66] Steiger detected a more than 100 percent increase in MCA flow velocity compared to preoperative values in eight out of a series of 150 cases.[60] These findings were associated with severe headaches in these eight patients. Ackerstaff et al. reported an average increase in MCA velocity of greater than 150 percent over baseline in four patients who had postoperative intracerebral hemorrhages from a group of 250 carotid endarterectomies.[65] This velocity value was significantly higher than the value in patients who did not sustain intracerebral hemorrhages.

The success of carotid endarterectomy in preventing strokes and TIAs in large populations is highly dependent on maintaining a low complication rate. Monitoring of MCA velocities using TCD may provide additional information that can be used to achieve the lowest complication rate possible.

CONCLUSIONS

Transcranial Doppler can provide the clinician with information about the pathophysiology of individual patients with cerebrovascular disease not previously obtainable with noninvasive techniques. When properly used, TCD can reliably detect intracranial arterial stenosis as well as evaluate the distal effects of proximal arterial lesions. Hemodynamic effects of extracranial and intracranial vascular disease can be assessed using VMR testing, and autoregulation testing may provide additional information. Natural history studies are emerging which indicate a poor prognosis in untreated patients with absent hemodynamic reserve.[39] The importance of understanding the collateral capacity of each individual patient rather than classifying patients strictly according to arterial lesions is now being recognized. TCD should not be considered as an indirect test to evaluate the pressure drop across a carotid stenosis,[67] but rather as a direct test to evaluate the hemodynamic consequences of all the arterial lesions and the individual collateral capacity on the cerebral arteries distal to the circle of Willis. The use of TCD for detection of cerebral microemboli in patients with TIA and stroke holds promise to provide a better understanding of the pathophysiology of these conditions that may lead to more rational, physiologically based treatments.

REFERENCES

1. Aaslid R, Markwalder T-M, Nornes H: Noninvasive transcranial Doppler ultrasound re-

cording of flow velocity in basal cerebral arteries. *J Neurosurg* 57:769–774, 1982.
2. Satomura S, Kaneko Z: Ultrasonic blood rheograph. *Proc 3rd Int Conf on Medical Electronics* 254–258, 1960.
3. Kaneko Z: First steps in the development of the Doppler flowmeter. *Ultrasound Med Biol* 12:1877–195, 1986.
4. Aaslid R: Developments and principles of transcranial Doppler, in Newell DW, Aaslid R, (eds): *Transcranial Doppler.* New York, Raven, chap 1, pp 1–8, 1992.
5. Fujioka KA, Douville CM: Anatomy and freehand examination techniques, in Newell DW, Aaslid R, (eds): *Transcranial Doppler.* New York, Raven, chap 2, pp 9–31, 1992.
6. Seiler RW, Newell DW: Subarachnoid hemorrhage and vasospasm, in Newell DW, Aaslid R (eds): *Transcranial Doppler.* New York, Raven, chap 9, pp 101–107.
7. Lindegaard K-F: Intracranial artery stenosis, in Newell DW, Aaslid R (eds): *Transcranial Doppler.* New York, Raven, chap 15, pp 161–166, 1992.
8. Ringelstein ER, Otis SM: Physiological testing of vasomotor reserve, in Newell DW, Aaslid R, (eds): *Transcranial Doppler.* New York, Raven, chap 8, pp 83–99.
9. Aaslid R, Lindegaard K-F, Sorteberg W, Nornes H: Cerebral autoregulation dynamics in humans. *Stroke* 20:45–52, 1989.
10. Aaslid R: Visually evoked dynamic blood flow response of the human cerebral circulation. *Stroke* 20:1005–1011, 1989.
11. Spencer MP: Detection of cerebral arterial emboli, in Newell DW, Aaslid R, (eds): *Transcranial Doppler.* New York, Raven, chap 19, pp 215–230, 1992.
12. Russell D: The detection of cerebral emboli using Doppler ultrasound, in Newell DW, Aaslid R, (eds): *Transcranial Doppler.* New York, Raven, chap 18, pp 207–213, 1992.
13. Siebler M, Sitzer M, Steinmetz H: Detection of intracranial emboli in patients with symptomatic extracranial carotid artery disease. *Stroke* 23:1652–1654, 1992.
14. Grolimund P: Transmission of ultrasound through the temporal bone, in Aaslid R (ed), *Transcranial Doppler Sonography.* New York, Springer-Verlag, 1986, pp 10–21.
15. Katz ML, Whisler GD: Examination using transcranial Doppler mapping, in Newell DW, Aaslid R, (eds): *Transcranial Doppler.* New York, Raven, chap 3, pp 33–39, 1992.
16. Bogdahn U, Becker G, Winkler J, et al: The transcranial color-coded real-time sonography in adults. *Stroke* 21:1680–1688, 1990.
17. Becker G, Greiner K, Kaune B, et al: Diagnosis and monitoring of subarachnoid hemorrhage by transcranial color-coded real-time sonography. *Neurosurgery* 28:814–820, 1991.
18. Schoning M, Walter J: Evaluation of the vertebrobasilar-posterior system by transcranial color duplex sonography in adults. *Stroke* 23:1280–1286, 1992.
19. Lindegaard KF, Bakke SJ, Aaslid R, Nornes H: Doppler diagnosis of intracranial artery occlusive disorders. *J Neurol Neurosurg Psychiatry* 49(5):510–518, 1986.
20. Ley-Pozo J, Ringelstein EB: Noninvasive detection of occlusive disease of the carotid siphon and middle cerebral artery. *Ann Neurol* 26:640–647, 1990.
21. von Reutern GM, Budingen HJ: Ultraschalldiagnostik der hirnversorgenden arterieu. Stuttgart, Thieme, 1989, pp 260–279.
22. Mattle H, Grolimund P, Huber P, et al: Transcranial Doppler sonographic findings in the middle cerebral artery disease. *Arch Neurol* 45(3):289–295, 1988.
23. de Bray JM, Joseph PA, Jeanvoine H, et al: Transcranial Doppler evaluation of middle cerebral artery stenosis. *J Ultrasound Med* 7(11): 611–616, 1988.
24. Spencer MP, Whisler D: Transorbital Doppler diagnosis of intracranial arterial stenosis. *Stroke* 17:916–921, 1986.
25. Call GK, Fleming MC, Sealfon S, et al: Reversible cerebral segmental vasoconstriction. *Stroke* 19(9):1159–1170, 1988.
26. Toole JF: Middle cerebral artery stenosis—a neglected problem? *Surg Neurol* 7(1):44–46, 1987.
27. Adams RJ, McKie V, Nichols F, et al: The use of transcranial ultrasonography to predict stroke in sickle cell disease. *N Engl J Med* 326:605–610, 1992.
28. Bogousslavsky J, Barnett HJM, Fox AJ, et al: Atherosclerotic disease of the middle cerebral artery. *Stroke* 17:1112–1120, 1986.

29. Leung SY, Ng THK, Yuen ST, et al: Pattern of cerebral atherosclerosis in Hong Kong Chinese. *Stroke* 24:779–786, 1993.
30. Schneider PA, Rossman ME, Bernstein EF, et al: Effect of internal carotid occlusion on intracranial hemodynamics. *Stroke* 19:589–593, 1988.
31. Ringelstein EB, Sievers C, Ecker S, et al: Noninvasive assessment of CO_2-induced cerebral vasomotor response in normal individuals and patients with internal carotid artery occlusions. *Stroke* 19:963–969, 1988.
32. Padget DH: The circle of Willis: Its embryology and anatomy, in Dandy WE (ed), *Intracranial Arterial Aneurysms*. New York, Comstock, 1944, pp 67–90.
33. Lassen NA: Cerebral blood flow and oxygen consumption in man. *Physiol Rev* 39:183–238, 1959.
34. Strandgaard S, Paulson OB: Cerebral autoregulation. *Stroke* 15(3):413–416, 1984.
35. Sorteberg W: Cerebral artery blood velocity and cerebral blood flow, in Newell DW, Aaslid R, (eds): *Transcranial Doppler.* New York, Raven, chap 6, pp 57–66, 1992.
36. Huber P, Haneda J: Effect of contrast material, hypercapnia, hyperventilation, hypertonic glucose and papaverine on the diameter of the cerebral arteries—angiographic determination in man. *Invest Radiol* 2:17–32, 1967.
37. Giller CA, Bowman G, Dyer H, et al: Cerebral arterial diameters during changes in blood pressure and carbon dioxide during craniotomy. *Neurosurgery* 32:737–742, 1993.
38. Bishop CC, Powell S, Rutt D, Browse NL: Transcranial Doppler measurement of middle cerebral artery blood flow velocity: A validation study. *Stroke* 17(5):913–915, 1986.
39. Kleiser B, Widder B: Course of carotid artery occlusions with impaired cerebrovascular reactivity. *Stroke* 23:171–174, 1992.
40. Kontos HA: Validity of cerebral arterial blood flow calculations from velocity measurements. *Stroke* 20:1–3, 1989.
41. Aaslid R, Newell DW, Stooss R, et al: Simultaneous arterial and venous transcranial Doppler assessment of cerebral autoregulation dynamics. *Stroke* 22:1148–1154, 1991.
42. Newell DW, Aaslid R, Lam A, et al: Comparison of flow and velocity during dynamic autoregulation testing in humans. *Stroke* 25:793–797, 1994.
43. Spencer MP, Campbell SD: Development of bubbles in venous and arterial blood during hyperbaric decompression. *Bull Mason Clin* 22(1):26–32, 1968.
44. Spencer MP, Lawrence GH, Thomas GI, Sauvage LR: The use of ultrasonics in the determination of arterial aeroembolism during open-heart surgery. *Ann Thorac Surg* 8(6):489–497, 1969.
45. Maroon JC, Albin MS: Air embolism by Doppler ultrasound. *Anes Analg* 3:399–402, 1974.
46. Padayachee TS, Parsons S, Theobold R: The detection of microemboli in the middle cerebral artery during cardiopulmonary bypass: A transcranial Doppler ultrasound investigation using membrane and bubble oxygenation. *Ann Thorac Surg* 44:298–302, 1987.
47. Harrison MJG, Pugsley W, Newman S, et al: Detection of middle cerebral emboli during coronary artery bypass surgery using transcranial Doppler sonography. *Stroke* 21(10):1512, 1990.
48. Albin MS, Hantler CB, Bunegin BS, et al: Intracranial air embolism is detected by the transcranial Doppler (TCD) during cardiopulmonary bypass procedures. *J Neurosurg Anesth* 2:223, 1990.
49. Spencer MP, Thomas GI, Nicholls SC, Sauvage LR: Detection of middle cerebral artery emboli during carotid endarterectomy using transcranial Doppler ultrasonography. *Stroke* 21:415–423, 1990.
50. Russell D, Madden KP, Clark WM, et al: Detection of arterial emboli using ultrasound in rabbits. *Stroke* 22:253–258, 1991.
51. Markus HS, Brown MM: Differentiation between different pathological cerebral embolic materials using transcranial Doppler in an in vitro model. *Stroke* 24:1–5, 1993.
52. Tegeler CH, Hitchings LP, Eicke M, et al: Microemboli detection in stroke associated with atrial fibrillation. *J Cardiovasc Tech* 9:283–284A, 1990.
53. Berger M, Davis D, Lolley D, et al: Detection of subclinical microemboli in patients with prosthetic aortic valves. *J Cardiovasc Tech* 9:282–283A, 1990.
54. Lash SR, Newell DW, Mayberg M, et al: Artery-to-artery cerebral emboli detection with

transcranial Doppler: Analysis of eight cases. *J Stroke Cerebrovasc Dis* 3:15–22, 1993.
55. Markus H, Loh A, Israel D, et al: Microscopic air embolism during cerebral angiography and strategies for its avoidance. *Lancet* 342:784–787, 1993.
56. Donnan GA: Cerebral angiography. *Lancet* 341:796, 1993.
57. Di Tullio M, Socco RL, Venketasubramanian N, et al: Comparison of diagnostic techniques for the detection of a patent foramen ovale in stroke patients. *Stroke* 24:1020–1024, 1993.
58. Stump DA, Tegeler CH, Rogers AT, et al: Neuropsychological deficits are associated with the number of emboli detected during cardiac surgery. *Stroke* (in press) 1994.
59. Tegeler CH, Burke GL, Dalley GM, Stump DA: Carotid emboli predict poor outcome in stroke. *Stroke* 24:98A, 1993.
60. Steiger HJ: Monitoring for carotid surgery in Newell DW, Aaslid R, (eds) *Transcranial Doppler.* New York, Raven, chap 17, pp 197–205, 1992.
61. Schneider PA, Ringelstein EB, Rossman ME, et al: Importance of cerebral collateral pathways during carotid endarterectomy. *Stroke* 19:1328–1334, 1988.
62. Halsey JH, McDowell HA, Gelman S: Transcranial Doppler and rCBF compared in carotid endarterectomy. *Stroke* 17:1206–1208, 1986.
63. Spencer MP, Thomas GI, Mochring MA: Relation between middle cerebral artery blood flow velocity and stump pressure during carotid endarterectomy. *Stroke* 23:1439–1445, 1992.
64. Halsey JH Jr: Risks and benefits of shunting in carotid endarterectomy. *Stroke* 23:1583–1587, 1992.
65. Ackerstaff RGA, Jansen C, Noll FL, et al: The significance of intra-operative TCD monitoring to predict intracerebral hemorrhage after carotid endarterectomy. *Stroke* 24:500A, 1993.
66. Powers AD, Smith RR: Hyperfusion syndrome after carotid endarterectomy: a transcranial Doppler evaluation. *Neurosurgery* 26:56–60, 1990.
67. Cantelmo NL, Babikian VL, Johnson WC, et al: Correlation of transcranial Doppler and noninvasive tests with angiography in the evaluation of extracranial carotid disease. *J Vasc Surg* 11:786–792, 1990.

13

Computed Tomography and Magnetic Resonance Imaging

Richard R. Keen
William H. Pearce

Imaging of the central nervous system has undergone remarkable changes since the surgical treatment of cerebrovascular disease began 40 years ago. Today, the management of patients with cerebrovascular disease is integrally dependent on both established and evolving applications of computed tomography (CT) and magnetic resonance imaging (MRI).

The care of patients with neurologic manifestations of cerebrovascular disease was revolutionized in 1973 by the introduction of cerebral CT by Godfrey Hounsfield[1] and MRI by Paul Lauterbur.[2] CT and MRI now have well-established roles in the diagnosis and management of cerebrovascular disease. Currently, CT and MRI can confirm the diagnosis of stroke and determine the presence of intracranial hemorrhage. CT and MRI also define the anatomic extent of both acute and chronic infarcts. The results of cerebral CT and MRI guide the timing of subsequent diagnostic and therapeutic interventions. Determination of the optimal time to perform cerebral angiography and carotid endarterectomy in patients with significant, symptomatic cerebrovascular disease often is based on both the resolution of neurologic symptoms and the results of cerebral imaging.[3]

CT is most useful in patients who present with the acute onset of neurologic symptoms consistent with stroke (Table 13-1). A patient who sustains a stroke secondary to carotid bifurcation disease, and who experiences significant neurologic recovery with a large ischemic infarct on CT, is at increased risk for perioperative stroke if carotid surgery is performed within two weeks, as compared to delaying operation until four to six weeks following the stroke.[4] Conversely, a patient who has had a hemispheric stroke with little residual deficit and no evidence on CT of a major infarct may undergo early carotid revascularization without increased risk of a perioperative neurologic event.[5]

MRI is most useful in patients who present with nonacute neurologic findings (Table 13-1).[6] Vertebrobasilar symptoms, visual disturbances, and progressive neurologic findings not typical of carotid hemispheric events also are best evaluated by MRI. Several centers have directed considerable effort toward the development of clinically useful magnetic resonance angiography (MRA).[7,8] The impetus behind the development of MRA for the evaluation of extracranial cerebrovascular disease is the small but real risk of stroke associated with intraarterial cerebral angiography (Chap. 14). The cervical carotid artery is well-suited for MRA because of its anatomic location in a single plane in the neck, the high rate of carotid artery laminar flow, and the availability of small, high sensitivity magnetic coils.[9] MRA does not require the use of intravenous contrast agents, thus avoiding the potential complications of nephrotoxicity and allergic reactions. MRA, combined with duplex imaging (Chap. 11), may eventually replace contrast arteriography in the angiographic evaluation of cerebrovascular disease.

As CT and MRI play an increasing role in the evaluation of patients with extracranial cerebrovascular disease, proper utilization of these imaging techniques requires an understanding of the strengths and limitations of each technology. This chapter provides an

Table 13-1 Indications for Cranial CT and MRI in Patients with Extracranial Cerebrovascular Disease

Diagnosis	Imaging technique
Classic presentations	
Acute hemispheric stroke	Noncontrast CT on day 0 and day 5 MRI if (−) CT
Subacute hemispheric stroke	Noncontrast and contrast CT or MRI
Hemispheric TIA (hemiparesis, aphasia)	Noncontrast CT; MRI if (−) CT
Hemispheric RIND	Noncontrast CT; MRI if (−) CT
Amaurosis fugax	Noncontrast CT; MRI if (−) CT
Vertebrobasilar TIA (diplopia, ataxia, and vertigo)	MRI
Atypical symptoms	
Progressive neurologic loss	MRI
Visual loss	MRI
Isolated dizziness, vertigo, ataxia, or drop attacks	MRI
Asymptomatic	None
Postoperative change in neurologic exam	Noncontrast CT; MRI if (−) CT

overview of the principles of CT, MRI, and cerebrovascular MRA. In addition, the characteristic CT and magnetic resonance images observed during different stages of cerebral infarction and the role that CT, MRI, and MRA play in the diagnosis and management of extracranial cerebrovascular disease are examined.

COMPUTED TOMOGRAPHY

Principles

The penetration of radiation through tissue is inversely proportional to the tissue density. The basic principle of CT imaging, as with standard x-rays, is the variable ability of radiation to penetrate tissues of different density. CT imaging measures the attenuation of an x-ray beam transmitted through a small volume of tissue. Transmission CT uses a finely collimated x-ray beam, sensitive detectors, and a computer to translate measurements of x-ray transmission through tissue into an image representing the structure being traversed by the beam. The x-ray tube directs a beam of photons that interact with electrons in the tissue, changing the strength of the beam.[10]

Tissue density is dependent on variations in the type and number of atoms within it, and this density determines the degree to which the x-ray beam is attenuated. The photoelectric effect, whereby the energy of a photon is completely absorbed by an atom's electron, accounts for most of the weakening of the x-ray beam as the beam travels. Since an increased number of electrons increases the likelihood that a photon and electron will interact, the photoelectric effect depends on the number of protons in the nucleus of the atom.

Measuring the degree of attenuation of the original x-ray beam is the next step in CT imaging. The thin CT x-ray beam strikes a reusable, sensitive, high pressure xenon detector, which converts the transmitted beam into an electric signal. These electric signals constitute the data from which the computer reconstructs the CT image. The CT scanner computer is able to create a two-dimensional image of the brain by collating all of the detector signals. For intracranial CT imaging, many contiguous scans through volumes the same size as the x-ray beam are taken by rotating the x-ray tube and detector around the patient's head. Each image is derived from signals resulting from the beam's transmission through the same volume at different angles. Reconstructing the image requires generating a matrix—a rectangular array of elements consisting of rows and columns. Each intersection between two readings represents a small volume, and the specific attenuation of these volume elements or voxels is determined by analyzing all intersections using a complex algorithm. The physical position of the intersection determines its position in the matrix. After determining the value for each voxel, the computer assigns a gray-scale intensity from black to white to each value. The composite CT image is synthesized from picture elements, or pixels, which represent two-dimensional images of the three-dimensional information for each voxel. The intensity of the CT image displayed on the computer monitor is measured in Hounsfield units, which are defined as −1000 for air, 0 for water, and +1000 for metal.

Pathologic events that change the brain's tissue density, such as hemorrhage, edema, or necrosis, augment or attenuate the strength of the detected x-ray beam and generate a change from the normal pattern of the CT image. Infusion of contrast agents such as iodinated dye or xenon is used to enhance these differences. Disadvantages of CT include nephrotoxicity and potential allergic reactions associated with intravenous contrast media. Radiation exposure from CT scanning is also not insignificant. While the exact radiation dose is difficult to calculate, cranial CT delivers from three to six rads to the brain and

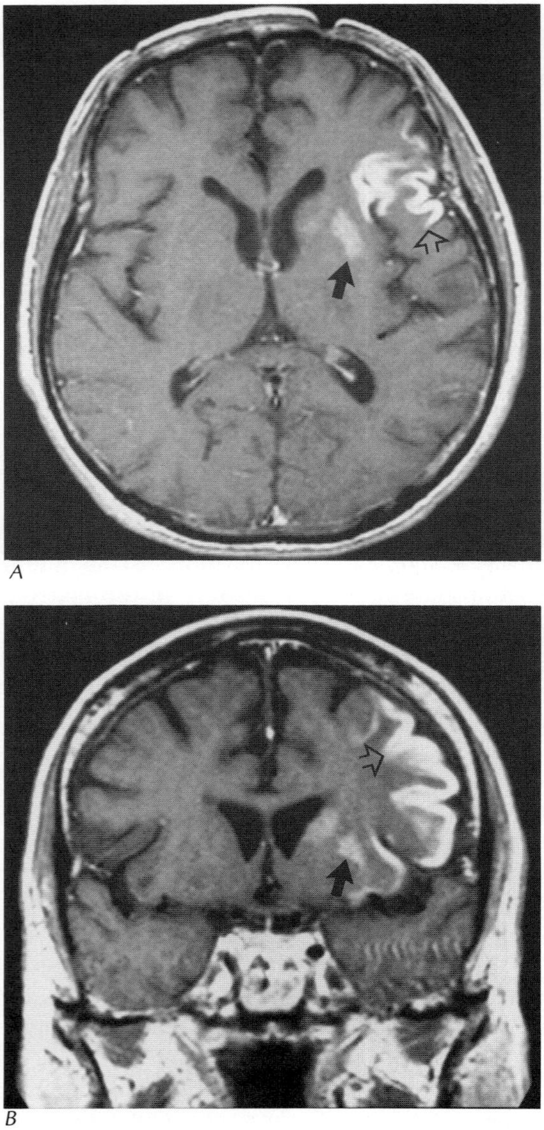

Figure 13-1. T_1-weighted MRI of a subacute ischemic infarction in the distribution of the left middle cerebral artery. Gyral (*open arrow*) and ganglionic enhancement (*solid arrow*) is observed on *A* axial and *B* coronal images. (TR, 700 msec; TE, 16 msec).

lenses of the eyes. To put this in perspective, natural radiation exposure is only 0.1 to 0.2 rads per year, and the radiation dose from a standard chest x-ray is less than 0.1 rads. Thus, while the radiation dose from cranial CT is small, it is not negligible.

MAGNETIC RESONANCE IMAGING

Principles

Magnetic resonance scanners obtain data by measuring the behavior of hydrogen nuclei subjected to a strong magnetic field. MRI instruments consist of a powerful 0.3 to 2.0 Tesla magnet, a series of sensors, and a computer for synthesizing and transforming the magnetic resonance signals into the final image.[10,11] Unlike CT, MRI provides anatomic detail without radiation exposure or intravenous contrast. The harmful effects of high magnetic fields do not appear to occur with magnetic fields up to 2.0 Tesla (the upper limit of magnetic strength of magnetic resonance scanners in use today). However, artifacts produced by metal objects on CT can be much greater on MRI. Patients with large metallic implanted objects, such as stainless steel rods or pacemakers, are ineligible for MRI. Some patients cannot tolerate the relatively long imaging time needed for MRI, and MRI also requires that the patient not move. MRI can reconstruct images in the coronal and sagittal planes, not just the transaxial plane used for CT reconstructions (Fig. 13-1). This capacity for multiplanar reconstruction can be used to visualize blood vessels that lie in a single plane and is the framework behind MRA.

While the detailed physics of MRI are beyond the scope of this chapter, an overview of the basic principles of magnetic resonance signal generation is appropriate (Fig. 13-2). By changing the acronym from "MRI" to "MRR" for *Magnetization, Radio-frequency pulse,* and *Relaxation,* one can better visualize and remember the three chronological steps of MRI.[12] These three separate, chrono-

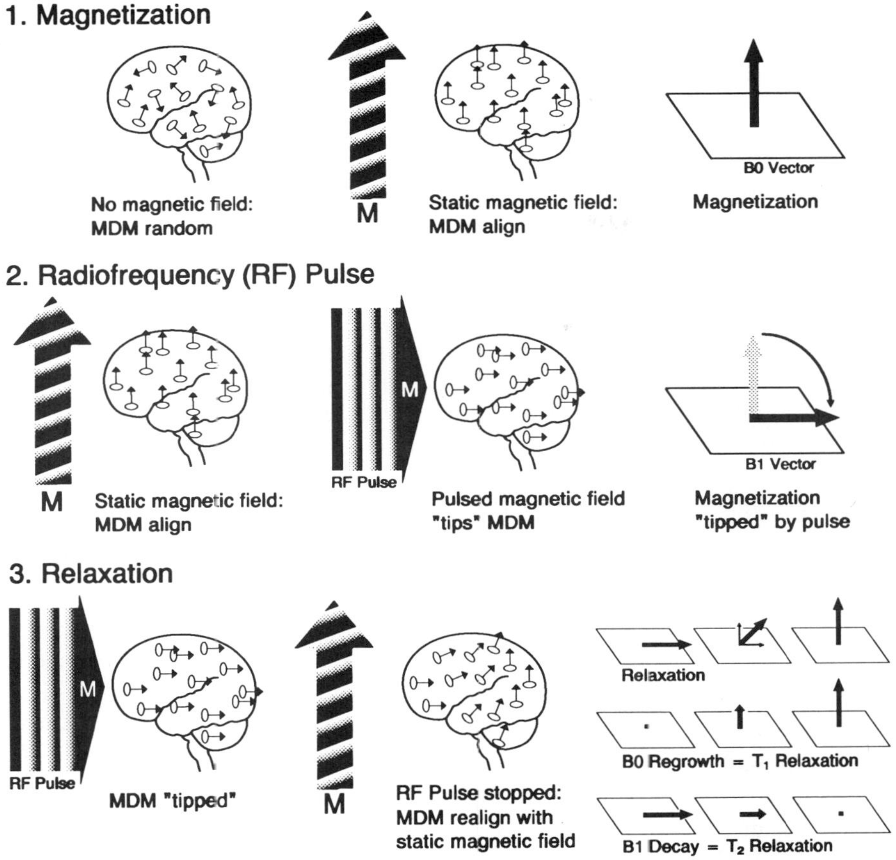

Figure 13-2. Steps in magnetic resonance signal generation.

logical events take place each time a magnetic resonance signal is generated.

Magnetization In the first step of MRI, the tissue to be imaged is placed in a static magnetic field, and the initial magnetization is measured. Initial magnetization is the measurable magnetic field produced by the tissue in response to the static magnetic field. The tissue produces its own magnetic field in response to the static magnetic field for the following reasons. Hydrogen nuclei, which are positively charged and spinning (i.e., moving), produce small magnetic fields. The magnetic fields produced by spinning hydrogen nuclei are called "magnetic dipole moments" or MDM. The MDM act like small magnets and align with the static magnetic field. The MDM, having magnitude and direction, are represented by vectors, which are additive. The summation of the tissue hydrogen MDM is the tissue magnetization. When the tissue is not exposed to a static magnetic field, the MDM are randomly oriented, and tissue magnetization, representing the sum of hydrogen MDM, is zero. The initial magnetization that is measured when the tissue is placed in the static magnetic field is represented by the B_0 vector. The B_0 vector is oriented by convention along the *z*-axis.

Radio-Frequency (RF) Pulse In the second step of MRI, a pulsed magnetic field is produced by the application of a short burst of electric current. The pulsed magnetic field is oriented perpendicular to the original static magnetic field. The new tissue magnetization is determined by the combined effects of both the static and pulsed magnetic fields. Because the pulsed magnetic field has a direction that differs from the static magnetic field by 90°, the MDM change direction by 90°. Thus, the RF pulse causes the MDM to "tip" from the *z*-axis to the *x-y* axis plane. The new tissue magnetization, represented by the B_1 vector, is oriented in the *x-y* plane.

Relaxation In the third step of MRI, the RF pulse is terminated, and relaxation occurs. Relaxation refers to the measurable changes in the tissue's magnetization that take place after the RF pulse is stopped. Relaxation has two components, termed T_1 and T_2 relaxation, which occur simultaneously once the RF pulse is stopped. As soon as the RF pulse is terminated, the pulsed magnetic field is no longer present. The hydrogen nuclei MDM "relax" as they "untip" from the *x-y* plane of the pulsed magnetic field and begin to realign with the original static magnetic field along the *z*-axis. The rate at which tissue magnetization increases along the *z*-axis is called T_1 relaxation. The magnitude of the magnetic resonance signal generated from T_1 relaxation is reflected by how quickly the B_0 vector increases in size. As the hydrogen nuclei MDM relax and untip from the *x-y* plane of the pulsed magnetic field, the number of MDM oriented in the *x-y* plane decreases, resulting in a decrease in the tissue magnetization in the *x-y* plane. The rate at which tissue magnetization in the *x-y* plane decays is called T_2 relaxation. The magnitude of the magnetic resonance signal generated from T_2 relaxation is reflected by how quickly the B_1 vector decreases in size.

The T_1 and T_2 relaxations are constant for each type of tissue, and provide the ultimate basis for tissue differentiation. However, the operator-adjustable imaging parameters, time to repetition (TR) and time to echo (TE), strongly affect the role that each relaxation time plays in generating an image. This permits generating images that are "T_1-weighted" or "T_2-weighted." Time to repetition is the time between two successive RF pulses, and can range from a few hundred milliseconds to several seconds. Time to echo is the time interval between the initial RF pulse and the reading of the radio signal generated by the pulsed tissue. The TE is much shorter than the TR. Standard values for TE are between 15 and 100 milliseconds, as opposed to hundreds of milliseconds or seconds for TR. To produce T_1-weighted images, one uses a short TR (approximating 500 msec) and a short TE (approximating 20 msec). Since fat has a short T_1 relaxation time, and water has a longer T_1 relaxation time, fat will appear brighter than water on T_1-weighted scans. To produce T_2-weighted images, one generally uses a long TR (exceeding 2000 msec) and a long TE (exceeding 80 msec). On T_2-weighted images, tissues with a longer T_2 relaxation time, such as water, will appear bright, while tissues possessing a short T_2 relaxation time, such as protein, will have lost their energy and appear dark. For example, the increased water content (edema) in acute ischemic infarcts causes these infarcts to appear bright on T_2-weighted images.

Multiple excitations of each tissue slice yield measurements in the form of generated radio signals which the receiving coils record and pass on to the computer workstation. Complex algorithms involving Fourier transformations convert this information from the form of a wave into a matrix. This matrix receives gray-scale values in a manner similar to CT, producing a recognizable video image.

THE ROLE OF CRANIAL CT AND MRI IN CEREBROVASCULAR DISEASE

The radiologic evaluation of intracranial manifestations of cerebrovascular disease relies primarily on CT and cerebral angiography. MRI and MRA play an evolving role that will most likely become more prominent with time. Cerebral imaging by CT or MRI is recommended in all patients with symptomatic cerebrovascular disease (Table 13-1). While CT is more appropriate in patients with acute, hemispheric symptoms, MRI is indicated as the imaging technique of choice in patients with progressive neurologic findings, vertebrobasilar symptoms, visual disturbances, or other atypical symptoms.

When evaluating a patient with acute neurologic findings consistent with stroke, there are two specific questions to be answered: (1) Was there a stroke? and (2) Is there intracranial bleeding? Both CT and MRI can confirm the diagnosis of stroke. However, only CT can reliably determine the presence of acute hemorrhage. Thus, for practical purposes, CT is the initial cerebral imaging study of choice in patients presenting with acute neurologic symptoms suggesting stroke. In patients with a clinical diagnosis of stroke not confirmed by the initial CT scan, MRI should be performed.

CT in Ischemic Infarction

The role of CT scanning in the early evaluation of cerebral infarction is well established.[13] CT scanning reliably distinguishes cerebral infarction from hemorrhage. Infarction is identified by the location and shape of the lesion, which can be correlated with the clinical findings. Even if the initial CT scan does not demonstrate an infarction, serial scans will demonstrate a well-described temporal sequence of changes that confirm the diagnosis and reflect the evolution of the cerebral lesion (Fig. 13-3). Eventually, cerebral infarction results in a positive CT scan in up to 98 percent of cases.[14] Changing density resulting in different attenuation, mass effect, cerebral atrophy, and specific patterns of contrast enhancement are observed at different stages in the natural history of the event. However, the greatest limitation of CT in the evaluation of acute neurologic deficits is its limited sensitivity in the first several days following infarction (Table 13-2 and Fig. 13-3*A*).

Cerebral infarction is classified into three evolutionary stages: acute (ictus to 7 days); subacute (7 to 21 days after ictus); and chronic (after 21 days).[15] The acute stage is further divided into the first 24 h (Phase I) and 24 h through 7 days after ictus (Phase II). The changes seen on cranial CT following ischemic infarction depend on the chronologic stage of the infarction as summarized in Table 13-2.

Successful detection of an acute infarction in the first 24 h following the ischemic event depends on the size of the lesion, its location, and the degree of ischemia.[16] Overall, CT is positive in approximately 50 percent of patients imaged within the first 24 h.[17] There are several reasons that explain why cerebral infarction is not imaged by the CT scan. First, the lesion may be too small to be detected. Second, alterations in the attenuation of the x-ray beam may be too subtle to be resolved. Third, low density edema can be canceled by high-density petechial hemorrhage. The earliest evidence of bland (nonhemorrhagic) cerebral infarction may be seen on cranial CT within three hours of the event. The hyperacute loss of gray-white discrimination in the area of the infarction is related to early inracellular edema. Within six hours, these changes progress to focal hypodense regions with indistinct margins that usually extend to

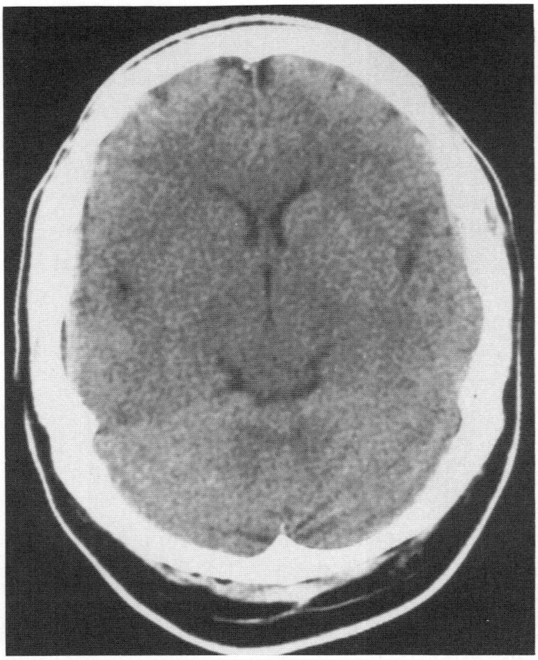

A

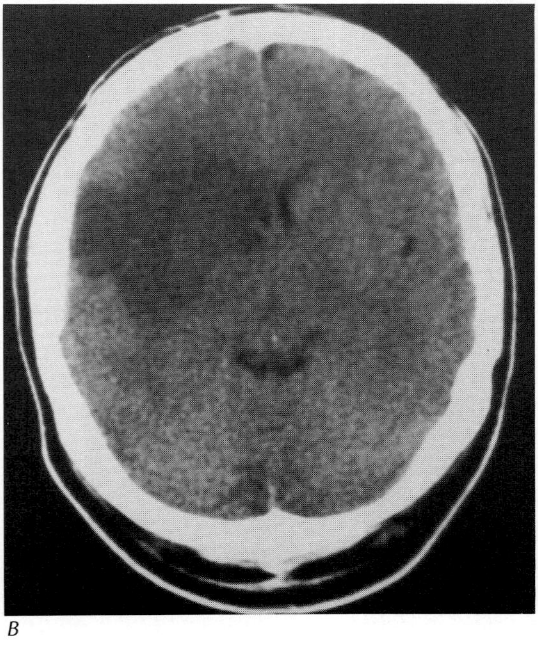

B

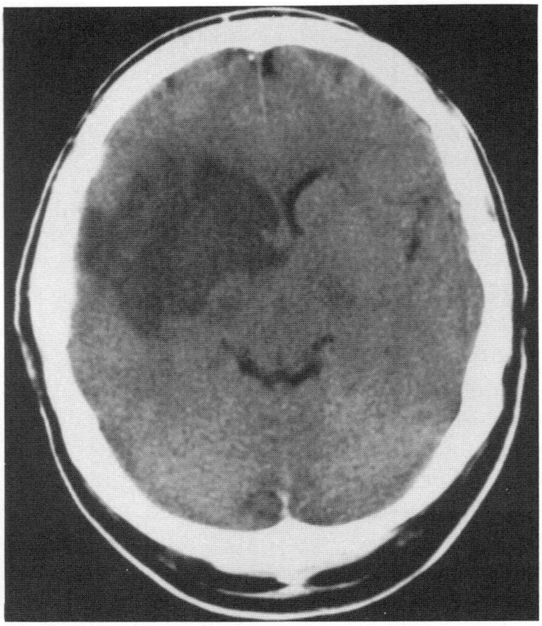

C

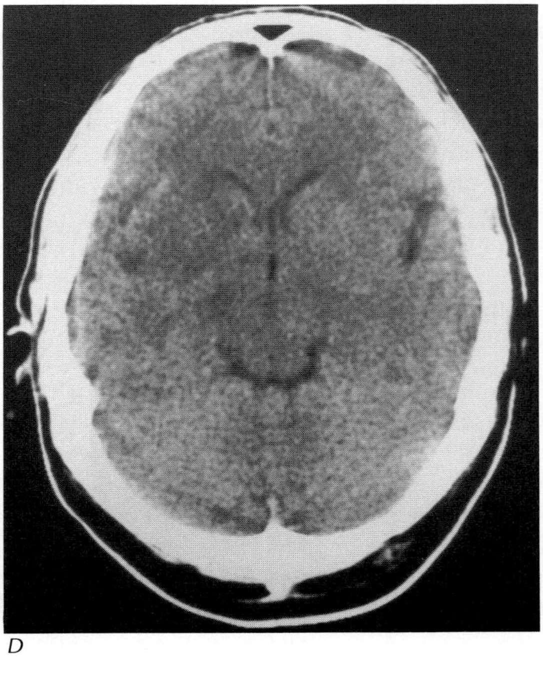

D

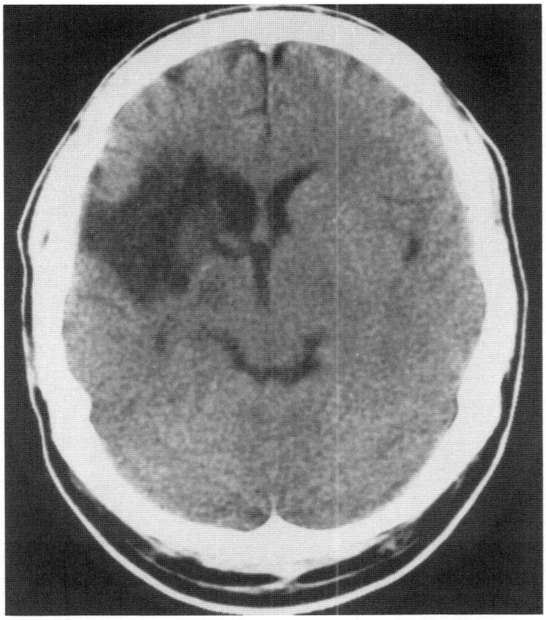

E

Figure 13-3. Evolution of an ischemic infarction in a 48-year-old man: *A.* Day 0 (Acute-phase I): Noncontrast CT is normal. *B.* Day 2 (Acute-phase II): Noncontrast CT demonstrates a large hypodense area in the distribution of the right middle cerebral artery (MCA). Note significant edema compressing the right ventricle and the indistinct margins of the infarct. *C.* Day 5 (Acute-Phase II): Noncontrast CT shows less edema and clearer margins in the area of the infarct. *D.* Day 21 (Subacute): The region of the infarct is now isodense (fogging) on noncontrast CT. *E.* Day 125 (Chronic): Noncontrast CT shows developing encephalomalacia. The chronic infarct is homogeneous with sharp margins.

the cortex. The margins become sharper and the region more hypodense in the following 12 to 24 h. Hypodensity may or may not be accompanied by a mass effect. During Phase I of the acute stage of stroke (up to 24 h after ictus) the administration of intravenous contrast medium is not indicated.

The sensitivity of CT in detecting ischemic infarction increases rapidly after the first 24 h. The hypodense region becomes more attenuated secondary to tissue necrosis. The area of low attenuation usually corresponds to part or all of the arterial segment involved and can extend to the border "watershed" zones between arterial distributions. Local edema produces effacement of cerebral sulci and cisternal spaces. More significant edema associated with larger infarcts will produce shifting and compression of the ventricles and displacement of the pineal gland and choroid plexus (Fig. 13-4). Maximal cerebral edema usually peaks from the third to fifth days.[18] While contrast enhancement is not usual before the third day, its usefulness increases rapidly thereafter. Noncontrast CT scans are performed prior to contrast-enhanced CT, because the contrast will mask an area that would have appeared hypodense. If contrast is used prior to the noncontrast CT, an acute stroke may be missed (Fig. 13-4).

During the subacute stage (7 to 21 days after cerebral infarction), approximately 90 percent of infarcts are seen on CT.[17] The areas of de-

Table 13-2 CT Findings in Cerebral Infarction

Stage	Time period	% Positive CT scans
Acute	Ictus to 7 days	60
Phase I	First 24 h	50
Phase II	24 h to 7 days after ictus	86
Subacute	7 to 21 days after ictus	90
Chronic	After 21 days	98

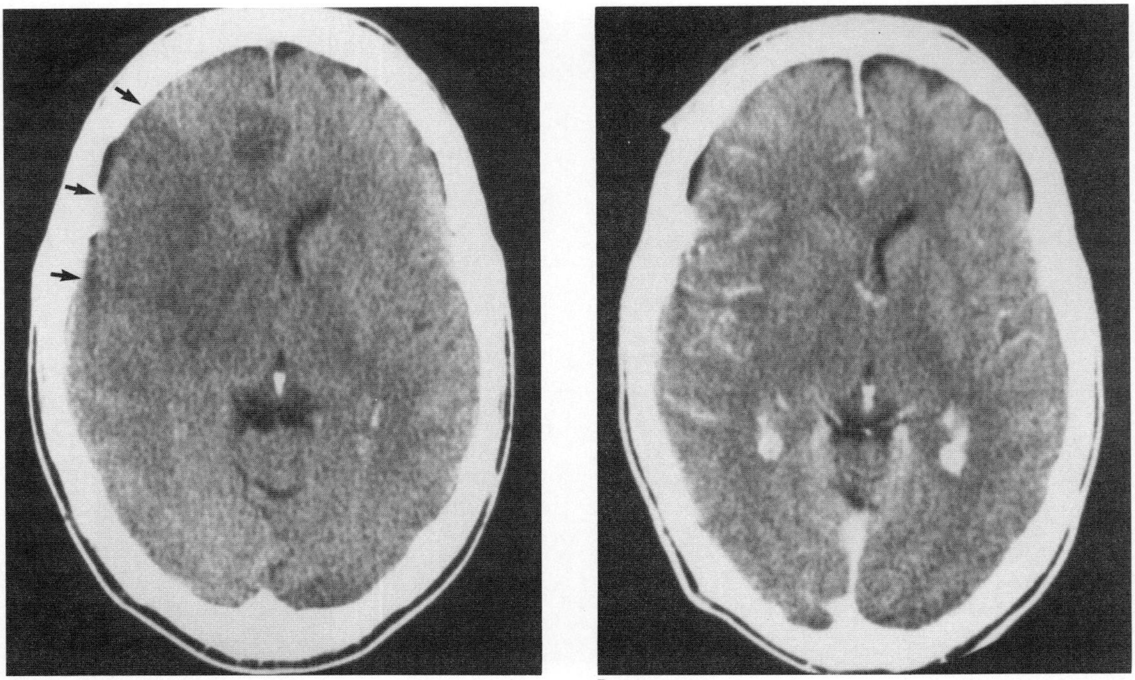

A B

Figure 13-4. *A.* Acute ischemic infarction: Non-contrast CT demonstrates an acute (day 3) infarction (arrows) in the distribution of the right internal carotid artery. *B.* Contrast-enhanced CT in the same patient. Intravenous contrast causes the acutely infarcted tissue to appear isodense with the surrounding tissue and masks the area of the infarct. Note the moderate edema compressing the right ventricle in both scans.

creased density become more homogeneous and the margins more sharply defined. Contrast enhancement of hypodense or isodense ischemic infarction occurs if the ischemic area is surrounded by a region of petechial hemorrhagic infarction (Fig. 13-5). A marked decrease in the mass effect accompanies the resorption of necrotic tissue and the resolution of edema in the area of the infarct. At the beginning of the second week, the hypodense lesion becomes isodense on noncontrast CT. This "fogging effect," believed to be due to incomplete coagulation necrosis and edema resolution, may occur uniformly in the lesion or in isolated areas of the infarct.[15] Contrast enhancement is usually present in cases of fogging on noncontrast CT, and intravenous contrast is essential for CT scans performed during the subacute stage (Fig. 13-6). Contrast enhancement that occurs on the seventh to the 18th days after ictus is believed due to both disruption of the blood-brain barrier and to neovascularity.

Chronic ischemic infarcts, defined as exceeding 21 days, continue to image on noncontrast CT as low-density areas. However, mature infarcts tend to be more homogeneous and to have sharper margins, and the mass effect has resolved (Fig. 13-3*E*). The size of the infarct decreases after eight weeks. The infarct appears to contract because of resorption of necrotic material. The development of ce-

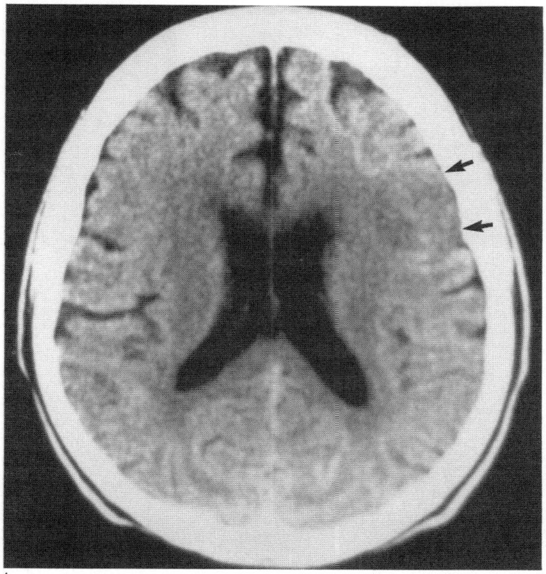

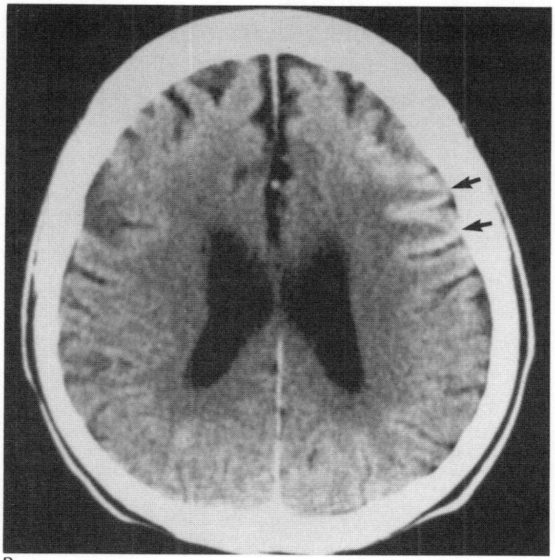

A *B*

Figure 13-5. *A.* Noncontrast CT of subacute ischemic infarction reveals loss of gray density in the cortex with effacement of gyri (*arrows*) in the region of the left middle cerebral artery. *B.* Contrast-enhanced CT shows gyral enhancement (*arrows*) in same region.

rebral atrophy (encephalomalacia) varies with the magnitude of the initial infarct. Thinning of gyri, dilation of contiguous sulci and cisternal spaces, and enlargement of ipsilateral ventricles also may be seen. Contrast enhancement usually declines after the third week, but may persist for up to seven weeks. There is currently no means for using CT to determine the exact age of chronic ischemic infarcts.

MRI in Ischemic Infarction

The specific indications for cranial MRI in the setting of symptomatic cerebrovascular disease reflect the ability of MRI to overcome the limitations of cranial CT. These include the failure of CT to detect small infarcts, decreased sensitivity in imaging very early infarctions, and limitations of CT in evaluating the cerebellum and brain stem. Fortunately, MRI can often detect each of these types of lesions when CT cannot. MRI is more sensitive than CT in detecting most cerebral pathology, including ischemic infarction.[19,20] MRI can often confirm the presence of an early, large infarct that CT does not image (Fig. 13-7). Salgado compared MRI to CT in 60 patients who presented with a clinical diagnosis of transient ischemic attack (TIA), amaurosis fugax, or infarction. While 88 percent of all MRI scans revealed focal parenchymal changes, only 67 percent of all CT scans were positive. The difference was most marked in patients with TIAs and amaurosis fugax (84 percent positive MRI versus 42 percent positive CT, $p<.01$). Small infarcts that would otherwise have been missed because of negative CT scans often image on MRI (Fig. 13-8). CT also may fail to detect infarcts of the cerebellum and brain stem because of interference from skull streak artifacts in this area. Fortunately, MRI can readily detect infarcts in the cerebel-

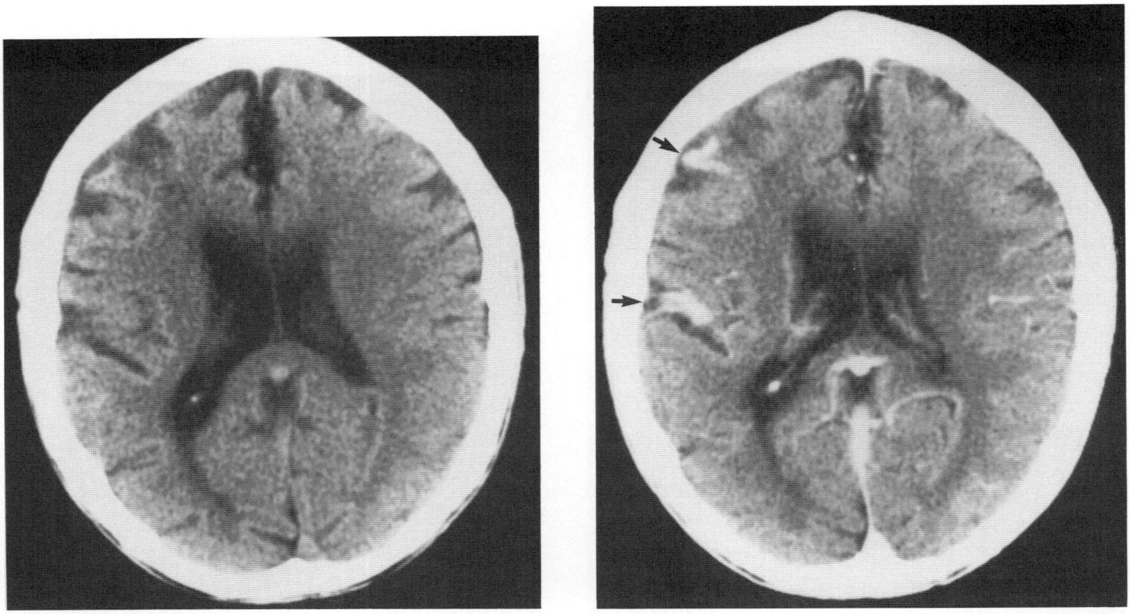

A *B*

Figure 13-6. A 56-year-old man presented two weeks following the abrupt onset of left arm weakness. *A.* Noncontrast CT of subacute ischemic infarction: The infarct is not visualized secondary to fogging. *B.* Contrast-enhanced CT demonstrates cortical enhancement (*arrows*) in this right temporal and parietal lobe infarction.

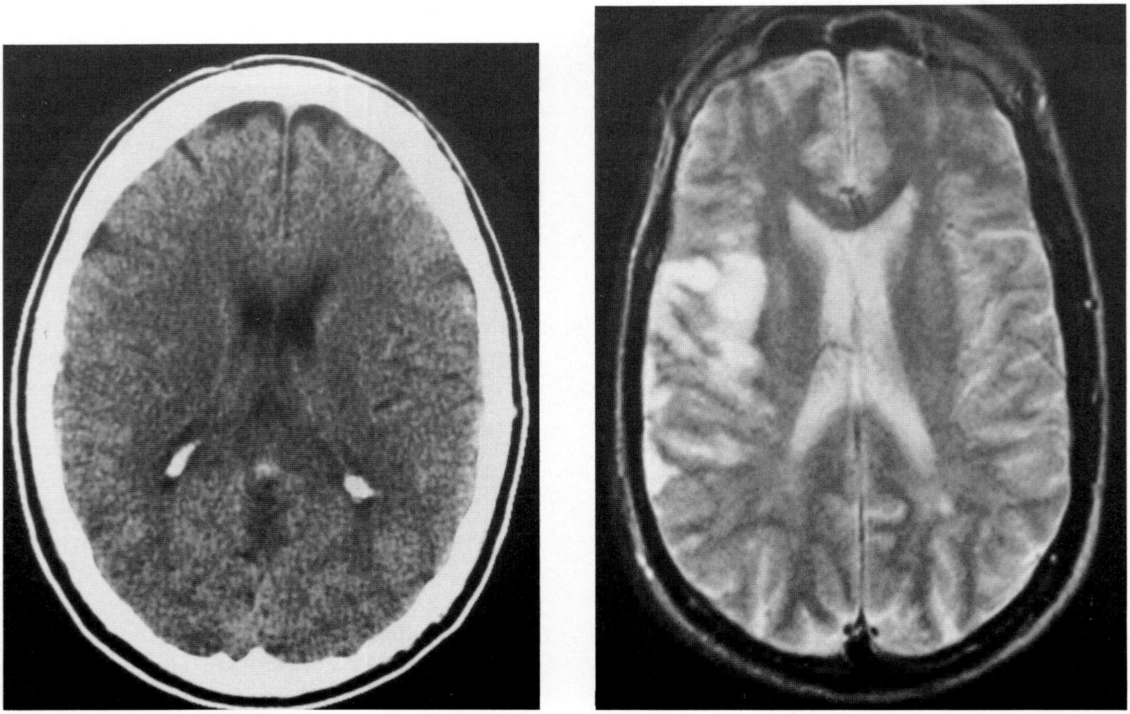

A *B*

Figure 13-7. *A.* A 60-year-old man presented with the acute onset of slurred speech and left arm weakness. Noncontrast CT fails to image the infarct. *B.* T_2-weighted MRI reveals a large acute ischemic infarct in the territory of the right middle cerebral artery (TR, 2000 msec; TE, 100 msec).

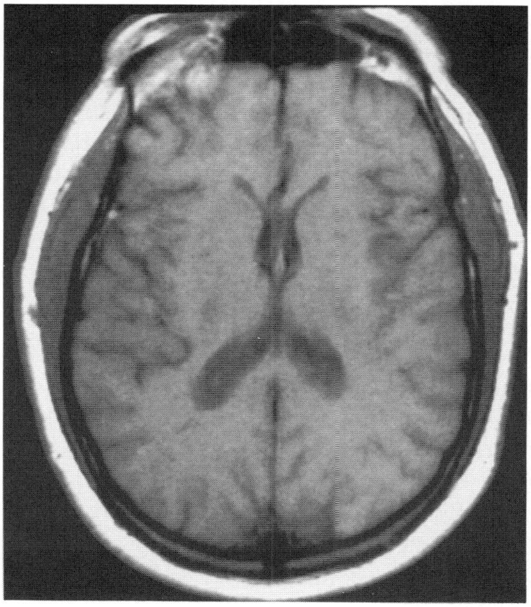

A

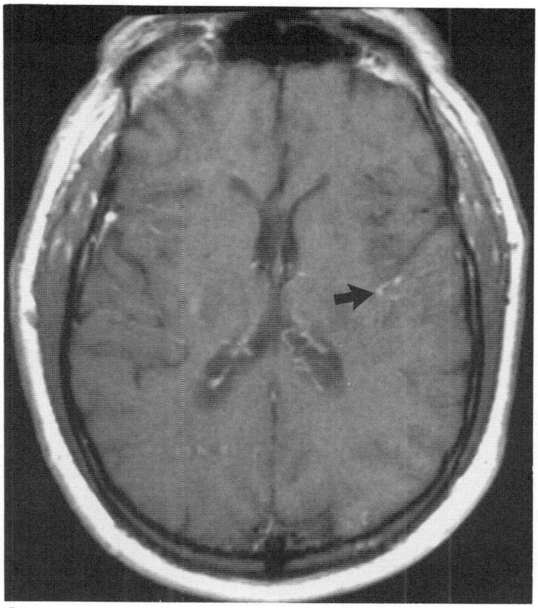

C

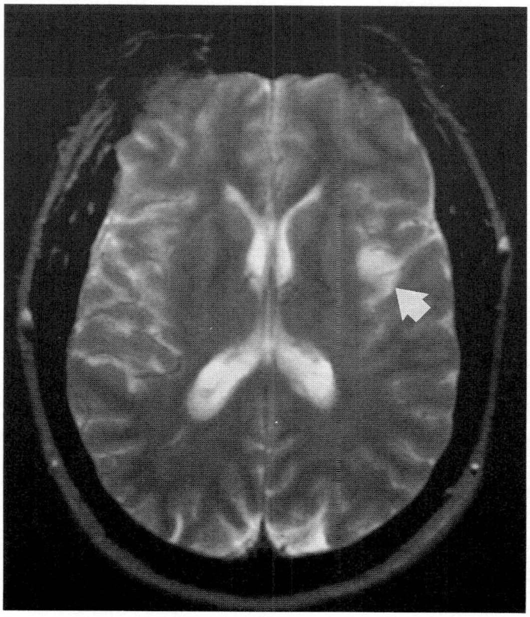

B

Figure 13-8. *A.* A 57-year-old man presented with the sudden onset of right arm weakness that fully resolved. CT scan was negative for infarction. T_1-weighted MRI without contrast does not demonstrate an infarction. *B.* T_2-weighted MRI demonstrates a high-intensity signal (*arrow*) representing an acute left sylvian cortical infarct (TR, 2400 msec; TE, 80 msec). *C.* Intravascular enhancement sign: T_1-weighted MRI following the infusion of gadopentetate dimeglumine (Gd-DTPA) demonstrates intravascular enhancement of the intracranial sylvian branch of the left middle cerebral artery (*arrow*).

lum and posterior fossa that are not imaged well on CT scan (Fig. 13-9).[21]

Because of its increased sensitivity, MRI is useful in evaluating patients who present with a clinical diagnosis of stroke not confirmed on the initial CT scan.[22] MRI is more sensitive than CT in detecting acute and small infarcts because infarction causes an increase in the water content of the ischemic cerebral tissue. Following the acute onset of brain tissue ischemia, the earliest changes seen reflect increased intracellular edema, followed by the extracellular edema that accompanies breakdown of the blood-brain barrier. MRI also detects changes as early as 30 min following experimental middle cerebral artery occlusion in animals.[23,24] MRI can detect infarcts that produce sufficient edema to alter relaxation values so that magnetic resonance signal intensity is altered. However, this same amount of edema may not be sufficient to alter the tissue density enough to see changes on early CT scans.[25] Since water has a longer T_2 relaxation time, acute ischemia and acute infarctions image as bright signals on T_2-weighted images (Table 13-3; Figs. 13-7 to 13-9).

Paramagnetic contrast agents have been introduced for use in MRI. These agents may prove useful in the accurate temporal staging of acute and subacute ischemic infarctions.[26] Gadopentetate dimeglumine (Gd-DTPA) is a magnetic resonance contrast agent that produces enhancement on T_1-weighted images.[27] Gd-DTPA does not cross the blood-brain bar-

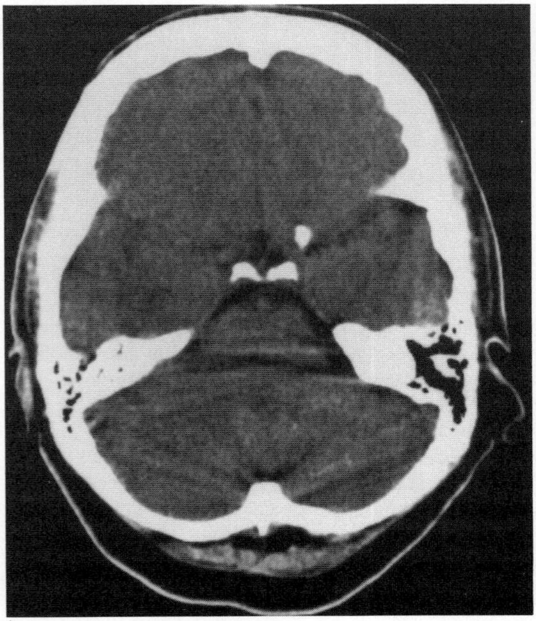

A

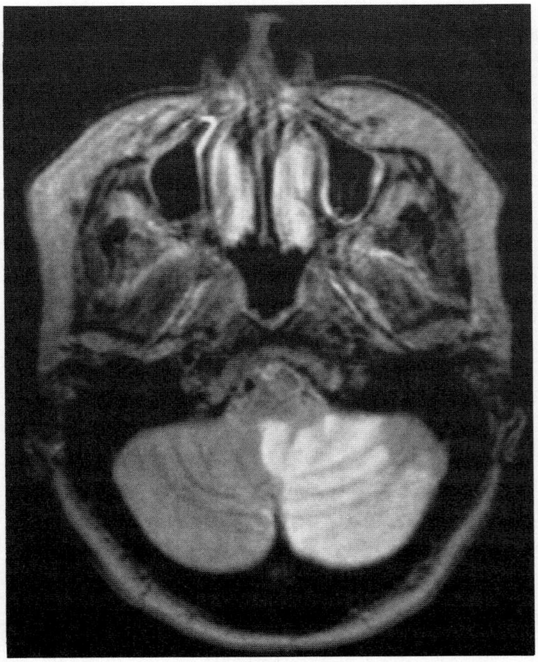

B

Figure 13-9. *A.* A 61-year-old woman presented with ataxia. Noncontrast CT fails to demonstrate the infarction. *B.* T_2-weighted MRI performed the following day reveals a large left cerebellar infarction (TR, 2500 msec; TE, 70 msec).

Table 13-3 MRI Contrast in Cerebrovascular Disease

Infarct stage	Acute	Subacute	Chronic
Ischemic infarction	T_2-weighted T_1-weighted + Gd-DPTA	$T_1 + T_2$	$T_1 + T_2$
Hemorrhagic infarction	T_1-weighted	$T_1 + T_2$	$T_1 + T_2$

SOURCE: Adapted from Deveshwar et al. *Current Therapy in Vascular Surgery,* 2d ed. Ernst CB, Stanley JC (eds), Philadelphia, BC Decker, 1989.

rier. During the subacute stage of ischemic infarction when the blood-brain barrier is disrupted, infusion of Gd-DTPA produces enhancement of the infarct on T_1-weighted images.[28] More recently, Gd-DTPA was found to produce intravascular enhancement of infarcts during the acute phase before the appearance of classic parenchymal enhancement.[29] This finding, called the "intravascular enhancement" sign, is due to decreased blood flow velocity in the intracranial arteries feeding the region of the recent infarct (Fig. 13-8*B* and *C*). The intravascular enhancement sign is positive in 77 percent of ischemic infarcts one to three days old.[29] This finding is specific for acute infarcts, as the intravascular enhancement sign is no longer seen seven days after ictus.

MRI is useful in confirming ischemic infarction during the subacute stage when CT images of the stroke are isodense with the normal surrounding tissue (i.e., fogging). In this situation, MRI reveals a rim of hyperintensity in T_2-weighted images surrounding a darker zone representing the infarct. This rim may reflect either persistent ischemia or Wallerian degeneration.[15]

CT and MRI in Hemorrhagic Infarction

While MRI is more sensitive than CT in detecting ischemic cerebral lesions, MRI does not currently offer any major advantages over CT in the evaluation of patients with acute stroke.[19] The impact of MRI on clinical decision-making in stroke patients is limited by the relative inability of MRI to reliably detect early hemorrhagic infarction. MRI has greater difficulty than CT in detecting blood during the first 48 h after intracranial bleeding.[30,31] The capacity to differentiate bland infarcts from hemorrhagic infarcts is critical in determining the use of systemic anticoagulation. Hemorrhagic infarction occurs in approximately 20 percent of all cerebral infarctions. CT scanning is very sensitive in detecting acute intracerebral hemorrhages and hemorrhagic infarcts.[32,33] While ischemic infarcts appear as hypodense areas on CT, hemorrhagic infarcts appear in noncontrast studies as isodense or hyperdense areas because freshly clotted blood has a higher attenuation than the surrounding cerebral tissue (Fig. 13-10). Hemorrhagic infarcts predominantly involve the cerebral cortex, which is well visualized on CT. Acute hemorrhagic infarcts lack sharp margins and, like acute ischemic infarcts, usually appear heterogeneous. This characteristic appearance of increased density on noncontrast CT may not be observed if contrast is given prior to obtaining a baseline, nonenhanced examination.

While MRI has limited applications in the evaluation of acute hemorrhagic infarctions, MRI can evaluate hemorrhagic infarction beyond the acute stage. The evolution and appearance of intracranial hemorrhage as detected by MRI is complex. MRI is very sensitive in differentiating oxygenated from deoxygenated hemoglobin and methemoglobin, and this evolutionary change in the hemorrhage can be used to stage these infarcts.[34] Within hours of the hemorrhage, oxygen within the hematoma is metabolized, precipitating the formation of deoxyhemoglobin. At this stage, the acute intracerebral hemorrhage

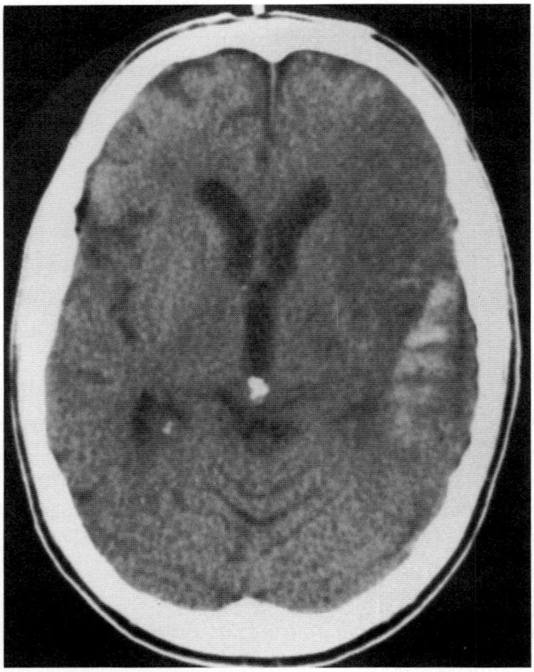

Figure 13-10. Noncontrast CT performed in a 72-year-old man demonstrates hemorrhagic infarction in the region of the left middle cerebral artery. An ischemic infarction extending into the distribution of the left anterior cerebral artery is also observed.

is isodense to brain tissue on both T_1- and T_2-weighted images. The low oxygen tension within the hemorrhage facilitates the conversion of deoxyhemoglobin to methemoglobin. This process begins within 48 h of hemorrhage. Methemoglobin within the hematoma causes a high intensity signal on T_1-weighted images (Table 13-3).

The Role of CT in the Timing of Cerebrovascular Operations

Difficult decisions arise in the management of patients who present with an acute, completed stroke secondary to a hemodynamically significant carotid artery stenosis.[35] In these patients, the risk of a recurrent stroke within one month of the initial event is high (20 percent in one series).[36] Therefore, early carotid surgery is prudent if the chance for neurologic recovery is good and the operation can be performed safely. Patients who show no evidence of significant neurologic recovery and have a profound deficit are not candidates for early carotid surgery. Patients who have resolution of their neurologic symptoms with little or no residual deficit are candidates for early carotid endarterectomy. The key step in this algorithm is identifying those patients who have recovered quickly but still have a prohibitively high risk of experiencing a perioperative stroke if carotid surgery is performed within the first two weeks after the ictus.[37,38] The perioperative stroke risk following carotid surgery in patients who have experienced a previous stroke is about 4 percent.

A CT scan obtained during the acute stage of a stroke appears to help identify patients who will have an increased risk of perioperative stroke. If the CT scan obtained during the acute phase is positive for a visible ischemic infarct, the risk of perioperative stroke is increased. Graber and coworkers observed that patients who had sustained a stroke that was imaged by CT at five days after ictus had a larger number of perioperative and postoperative strokes, even if they had resolution of symptoms at the time of operation.[4] This retrospective series of 110 patients who underwent carotid endarterectomy and also had preoperative CT reported an eightfold increase in postoperative stroke (12 percent versus 1.5 percent), and a threefold increase in transient postoperative deficits (10 percent versus 3 percent), in patients with a positive preoperative CT scan.

A negative CT scan in this same group of patients appeared to identify those who could safely undergo the operation within two weeks of the event without experiencing an increased perioperative stroke risk.[4,5] The perioperative and postoperative stroke rate following carotid endarterectomy in patients who had mild preoperative neurologic deficits and negative CT scans was not increased (0.9 percent stroke rate).[36]

Therefore, in patients who present with a stroke and have hemodynamically significant carotid disease, a CT scan should be performed both on presentation and at four to six days following the stroke. These CT scans should be able to document the ischemic event in the appropriate intracranial arterial distribution. Also, CT should exclude the possibility of an unsuspected late cerebral hemorrhage that could progress following the intraoperative administration of heparin.[35] Those patients who have a large ischemic infarct imaged by CT on either day 1 or day 5, even with significant neurologic recovery, will benefit from at least four to six weeks of medical therapy, including heparin and warfarin (if no contraindication exists).

Patients with severe, fixed neurologic deficits usually demonstrate an infarct on CT by the fifth day. If the CT at day 5 is negative or inconclusive, MRI should be performed (Table 13-1). MRI will usually provide radiologic confirmation of an infarct. If significant clinical improvement occurs after a four- to six-week waiting period, operative therapy is recommended.

The role of MRI in evaluating patients with negative CT scans and mild residual neurologic deficits, or deficits that quickly resolve, is not established. Because MRI has greater sensitivity in detecting infarction compared to CT, MRI should identify some patients with significant infarcts that were not imaged on CT at 5 days following the initial event. If the infarct cannot be seen on CT by 5 days, then the stroke may not be severe enough to warrant a delay in operative intervention. Whether patients with small cerebral infarctions that are identified on MRI but not seen on CT actually have a worse clinical outcome with early operative intervention is not currently known.

Accompanying the high sensitivity of cerebral MRI is a lack of specificity. An abnormal MRI alone in a patient with a negative CT is not a contraindication to early carotid revascularization. Awad and coworkers utilized both CT and MRI to prospectively examine 22 patients who presented with TIAs but without a prior history of stroke.[39] MRI was more sensitive, as 32 percent of CT scans (7/22 patients) and 77 percent of MRI scans (17/22 patients) had focal abnormalities. Among the 15 patients who presented with unilateral carotid TIAs, CT detected focal abnormalities within the vascular territory of the transient ischemia in only four cases. MRI was more sensitive, but also less specific; MRI detected focal abnormalities in the appropriate hemisphere in 11 of 15 patients. However, bilateral cerebral abnormalities were found in seven of these 11 patients who had positive MRI scans. The authors coined the term "UBO's" for "unidentified bright objects," whose clinical significance on MRI is not known. Care needs to be taken in interpreting MRI scans in this setting so that the lesion imaged as an acute infarct correlates anatomically with the patient's symptoms.

In patients with asymptomatic but hemodynamically significant extracranial cerebrovascular disease, neither CT nor MRI is required prior to operation (Table 13-1). In patients who present with atypical neurologic symptoms and hemodynamically significant carotid or vertebral artery disease, MRI should be performed in order to rule out other causes for these symptoms, such as malignancy, arteriovenous malformation, cerebral aneurysm, or brain abscess.[40] MRI is the imaging study of choice in patients who present with visual symptoms or isolated vertigo. Symptoms that could be attributed to vertebrobasilar insufficiency are also best evaluated by MRI.[6]

MAGNETIC RESONANCE ANGIOGRAPHY

MRA has developed in response to the need for a noninvasive, outpatient method for evaluating the entire cerebrovascular system. Both symptomatic and asymptomatic patients with significant extracranial cerebrovascular disease are subject to a real risk of stroke occurring as a result of cerebral angiography. In 600 patients with asymptomatic carotid stenosis, a prospective study of the risk of stroke following cerebral angiography revealed a stroke rate of 0.4 percent.[41] The risk of stroke following cerebral angiography in symptomatic patients is higher, ranging from 0.6[42] to 5.4 percent.[43] While intra-arterial digital subtraction angiography (DSA) reduces the risk of cerebral angiography, these complications are not completely eliminated.

Duplex scanning is reliable for the carotid bifurcation, but a significant proportion of all surgically accessible stenoses of the carotid and vertebral arteries occur at sites other than the carotid bifurcation. Because of its ability to image the entire length of the carotid and vertebral arteries from the aortic arch to the circle of Willis, MRA could be useful in screening patients for surgically treatable cerebrovascular lesions. MRA is similar to contrast arteriography in that MRA forms an image of the flowing blood within the artery that can be interpreted by the surgeon. MRA is essentially a subtraction technique, where flowing protons are made to appear more intense or less intense than the surrounding tissue.[44] Three techniques of MRA are presently in use: phase contrast; two-dimensional time-of-flight (2-d TOF); and three-dimensional time-of-flight (3-d TOF). The detailed physics of MRA are beyond the scope of this chapter, but a brief overview will be presented.

Phase Contrast

Since the hydrogen atoms within the bloodstream are moving in relation to the static magnetic field and the pulsed magnetic field, flowing hydrogen atoms will respond differently to these external forces than the surrounding stationary hydrogen atoms. This variability in response to pulsed external magnetic fields causes a loss of coherence or "dephasing." Dephasing depends on the distance the blood moves and its direction. Since stationary tissue maintains its coherence or "phase," subtraction images of flowing blood are created by measuring the difference in phase between the moving blood and the stationary surrounding tissue. While phase contrast was the first technique of MRA to be developed, its applications are limited, and it is used predominantly for imaging the intracranial carotid artery.[45]

Time-of-Flight

Time-of-flight (TOF) is the technique most commonly used to image the extracranial carotid arteries, including the carotid bifurcation. TOF is based on the flow into and out of the region being imaged. The area of interest is subjected to rapid RF excitations that selectively saturate portions of the vascular tree. The magnetization of the stationary tissue is suppressed while the magnetization of the intraluminal blood is replenished. The result is high contrast between the flowing blood and the stationary tissue.

TOF MRA can be performed in two dimensions and the individual slices stacked sequentially to form a three-dimensional image, or it can be performed initially in three dimensions (i.e., volumetric) (Figure 13-11). Manipulation of several parameters including TE, the saturation of pulses, and the volume imaged (voxels) determine the quality of images.

Though its future is promising, MRA has significant limitations. Signal loss from turbulent flow at branch points or from slow moving blood can cause inaccurate delineation of the vascular anatomy. As a result, the resolution of MRA is at present inferior to that of both conventional and digital subtraction arteriography (Fig. 13-12). A stenosis may be overestimated owing to turbulence distal to the stenosis. Very severe stenoses may cause low flow velocities, leading to poor flow contrast. Two-dimensional and 3-d TOF MRA each have specific advantages that make the tech-

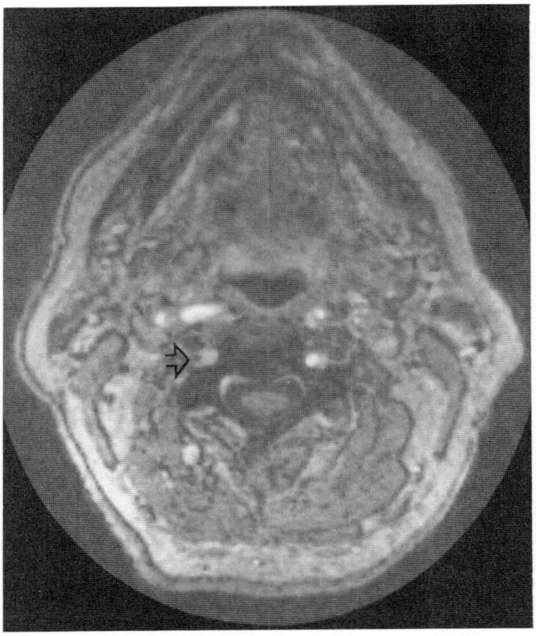

A

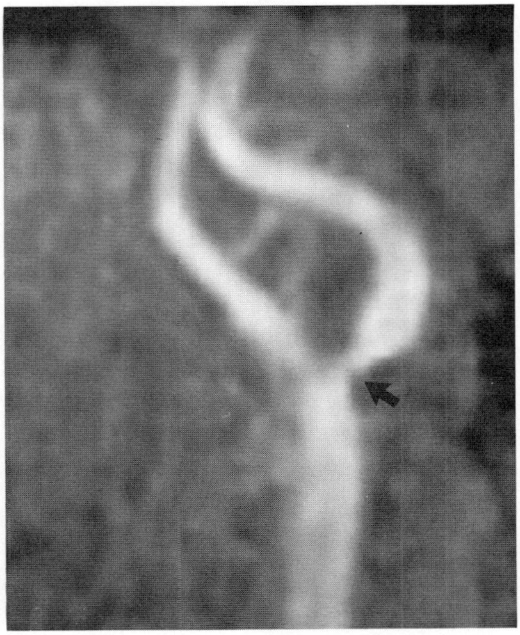

C

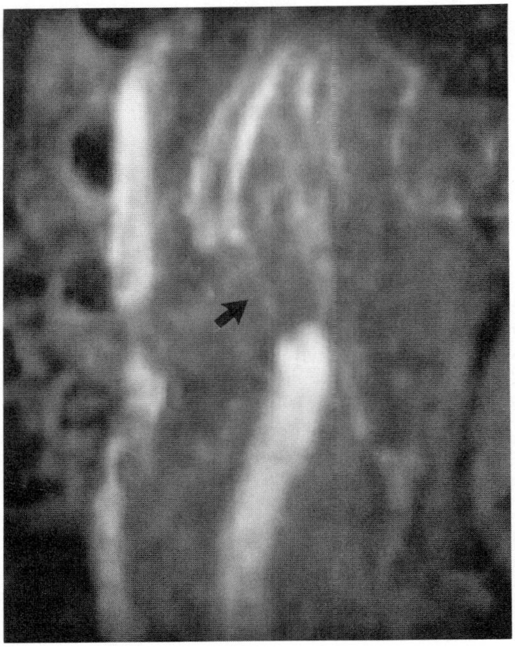

B

Figure 13-11. *A.* A 79-year-old woman presented with vertebrobasilar TIAs. Maximum intensity projection reconstruction of intracranial 2-d TOF MRA demonstrates high intensity signals in the patent right and left internal carotid arteries and the patent left vertebral artery. The occluded right vertebral artery (*arrow*) does not image with a high intensity signal. *B.* Extracranial 3-d TOF MRA of the left cervical arteries in the same patient reveals a severe stenosis of the proximal left internal carotid artery (ICA) (*arrow*). A high intensity signal in the ICA distal to the stenosis signifies a patent artery beyond the stenosis. The patent left vertebral artery is also visualized. *C.* Extracranial 3-d TOF MRA of the right cervical arteries demonstrates a severe stenosis of the proximal right ICA (*arrow*). The occluded right vertebral artery is not seen.

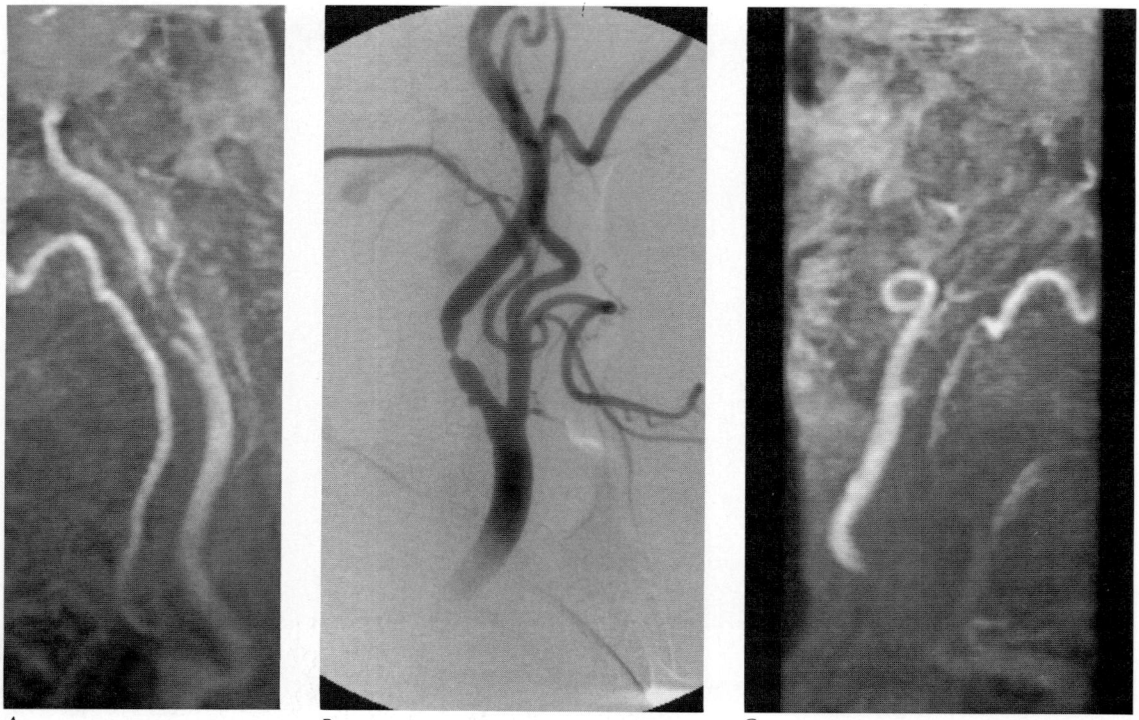

A B C

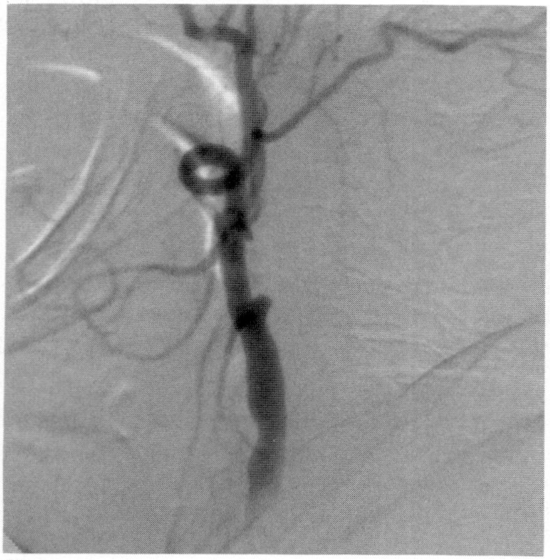

D

Figure 13-12. *A.* A 77-year-old woman with a history of a left hemispheric stroke 12 years ago is found on routine duplex imaging to have an occlusion of the left internal carotid artery and an 80 to 99 percent stenosis of the right internal carotid artery. 3-d TOF MRA demonstrates a critical stenosis of the right internal carotid artery and a patent right vertebral artery. The innominate and subclavian arteries are also imaged. *B.* Intra-arterial digital subtraction angiogram (DSA) confirms the critical stenosis of the right internal carotid artery. *C.* 3-d TOF MRA demonstrates occlusion of the left internal carotid artery at its origin and a coiled external carotid artery. A small left vertebral artery is also imaged. *D.* Intra-arterial DSA confirms the occlusion of the left internal carotid artery at its origin.

niques complementary. Two-dimensional TOF is more sensitive to slow flow.[46] On the other hand, 3-d TOF has better resolution for visualization of tortuous vessels and bifurcations.[47] Current trends suggest that 2-d and 3-d TOF techniques will be used in combination.[48]

Several initial trials have demonstrated the efficacy of MRA in both detecting and confirming high-grade carotid stenosis. MRA has been studied in both symptomatic and asymptomatic patient populations. Turnipseed and coworkers prospectively evaluated MRA in 20 symptomatic patients.[49] Phase contrast MRA was used for intracranial vascular imaging, while 2-d TOF MRA was used to evaluate the carotid bifurcation. Compared with conventional angiography, MRA was 91 percent accurate, versus 86 percent for duplex scanning. MRA was 100 percent sensitive for confirming critical levels of stenosis and for detecting complete internal carotid occlusion.

Wesbey and associates compared 3-d TOF MRA with duplex scanning and conventional cerebral angiography for examining 182 internal carotid arteries in 128 patients with both symptomatic and asymptomatic disease.[50] An exact correlation among the imaging methods was observed for the severity of stenosis in 75 percent of the arteries imaged. The degree of stenosis imaged on MRA matched the operative findings in 39 of 40 patients.

Pan and coworkers[48] combined 2-d and 3-d TOF MRA of the extracranial carotid arteries to demonstrate that MRA was comparable to conventional angiography in determining all degrees of carotid stenosis. They examined the proximal four centimeters of 61 internal carotid arteries in 42 patients, and classified the diameter stenosis as none (0 percent), mild (1 to 39 percent), moderate (40 to 59 percent), severe (60 to 79 percent), critical (80 to 99 percent), and total (100 percent).[48] The degree of stenosis classified within these percentage increments on MRA correlated exactly with the images obtained by conventional angiography in 42 of 61 arteries examined (69 percent). In 19 arteries, while the degree of stenosis observed on MRA did not correlate exactly with angiography, the calculated degree of stenosis was off by only one category (i.e., mild versus moderate).

A previous criticism of MRA was that this technique would incorrectly identify severe stenoses as total occlusions. However, this criticism may no longer be valid.[46,50] MRA confirmed carotid artery occlusion in five out of five cases in the study by Pan and coworkers and did not incorrectly image any patent arteries as being occluded. In that study, MRA did tend to overestimate the degree of stenosis (16/19 cases) as opposed to underestimate the degree of stenosis (3/19 cases) in nonoccluded internal carotid arteries.[48]

Patient motion and metallic artifacts (including surgical clips) continue to be significant limitations to the widespread application of MRA to the extracranial carotid arteries.[51] Metallic clips can produce an artifact that causes a completely normal internal carotid artery to appear severely stenosed on MRA. For this reason, plain x-rays of the neck are required prior to carotid MRA in all patients with a history of neck surgery.[50] Both two- and three-dimensional TOF will fail if patient motion is continuous, although two-dimensional TOF is more tolerant of small amounts of patient movement. Satisfactory MRA cannot be obtained in approximately 14 percent of patients.[48]

Another major weakness of MRA is that none of the current MRA techniques are sensitive enough to detect ulcerative plaques at the carotid bifurcation.[46] Once familiarity with the technique is achieved, MRA tends to take about 35 min to perform, with 15 min for post-processing and photography.[48] Since MRA does not depend on the use of intravenous contrast, MRA has neither allergic nor nephrotoxic complications. Since MRA is noninvasive, the risk of embolic stroke secondary to the imaging procedure is eliminated.

This latter advantage makes MRA especially appealing for use in confirming high-grade stenoses in patients without cerebrovascular symptoms. While the current literature suggests that MRA can play an important role in the evaluation of both symptomatic and asymptomatic patients, the greatest immediate utility of MRA probably will be in the evaluation of patients with no symptoms but hemodynamically severe carotid artery stenoses on duplex imaging.[47] Thus, the ultimate role for MRA will most likely be complementary to that of duplex imaging. Eventually, MRA probably will replace conventional cerebral angiography in the evaluation of patients with both symptomatic and asymptomatic cerebrovascular disease.

ACKNOWLEDGMENTS

We thank Dr. Eric Russell, Department of Neuroradiology, Northwestern University Medical School, for assistance in providing cerebral CT and magnetic resonance scans. We also thank Dr. José Biller, Department of Neurology, Northwestern University Medical School, for reviewing the manuscript.

REFERENCES

1. Hounsfield GN: Computerized transverse axial scanning (tomography): Part I. Description of system. *Br J Radiol* 46:1016, 1973.
2. Lauterbur PC: Image formation by induced local interactions: Examples employing nuclear magnetic resonance. *Nature (Lond)* 247:190, 1973.
3. McIntyre KE, Goldstone J: Carotid surgery for crescendo TIA and stroke in evolution, in Bergan JJ, Yao JST (eds): *Cerebrovascular Insufficiency*. New York, Grune & Stratton, pp. 213–226, 1983.
4. Graber JN, Vollman RW, Johnson WC, et al: Stroke after carotid endarterectomy: Risk as predicted by preoperative computerized tomography. *Am J Surg* 147:492, 1984.
5. Pitrowski JJ, Bernhard VM, Rubin JR, et al: Timing of carotid endarterectomy after acute stroke. *J Vasc Surg* 11:45, 1990.
6. Hyman RA, Gorey MT: Imaging strategies for MR of the brain. *Radiol Clin North Am* 26:471, 1988.
7. Riles TS, Litt AW: Magnetic resonance angiography, in Yao JST, Pearce WH (eds): *Technologies in Vascular Surgery*. Philadelphia, WB Saunders, pp 81–95, 1991.
8. Masaryk TJ, Ross JS, Modic MT, et al: Carotid bifurcation: MR imaging. *Radiology* 166:461, 1988.
9. Anderson CM, Saloner D, Lee RE, Fortner A: Dedicated coil for carotid MR angiography. *Radiology* 176(3):868, 1990.
10. Pearce WH, Salyapongse AN, Fitzgerald SW, Nemcek A: Computed tomographic scanning and vascular disease, in Callow AD (ed): *Textbook of Vascular Surgery*. Norwalk, CT, Appleton & Lange, 1993, in press.
11. Pearce WH, Salyapongse AN, Fitzgerald SW: Computed tomography (CT) and magnetic resonance imaging (MRI) in vascular disease, in: Rutherford RB (ed): *Vascular Surgery,* 4th Ed. Philadelphia, WB Saunders, 1993, in press.
12. Horowitz AL: *MRI Physics for Physicians*. New York, Springer-Verlag, 1989.
13. Vollman RW, Eldrup-Jorgensen J, Hoffman MA: The role of cranial computed tomography in carotid surgery. *Surg Clin North Am* 66(2): 255, 1986.
14. Kinkel WR, Jacobs L: Computerized axial transverse tomography in cerebrovascular disease. *Neurology* 26:924, 1976.
15. Jarenwattananon A, Khandji A, Brust JCM: Diagnostic neuroimaging in stroke, in Theodore WH (ed): *Clinical Neuroimaging*. New York, Alan Liss, pp 11–47, 1988.
16. Wall SD, Brant-Zawadzki M, Jeffrey RB, et al: High-frequency CT findings within 24 hours after cerebral infarction. *Am J Radiol* 138:307, 1982.
17. Inoue Y, Takemoto K, Miyamoto T, et al: Sequential computed tomography scans in acute cerebral infarction. *Radiology* 135:655, 1980.
18. Theodore WH: Introduction, in Theodore WH (ed): *Clinical Neuroimaging*. New York, Alan Liss, pp 1–9, 1988.
19. Salgado ED, Weinstein M, Furlan AJ, et al:

Proton magnetic resonance imaging in ischemic cerebrovascular disease. *Ann Neurol* 20:502, 1986.
20. Brant-Zawadzki M, Weinstein PR, Bartkowski H, Moseley M: MR imaging and spectroscopy in clinical and experimental cerebral ischemia: A review. *Am J Radiol* 148:579, 1987.
21. Cormier PJ, Long ER, Russell EJ: MR imaging of posterior fossa infarctions: Vascular territories and clinical correlates. *Radiographics* 12: 1079, 1992.
22. Deveshwar R, Welch KMA, Ramadan N, Levine SR: Magnetic resonance imaging and positron emission tomography in assessment of cerebrovascular disease, in Ernst CB, Stanley JC (eds): *Current Therapy in Vascular Surgery,* 2d ed. Philadelphia, BC Decker, pp 33–43, 1989.
23. Brant-Zawadzki M, Solomon M, Newton TH, et al: Basic principles of magnetic resonance imaging in cerebral ischemia and initial clinical experience. *Neuroradiology* 27:517, 1985.
24. Spetzler RF, Zabramski JM, Kaufman B, et al: Acute NMR changes during MCA occlusion: A preliminary study in primates. *Stroke* 14:185, 1983.
25. Unger E, Littlefield J, Gado M: Water content and water structure in CT and MR signal changes; possible influence in detection of early stroke. *Am J Neuroradiol* 9:687, 1988.
26. McNamara MT, Brant-Zawadzki M, Berry I, et al: Acute experimental ischemia: MRI enhancement using Gd DTPA. *Radiology* 158: 701, 1986.
27. Russell EJ, Schaible TF, Dillon W, et al: Multicenter double-blind placebo-controlled study of gadopentetate dimeglumine as an MR contrast agent: Evaluation in patients with cerebral lesions. *Am J Neuroradiol* 10:53, 1989.
28. Virapongse C, Mancuso A, Quisling R: Human brain infarcts: Gd DTPA-enhanced MR imaging. *Radiology* 161:785, 1986.
29. Elster AD, Moody DM: Early cerebral infarction: Gadopentetate dimeglumine enhancement. *Radiology* 177:627, 1990.
30. Gomori JM, Grossman RI, Goldberg HI, et al: Intracranial hematoma: Imaging by high-field MR. *Radiology* 157:87, 1985.
31. Hecht-Leavitt C, Gomori JM, Grossman RI: High-field MRI of hemorrhagic cortical infarction. *Am J Neuroradiol* 7:581, 1986.
32. Dolinskas C, Bilaniuk L, Zimmerman R, et al: Computed tomography of intracerebral hematomas. I. Transmission. CT observations on hematoma resolution. *Am J Radiol* 129:681, 1977.
33. Loes DJ, Smoker WRK, Biller J: Nontraumatic lobar intracerebral hemorrhage: CT/angiographic correlation. *Am J Neuroradiol* 8: 1027, 1987.
34. Barkovich AJ, Atlas SW: Magnetic resonance imaging of intracranial hemorrhage: Imaging in Neuroradiology. *Radiol Clin North Am* 26:801, 1988.
35. Hertzer NR: Management of totally and nearly occluded extracranial internal carotid arteries, in Ernst CB, Stanley JC (eds): *Current Therapy in Vascular Surgery,* 2d ed. Philadelphia, BC Decker, pp 70–76, 1989.
36. Dosick SM, Whalen RC, Gale SS, Brown OW: Carotid endarterectomy in the stroke patient: Computerized axial tomography to determine timing. *J Vasc Surg* 2:214, 1985.
37. Sandmann W, Kniemeyer HW, Jaeschock R, Aulich A: Indication for carotid artery reconstruction in patients with established stroke, in Greenhalgh RM (ed): *Indications in Vascular Surgery*. Philadelphia, WB Saunders, pp 25–32, 1988.
38. Rubin JR, Goldstone J, McIntyre KE, et al: The value of carotid endarterectomy in reducing the morbidity and mortality of recurrent stroke. *J Vasc Surg* 4:443, 1986.
39. Awad I, Modic M, Little JR, et al: Focal parechymal lesions in transient ischemic attacks: correlation of computed tomography and magnetic resonance imaging. *Stroke* 17(3):399, 1986.
40. Elster AD: Cerebral vascular diseases and disorders, in Elster AD (ed): *Cranial Magnetic Resonance Imaging*. New York, Churchill Livingstone, pp 151–182, 1988.
41. Hobson RW, Song IS, George AM, Weiss DG: Results of arteriography for asymptomatic carotid stenosis. *Stroke* 20(1):135, 1989.
42. Earnest F, Forbes G, Sandok B, et al: Complications of cerebral angiography: prospective assessment of risk. *Am J Roentgenol* 142:247, 1984.

43. Faught E, Trader SD, Hanna GP: Cerebral complications of angiography for transient ischaemia and stroke: Prediction of risk. *Neurology* 29:4, 1979.
44. Edelman RR, Mattle HP, Wallner B, et al: Extracranial carotid arteries: evaluation with "black blood" MR angiography. *Radiology* 177: 45, 1990.
45. Pernicone JR, Seibert JE, Potchen EJ, et al: Three dimensional phase-contrast MR angiography in the head and neck: Preliminary report. *Am J Neuroradiol* 11(3):457, 1990.
46. Litt AW, Eidelman EM, Pinto RS, et al: Diagnosis of carotid artery stenosis: Comparison of 2DFT time of flight MR angiography with contrast angiography in 50 patients. *Am J Radiol* 156:611, 1991.
47. Masaryk AM, Ross JR, DiCello MC, et al: 3DFT MR angiography of the carotid bifurcation: Potential and limitations as a screening examination. *Radiology* 179:797, 1991.
48. Pan XM, Anderson CM, Reilly LM, et al: Magnetic resonance angiography of the carotid artery combining two- and three-dimensional acquisitions. *J Vasc Surg* 16:609, 1992.
49. Turnipseed WD, Kennell TW, Turski PA, et al: Combined use of duplex imaging and magnetic resonance angiography for evaluation of patients with symptomatic ipsilateral high-grade carotid stenosis. *J Vasc Surg* 17:832, 1993.
50. Wesbey GE, Bergan JJ, Moreland SI, et al: Cerebrovascular magnetic resonance angiography: A critical verification. *J Vasc Surg* 16:619, 1992.
51. Anderson CM, Saloneer D, Tsuruda JS, et al: Artifacts in maximum-intensity-projection display of MR angiograms. *Am J Radiol* 154:623, 1990.

14

Angiography

John D. Harley
David R. Haynor

The role of carotid angiography in the work-up of extracranial carotid atherosclerosis is changing as ultrasound and magnetic resonance imaging and flow detection techniques are being developed and refined.[1] In the future, these or other techniques may replace angiography, but in 1994 the majority of patients who undergo carotid endarterectomy in the United States have a preoperative carotid angiogram.

Angiography is used to confirm the noninvasive evaluation of the carotid arteries and is particularly helpful in distinguishing between very high-grade stenosis and occlusion, which can be difficult by noninvasive means. Angiography also provides important information about concurrent intracranial vascular disease, disease at the origins of the brachiocephalic vessels, collateral vascular pathways, and unsuspected vascular anomalies. Because of the small but real risks, only patients who are candidates for surgical revascularization or in whom therapy would be modified by the findings of the procedure should undergo angiography.

TECHNIQUE

The following is a description of the angiographic work-up of cerebrovascular insufficiency as it is currently practiced at the University of Washington Affiliated Hospitals. Practice elsewhere is similar.

Patient Preparation

The goal of carotid angiography is to visualize the extracranial and intracranial cerebral circulations. In order to do this as safely and efficiently as possible, it is essential that, prior to performing the study, the radiologist be familiar with the patient's clinical problem, relevant medical history, and the results of noninvasive tests. Particular attention is paid to a history of contrast allergy or renal failure. All patients are vigorously hydrated before the procedure. Patients with a history of allergy to contrast media are pretreated with steroids and antihistamines, and a nonionic contrast medium is used.[2] In patients with renal failure (creatinine > 1.6 mg/dl) in whom carotid angiography is indicated, the volume of contrast medium is minimized by limiting the number of injections, nonionic contrast is used exclusively, and mannitol is given before and after the procedure to decrease further the risk of renal failure.[3,4]

Imaging

Depending on institutional preferences and equipment availability, a mixture of conventional ("cut film") and digital subtraction angiography is used to image the brachiocephalic circulation.

Digital Subtraction Angiography (DSA) Digital subtraction angiography is a technique of image acquisition wherein fluoroscopic images of opacified blood vessels are digitized into picture elements (pixels) arranged in a 512 × 512 or 1024 × 1024 matrix.[5] A similar image of the same body region made just before injection of the contrast medium (the subtraction mask) is subtracted electronically from the images of contrast opacified vessels. (Fig. 14-1*A* and *B*). Assuming that the patient has not moved, all structures common to both the mask image and the subsequent images, such as bones and soft tissues, will be subtracted out, resulting in final images that display only the opacified vessels.[5]

The spatial resolution of DSA images is limited by the size of the pixel matrix and is poorer than that of conventional film images for high-contrast objects. DSA images are also subject to degradation by certain artifacts inherent in the subtraction process, particularly patient motion, which causes misregistration between the subtraction mask image and subsequent images (Fig. 14-1*C*). However, DSA is much superior to conventional filming in detection of low contrast objects.[5,6] In practice, this means that DSA images may be obtained with reduced volumes and concentrations of contrast medium as compared to those required for conventional film angiography.

Direct comparisons of intraarterial DSA and conventional film angiography using phantoms and clinical studies have shown that DSA is equal or superior to film angiography, except for the uncommon situation in which details of very small (< 0.2 mm) blood vessels must be visualized.[6] In the evaluation of carotid occlusive disease, modern intraarterial DSA is diagnostically equivalent to film angiography except when patients cannot hold still during the ten second filming sequence.[7] This, combined with the other advantages of DSA, which include speed and ease of examination, reduced volumes and concentrations of contrast medium injections, reduced film cost, and the ability to electronically manipulate and enhance the images, explains its popularity. At the University of Washington Affiliated Hospitals some cerebrovascular angiographic studies are performed entirely with digital imaging while others are performed with a mixture of conventional and digital imaging, depending on available equipment.

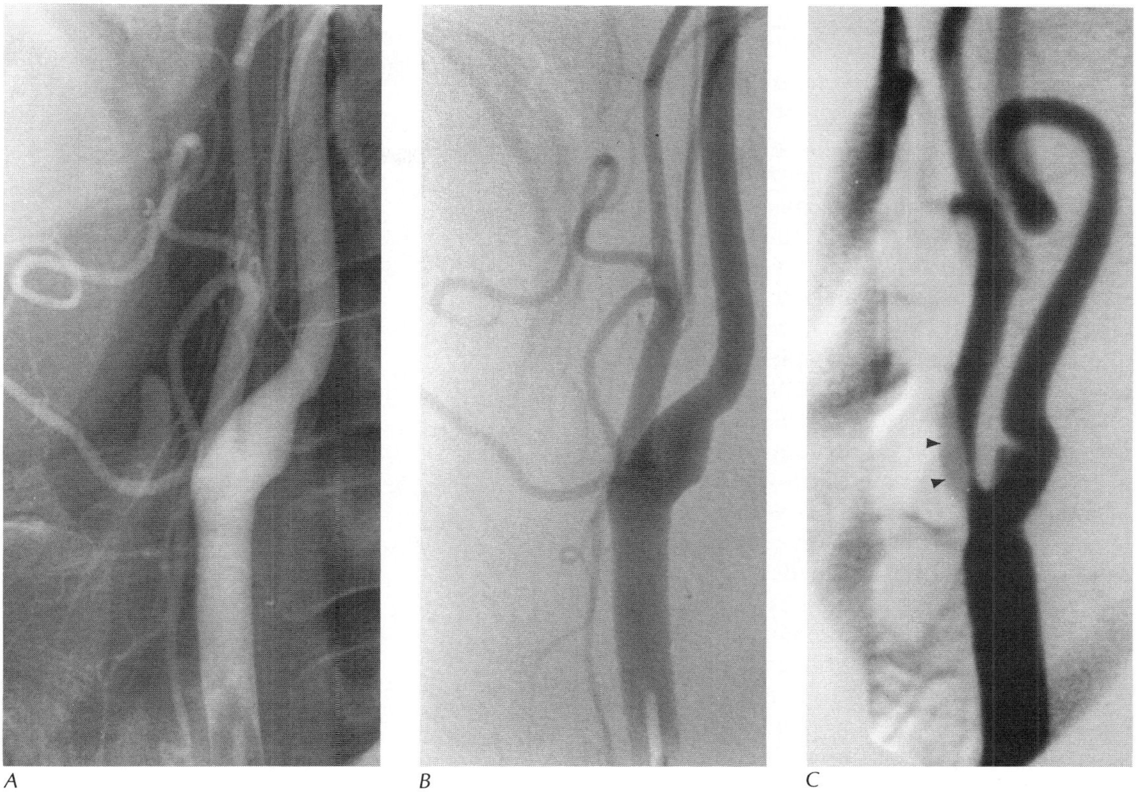

Figure 14-1. Intraarterial digital subtraction angiography (DSA). *A.* Unsubtracted digital fluoroscopic image of a normal carotid bifurcation in lateral projection made with 1024 line resolution. *B.* Electronically subtracted rendition of same image. Note virtually complete elimination of bone and soft tissue shadows in the subtracted image and excellent vascular detail. *C.* Subtracted lateral view of the carotid bifurcation of another patient made with 512 line resolution. Vascular detail is slightly less sharp. There is a weblike stricture at the anterior margin of the carotid bulb. A subtraction artifact produced by movement of the air-filled hypopharynx during swallowing partially obscures the anterior margin of the proximal external carotid artery, simulating a long smooth stenosis. The normal vessel margin can still be faintly seen (*arrowheads*). Review of unsubtracted images and additional projections will usually readily discriminate artifact from real abnormality unless there is gross patient motion.

Intravenous Digital Subtraction Angiography When DSA first became practical in the early 1980s, it was hoped that the ability of DSA to image very low concentrations of contrast medium would allow diagnostic angiography of the brachiocephalic vasculature with intravenous injection (IVDSA). Potential advantages of IVDSA include the ability to perform the procedure on outpatients and elimination of the complications associated with arterial catheterization. However, after an initial flurry of enthusiasm, reports of patient series comparing IVDSA with film angiography showed that IVDSA had significant limitations.[8,9,10]

IVDSA requires injection of a 40 to 60 cc bolus of high-concentration contrast medium into either a peripheral vein or a catheter placed in the vena cava or right atrium. The contrast medium circulates through the lungs to the systemic circulation, arriving at the cervical and cerebral vasculature considerably more diluted than with an intraarterial injection. While the digital subtraction technique can produce images from this diluted contrast, the signal-to-noise ratio is lower than with intraarterial studies, and vascular definition is poorer. In patients with reduced cardiac output, the contrast medium bolus is temporally elongated, further diluting the contrast medium and reducing the conspicuity of the brachiocephalic vessels. Since all the brachiocephalic vasculature is opacified simultaneously, imaging in multiple projections is required to achieve an appropriate display of the vessels of interest and to minimize overlap of vessels (Fig. 14-2). Each projection requires a separate injection of contrast medium.

Motion artifacts, particularly those due to swallowing, are more common with IVDSA than with intraarterial studies. In some patients, vessel tortuosity may make it impossible to obtain optimal projection of a vessel segment without superimposition of other vessels. For these reasons, about 20 percent of patients referred for IVDSA will have technically unsatisfactory examinations.[8,9] Even with good quality examinations, IVDSA has been shown to both over- and underestimate carotid stenoses as compared to selective catheter angiography and to be insensitive to intracranial lesions.[8,9]

With respect to identification of hemodynamically significant carotid bifurcation lesions (stenosis greater than 50 percent diameter reduction), Crocker, in a study of 87 patients, reported the sensitivity of IVDSA to be 85 percent, the specificity 94 percent, and the overall accuracy 92 percent using selective catheter angiography as the "gold standard."[8] However, IVDSA failed to identify eight of 11 intracranial lesions, and surgical therapy planned on the basis of the IVDSA was modified in 12 of the 87 patients (14 percent) based on subsequent selective angiographic findings.

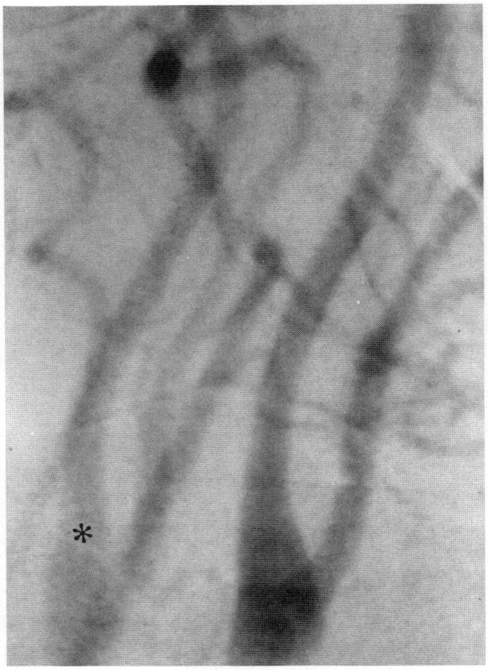

Figure 14-2. Right anterior oblique (RAO) view of the carotid bifurcation from an IVDSA study of normal brachiocephalic vessels. Contrast medium opacification of the vasculature is less dense than that seen with intraarterial injection (see Fig. 14-1), vascular margins are not sharp, and all vessels are simultaneously opacified. The right internal carotid artery (*asterisk*) is fairly well seen, but the right vertebral artery partially overlaps and obscures the external and common carotid arteries. The bulb of the left internal carotid artery points straight at the viewer and is foreshortened, causing it to appear artifactually dense, and the origins of the internal and external carotid arteries are superimposed. A significant lesion could be present in this portion of the left carotid; other projections are mandatory.

Although neurologic complications are reduced with IVDSA, systemic complications, primarily cardiovascular and presumably due to the rapid central venous injection of large volumes of contrast medium, are reported to occur in as many as 20 percent of patients.[10] Therefore, although IVDSA as a screening test or a follow-up examination still has a few proponents,[11] it has largely been abandoned as a substitute for preoperative selective catheter angiography.

Techniques of Selective Arterial Catheterization

Because lesions anywhere between the heart and the cerebral microcirculation are potential causes of strokes and transient ischemic attacks, the carotid arteries should be visualized throughout their entire length (arch to siphon) and the intracranial circulation also should be studied. The great majority (more than 95 percent) of all carotid angiograms are performed by the femoral approach, using the standard Seldinger technique.[12] Occasionally, because of bilateral iliac occlusion or stenosis, a study is done via the right axillary artery. A sheath is used if the iliac or femoral arteries are tortuous or if an aortofemoral bypass graft must be directly punctured. We do not routinely heparinize patients, although 1000 units of heparin are added to each 500 cc of flush solution or nonionic contrast medium. Other authors have suggested routine systemic heparinization.[13]

Most studies are begun with an examination of the aortic arch using an end-hole catheter with a small hockey-stick distal curve. If the patient has had previous coronary artery surgery, the study is begun with a pigtail catheter, exchanging this for an endhole catheter after the arch study is done. A digital subtraction angiogram of the aortic arch is performed, usually in the left anterior oblique (LAO) projection (Fig. 14-3*A*). A contrast medium injection rate of 12 cc/sec, with a total volume of 25 cc, is adequate for visualization of the great vessels from their origins up to the level of the carotid bifurcations. The images are studied with particular attention to the following points: (a) proximal stenoses of the great vessels, including the possibility of carotid or subclavian occlusion; (b) appearance and relative size of the vertebral arteries; (c) level of the carotid bifurcations, which in rare cases can be as low as C7–T1; and (d) anatomic variants that may make catheterization more difficult, such as unusually tortuous vessels (a frequent finding in patients with carotid disease) or a common origin of the brachiocephalic and left common carotid arteries ("bovine" arch), which can make catheterization of the left carotid more difficult.

After the arch study, the carotid arteries are selectively evaluated, beginning with the side of maximum clinical interest. In most cases, the common carotid arteries can be adequately catheterized using the hockey-stick shaped catheter and hydrophilic guide wires (Glidewire, Terumo). In patients with unusually tortuous vessels or a bovine arch, a reverse curve (Simmons) catheter sometimes must be used. The tip of the catheter is placed at about the level of C6, taking care not to traverse the carotid bifurcation with either the catheter or the guide wire. The cervical and intracranial circulations may now be studied with cut-film or digital techniques, or with a combination of both (Fig. 14-3*B–D*).

If the cut-film technique is used, a biplane study is done using a field of view that captures the entire head and neck down to the level of the carotid bifurcations on each set of films in anteroposterior (AP) and lateral projections. This biplane study is usually supplemented with oblique DSA studies of the carotid bifurcation (usually LAO for the left carotid, RAO for the right carotid). For an all-digital study, each of the planes (AP and lateral) must be imaged separately, unless biplane digital angiography is available.

If the digital field of view is not large enough to obtain both the head and neck on the same image, five contrast injections (AP head, AP neck, lateral head, lateral neck, oblique neck) may be needed for each side, as opposed to the two injections needed for the biplane cut-film/digital hybrid technique. Approximately 12 cc of contrast (at 8 cc/sec) is injected for each cut-film run and 7 to 10 cc (at 5 to 7 cc/sec) for each digital sequence. The filming sequence for the head is that routinely used for cerebral angiography (with cut-films, for ex-

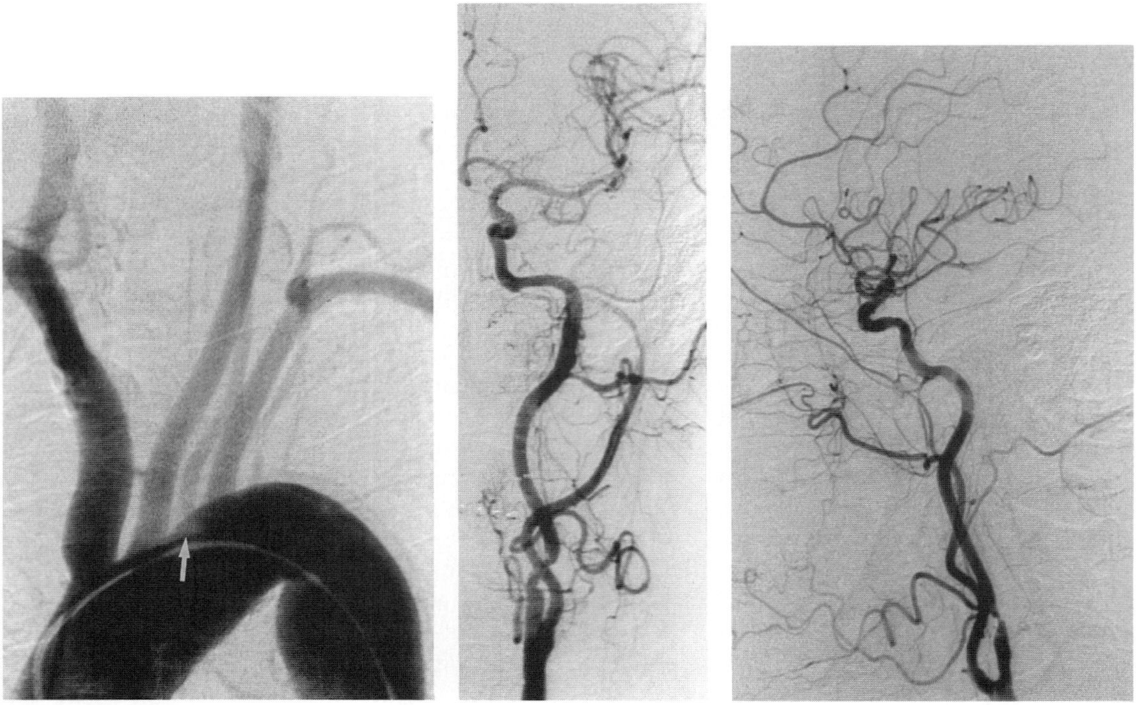

A B C

Figure 14-3. Intraarterial DSA of the brachiocephalic vasculature made with a large (14-in) field of view image intensifier and 1024 line resolution. *A.* Arch aortogram in left anterior oblique (LAO) projection shows minor smooth narrowing of the origin of the innominate artery. The left vertebral artery (*arrow*) arises directly from the aorta, a normal variant. Optimal visualization of the origins of the right vertebral and common carotid arteries would require additional views. *B.* Anteroposterior (AP) and (*C*) lateral views of the head and neck following selective injection of contrast medium into the left common carotid artery show normal intracranial circulation and a high grade (80 percent by NASCET criteria) stenosis of the proximal internal carotid artery. The external carotid artery overlaps and partly obscures the lesion in both views, particularly the AP view. *D.* A LAO view of the bifurcation best demonstrates the internal carotid lesion (*arrow*). Selective right carotid angiography (not shown) was normal.

ample, 2 to 3 films/second for 3 seconds, then 1 film/second for 3 seconds, then 1 film every other second for two more films); digital filming of the neck is limited to the arterial phase only.

Images are reviewed with particular attention to (a) degree and location of carotid stenosis and its effect on the filling of the internal carotid artery and its branches; (b) presence of ulceration; (c) adequacy of collateral circulation in cases of high-grade lesions (external carotid artery branches, circle of Willis); (d) presence of intracranial stenoses; and (e) other abnormalities (for example, dissection, aneurysm, or fibromuscular dysplasia).

Additional studies of the head may be required if an intracranial abnormality is visualized. The most common abnormality (2 percent of cases) is a clinically unsuspected cerebral aneurysm. Attention is then turned to the vertebral arteries. These are studied if there is either clinical suspicion of vertebral

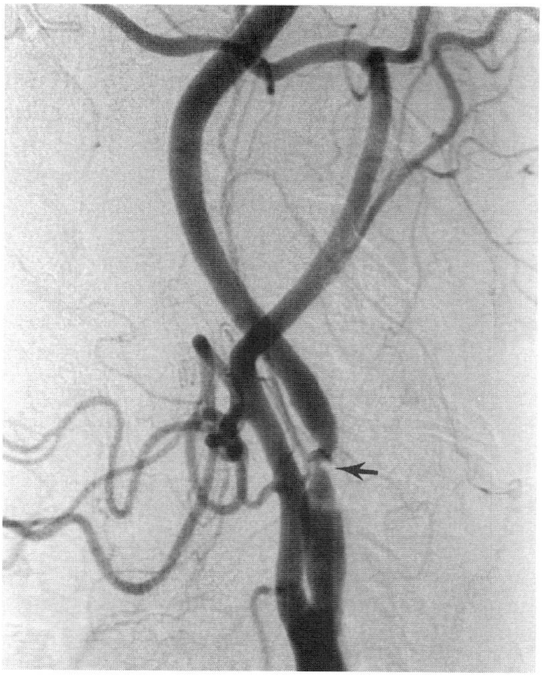

D

Figure 14-3. (*Continued*)

disease (e.g., posterior fossa symptoms) or the extent of collateral blood supply from the vertebrobasilar system to a compromised anterior circulation is of interest. We routinely study only a single vertebral artery, usually the dominant one (or the left vertebral if they are approximately equal in size). If the vertebral orifice is widely patent and the vessel does not appear to be diseased proximally, the catheter may be placed gently in the orifice of the vertebral artery. Otherwise, the tip of the catheter is placed in the subclavian artery just distal to the vertebral origin, and a blood pressure cuff is inflated to greater than systolic pressure on the ipsilateral arm. With appropriate contrast injection rates (8 cc/sec, total 15 cc for subclavian injections; 5 cc/sec, total 10 cc for vertebral injections), adequate visualization of the posterior circulation is achieved using digital filming of the head.

The catheter is then withdrawn and hemostasis obtained. Routine postprocedure orders include adequate hydration, 6 h of strict bed rest, and frequent checks of femoral and distal pulses.

COMPLICATIONS

The most significant, although fortunately uncommon, complication of cerebral angiography is stroke, usually the result of periprocedure cerebral emboli. These emboli are presumed to be either small fragments of atherosclerotic plaque or mural thrombus dislodged by the catheter or guide wire, or small blood clots that formed in or on the catheter or on the guide wire. Catheter- or guide wire-induced carotid dissection and occlusion also may occur, but are rare.

Hankey recently reviewed eight prospective and seven retrospective studies of the neurologic complications of cerebral angiography.[14] The total neurologic complication rate estimated from pooling the eight prospective studies was 4.1 percent (95 percent confidence range, 3.3 to 5 percent), with a permanent complication (i.e., stroke) rate of 1 percent (0.6 to 1.5 percent) and a mortality rate of 0.06 percent (0 to 0.18 percent). The pooled estimated complication rates from the retrospective studies were 1.9, 0.6, and 0.6 percent for the same three categories. The discrepancy between the two estimates of total complication rates was attributed to the under-reporting of nonlethal complications typical in retrospective studies. Since some of these studies considered any neurologic event occurring within 24 h of angiography to be an angiographic complication, an unknown proportion of these complications were due to the underlying disease rather than to the angiographic procedure itself. No studies have permitted definitive determination of risk factors for complications of cerebral angiography, although age and health of the patient, angiographer experience, and duration of the procedure have all been suggested by one or more studies as possibly being of importance.

Other potential complications of cerebral angiography include contrast reaction, puncture site infection or vascular injury, and contrast medium-induced reduction in renal function. The risk of permanent impairment of renal function due to radiographic contrast medium depends on the total dose of contrast injected and is thought to be increased by preexisting renal failure (creatinine $>$ 1.6 mg/dl), dehydration, diabetes (especially with renal failure), heart disease, and advanced patient age.[4] Compared with some other radiologic investigations, the amount of contrast medium used in cerebral angiography (normally $<$ 125 cc) is relatively small. Worsening of renal function in high-risk patients may be minimized by vigorous hydration prior to and immediately after angiography, minimizing contrast medium volume and concentration, use of nonionic contrast medium, and administration of mannitol (12 to 25 g) during or immediately after the procedure.[3,4]

INTERPRETATION

Accurate interpretation of brachiocephalic angiograms requires technically good quality angiography in at least two planes. The angiographer must be aware of image artifacts produced by the DSA technique and those related to arterial catheterization, including catheter- or guide wire-induced vasospasm or intimal dissection and contrast medium layering or incomplete mixing in slow-flow situations.

Quantification of Stenoses

Although contrast angiography is considered to be the standard against which all other methods for detection and characterization of atherosclerotic disease are compared, there is surprising variability in the reported measurement techniques. An awareness of these variations is important for proper understanding of radiographic reports and is particularly important for interpretation of large, multicenter studies and the application of their results to a given patient or institution. Absolute measurement of lumen cross section with atherosclerotic lesions is impractical owing to variations in anatomy and lesion morphology, the limited number of radiographic projections, and variable radiographic magnification. Therefore, by convention, atherosclerotic stenoses are reported as a percentage reduction in luminal diameter. However, this method can potentially over- or underestimate the significance of the irregularly shaped or very eccentric lesion and is not as simple and straightforward as it might seem.

Determination of the percentage reduction in luminal diameter requires precise measurement of the diameter of the stenotic segment (the numerator) and measurement or estimation of a normal or reference vessel diameter (the denominator). Expressed as an equation: % stenosis = [1 − (narrowest vessel diameter/"normal" vessel diameter)] × 100 percent. The luminal diameter at the stenotic site is taken as the smallest measurement from at least two views of the lesion.[15] Determination of the luminal diameter of the "normal" or reference vessel is more problematic—especially for internal carotid lesions involving the carotid bulb, which may have a normal diameter up to twice that of the more distal carotid artery (Fig. 14-4*A*).

The European Carotid Surgery Trial used estimated normal carotid bulb diameter in calculating percentage stenosis of internal carotid artery (ICA) lesions, and the duplex imaging criteria for determining ICA stenosis developed at the University of Washington are also based on this measurement method.[16,17] However, the large and ongoing North American Symptomatic Carotid Endarterectomy Trial (NASCET) uses the diameter of an unaffected segment of the ICA distal to the carotid bulb as the reference diameter.[15] This method also was used in the Veterans Affairs Cooperative Trial and by the Asymptomatic Carotid Atherosclerosis Study Group.[18,19] The Committee on Standards for Noninvasive Vascular Testing of the Joint Council of the Society for Vascular Surgery and the North American Chapter of the International Society for Cardiovascular Surgery has recommended a slightly different measurement technique in which the reference vessel diameter is taken as the diameter of the normal ICA immediately distal to the diseased area.[20] This diameter could be located within the bulb or distal to the bulb, depending on the location and linear extent of the lesion.

Methods that directly measure both the stenotic and reference vessel luminal diameters are technically easier and potentially more precise than those that require an estimation of normal carotid bulb diameter, since angiography does not directly visualize the vessel wall, only the opacified lumen. However, use of the distal ICA as the reference vessel results in significant underestimation of stenotic lesions involving the carotid bulb.[21] For example, a proximal ICA lesion with a measured 5 mm minimal lumen diameter, a normal bulb diameter of 13 mm, and a distal ICA diameter of 6 mm has a 62 percent diameter-reducing lesion using the bulb diameter as a reference, but only a 17 percent diameter reduction using the distal ICA diameter (NASCET technique) (Fig. 14-4*B*). The same calculations applied to more severe stenoses result in less disparity between the two methods. Reproducibility of the two methods is similar. Moneta found good agreement (kappa = 0.93) between two independent observers asked to classify angiographically demonstrated common or internal carotid lesions as greater than or less than 70 percent by the NASCET criteria.[21] Chikos obtained equally good intra- and interobserver agreement in a study of the ability of three radiologists to classify angiographically demonstrated carotid stenoses using a measurement

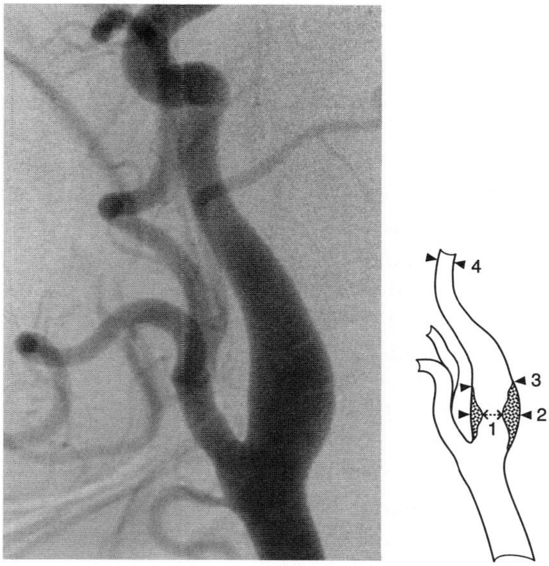

A *B*

Figure 14-4. Measurement of atherosclerotic stenoses of the proximal internal carotid artery. *A.* DSA image of a normal carotid bifurcation. In this patient the diameter of the carotid bulb is 2.2 times the diameter of the post-bulbar internal carotid artery. *B.* Diagramatic representation of a carotid bifurcation with an atherosclerotic lesion (*stippled area*) confined to the proximal carotid bulb. Calculation of the degree of stenosis by the formula, percent stenosis = [1 − (narrowest vessel diameter/"normal" vessel diameter)] × 100%, requires measurement of the lumen diameter at the point of maximum narrowing, measurement (*1*), and a "normal" or reference diameter which may be measurement (*2*), (*3*), or (*4*) depending on the method employed. Using estimated bulb diameter, measurement (*2*) in this example, as the reference diameter yields a calculated stenosis of 59 percent. Using the NASCET method and the diameter of the normal internal carotid artery distal to the bulb, measurement (*4*), as the reference diameter, there is 0 percent calculated stenosis. Using the diameter of the internal carotid artery immediately distal to the lesion, measurement (*3*), (still within the expansion of the carotid bulb) as the reference diameter, yields a 50 percent stenosis. Note that direct measurement of the normal width of the carotid bulb in the presence of an atherosclerotic lesion as shown in this artist's rendition is not possible from an angiogram, since the vessel wall is not visualized on a contrast angiogram unless it is heavily calcified. Bulb width must be estimated based on a projection of expected contour or the diameter of a contralateral normal bulb.

technique that involved estimation of carotid bulb diameter.[22] In that study, 128 carotid angiograms were read twice by three radiologists. For the internal carotid artery the intraobserver and (interobserver) agreement rates were 96 percent (93 percent) for stenosis of less than 50 percent diameter reduction, 90 percent (85 percent) for 50 percent or greater stenosis, and 97 percent (97 percent) for 100 percent stenosis.

It is clear that there is no consensus on the best method for measuring stenoses of the proximal ICA. The adoption of the diameter of the distal ICA as the denominator in calculation of ICA stenosis in the NASCET appears to have established this as the current standard, but the reader is urged to pay careful attention to the measurement method employed in reported studies and at their own institution. Whatever measurement protocol is adopted, it is important to use a meticulous direct measurement technique that includes use of calipers or loupe magnification.[21,22] Pelz has shown that "eyeball" estimation of percentage stenosis using the NASCET criteria, even in the hands of experienced readers, is inaccurate compared with carefully obtained direct measurements and unreliable as a method of assigning patients to proper treatment groups.[23]

The Nearly Occluded Carotid Artery (Pseudo-Occlusion)

The clinically important distinction between complete occlusion and very high-grade stenosis (pseudo-occlusion) of the carotid artery can be made only by angiography.[24,25] Patients with highly stenotic lesions may benefit from carotid endarterectomy, whereas those with complete occlusions will not.[26] Noninvasive techniques are often insensitive to the very slow trickle of blood past a near total occlusion and, even at angiography, the findings may be subtle. The cardinal angiographic finding is the so-called "string" or "slim" sign, a thin layer of contrast medium accumulating along the posterior wall of the poststenotic carotid and progressing slowly toward the base of the skull on late films (Figs. 14-5 and 14-6). This appearance is the result of dependent layering of the high specific gravity contrast medium in a stagnant column of blood and possibly to the lowered blood pressure and diminished size of the vessel distal to the lesion.

A special angiographic technique consisting of injecting a larger than usual volume of contrast medium over a longer period (e.g., 16 cc over 4 sec) proximal to the lesion with a longer filming sequence may be needed to identify the very slow blood flow across a subocclusive stenosis.[27] Therefore, the possibility of a pseudo-occlusion should be considered in any patient with symptoms referable to a carotid artery presumed occluded on the basis of noninvasive testing or a standard angiogram. An additional reported angiographic clue to this condition is a long, tapered proximal "stump" at a presumed occlusion site.[28] Uncommon differential considerations for the angiographic "string" sign are carotid dissection, congenital hypoplasia, and radiation-associated carotid disease.[29]

Lesion Morphology

In addition to the degree of stenosis, atherosclerotic lesions are typically characterized angiographically as smooth, irregular, or frankly ulcerated (Fig. 14-7). A sharply marginated or undermined niche seen in profile or *en face* within an atheroma, an irregularly marginated plaque, and delayed wash-out of contrast medium from areas of irregularity have been suggested as signs of ulceration.[30] The likelihood of detecting ulcerations and asymmetric atheromata increases with the number of radiographic projections made.[22,31] It has been shown by in vitro experiments that complete radiographic characterization of filling defects in tubular structures requires at least three projections.[32] Most institutions and

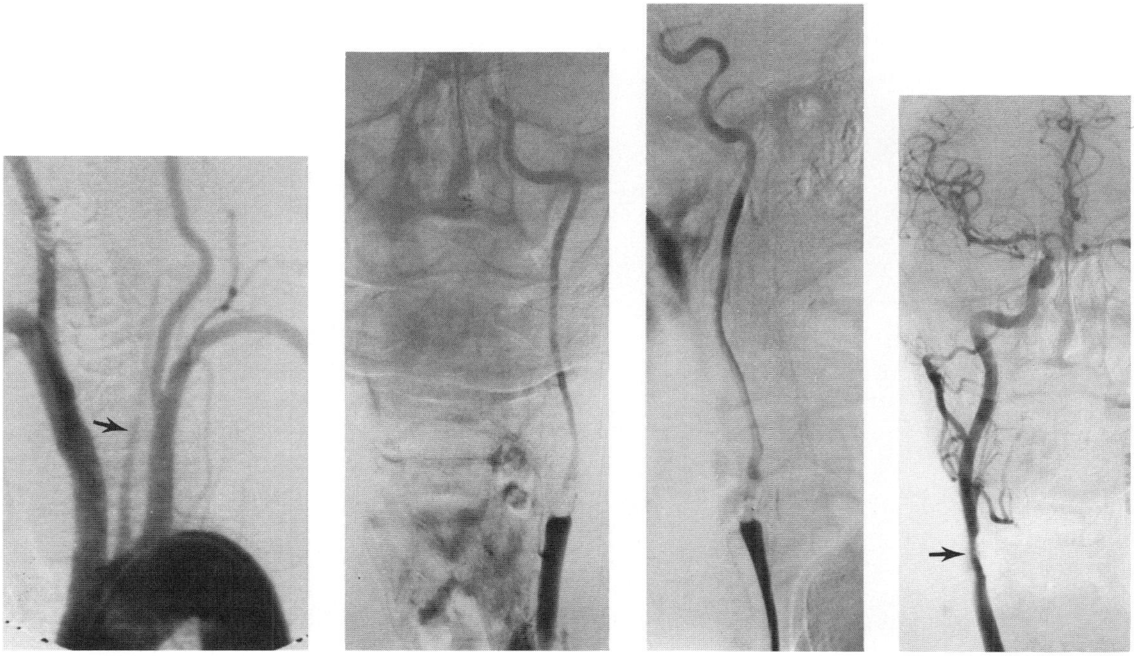

A B C D

Figure 14-5. Nearly occluded internal carotid artery (ICA). *A.* Digital subtraction arch aortogram in LAO projection demonstrates faint opacification of the proximal left common carotid artery (CCA) (*arrow*) without apparent distal flow. *B.* AP and (*C*) lateral projections of late films from a selective left CCA angiogram demonstrate a stagnant column of contrast medium in the CCA, occlusion of the external carotid artery (ECA), and faint opacification of the ICA distal to a very high-grade proximal stenosis. Note the small caliber of the ICA with layering of the contrast medium along the posterior margins of the vessel and dilution of the contrast medium at the carotid-middle cerebral artery junction due to "washout" by unopacified collateral blood flow. *D.* AP projection of the right CCA angiogram demonstrates collateral blood flow to the left middle cerebral artery. There is a moderate stenosis of the right carotid bifurcation (arrow), better seen on other projections not illustrated.

reported studies utilize two views of the carotid artery, with supplementary additional views as necessary to accommodate unusual anatomy or to clarify a complex lesion. Choice of angulation of supplementary views must be individualized because of variations in the position of the external carotid artery relative to the ICA.[33]

Jeans reported 135 patients routinely studied with three views of the carotid bifurcation (lateral and both anterior oblique views).[31] Atheromata were seen on only one view in 44 percent of 181 patent but diseased carotid arteries. No single projection was superior to the others in identifying disease. As would be expected, atheromata seen on only one view tended to be less severe than lesions seen on more than one view. Chikos showed that the addition of two oblique views to the AP and lateral projections had no statistical effect on the estimate of the percentage stenosis but increased the frequency of diagnosis of irregularity and ulceration.[22]

Unfortunately, there is a poor correlation between radiologically identified ulcerations and surgical findings, especially for irregular

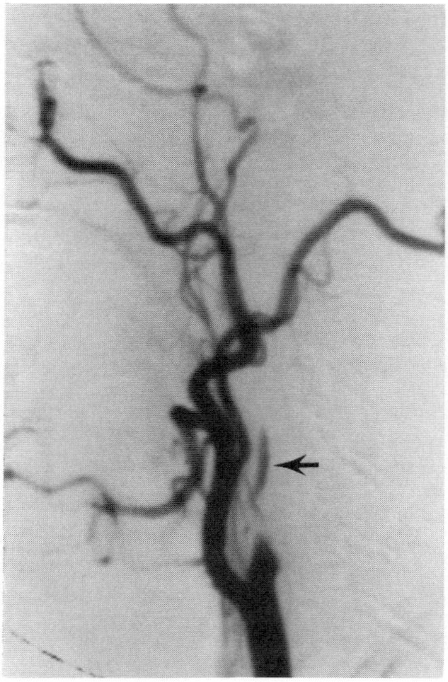

A

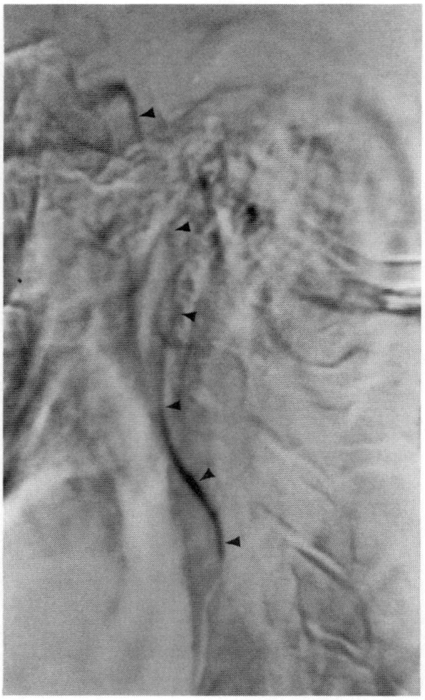

B

Figure 14-6. Early and late lateral projections of a selective CCA DSA in another patient demonstrate more subtle findings in a very high-grade, subocclusive ICA stenosis. *A.* Early arterial phase DSA image demonstrates a normal ECA, a truncated carotid bulb with a pointed distal profile, and a short linear contrast medium accumulation (*arrow*) in the post-bulbar ICA which could be easily confused with an ECA branch vessel or artifact. *B.* A very late image demonstrates contrast medium in dependent portions of the distal ICA and carotid siphon (*arrowheads*). The subtracted image is degraded due to patient motion during the long filming sequence.

Figure 14-7. DSA images of five different carotid bifurcations with atherosclerotic lesions of the proximal ICA. *A.* Smoothly marginated circumferential plaque at the origin of the ICA produces a 55 percent stenosis by NASCET criteria. *B.* Nearly smooth plaque on the posterior wall of the distal bulb. No measurable stenosis by NASCET criteria. A slight indentation in the plaque (*arrow*) is indeterminant for ulceration. *C.* Smoothly marginated posterior bulb plaque with undulating margin produces no stenosis by NASCET criteria. It cannot be determined angiographically whether the central contrast medium collection (*arrow*) represents a shallow ulceration or simply an undulating profile of an endothelialized plaque. *D.* Long irregular stenosis of the distal bulb and post-bulbar carotid. By NASCET criteria, there is a 64 percent stenosis. A small, sharply marginated, niche-like, contrast medium collection in the central portion of the stricture (*arrow*) is suggestive of ulceration. *E.* Complex lesion involving the entire carotid bulb. There is a 65 percent stenosis by NASCET criteria. The large, irregular posterior contrast collection (*arrow*) almost certainly represents a large undermining ulcer in the center of a large posterior atherosclerotic plaque.

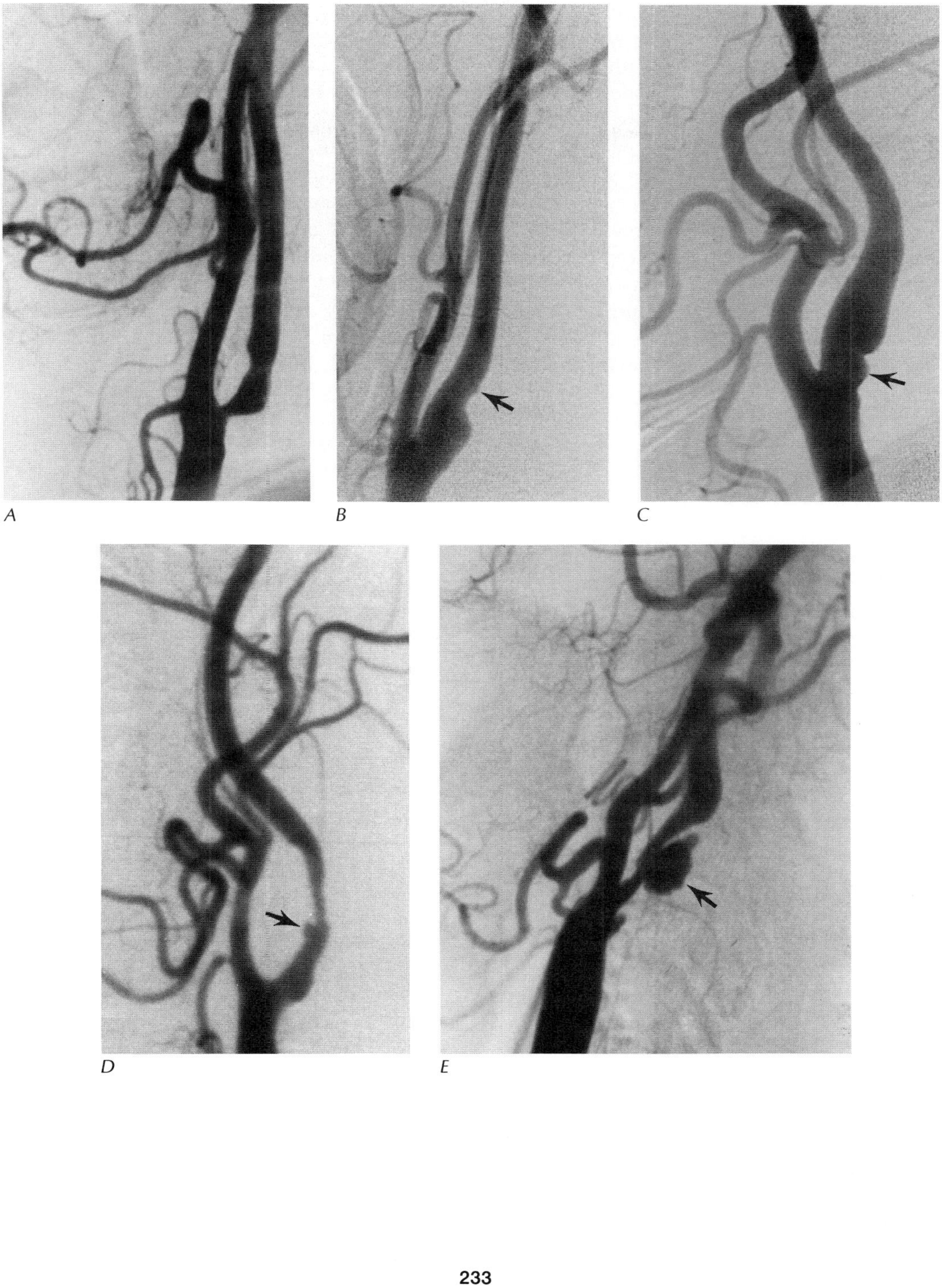
A
B
C
D
E

plaques and shallow ulcerations. In a prospective comparison of angiography with findings at surgery in 45 patients who underwent 50 carotid endarterectomies, Blaisdell found an overall accuracy for angiography of 86 percent for diagnosis of ulceration, with no false-negatives.[30] In that series, when a lesion was more than 30 percent occlusive, ulceration was present at surgery in 80 percent of the lesions. More recently, Streifler reported on a cohort of 500 operated patients recruited for the NASCET.[34] Ulcerated plaques were observed by surgeons in 290 cases (58 percent). Of these, ulceration was diagnosed independently by both the original radiologist and the study neuroradiologist in only 142 (49 percent). In 26 percent of cases with proved ulceration there was interobserver disagreement, and in 35 percent of "agreed" cases both radiologists reported a false-negative diagnosis of no ulcer. Edwards, in a study of 50 operated carotid bifurcations, found ulcerations at surgery in 20 (40 percent).[35] Only 12 (60 percent) were demonstrated angiographically and four (20 percent) were found in angiographically smooth plaques. Of the 30 ulcer-free carotids, 17 (57 percent) were incorrectly diagnosed as ulcerated at angiography. In 10 of these 17 patients, intramural hemorrhage and subintimal hematoma were thought to account for the false-positive angiographic findings.

This poor pathologic-angiographic correlation no doubt relates to the impossibility of determining the presence or absence of an endothelial covering over an atheroma by angiographic means, no matter what its morphology may be. Gross irregularities may be covered by endothelium, and small or shallow ulcerations may not be detected. Indeed, Hertzer has suggested that microscopic ulcerations and thrombi on the order of 100 to 600 μm occur on carotid bifurcation atheromata undetectable by both angiography and direct inspection but of sufficient size to produce symptomatic emboli.[36] Therefore, while angiography may demonstrate quite exquisitely the morphology of a carotid bifurcation lesion, the angiographic diagnosis of true pathologic ulceration (i.e., loss of intima or endothelium) is not reliable.

An intraluminal thrombus associated with an atherosclerotic plaque may occasionally be identified angiographically.[37] Mural thrombi usually occur immediately distal to a high-grade stricture and appear as smooth-surfaced, elongated filling defects in the contrast column. A thrombus may have a broad attachment to the vessel wall, but on at least one projection its margin will be convex, and contrast medium will be seen to extend between the thrombus and the vessel wall.

REFERENCES

1. Wolpert SM, Caplan LR: Current role of cerebral angiography in the diagnosis of cerebrovascular diseases. *AJR* 159:191, 1992.
2. Lasser EC, Berry CC, Talner LB, et al: Pretreatment with corticosteroids to alleviate reactions to intravenous contrast material. *N Engl J Med* 317:845, 1987.
3. Anto HR, Chou S-Y, Porush JG, Shapiro WB: Infusion intravenous pyelography and renal function. Effects of hypertonic mannitol in patients with chronic renal insufficiency. *Arch Intern Med* 141:1652, 1981.
4. Katholi, RE, Taylor GJ, Woods WT, et al: Nephrotoxicity of nonionic low-osmolality versus ionic high-osmolality contrast media: A prospective double-blind randomized comparison in human beings. *Radiology* 186:183, 1993.
5. Kruger RA, Riederer SJ: *Digital Subtraction Angiography,* Boston, GK Hall Medical Publishers, 1984.
6. Brant-Zawadzki M, Gould R, Norman D, et al: Digital subtraction cerebral angiography by intraarterial injection: Comparison with conventional angiography. *AJR* 140:347, 1983.
7. Lipchik EO, Mewissen MW: A comparison of normal intraarterial digital subtraction angiography with standard angiography in patients

with symptomatic cerebrovascular ischemia. *AJNR* 11:837, 1990.
8. Crocker EF Jr, Tutton RH, Bowen JC: The role of intravenous digital subtraction angiography in the evaluation of extracranial carotid artery disease: Can the decision for carotid artery surgery be made solely on the basis of its findings? *J Vasc Surg* 4:157, 1986.
9. Earnest F, Houser OW, Forbes GS, et al: The accuracy and limitations of intravenous digital subtraction angiography in the evaluation of atherosclerotic cerebrovascular disease: Angiographic and surgical correlation. *Mayo Clin Proc* 58:735, 1983.
10. Aaron JO, Hesselink JR, Oot R, et al: Complications of intravenous DSA performed for carotid artery disease: A prospective study. *Radiology* 153:675, 1984.
11. Stevens JM: Where you are doubtful of doing good, be sure of doing no harm. *Radiology* 173:880, 1989.
12. Osborn AG, Maack JC, Nelson BR: *Introduction to Cerebral Angiography*. Hagerstown MD, Harper & Row, 1980.
13. Miller DL: Heparin in angiography: Current patterns of use. *Radiology* 172:1007, 1989.
14. Hankey GJ, Warlow CP, Sellar RJ: Cerebral angiographic risk in mild cerebrovascular disease. *Stroke* 21:209, 1990.
15. North American Symptomatic Carotid Endarterectomy Trial (NASCET) Steering Committee: North American Symptomatic Carotid Endarterectomy Trial: Methods, patient characteristics, and progress. *Stroke* 22:711, 1991.
16. European Carotid Surgery Trialist's Collaborative Group: MRC European Carotid Surgery Trial: Interim results for symptomatic patients with severe (70–99%) or with mild (0–29%) carotid stenosis. *Lancet* 337:1235, 1991.
17. Roederer GO, Langlois YE, Chan ATW, et al: Ultrasonic duplex scanning of the extracranial carotid arteries: Improved accuracy using new features from the common carotid artery. *J Cardiovasc Ultrasonography* 1:373, 1982.
18. A Veterans Administration Cooperative Study: Role of carotid endarterectomy in asymptomatic carotid stenosis. *Stroke* 17:534, 1986.
19. The Asymptomatic Carotid Atherosclerosis Study Group: Study design for randomized prospective trial of carotid endarterectomy for asymptomatic atherosclerosis. *Stroke* 20:844, 1989.
20. Thiele BL, Jones AM, Hobson RW, et al: Standards in noninvasive cerebrovascular testing: Report from the Committee on Standards for Noninvasive Vascular Testing of the Joint Council of the Society for Vascular Surgery and the North American Chapter of the International Society for Cardiovascular Surgery. *J Vasc Surg* 15:495, 1992.
21. Moneta GL, Edwards JM, Chitwood RW, et al: Correlation of North American Symptomatic Endarterectomy Trial (NASCET) angiographic definition of 70% to 99% internal carotid artery stenosis with duplex scanning. *J Vasc Surg* 17:152, 1993.
22. Chikos PM, Fisher LD, Hirsch JH, et al: Observer variability in evaluating extracranial carotid artery stenosis. *Stroke* 14:885, 1983.
23. Pelz DM, Fox AJ, Eliasziw M, Barnett HMJ: Stenosis of the carotid bifurcation: Subjective assessment compared with strict measurement criteria. *Can Assoc Radiol J* 44:247, 1993.
24. Ammar AD, Turrentine MW, Farha SJ: The importance of arteriographic interpretation in occlusion or pseudo-occlusion of the carotid artery. *Surg Gynecol Obstet* 167:119, 1988.
25. O'Leary DH, Gibbons GW, Pine DF: Limitations of noninvasive testing in assessing the "occluded" carotid artery. *AJNR* 4:759, 1983.
26. North American Symptomatic Carotid Endarterectomy Trial Collaborators: Beneficial effect of carotid endarterectomy in symptomatic patients with high-grade carotid stenosis. *N Engl J Med* 325:445, 1991.
27. Countee RW, Vijayanathan T: Reconstitution of "totally" occluded internal carotid arteries. *J Neurosurg* 50:747, 1979.
28. Gabrielson TO, Seeger JF, Knake JE, et al: The nearly occluded internal carotid artery: A diagnostic trap. *Radiology* 138:618, 1981.
29. Mehigan JT, Olcott C: The carotid "string" sign. *Am J Surg* 140:137, 1980.
30. Blaisdell FW, Glickman M, Trunkey DD: Ulcerated atheroma of the carotid artery. *Arch Surg* 108:491, 1974.
31. Jeans WD, Mackenzie S, Baird RN: Angiography in transient cerebral ischaemia using three

views of the carotid bifurcation. *Br J Radiol* 59:135, 1986.
32. Berne FA, Lawrence WP, Carlton WH: Roentgenographic measurement of arterial narrowing. *AJR* 110:757, 1970.
33. Trigaux JP, Delchambre F, Van Beers B: Anatomical variations of the carotid bifurcation: Implications for digital subtraction angiography and ultrasonography. *Br J Radiol* 63:181, 1990.
34. Streifler JY, Benavente OR, Fox AJ: The accuracy of angiographic detection of carotid plaque ulceration: Results from the NASCET study (abstr). *Stroke* 22:149, 1991.
35. Edwards JH, Kricheff II, Riles T, Imparanto A: Angiographically undetected ulceration of the carotid bifurcation as a cause of embolic stroke. *Radiology* 132:369, 1979.
36. Hertzer NR, Beven EG, Benjamin SP: Ultramicroscopic ulcerations and thrombi of the carotid bifurcation. *Arch Surg* 112:1394, 1977.
37. Roberson GH, Scott WR, Rosenbaum MD: Thrombi at the site of carotid stenosis. *Radiology* 109:353, 1973.

Part Four

Therapeutic Approaches and Randomized Clinical Trials

15

Antithrombotic Therapies to Prevent Stroke

Diane H. Solomon
Robert G. Hart

Antithrombotic medications include anticoagulants, antiplatelets agents, and medications that enhance fibrinolysis. These agents are effective and important in the management of many patients with threatened stroke. Postmortem observations of thrombotic cerebral arterial occlusion and clinical case reports in the 1950s and 1960s[1,2] suggested that antithrombotic agents might be useful for preventing ischemic stroke. Enthusiasm for warfarin anticoagulation waxed and then waned as antiplatelet agents were shown to be effective for stroke prevention in several randomized clinical trials during the past decade.[3] While warfarin has been established as effective for prevention of cardiogenic brain embolism,[4] its value has not been proved for patients with intrinsic cerebrovascular diseases. Antiplatelet agents are the current mainstay of prophylactic therapy for primary atherosclerotic cerebrovascular disease. However, specific patient management requires consideration of the diverse causes of stroke.

Ischemic stroke is a syndrome caused by several common and many uncommon disorders which lead to occlusion of cerebral arteries (Figs. 15-1 and 15-2). Severe carotid artery stenosis is present in 20 percent or less of patients with brain ischemia. Hence, medical therapies and risk factor modification are far more valuable than carotid endarterectomy for most patients with threatened stroke. Nonstenotic atherosclerotic plaques can cause transient ischemic attack (TIA) and stroke by acting as sources of arteriogenic emboli that obstruct distal vessels. Primary occlusive disease of the penetrating arteries leads to small subcortical infarcts ("lacunae") by fibrinoid necrosis, a process distinct from atherosclerosis. Minor differences and fluctuations in the tendency to thrombosis probably act in synergy with underlying structural disease to precipitate stroke. The efficacy of antithrombotic prophylaxis in each of these major subtypes of primary cerebrovascular disease is likely to be different.

Until recently, clinical trials of antithrombotic therapy have considered patients with these differing pathologies together, owing to the difficulty of defining the specific etiology of threatened stroke in individual patients. Hence, estimates of the efficacy of antithrombotic agents for stroke prevention were based on a diverse group of pathologic mechanisms that may or may not respond identically. This has been a major limitation in identifying highly effective antithrombotic regimens for stroke prevention.

Antithrombotic agents have competing beneficial and potentially adverse effects in patients with cerebrovascular disease. By inhibiting clot formation they can reduce in situ thrombotic occlusion, inhibit propagating thrombosis in low-flow areas distal to occlusions of any cause, and reduce the occurrence of arteriogenic emboli. Hypothetically, these agents can worsen intraplaque hemorrhage in atherosclerotic lesions, a phenomenon of uncertain clinical importance.[5,6] Anticoagulation to conventional intensities increases the risk of intracerebral hemorrhage and, to a lesser degree, so does aspirin.[7,8] The clinical effect of

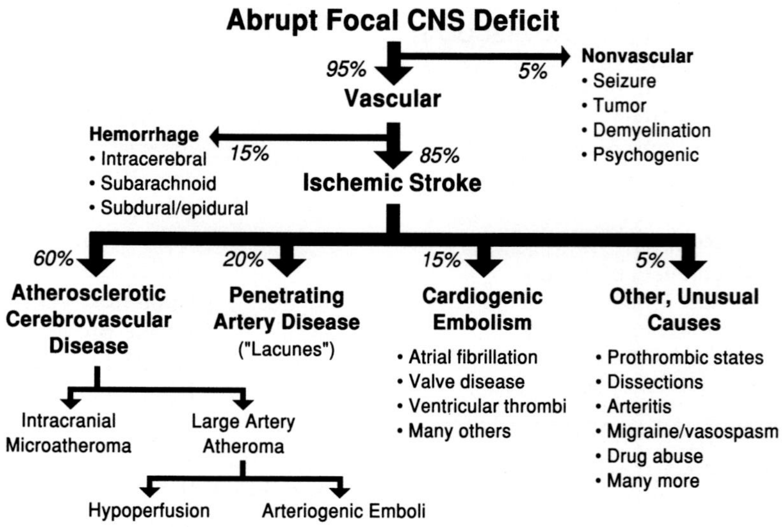

Figure 15-1. Differential diagnosis of ischemic stroke.

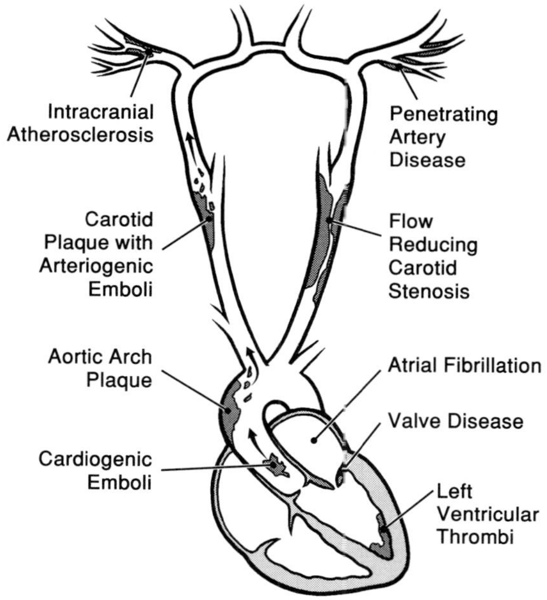

Figure 15-2. Pathophysiology of common causes of ischemic stroke.

antithrombotic agents on endothelial reparative processes in cerebrovascular atherosclerosis has not been well defined.[9,10] Hence, the risk/benefit balance of chronic antithrombotic therapies is a complex and difficult problem.

Assessing the risks and benefits of chronic antithrombotic therapies for stroke prevention is made more complicated by frequent concomitant illnesses in the elderly, stroke-prone population. Some clinical trials have shown that antithrombotic therapies that theoretically should be beneficial are actually ineffective or even harmful. There is no substitute for randomized clinical trials with carefully defined objectives, despite their organizational complexity, length, expense, and limitations. In this chapter, we will focus on sound and durable antithrombotic management justified by randomized clinical trials. We offer guidelines for antithrombotic therapy for each of the major clinical settings in ischemic cerebrovascular disease, acknowledging a range of acceptable management strategies based on current clinical science and common sense (Table 15-1).

PLATELETS AND THE PATHOGENESIS OF THROMBOSIS

Platelet aggregation is an integral part of thrombus formation, and arterial thrombi are the most common mechanism of ischemic stroke, whether their occlusive effect occurs at the site of formation or distally as emboli. Platelets adhere to abnormal vessels and re-

Table 15-1 Antithrombotic Therapy in Cerebrovascular Diseases

Clinical situation	Recommended therapy	Acceptable options
TIA or stroke[a]	ASA 325 mg/day[b]	ASA 75–1300 mg/day Ticlopidine 250 mg bid
TIA or stroke[a] during ASA	Ticlopidine 250 mg bid	ASA 75–1300 mg/day Warfarin INR 2–3
Atrial fibrillation		
Primary prevention	ASA 325 mg/day or warfarin INR 2–3[c]	Warfarin INR 1.5–4
Secondary prevention	Warfarin INR 2–3	Warfarin INR 1.5–4 ASA 325 mg/day
Asymptomatic carotid stenosis	ASA 325 mg/day	ASA 75–1300 mg/day no antithrombotic Rx
Asymptomatic people > 60 years old	No Rx	ASA 75–325 mg/day if risk factors

[a]Carotid endarterectomy for TIA or minor stroke associated with 70 to 99 percent ipsilateral stenosis unless contraindicated.
[b]Experts disagree about whether ≥ 975 mg of ASA offers more benefits than lower doses.
[c]See risk factors for thromboembolism for identification of high-risk subgroups.[71]

lease vasoactive and platelet-stimulatory substances to recruit further platelet aggregation. These aggregates mix with fibrin to form whitish-gray, platelet-rich thrombi. There are three major pathways of platelet aggregation: (1) activation of thromboxane A_2 by cyclooxygenase; (2) direct platelet aggregation by adenosine diphosphate; and (3) stimulation of thrombin by phospholipases A and C. Leukocytes or damaged endothelial cells can also directly activate platelets by stimulation of platelet-activating factor.[11] Additionally, catecholamines are weak direct platelet agonists that can augment platelet aggregability, opposing natural antiplatelet agents such as prostacyclin and partly overcoming the antiplatelet effect of aspirin.[12]

As the pathogenesis of thrombosis has become better understood, drugs have been identified that alter specific steps in platelet aggregation. The most promising have been tested in clinical trials of stroke prevention. These agents include aspirin, dipyridamole, sulfinpyrazone, and ticlopidine.

ASPIRIN IN CEREBROVASCULAR DISEASE

Mechanism of Action

Aspirin (acetylsalicylic acid, ASA) is the most studied and widely used antiplatelet agent. Its use is based on its ability to block the thromboxane A_2 pathway of platelet aggregation. Aspirin permanently inhibits the rate-limiting enzyme cyclooxygenase for the life of the platelet, thus preventing the production of thromboxane A_2 with its attendant excitatory effect on platelet aggregation and potent vasoconstriction.[13] Aspirin does not affect the other known major pathways of platelet aggregation, although it may affect platelet function in additional ways not yet well understood. Doses of 325 mg/day or more prolong the bleeding time to about twice baseline level.[11] At doses greater than 40 mg/day, aspirin inhibits prostacyclin, a vasodilator and platelet antiaggregant secreted by the vascular endothelium.[14]

Clinical Trials

There have been more than ten randomized clinical trials comparing aspirin to placebo for stroke prevention in patients with TIA, and minor or major stroke (Chap. 16, 17).[15–26] Metanalysis (pooled results) indicates an overall 22 percent reduction in nonfatal stroke and a 25 percent reduction in the constellation of nonfatal stroke, myocardial infarct, or vascular death.[3,27]

While a 20 to 25 percent risk reduction in stroke by aspirin is generally accepted, based on the highly statistically significant results of pooled data, the variable results of individual clinical trials warrant comment. Inconsistencies between trials may be in part methodological, such as insufficient sample size (with Type II error) and differences in defining endpoints. It is likely that differences in patient population and perhaps in the type and dose of antiplatelet medication also contribute. Hypothetically, there may be subsets of patients more (or less) likely to respond to aspirin. Greater stroke reduction with aspirin may be obtained if the "aspirin-responsive" subsets of patients can be identified and treated, with alternative therapies found for other patients. Based on the hypothesis that antiplatelet agents are more effective for some patients with threatened stroke than for others, stroke trials are now beginning to stratify patients into key pathogenetic and demographic subgroups. Most of the work in this area to date has involved secondary analyses and has been limited by small numbers of patients.

Gender and Aspirin Efficacy

Two early studies showed a sex difference in the effectiveness of aspirin for secondary stroke prevention.[16–18] These studies did not show a benefit of aspirin in women, but it is now accepted that this apparent sex difference was most likely an artifact due to the small number of women entered into the trials and the inherently lower event rate among women.[28,29] Several more recent clinical trials have confirmed that aspirin is beneficial for preventing stroke in both men and women.[15,26,30,31] The recent collaborative overview of randomized trials of antiplatelet treatment found no difference in benefit from aspirin in those with increased risk for all types of occlusive vascular disease regardless of sex.[3]

Aspirin in Lacunar Stroke

It is likely that the effect of antiplatelet agents varies with specific stroke subtypes (Figs. 15-1, 15-2). Lacunar strokes are small, subcortical infarcts usually associated with characteristic clinical syndromes such as pure hemisensory loss or isolated hemiparesis (Fig. 15-3). Diagnosis requires visualization by CT or MRI (Chap. 13) or, if no such lesion is visible, documenting the absence of cortical ischemia. Recurrence is common, and secondary prevention is important in management. Lacunar strokes are uncommonly caused by emboli from large arteries or cardioembolic sources; they are most often the result of small vessel occlusive disease or microatheroma. Diabetic and hypertensive patients are particularly predisposed to disease of the small cerebral vessels.

In the 1970s, Fisher identified a distinct pathophysiology of lipohyalinosis underlying occlusion of the deep penetrating artery branches, in contrast to the thrombus formation of large vessel disease.[32] More recently, Hess and others have noted that the endothelial cells of small vessels differ from those of large vessels. Because endothelial cells regulate prostaglandin synthesis and thrombogenicity, local coagulation may be regulated differently, depending on vessel size.[33] Based on this information, interest has developed in

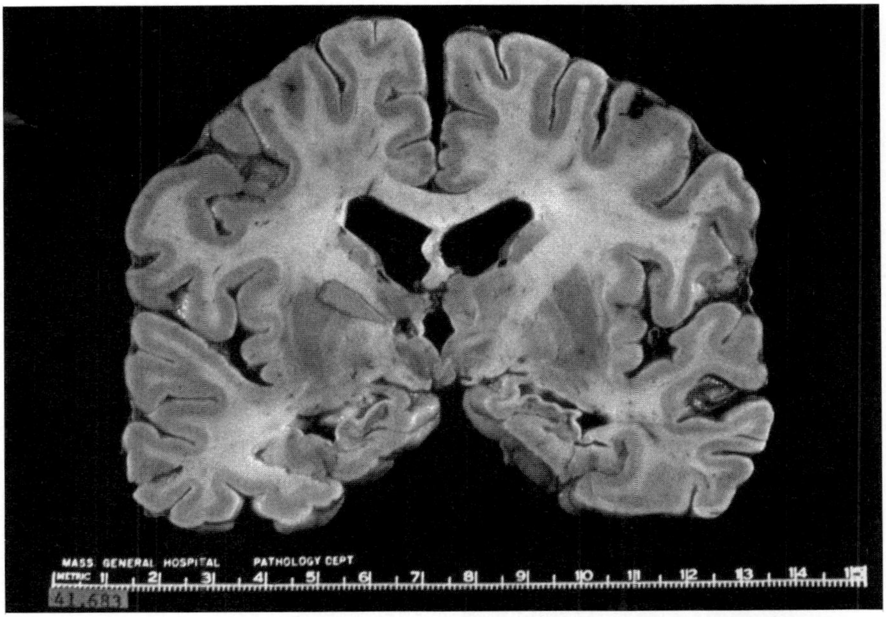

Figure 15-3. Gross coronal section showing a thalamic lacunar infarct (*arrow*).

evaluating antithrombotic therapy for prevention of lacunar infarcts separately from stroke due to large artery disease.

The efficacy of aspirin in lacunar stroke has not been definitively assessed, but there is a suggestion from three clinical studies that aspirin may be especially beneficial in this common stroke subtype. Chimowitz and coworkers found a low frequency of lacunar infarction (11.5 percent) in 47 patients sustaining an ischemic stroke while taking aspirin.[34] In the Ticlopidine Aspirin Stroke Study, only 17 (8 percent) of 212 recurrent strokes in aspirin-treated patients were lacunar.[35] Since there were no concomitant control groups in these two studies, it is not possible to be certain that these low prevalences of lacunae (which usually comprise 20 to 25 percent of brain infarcts) were a direct result of aspirin treatment. However, in the randomized AICLA trial, group subanalysis showed a 10 percent incidence of recurrent stroke in patients with lacunar infarcts treated with aspirin compared with 26 percent in the placebo group (a risk reduction of 62 percent).[15] It is not always possible to identify accurately the etiology of stroke, and often there are multiple possible etiologies in a given patient. Nevertheless, future studies may confirm a greater benefit of aspirin treatment for this subtype of stroke and stimulate improved diagnosis.

Optimal Dose of Aspirin

At present, there is ongoing controversy regarding the optimal dose of aspirin for stroke prevention. Interestingly, recommendations tend to be regional, with European authorities favoring low doses (30–75 mg/day), Canadians advocating high doses (> 1000 mg/day), and most Americans opting for doses in between. Clinical data supporting all three choices exist. The strongest argument against using high doses of aspirin is that gastrotoxicity is clearly dose-dependent. Aspirin probably also slightly increases the risk of intracerebral hemorrhage, but it is not clear whether this effect is dose-related.[7,8]

Several unresolved pharmacologic issues contribute to the aspirin dose controversy. Considerable individual variability in response to aspirin occurs. Doses as low as 20 mg/day have been shown to completely inhibit platelet aggregation in some patients,[36] but 16 percent of patients taking less than 650 mg/day in one study did not achieve complete inhibition.[37] Even 1300 mg/day may not result in complete acetylation of cyclooxygenase in a small percentage of patients.[38] The effect of low-dose aspirin on platelet aggregability may depend on the strength of the trigger for thrombogenesis.[39] It is not clear whether the in vitro measurement of aspirin effect on platelet aggregation correlates with prevention of cerebral ischemia.[38]

Another pharmacologic issue revolves around preservation of the strong, naturally occurring vasodilator, prostacyclin. Aspirin doses of 40 mg or less do not inhibit endothelial prostacyclin and would theoretically be beneficial.[14] Yet, the importance of sparing prostacyclin inhibition has not been established clinically.[40] There is some evidence that endothelial prostacyclin may be elevated in patients with severe atherosclerosis.[41]

Prevention of platelet hyperreactivity to shear stress is dose-related and may be important in stroke reduction, especially following carotid endarterectomy. Ratnatunga and colleagues found that platelet hyperreactivity to shear stress was present in patients taking 75 mg/day of aspirin after coronary bypass.[42] Platelet reactivity to shear stress was significantly reduced by 300 mg/day, and it may be further reduced by higher doses.

Clinical trials have established the efficacy of a broad range of doses but have not identified an optimal aspirin dose. Most earlier stroke studies used doses of 900 mg to 1500 mg daily, but recent trials have evaluated lower doses. The Dutch TIA trial randomized 3131 patients with TIA or minor stroke to either 30 mg or 283 mg of aspirin daily.[40] There was no significant difference in vascular death, stroke, or myocardial infarction (MI) between the two low-dose groups (14.7 percent in the 30-mg group and 15.2 percent in the 283-mg group). As expected using these low doses, major bleeding complications were infrequent (2.6 percent in the 30-mg group and 3.2 percent in the 283-mg group). The Swedish Aspirin Low-Dose Trial was the first to show a beneficial effect with a daily aspirin dose of less than 300 mg as compared to placebo.[26] A dose of 75 mg/day provided a 17 percent risk reduction (95 percent CI, 0 to 30 percent) for vascular death, stroke, or MI in symptomatic patients. The prevalence of severe bleeding was again low (3 percent), but significantly higher than in the placebo group (1.3 percent). While considerably safer than high doses, low-dose aspirin does not eliminate the risk of hemorrhagic side effects.

The UK-TIA trial is the only stroke study to date that has directly compared medium-dose aspirin (300 mg/day) to high-dose (1200 mg/day).[23] The two doses appeared equally effective for stroke prevention. There was increased gastrointestinal bleeding in those receiving 1200 mg/day of aspirin (5 percent for the 1200-mg group and 3 percent for the 300-mg group). The results of this study do not justify the added risk of GI bleeding associated with high aspirin doses.

The Physicians' Health Study was a primary stroke prevention trial in which 22,071 male physicians received either 325 mg of aspirin every other day or placebo for five years.[43] There was no reduction in the occurrence of stroke in those given aspirin. The lack of effect of aspirin in this study has been attributed by some to the low aspirin dose; however, it seems more likely that the characteristics of the study population were responsible. The dose of aspirin that was ineffective for stroke prevention in the younger, healthier men of the Physicians' Health Study may not be relevant to that used in the secondary prevention trials, which treated patients with established vascular disease. The mechanisms of stroke probably differed considerably, and it may be that aspirin at any dose is less effective in preventing strokes in young people without manifest vascular disease.

The Antiplatelet Trialists' Collaboration identified four clinical trials with at least 1000 patients which directly compared doses of aspirin less than or equal to 325 mg/day with doses greater than 325 mg/day in patients with cardiovascular or cerebrovascular disease.[3] No significant difference between the aspirin doses was found. This respected group of collaborators also made indirect comparisons of 122 trials evaluating a particular dose of aspirin versus placebo. They found a nonsignificant trend toward a greater effect using lower daily doses. Many of these trials included cardiac patients, and extrapolation to stroke patients must be made with caution, since there are many differences between the heart and the brain with regard to pathophysiology, risk factors, and complications.

Considering available data, an aspirin dose of 325 mg/day can be recommended for secondary stroke prevention. This dose has been shown to be effective in clinical trials, fulfills most of the concerns raised by pharmacologic studies, and importantly decreases the gastrotoxicity of higher doses.

TICLOPIDINE

Mechanism of Action

Ticlopidine hydrochloride is an effective antiplatelet agent unrelated to aspirin that has been available in the United States since December 1991. Unlike aspirin, ticlopidine does not inhibit the thromboxane A_2 pathway of platelet aggregation, nor does it affect production of prostacyclin by the endothelium. Ticlopidine's antiplatelet aggregating action occurs through inhibition of the direct adenosine diphosphate pathway. Bleeding time is prolonged in a dose-dependent manner and to a greater extent than with aspirin. Ticlopidine appears to decrease platelet adhesion and reduce blood viscosity.[44,45] It has no analgesic properties.[46] The maximum platelet antiaggregation effect requires about five days, with recovery of normal platelet activity after ticlopidine withdrawal within four to eight days.[47]

Clinical Trials

Two large, double-blind clinical trials have evaluated the effectiveness of ticlopidine for the secondary prevention of stroke.[35,48] While both showed it to be an effective prophylactic agent, only one compared ticlopidine to aspirin. In the Ticlopidine Aspirin Stroke Study (TASS), 3069 patients with TIA or minor ischemic stroke were assigned to ticlopidine or aspirin.[35] Over three years, stroke recurred at rates of 13 percent in patients taking 1300 mg/day of aspirin and 10 percent in patients taking 500 mg/day of ticlopidine, for a relative risk reduction of 21 percent, and an absolute ischemic stroke reduction of 1 percent/year with ticlopidine therapy as compared with aspirin therapy.[49] Many of the patients who later participated in TASS had been taking aspirin at the time of their qualifying event. The randomization of these "aspirin failures" to aspirin or ticlopidine may have introduced a bias against aspirin.

The Antiplatelet Trialists' Collaboration analyzed the three trials that have directly compared ticlopidine with aspirin, including TASS.[3] They found no significant difference in the occurrence of MI, stroke, or vascular death. Similarly, when 29 ticlopidine trials were indirectly compared to the results of 45 aspirin trials, there was no significant benefit of ticlopidine in preventing the same major vascular events.

The impact of ticlopidine on MI and vascular death must be considered when evaluating its role in the management of patients with cerebrovascular disease. Surprisingly, the major effect of ticlopidine on death, relative to aspirin, involved nonvascular deaths. When all vascular events (ischemic strokes, MI, and vascular deaths) are pooled, the TASS results demonstrate only a slight advantage for ticlopidine over aspirin (3 percent relative risk reduction).[50] There appears to be no advantage of ticlopidine over aspirin for MI prophylaxis. Both agents are effective, but a 9 percent increase in all cholesterol fractions has been associated with ticlopidine use.[51,52] It is not known whether this will have an adverse effect on MI and vascular death in the long-term.[53]

Survivors of major disabling stroke had fewer recurrences while taking ticlopidine than placebo.[48] No study has yet directly compared ticlopidine with aspirin for secondary stroke prevention in this setting. In fact, aspirin's effectiveness in such patients has not been proved.[20]

Combination Therapy

A small study compared low-dose combination therapy (aspirin 81 mg/day, ticlopidine 100 mg/day) with either aspirin (300 mg/day), ticlopidine (200 mg/day), or placebo.[54] The combination markedly inhibited platelet aggregation by ADP, arachidonate, and platelet activating factor, and decreased plasma concentration of platelet factor IV and beta-thromboglobulin. This represented an additive antiplatelet effect. The bleeding time was also more prolonged with the combination than with either agent alone. If platelets are profoundly suppressed, there could be a major risk of bleeding, including possible intracranial hemorrhage.[55] Until the safety and efficacy of using both medications is established, their combination is not recommended.

Adverse Effects

Ticlopidine has considerable side effects, including a 2.4 percent incidence of neutropenia. Other minor but more common problems include diarrhea (occurring in about 20 percent of patients) and rash (occurring in about 10 percent).[35,48] Gastrointestinal intolerance occurs more commonly with high-dose aspirin (1 g/day or more) than with ticlopidine. However, patients should be cautioned to avoid nonsteroidal anti-inflammatory drugs during ticlopidine therapy because of the potentially additive effect on bleeding time and increased hemorrhagic risk. A few patients (1 percent) have developed cholestatic jaundice. In one large study, 12 percent of patients discontinued treatment before the end of the study because of side effects.[35]

Of the 2048 patients treated with ticlopidine who participated in two large clinical trials, 50 patients (2.4 percent) developed an absolute neutrophil count (ANC) less than 1200 neutrophils/mm^3. Most cases occurred during the first three months of therapy; in cases considered severe enough to warrant withdrawal from ticlopidine, neutrophil counts returned to normal within three weeks. After the first three months of therapy, the incidence of mild and moderate neutropenia (ANC between 451 and 1200 neutrophils/mm^3) were similar for ticlopidine, aspirin, and placebo.

It is not possible to predict which patients will develop neutropenia. Complete blood counts and white cell differential counts must be performed every two weeks, starting from the second week to the end of the third month of ticlopidine therapy. More frequent monitoring is necessary for patients whose granulocyte counts have been consistently declining or are 30 percent less than the baseline count. If clinical evaluation and monitoring confirm neutropenia (fewer than 1200 neutrophils/mm^3), ticlopidine should be discontinued. Following three months of ticlopidine therapy, blood counts need to be obtained only in patients with signs or symptoms of infection.[56]

Recommendations

Ticlopidine is slightly more effective than aspirin for secondary stroke prevention. However, the newer antiplatelet agent may cause life-threatening neutropenia and costs approximately \$80/month compared with \$1/month for aspirin. The additional cost of blood work and monitoring also must be considered. An absolute risk reduction of one stroke per 100 patients per year probably does not warrant the use of a more dangerous and more expensive treatment for many patients. It is most practical, in terms of both risk/benefit profile and cost containment, to reserve ticlopidine for patients intolerant of aspirin and those experiencing TIA or stroke during aspirin therapy ("aspirin failures").[49,57] Ticlopidine can be considered a first-line choice following disabling noncardioembolic major stroke, primarily because it has been proved effective in this setting and aspirin has not.[48] The higher risk of recurrent stroke following major stroke further supports the use of ticlopidine for initial therapy in these patients.

OTHER ANTIPLATELET AGENTS

Other antiplatelet agents evaluated in clinical trials include dipyridamole and sulfinpyrazone. Dipyridamole (Persantine) inhibits phosphodiesterase rather than cyclooxygenase. One early study randomized 169 patients with TIA and stroke to dipyridamole or placebo and showed no benefit after two years.[58] Since then, three trials have evaluated the combination of aspirin with dipyridamole against aspirin alone. Despite a theoretical potential for added benefit due to the different mechanisms of the two agents, none was found.[15,30,59] While dipyridamole may be effective for preventing emboli from mechanical heart valves, there is no evidence to support its use in patients with primary cerebrovascular disease.

Sulfinpyrazone is a weak competitive inhibitor of cyclooxygenase. It decreases platelet adhesion and prolongs platelet survival. It has a slow onset of action and must be administered in multiple daily doses. Sulfinpyrazone versus aspirin was studied in 127 patients with TIA, and no difference was found.[60] When sulfinpyrazone with aspirin was compared with aspirin alone in the Canadian Cooperative Stroke Study, there was no added benefit of sulfinpyrazone.[16] Hence, there is little support for its use to prevent stroke.

ANTICOAGULATION FOR CEREBROVASCULAR DISEASE

There has been resurgent interest in a potential role for chronic oral anticoagulation to prevent stroke in patients with primary cerebrovascular disease (i.e., noncardioembolic brain ischemia). This interest has been kindled by: (1) evidence that low (safer) intensities of anticoagulation are effective in several clinical situations (e.g., atrial fibrillation, deep venous thrombosis); (2) randomized trials testing anticoagulation in elderly patients with atrial fibrillation, showing a relatively low risk of major bleeding in these selected patients; (3) reproducible monitoring using the international normalized ratio (INR); and (4) the limitations of antiplatelet agents, as some 75 percent of strokes are not prevented by antiplatelet therapy.

Oral anticoagulants are vitamin K antagonists, which interfere with hepatic synthesis of coagulation proteins.[61] Warfarin is the most widely used oral anticoagulant in North America. Optimal anticoagulation requires monitoring with the INR, which corrects for differing sensitivities of commercial laboratory thromboplastins. An INR range of 2.0 to 3.0 approximates a prothrombin time ratio of 1.3 to 1.6, but this varies depending on thromboplastin sensitivity. Because of the narrow therapeutic range and frequent drug interactions, safe oral anticoagulation requires monitoring by those with special expertise. Bleeding is the only common complication of oral anticoagulation. Serious bleeding requiring hospitalization occurs in 1 to 4 percent yearly of elderly patients anticoagulated to INRs of 2 to 4. The risk of intracerebral hemorrhage is also increased about eightfold and is associated with increasing patient age (especially over age 75) and prior cerebral infarction.

Whether chronic oral anticoagulation is of value in patients with threatened stroke due to primary cerebrovascular disease is unknown. Initial clinical studies were carried out nearly 30 years ago, antedating application of modern clinical trial methodology. These trials were small, with vague entry and event criteria and short or incomplete follow-up. Further confounding interpretation of these early trials, higher intensities of anticoagulation were employed, blood pressure management was suboptimal, and CT imaging was not available to identify hemorrhagic strokes reliably. Three small randomized trials carried out more recently compared anticoagulation (approximate INR 1.7 to 4.0) to platelet antiaggregants in patients with TIA and stroke without residual deficits.[62–64] No clear benefit of anticoagulation was demonstrated, but the small number of stroke events makes Type II error (missing true benefit) a concern and aggregate results inconclusive.

At present chronic oral anticoagulation should not be the initial therapy for unselected patients with cerebrovascular disease, as no advantage over the safer and proven-effective platelet antiaggregation agents has yet been demonstrated in clinical studies. Some physicians empirically use oral anticoagulants in patients who have TIA or stroke while taking aspirin. Ticlopidine is a better validated alternative in this situation. Others occasionally recommend anticoagulation for patients with severe symptomatic, inoperable carotid or vertebrobasilar stenosis. Selective anticoagulation of such high-risk patients is within the range of acceptable management, but remains unsupported by adequate clinical studies. Combinations of very low-intensity anticoagulation (INR < 1.5) with low doses of aspirin are being tested in patients with coronary artery disease, but relative efficacy and particularly safety in patients with cerebrovascular disease has not yet been assessed.

CARDIOGENIC EMBOLISM

Antithrombotic therapies are highly effective for prophylaxis of cardiogenic embolism, and hence cardioembolic strokes are among the most preventable causes of brain ischemia. About one ischemic stroke in six is due to cardiogenic embolism.[65] Antithrombotic prophylaxis for cardiogenic embolism depends on the specific cardiac disorder (Fig. 15-4).[4]

Advances in cardiac imaging techniques, particularly ultrasonography, have resulted in more reliable identification of cardioembolic sources. With transesophageal echocardiography (TEE), the ultrasound transducer is placed in the esophagus adjacent to the left atrium, affording improved visualization of the atrium, its appendage, and the ascending aorta. Compared with conventional transthoracic echocardiography, TEE more sensitively detects abnormalities of the interatrial septum (atrial septal aneurysms, patent foramen ovale, atrial septal defects), atrial appendage thrombi associated with atrial fibrillation, and the mitral valvular vegetations of infective endocarditis and nonbacterial thrombotic endocarditis.[66] Atherosclerotic lesions of the ascending aorta with overlying thrombi can be detected by biplanar TEE.[67] About 20 percent of patients with ischemic stroke will have one or more potentially embolic sources detected by TEE that would not be apparent by transthoracic echocardiography. At present, the management implications of detecting minor potential embolic sources are unclear, as longitudinal clinical studies are not available to define natural history or response to therapy.

Atrial fibrillation, even in the absence of

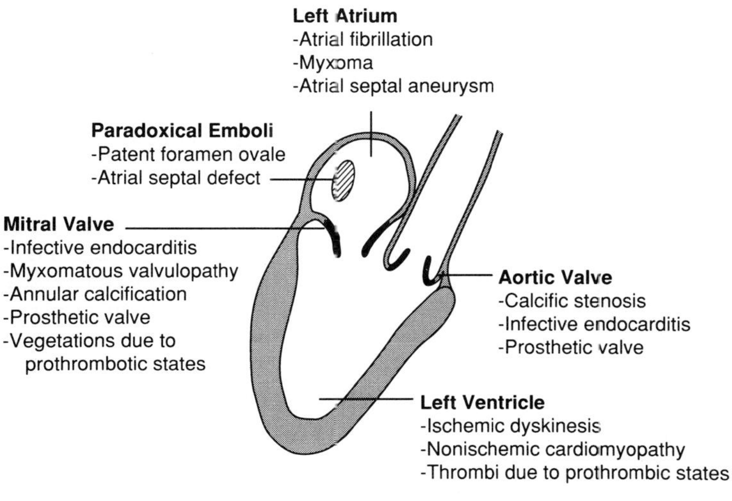

Figure 15-4. Sources of cardiogenic emboli leading to stroke. (*From Hart RG. Cardiogenic embolism to the brain. Lancet 339:589, 1992.*)

rheumatic heart disease, carries a substantially increased risk of ischemic stroke and is the most common source of cardiogenic embolism.[65] Particularly in elderly women, atrial fibrillation may be the most important predictor of disabling brain infarction. Atrial fibrillation is associated with perioperative stroke, perhaps mediated by a postoperative prothrombotic state contributing to formation of left atrial thrombi, a situation similar to perioperative deep venous thrombosis.[68]

Recently, five randomized clinical trials independently assessed the value of antithrombotic prophylaxis for patients with atrial fibrillation.[4] The rate of ischemic stroke among patients assigned to placebo averaged 5 percent/year. In the aggregate, warfarin anticoagulation (approximate INR 1.5 to 4.0) was shown to substantially (mean = 70 percent) reduce the risk of arterial thromboembolism.[4] The effect of aspirin studied in two trials was not uniform, with a substantial reduction (42 percent, $p = .02$) found in the large multicenter Stroke Prevention in Atrial Fibrillation (SPAF I) Study[69] using 325 mg/day, but with only a minimal, nonsignificant effect (16 percent reduction) in the Copenhagen AFASAK Study using 75 mg/day in relatively older patients.[70]

The absolute rate of ischemic stroke in patients with atrial fibrillation is critically influenced by coexistent cardiovascular disease. Characterization of subpopulations of patients with atrial fibrillation who have relatively high or low absolute rates of stroke determines which patients will gain greater or lesser benefit from prophylactic antithrombotic therapy. Multivariate analysis of the largest cohort of placebo-treated patients yielded three independent clinical predictors of an increased risk of arterial thromboembolism: a history of hypertension, recent (within three months) congestive heart failure, and prior TIA or stroke[71]; and two echocardiographic predictors: left atrial size > 4.6 cm, and impaired left ventricular function.[72] At present, chronic anticoagulation with warfarin (INR 2.0 to 3.0) is recommended for atrial fibrillation patients with one or more of these risk factors for thromboembolism. Recent reviews discuss specific prophylactic antithrombotic therapy for other, less common sources of cardiogenic embolism.[4,65]

REFERENCES

1. Kubik CS, Adams RD: Occlusion of the basilar artery: A clinical and pathological study. *Brain* 69:73–102, 1976.
2. Harrison MJG, Marshall J, Meadows JC, et al: Effect of aspirin in amaurosis fugax. *Lancet* 2:743–744, 1971.
3. Antiplatelet Trialists' Collaboration: Collaborative over-view of randomized trials of antiplatelet therapy, III: Reduction in venous thrombosis and pulmonary embolism by antiplatelet prophylaxis among surgical and medical patients. *BMJ* 308:235–246, 1994.
4. Hart RG: Cardiogenic embolism to the brain. *Lancet* 339:589–594, 1992.
5. Imparato AM, Riles TS, Mintzer R, et al: The importance of hemorrhage in the relationship between gross morphologic characteristics and cerebral symptoms in 376 carotid artery plaques. *Am Surg* 197:195–203, 1983.
6. Fisher M, Blumenfeld AM, Smith TW: The importance of carotid artery plaque disruption and hemorrhage. *Arch Neurol* 44:1086–1089, 1987.
7. Hart RG, Pearce LA: In vivo antithrombotic effects of aspirin: Dose vs. nongastrointestinal bleeding. *Stroke* 24:138–139, 1993.
8. Mayo NE, Levy R, Goldberg MS: Aspirin and hemorrhagic stroke. *Stroke* 22:1213–1214, 1991.
9. Volker W, Faber V: Aspirin reduces the growth of medial and neointimal thickenings in balloon-injured rat carotid arteries. *Stroke* 21 (suppl):44–45, 1990.
10. Ross R: The pathogenesis of atherosclerosis. *N Engl J Med* 314:488–500, 1986.
11. Weksler B: Platelet function and antiplatelet therapy in ischemic cerebrovascular disease in Barnett HJM, Mohr JP, Stein BM, Yatsu FM

(eds): *Stroke Pathophysiology, Diagnosis, and Management,* 2d ed. New York, Churchill Livingstone, chap 37, pp 913–928, 1992.
12. Ohlstein EH, Storer B, Nambi P, et al: Endothelin and platelet function. *Thromb Res* 57: 967, 1990.
13. Smith JB, Willis AL: Aspirin selectively inhibits prostaglandin production in human platelets. *Nature* 231:235–237, 1971.
14. Patrono C, Ciabattonni G, Patrignani P, et al: Clinical pharmacology of platelet cyclooxygenase inhibition. *Circulation* 72:1177–1184, 1985.
15. Bousser MG, Eschwege E, Haguenau M, et al: "AICLA" controlled trial of aspirin and dipyridamole in the secondary prevention of atherothrombotic cerebral ischemia. *Stroke* 14:5–14, 1983.
16. Canadian Cooperative Study Group: A randomized trial of aspirin and sulfinpyrazone in threatened stroke. *N Engl J Med* 299:53–59, 1978.
17. Fields WS, Lemak NA, Frankowski RF, Hardy RJ: Controlled trial of aspirin in cerebral ischemia. *Stroke* 8:301–315, 1977.
18. Fields WS, Lemak NA, Frankowski RF, Hardy RJ: Controlled trial of aspirin in cerebral ischemia. Part II. Surgical results. *Stroke* 9:309–319, 1978.
19. Sorenson PA, Pedersen H, Marquardsen J, et al: Acetylsalicylic acid in the prevention of stroke in patients with reversible cerebral ischemic attacks: A Danish cooperative study. *Stroke* 14:15–22, 1983.
20. Swedish Cooperative Study: High-dose acetylsalicylic acid after cerebral infarction. *Stroke* 18:325–334, 1987.
21. The ESPS Group: The European stroke prevention study (ESPS): Principal end-points. *Lancet* 2:1351–1354, 1987.
22. UK-TIA Study Group: United Kingdom transient ischaemic attack (UK-TIA) aspirin trial: Interim results. *Br Med J (Clin Res)* 296:316–320, 1988.
23. UK-TIA Study Group: United Kingdom transient ischaemic attack (UK-TIA) aspirin trial: Final results. *J Neurol Neurosurg Psychiatry* 54:1044–1054, 1991.
24. Ruether R, Dorndorf W: Aspirin in patients with cerebral ischemia and normal angiograms or nonsurgical lesions: The results of a double-blind trial, in Breddin K, Dorndorf W, Lowe D, et al (eds): *Acetylsalicylic Acid in Cerebral Ischemia and Coronary Heart Disease.* Stuttgart, Schattauer, pp 97–106, 1978.
25. Boysen G, Sorenson PS, Juhler M, et al: Danish very-low-dose aspirin after carotid endarterectomy trial. *Stroke* 19:1211, 1988.
26. The SALT Collaborative: Swedish aspirin low-dose trial (SALT) of 75 mg aspirin as secondary prophylaxis after cerebrovascular ischemic events. *Lancet* 338:1345–1349, 1991.
27. Antiplatelet Trialists' Collaboration: Secondary prevention of vascular disease by prolonged antiplatelet treatment. *BMJ* 296:320–321, 1988.
28. Sherman DG, Dyken ML, Fisher M, et al: Antithrombotic therapy for cerebrovascular disorders. *Chest* 102(Suppl):5295–5375, 1992.
29. Barnett HJM: Antithrombotic therapy in cerebral arterial disease, in Barnett HJM, Mohr JP, Stein BM, Yatsu FM (eds): *Stroke Pathophysiology, Diagnosis and Management,* 2d ed. New York, Churchill Livingstone, chap 38, pp 929–942, 1992.
30. American-Canadian Cooperative Study Group: Persantine aspirin trial in cerebral ischemia. Part II. Endpoint results. *Stroke* 16:406–415, 1985.
31. Sivenius J, Laakso M, Pentillä IM, et al: The European Stroke Prevention Study: Results according to sex. *Neurology* 41:1189–1192, 1991.
32. Fisher CM: The arterial lesions underlying lacunes. *Acta Neuropath* 12:1–15, 1969.
33. Hess DC, Sheppard JC, Adams RJ: Increased immunoglobulin binding to cerebral endothelium in patients with antiphospholipid antibodies. *Stroke* 24:994–999, 1993.
34. Chimowitz MI, Furlan AJ, Nayak S, Sila CA: Mechanism of stroke in patients taking aspirin. *Neurology* 40:1682–1685, 1990.
35. Hass WK, Easton JD, Adams HP Jr, et al: Ticlopidine Aspirin Stroke Study Group: A randomized trial comparing ticlopidine hydrochloride with aspirin for the prevention of stroke in high-risk patients. *N Engl J Med* 321:501–507, 1989.
36. Van Gijn J: Aspirin: Dose and indications in

modern stroke. *Neurologic Clinics* 10:193–207, 1992.
37. Ackerman RH, Newman KL: Incomplete antiplatelet effects in patients on aspirin compounds (abstrt). *Ann Neurol* 28:224, 1990.
38. Helgason CM, Tortorice KL, Winkler SR, et al: Aspirin response and failure in cerebral infarction. *Stroke* 24:345–350, 1993.
39. Tohgi H, Konno S, Tamura K, Kimura B, et al: Effects of low-to-high doses of aspirin on platelet aggregability and metabolites of thromboxane A2 and prostacyclin. *Stroke* 23:1400–1403, 1992.
40. The Dutch TIA Study Group: A comparison of two doses of aspirin (30 mg vs 283 mg a day) in patients after a transient ischemic attack or minor ischemic stroke. *N Engl J Med* 325:1261–1266, 1991.
41. Fitzgerald GA, Smith B, Pedersen AK, Brash AR: Increased prostacyclin biosynthesis in patients with severe atherosclerosis and platelet activation. *N Engl J Med* 310:76, 1984.
42. Ratnatunga CP, Edmondson SF, Rees GM, Kovacs IB: High-dose aspirin inhibits shear-induced platelet reaction involving thrombin generation. *Circulation* 85:1077–1082, 1992.
43. Steering Committee of the Physicians' Health Study Research Group: Final report on the aspirin component of the ongoing physicians' health study. *N Engl J Med* 321:129–135, 1989.
44. McTavish D, Faulds D, Goa K: Ticlopidine: An updated review of its pharmacology and therapeutic use in platelet-dependent disorders. *Drugs* 40:238–259, 1990.
45. Robert S, Miller AJ, Fagan SC: Ticlopidine: A new antiplatelet agent for cerebrovascular disease. *Pharmacotherapy* 11:317–325, 1991.
46. Hass WK: Ticlopidine: A new drug to prevent stroke, in Norris JW, Hachinski VC (eds): *Prevention of Stroke*. New York, Springer-Verlag, chap 10, pp 127–138, 1991.
47. Lips JPM, Sixma JJ, Schiphorst ME: The effect of ticlopidine administration to humans on binding of adenosine diphosphate to blood platelets. *Thromb Res* 17:19–27, 1980.
48. Gent M, Blakeley JA, Easton JD and the CATS Group: The Canadian-American Ticlopidine Study (CATS) in thromboembolic stroke. *Lancet* 1:1215–1220, 1989.
49. Rothrock JF, Hart RG: Ticlopidine use and threatened stroke: A clinical perspective. *Western J Med* 160:43–47, 1994.
50. Warlow C: Ticlopidine, a new antithrombotic drug: But is it better than aspirin for long-term use? *J Neurol Neurosurg Psychiatry* 53:185–187, 1990.
51. Janzon L, Bergquist D, Boberg J, et al: Prevention of myocardial infarction and stroke in patients with intermittent claudication: Effects of ticlopidine. Results from STIMS, the Swedish Ticlopidine Multicentre Study. *J Intern Med* 227:301–308, 1990.
52. Berglund U, Wallentin L: Influence on lipoprotein metabolism of the platelet inhibitory drug ticlopidine. *Atherosclerosis* 59:241–246, 1986.
53. Hart RG: Comparison of ticlopidine and aspirin for the prevention of stroke (letter). *N Engl J Med* 322:404–405, 1990.
54. Uchiyama S, Sone R, Nagayama T, et al: Combination therapy with low-dose aspirin and ticlopidine in cerebral ischemia. *Stroke* 20:1643, 1989.
55. De Caterina R, Sicari R, Bernini W, et al: Benefit/risk profile of combined antiplatelet therapy with ticlopidine and aspirin. *Thromb Haemost* 65:504–510, 1991.
56. Gardner FH: Ticlopidine-induced neutropenia: Recognition and management. *IM Hematology* 12:35–41, 1991.
57. Haynes RB, Sandler RS, Larson EB, et al: A critical appraisal of ticlopidine, a new antiplatelet agent: Effectiveness and clinical indications for prophylaxis of atherosclerotic events. *Arch Intern Med* 152:1376–1380, 1992.
58. Acheson J, Danta G, Hutchinson EC: Controlled trial of dipyridamole in cerebral vascular disease. *Br Med J* 1:614, 1969.
59. Guiraud-Chaumeil B, Rascol AD, Boneu B, et al: Prévention des récidives des accidents vasculaires cérébraux ischemiques par les anti-agrégates plaquettaires. *Rev Neurol (Paris)* 5:367, 1982.
60. Candelise L, Landi G, Perrone P, et al: A randomized trial of aspirin and sulfinpyrazone in patients with TIA. *Stroke* 13:175–179, 1982.
61. Hirsh J: Oral anticoagulant drugs. *N Engl J Med* 324:1865–1875, 1991.
62. Garde A, Samuelsson K, Fahlgran H, et al:

Treatment after transient ischemic attacks: A comparison between anticoagulant drug and inhibition of platelet aggregation. *Stroke* 14:677–681, 1983.
63. Olsson JE, Brechter C, Backlund H, et al: Anticoagulant vs. antiplatelet therapy as prophylactic against cerebral infarction in transient ischemic attacks. *Stroke* 11:4–9, 1980.
64. Buren A, Ygge J: Treatment program and comparison between anticoagulants and platelet aggregation inhibitors after transient ischemic attack. *Stroke* 12:578–580, 1981.
65. Cerebral Embolism Task Force: Cardiogenic brain embolism: The second report of the Cerebral Embolism Task Force. *Arch Neurol* 46: 727–741, 1989.
66. Pearson AC, Labovitz AJ, Tatineni S, Gomez C: Superiority of transesophageal echocardiography in detecting cardiac source of embolism in patients with cerebral ischemia of uncertain etiology. *J Am Coll Cardiol* 17:66–72, 1991.
67. Karalis DG, Chandrasekaran K, Victor MF, et al: The recognition and embolic potential of intra-aortic atherosclerotic debris. *J Am Coll Cardiol* 17:73–78, 1991.
68. Hart RG, Hindman BG: Mechanisms of perioperative cerebral infarction. *Stroke* 13:766–773, 1982.
69. Stroke Prevention in Atrial Fibrillation Investigators: The Stroke Prevention in Atrial Fibrillation Study: Final results. *Circulation* 84:527–539, 1991.
70. Petersen P, Boysen G, Godtfredsen J, et al: Placebo-controlled, randomized trial of warfarin and aspirin for prevention of thromboembolic complications in chronic atrial fibrillation: The Copenhagen AFASAK Study. *Lancet* 1: 175–179, 1989.
71. Stroke Prevention in Atrial Fibrillation Investigators: Predictors of thromboembolism in atrial fibrillation: Clinical features in patients at risk. *Ann Intern Med* 116:1–5, 1991.
72. Stroke Prevention in Atrial Fibrillation Investigators: Predictors of thromboembolism in atrial fibrillation: Echocardiographic features in patients at risk. *Ann Intern Med* 116:6–12, 1991.

16

Randomized Clinical Trials of Medical and Surgical Treatment for Symptomatic Carotid Stenosis

D. Eugene Strandness, Jr.

The relationship between atherosclerosis of the carotid bifurcation and cerebrovascular ischemic events was put on solid ground by C. Miller Fisher in 1951.[1] He clearly established that disease at this level could lead to transient ischemic attack (TIA) and stroke. In 1954 Eascott, Pickering, and Rob reported what is widely regarded as the first reconstructive surgical procedure for the treatment of carotid bifurcation disease (Chap. 1).[2] This initial success was followed by enthusiastic acceptance by many surgeons, who began to perform carotid endarterectomy in increasing numbers.

However, enthusiasm for the procedure was dampened by a series of reports pointing out that the perioperative morbidity and mortality rates were unacceptably high. One of the earliest community-based studies, by Easton and Sherman in 1977, reported on 228 consecutive carotid operations performed in Springfield, Illinois, in which the perioperative complication rate was in the range of 20 percent.[3] Thus, the two major issues in the controversy over carotid artery surgery became the safety of the operation and its long-term efficacy.

Later reports, while not showing the same high complication rates, still raised serious doubts about the role of carotid endarterectomy in preventing stroke. One of the first randomized clinical trials for symptomatic patients was published in 1970.[4] While carotid endarterectomy appeared to provide protection against stroke, the beneficial effects were largely negated by high perioperative and postoperative complication rates. Nonetheless, the procedure continued to be performed in increasing numbers. For example, the number of carotid endarterectomies done outside of Veterans Hospitals rose from 15,000 in 1971 to 107,000 in 1985.[5]

In the years during which the operation became more popular, neurologists expressed increasing concerns that the benefits of surgery in the prevention of stroke had not been proved. There also appeared to be rather marked geographical differences that included not just the complication rates but also the indications for the procedure.[6] As all the evidence began to accumulate, there were pleas for a more conservative approach to the treatment of carotid bifurcation disease and stroke. In addition, increasing numbers of clinicians wanted randomized clinical trials carried out to settle the issue once and for all.[7,8]

TRIAL DESIGN AND RESULTS

Three clinical trials in symptomatic patients have reported interim results, settling, at least in part, the current controversy over the role of carotid endarterectomy.[9–11] Before considering the results of these trials in detail, it is important to review some of the methods used to document the location and extent of carotid disease. While ultrasound methods were used, the testing procedures were not standardized, making this one of the weaker aspects of these trials.

With regard to documenting the severity of carotid bifurcation disease, it is helpful to review the arteriographic methods for estimating the degree of arterial narrowing. This is very important, since the two largest trials used different methods of measurement yet reported similar clinical results. Most arteriographers use the internal carotid artery distal to the bulb as the normal "reference" vessel. This might seem an intuitively sound method, but it must be recognized that it will only give a true estimate of the degree of narrowing for an artery that has no dilated areas, such as the carotid bulb, which may have a normal diameter of up to twice that of the more distal carotid artery (Chap. 14). An atheromatous lesion could occupy a large portion of the posterolateral aspect of the carotid bulb and still not interfere with blood flow.

In the North American Symptomatic Carotid Endarterectomy Trial (NASCET), which used the distal internal carotid as the normal reference site, such a lesion would be measured as a 0 percent stenosis.[9] In the European Carotid Surgery Trial (ECST), all estimates of stenosis severity were based on measurements made directly from the carotid bulb.[10] Thus, for the lesion just described as a 0 percent stenosis using the NASCET approach, the method used in the ECST could result in up to a 50 percent diameter-reducing stenosis. As will be discussed, both of these trials found that it was the 70 percent or greater diameter-reducing lesion that was the most dangerous clinically. However, a 70 percent diameter-reducing stenosis is clearly not exactly the same for the two trials.

Several aspects of these clinical trials make them different, even though they might appear similar. Obviously, for the results to be valid, the patients who enter the trial must be randomized to achieve similar groups in the various arms of the trial. In addition, it is important to establish clearly which specific symptoms will qualify a patient for admission to the trial and the manner in which participating clinicians are allowed to treat the study patients. Here again, the NASCET and ECST were very different.

The North American Symptomatic Carotid Endarterectomy Trial (NASCET)

A total of 50 centers were involved in this trial throughout the United States and Canada. At each center, a vascular surgeon or neurosurgeon and a neurologist were responsible for the study. In order to qualify for participation, all surgeons had to demonstrate that their perioperative morbidity and mortality rates were 5 percent or less. Patients with either a hemispheric TIA or stroke were eligible for randomization if the event had occurred within the previous 120 days. However, all stroke patients had to show enough improvement to be able to function independently.

Once the patient was deemed eligible for randomization, selective carotid arteriography was performed and the interpretation done using a jeweler's eyepiece to document the degree of stenosis relative to the normal distal internal carotid artery. Two levels of stratification based on the degree of narrowing were used in the analysis: 30 to 69 percent and 70 to 99 percent diameter reduction. If a 30 to 99 percent carotid stenosis appropriate to the neurologic symptoms was identified, the patient was randomly assigned to either medical or surgical therapy.

Between January 1988 and February 1991, 659 patients with a 70 to 99 percent carotid stenosis were randomized, 331 in the medical arm and 328 in the surgical arm of the study. The baseline characteristics for the two groups of patients are shown in Table 16-1. All patients in both arms of the trial were placed on aspirin at a dose of 1300 mg/day (or less if it was poorly tolerated). The best "current therapy" for all patients in both arms of the trial was provided and included, where appropriate, treatment of hypertension, hyperlipidemia, and diabetes. The specific surgical treatment employed was left up to the participating surgeon. Data on all patients considered eligible but not randomized were collected as well.

Table 16-1 Baseline Characteristics for the Patients Randomized to the Medical and Surgical Arms of the NASCET[b]

	Medical	Surgical
Median age (years)	66	65
Sex		
Male	69%	68%
Female	31%	32%
TIA at entry	69%	67%
Stroke at entry	31%	33%
Ipsilateral stenosis		
70–79%	43%	40%
80–89%	33%	38%
90–99%	24%	22%
Contralateral 70–99% stenosis	9%	8%
Race		
White	89%	93%
Black	4%	2%
Other	7%	5%
Antithrombotic medications	85%	85%

[a]There were 331 patients in the medical arm and 328 in the surgical arm of the study.[9]

The follow-up protocol for the NASCET was as follows:

1. For the patients in the surgical arm, the surgeons evaluated the immediate postoperative results by examination either at the time of hospital discharge or at 30 days, whichever occurred first.

2. Neurologic assessment was done by the participating neurologist at 30 days, and then every three months during year one and every four months in the ensuing years.

3. The management of coexisting cardiovascular problems was monitored centrally.

4. Duplex ultrasonography was repeated one month after operation and after any cerebrovascular event.

5. Repeat arteriography was done only if clinically indicated.

In February of 1991, after an average follow-up of 18 months, randomization of patients in the 70 to 99 percent stenosis category was terminated by invoking the preplanned stopping rule because of overwhelming evidence of treatment efficacy for patients in this group who underwent carotid endarterectomy. A Clinical Alert was promptly issued by the National Institutes of Health notifying physicians of the outcome. At the same time, those patients in the medical arm of the trial who had this degree of stenosis were counseled to have a carotid endarterectomy performed. This very unusual step emphasized the importance of these results and their implications for the management of patients with symptomatic high-grade carotid stenoses. Because the benefit of surgery for less severe degrees of carotid disease remained uncertain, randomization of symptomatic patients with carotid stenoses in the range of 30 to 69 percent was continued.

The early reduction in benefit due to perioperative complications in the surgical arm of the trial was rapidly overcome within the first three months by the added benefit observed among the surgical patients, which persisted for up to 30 months of follow-up. The total event rate for the surgical patients was 5.8 percent during the first 30 days after operation, as compared to 3.3 percent for the comparable first 32 days in the medically treated group. Since surgery was performed a median of two days after randomization, two days were added to the medical group for the latter comparison. When the analysis was restricted to major stroke and death, the perioperative event rates were 2.1 percent in the surgical group and 0.9 percent on the medical group.

Table 16-2 summarizes the clinical outcome for the patients in both arms of the NASCET. The cumulative risk of an ipsilateral stroke at two years was 9 percent for patients randomized to surgery and 26 percent for medically treated patients. This represented an absolute risk reduction of approximately 17 percent and a relative risk reduction of 65 percent. Similarly, the cumulative risk of a major or fatal ipsilateral stroke was 2.5 percent for the surgical patients and 13.1 percent for the medical patients, resulting in a relative risk reduction of 81 percent. For those patients who did not die or have a major stroke during the first month after randomization, the risk of stroke within two years was 12.2 percent in the medical group and 1.6 percent in the surgical group ($p<.00001$).

Another important finding in the NASCET was the relationship between the degree of risk reduction after surgery and the severity of carotid stenosis. The absolute risk reduction

Table 16-2 First Adverse Events for the Patients in the Two Arms of the NASCET at Two Years of Follow-up[9]

	Events (event rate, %)			
Event	Medical patients ($n=331$)	Surgical patients ($n=328$)	Absolute difference (% ± SE)	Relative risk reduction (%)
Any ipsilateral stroke	61 (26)	26 (9)	17 ± 3.5^b	65
Any stroke	64 (27.6)	34 (12.6)	15 ± 3.8^b	54
Any stroke or death	73 (32.3)	41 (15.8)	16.5 ± 4.2^b	51
Major or fatal ipsilateral stroke	29 (13.1)	8 (2.5)	10.6 ± 2.6^b	81
Any major or fatal stroke	29 (13.1)	10 (3.7)	9.4 ± 2.7^b	72
Any major stroke or death	38 (18.1)	19 (8.0)	10.1 ± 3.5^c	56

[a]Event rates were determined by Kaplan-Meier estimates for survival. "Death" refers to mortality from all causes. All events from the time of randomization to the first 30 days in the surgical group and 32 days in the medical group are included, along with subsequent events defining treatment failure.

[b] = $p<.001$ for the comparison of the treatment groups.

[c] = $p<.01$ for the comparison of the treatment groups.

(% ± SE) for all ipsilateral stroke at two years was 12 ± 4.8 percent for stenoses of 70 to 79 percent diameter reduction, 18 ± 6.2 percent for 80 to 89 percent stenoses, and 26 ± 8.1 percent for 90 to 99 percent stenoses. These results confirm once again how important the degree of carotid narrowing is in predicting the outcome after an initial ischemic event.

The European Carotid Surgery Trial (ECST)

As noted earlier, The ECST was different in many respects from the NASCET, but the conclusions and recommendations were nearly the same.[10] In this study, which involved 80 centers in 14 countries and spanned 10 years, a total of 2518 patients with carotid territory stroke, TIA, or retinal infarction were randomized to either medical or surgical therapy. The mean follow-up was nearly 3 years. For patients in the medical arm of the trial, the specific use of antithrombotic agents was left to the discretion of the treating physician—in contrast to the NASCET, where all patients were placed on aspirin regardless of treatment group. Other important differences between these two trials are as follows:

1. Whereas in the NASCET the qualifying neurologic event had to be within 120 days prior to randomization, in the ECST this period was six months.

2. In the ECST a delay of surgery for up to six weeks was permitted in some cases of recent stroke.

3. The ECST included only patients for whom the participating surgeon and neurologist agreed that there was substantial uncertainty about the benefit of operation, a policy not applicable to the NASCET.

4. The arteriographic methods for measuring the extent of stenosis were different, as previously discussed.

In May 1991 the interim results of the ECST were reported for the groups of symptomatic patients with 70 to 99 percent stenoses and 0 to 29 percent stenoses.[10] The results for the 778 randomized patients in the 70 to 99 percent stenosis group were as follows:

1. In the surgical arm of the trial the perioperative (30-day) morbidity and mortality rate was 7.5 percent.

2. During the three years of follow-up, the risk of an ipsilateral stroke was an additional 2.8 percent in the surgical group but 16.8 percent for the medically treated patients, which is a sixfold risk reduction ($p<.0001$).

3. At three years, the total risk of surgical death, surgical stroke, ipsilateral ischemic stroke, or any other stroke was 12.3 percent for patients in the surgical arm, compared with 21.9 percent for the medically treated patients. ($p<.01$).

4. For disabling events or death, the results at three years were an extra 1.1 percent for the surgical group and 8.4 percent for the medical group ($p<.0001$).

For carotid lesions in the range of 0 to 29 percent diameter-reduction there was no apparent benefit from operation, so further randomization of these patients was no longer recommended. For the intermediate grades of stenosis (30 to 69 percent diameter reduction) there were not enough data to support any definite conclusions. Consequently, as in the NASCET, randomization for this group of patients is continuing.

The Veterans Affairs Trial

The Department of Veterans Affairs Cooperative Studies Program also undertook a multicenter randomized trial of medical and surgical treatment for patients with symptomatic carotid disease, but this study was terminated in 1991 after the results of the other trials discussed above were reported.[11] This trial was relatively small, with only 189 patients being randomized among 16 university-affiliated Veterans Affairs medical centers, but the results were similar to the NASCET and ECST. The end-points for this trial also included TIA, which was not the case for the two larger trials. At a mean follow-up of only 11.9

months, the risk of a neurologic event for the surgical patients was 7.7 percent as compared with 19.4 percent for the medical patients ($p = .011$). This benefit appeared within two months of randomization.

CONCLUSIONS

The results of these clinical trials clearly establish the advantages of surgery over medical therapy for symptomatic patients with 70 percent or greater stenosis of the appropriate internal carotid artery. These studies also point out how ineffective medical therapy can be for this group of patients. With regard to antithrombotic medications, nearly 90 percent of the NASCET patients were being treated with aspirin at the time of randomization; however, corresponding information was not given in the ECST report. On the other extreme, there is no convincing evidence from these trials that symptomatic patients with less than 30 percent carotid stenosis will benefit from carotid endarterectomy. The numbers of symptomatic patients with stenoses in the 30 to 69 percent range has been insufficient to support any definitive conclusions regarding the benefit of surgery and, although recruitment of these patients continues, it may be difficult to obtain an adequate number of patients for randomization.[12]

Other important aspects of these trials need to be emphasized. While it might appear that the two major trials refer to similar degrees of carotid narrowing, this is not necessarily the case. As mentioned previously, the methods used for estimating the degree of stenosis by arteriography were different. If one applies the NASCET approach based on the normal distal internal carotid artery, then any degree of stenosis that does not compromise the channel through the bulb would be considered a 0 percent stenosis. A corresponding lesion assessed in relation to the normal carotid bulb, as done in the ECST, would be interpreted as a more severe lesion. However, application of these two methods to increasingly severe degrees of stenosis results in a lesser discrepancy between the estimates of diameter reduction.

Does the method used to assess carotid disease influence how physicians choose to treat symptomatic patients? Unfortunately, both the NASCET and the Veterans Affairs Trial concluded that carotid duplex scanning was not sufficiently accurate for screening purposes. However, in neither of these trials were the noninvasive methods or equipment standardized, making these conclusions unacceptable. Of 1062 NASCET patients undergoing ultrasonography and arteriography, it was reported that an ultrasound finding of less than 70 percent stenosis missed 12 percent of patients with high-grade stenoses by arteriography (sensitivity 88 percent), while an ultrasound result of greater than 70 percent stenosis was falsely positive in 40 percent of patients with lesser degrees of disease (specificity 60 percent).[13] The poor performance of ultrasonography in these trials is misleading, since the studies were not designed to determine the accuracy of carotid duplex scanning. Furthermore, the excellent results of careful validation studies, including comparisons with arteriography, cannot be ignored.[14] A modification of the widely used criteria for classifying carotid stenoses by duplex scanning has been proposed to accommodate the NASCET threshold of 70 percent diameter reduction.[15]

If arteriography is routinely obtained in the work-up of patients with symptomatic carotid artery disease, as was done in the randomized clinical trials discussed above, a small additional proportion of patients will have a serious or even fatal outcome from the diagnostic procedure. What is this risk? If one uses the most conservative figures, at least one patient out of every 100 subjected to arteriography will have a stroke.[16] Appropriate use of screening tests can avoid unnecessary arteriograms and reduce both the costs and risks of treating patients with carotid artery disease. The best answer to the critics of duplex scanning is that the method is accurate when performed by validated and standardized techniques. These issues are considered in more detail in Chaps. 11, 14, and 21.

REFERENCES

1. Fisher M: Occlusion of the internal carotid artery. *Arch Neurol Psychiat* 65:346–377, 1951.
2. Eastcott HHG, Pickering GW, Rob CG: Reconstruction of internal carotid artery in a patient with intermittent attacks of hemiplegia. *Lancet* 2:994–996, 1954.
3. Easton JD, Sherman DG: Stroke and mortality rate in carotid endarterectomy: 228 consecutive operations. *Stroke* 8:565–568, 1977.
4. Fields WS, Maslenikov V, Meyer JS, et al: Joint study of extracranial arterial occlusion: V. Progress report of prognosis following surgery or nonsurgical treatment for transient cerebral ischemic attacks and cervical carotid lesions. *JAMA* 211:1993–2003, 1970.
5. Pokras R, Dyken ML: Dramatic changes in the performance of endarterectomy for diseases of the extracranial arteries of the head. *Stroke* 10:1289–1290, 1988.
6. Brook R, Park E, Chassin M, et al: Carotid endarterectomy for elderly patients. Predicting complications. *Ann Intern Med* 113:747–753, 1990.
7. Chambers BR, Norris JW: The case against surgery for asymptomatic carotid stenosis. *Stroke* 15:964–967, 1984.
8. Barnett HJM, Plum F, Walton JN: Carotid endarterectomy: An expression of concern. *Stroke* 15:941–943, 1984.
9. North American Symptomatic Carotid Endarterectomy Trial Collaborators: Beneficial effect of carotid endarterectomy in symptomatic patients with high-grade carotid stenosis. *N Engl J Med* 325:445–463, 1991.
10. European Carotid Surgery Trialists' Collaborative Group: MRC European Carotid Surgery Trial. Interim results for symptomatic patients with severe (70–99%) or with mild (0–29%) stenosis. *Lancet* 337:1235–1243, 1991.
11. Mayberg MR, Wilson SE, Yatsu R, et al: Carotid endarterectomy and prevention of cerebral ischemia in symptomatic carotid stenosis. *JAMA* 266:3289–3294, 1991.
12. Strandness DE Jr: Carotid endarterectomy: Current status and effects of clinical trials. *Cardiovasc Surg* 1:311–316, 1993.
13. Haynes B, Thorpe W, Taylor W, et al: Poor performance of ultrasound in detecting high-grade carotid stenosis. *Can J Surg* 35:446 (abstrt), 1992.
14. Langlois YE, Roederer GO, Strandness DE Jr: Ultrasonic evaluation of the carotid bifurcation. *Echocardiography* 4:141–149, 1987.
15. Moneta GL, Edwards JM, Chitwood RW, et al: Correlation of North American Symptomatic Carotid Endarterectomy Trial (NASCET) angiographic definition of 70% to 90% internal carotid artery stenosis with duplex scanning. *J Vasc Surg* 17:152–159, 1993.
16. Mani RL, Eisenberg RL, McDonald EJ Jr, et al: Complications of catheter cerebral arteriography: Analysis of 5000 procedures. I. Criteria and incidence. *AJR* 131:861–865, 1978.

17

Randomized Clinical Trials on the Efficacy of Carotid Endarterectomy for Asymptomatic Carotid Stenosis

Robert W. Hobson II

Clinical indications for carotid endarterectomy have been reassessed in recent years because of three major factors: (1) some clinicians[1] questioned the increasing number of procedures and their efficacy; (2) reports of unacceptably high perioperative complication rates[2,3] were commonly generalized as being representative of practice throughout the country; and (3) lack of prospective analysis threatened the credibility of surgeons about the indications for operative intervention.

These concerns led to the planning and execution of several randomized clinical trials. Their advantages over retrospective analyses stem from an emphasis on nonbiased assignment of patients to treatment groups and the necessary requirement for uniform clinical follow-up, generally by both medical and surgical specialists. Although the randomized trials on the management of symptomatic patients with recent transient ischemic attack (TIA) or nondisabling stroke have resulted in definitive recommendations for carotid endarterectomy in patients with 70 percent or greater carotid stenoses (Chap. 16),[4–6] the indications for carotid endarterectomy in patients with high-grade asymptomatic carotid stenoses remain less clear. The purpose of this chapter is to review both information from the two published trials[7,8] and from potentially important results to be published in the near future from other sources.[9,10]

SIGNIFICANT CAROTID STENOSIS

An asymptomatic carotid bruit is associated with a relatively low risk of stroke as defined in population based studies.[11,12] Recognizing that bruits can occur with carotid stenoses as slight as 20 percent, Norris and coauthors[13] confirmed that within a group of patients with minimal stenoses the annual stroke rate is in the range of 1 percent per year or less. However, as the area-reduction of a stenosis increases from 50 to 75 percent and more, the incidence of TIA, stroke, and vascular death increases significantly (Table 17-1).

Consequently, there has been a shift in emphasis in recent years toward diagnosing severe or hemodynamically significant asymptomatic carotid stenoses. The threshold for a hemodynamically significant stenosis has been defined arteriographically as a 50 percent reduction in the luminal diameter or a calculated 75 percent reduction in the cross-sectional area of the artery (Fig. 17-1). The percentage of diameter stenosis is commonly determined by comparing the smallest transverse diameter at the stenosis with the diameter of the postbulbar internal carotid artery once its walls have become parallel. When coupled with positive results of such noninvasive tests as ocular pneumoplethysmography[14] or duplex scanning,[15] the 50 percent diameter stenosis or the 75 percent area stenosis becomes a recommended threshold stenosis for considering surgical intervention in asymptomatic patients.[16]

CLINICAL TRIALS

Two randomized clinical trials involving patients with asymptomatic carotid stenosis have published their results.[7,8] The selection of patients for randomization as well as an analysis of end-points in these trials have resulted in an incomplete consensus regarding the indications for carotid endarterectomy in this important group of patients.

The CASANOVA Study

The first publication of results from a randomized clinical trial on the efficacy of carotid endarterectomy for asymptomatic carotid stenosis was from the Carotid Artery Stenosis with Asymptomatic Narrowing: Operation Versus Aspirin (CASANOVA) study group. This multicenter trial included patients with asymptomatic 50 to 90 percent internal carotid stenoses confirmed arteriographically.[7] According to the design of the randomization protocol, 206 patients with unilateral or bilateral stenoses had carotid endarterectomy unilaterally or bilaterally as indicated. In a nonoperative group of 160 patients with unilateral stenosis, carotid endarterectomy was deferred until the stenosis progressed to exceed 90 percent, the development of bilateral internal carotid stenoses of greater than 50 percent (operation performed on the side with the most severe stenosis), the occurrence of a TIA ip-

Table 17-1 Annual Percentage Rate of Vascular Events over Period of Follow-up

Degree of stenosis (%)	TIA	Stroke	Cardiac	Vascular death
<50 (mild)	1.0	1.3	2.7	1.8
50–75 (moderate)	3.0	1.3	6.6	3.3
>75 (severe)	7.2	3.3	8.3	6.5

NOTE: TIA = transient ischemic attack
SOURCE: From Norris JW et al.[13] Reproduced by permission.

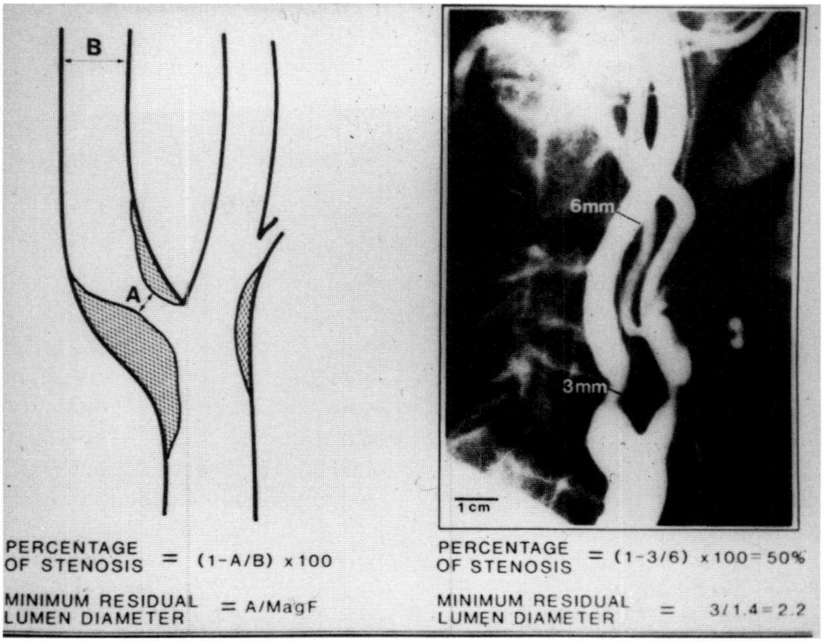

Figure 17-1. The percentage of stenosis is calculated by dividing the least transverse diameter of the internal carotid artery at the stenosis (*A*) by the diameter of the distal, uninvolved artery (*B*). The minimum residual lumen diameter is equivalent to the least transverse diameter (*A*) divided by the magnification factor (MagF) of the arteriogram. The example (*right*) illustrates a 50 percent stenosis by diameter and a minimum residual lumen diameter of 2.2. (*From Lynch TG et al.*[30] *Reproduced by permission.*)

silateral to a 50 percent or greater carotid stenosis, the development of an internal carotid stenosis greater than 50 percent contralateral to a previously operated side, or restenosis of greater than 50 percent following operation.

Most important, all patients with internal carotid stenoses of 90 percent or greater were excluded from the randomization protocol and referred primarily for operation. Since patients with high-grade stenoses constitute the group who might benefit significantly from operation, the authors' conclusion that no differences existed between treatment categories was not surprising, and these results should be regarded as inconclusive. Consequently, while surgeons should be aware of the CASANOVA study, its results should not influence surgical practice.

The Veterans Affairs Cooperative Study

The results of a second randomized clinical trial on asymptomatic carotid stenosis conducted by the Veterans Affairs Cooperative Studies Program[8] have provided additional insight into the management of these patients. This multicenter trial was conducted at 11 Department of Veterans Affairs medical centers to determine the effect of carotid endarterectomy on the combined incidence of neurological outcome events, including TIA, transient monocular blindness, and stroke.

Potential study patients were identified by noninvasive screening with ocular pneumoplethysmography or duplex scanning. A total of 444 adult male patients were recruited who had asymptomatic carotid stenosis shown arteriographically to reduce the diameter of the lumen by 50 percent or more. Patients were randomized to carotid endarterectomy with optimal medical management including aspirin therapy ($n = 211$) or optimal medical management and aspirin therapy alone ($n = 233$). The mean age of the study population was 64.5 years; the clinical characteristics of the randomized patients at entry are summarized in Table 17-2.

All patients were followed independently by a vascular surgeon and a neurologist at each participating center. Thirty-two percent of the randomized patients had a history of cerebral ischemic events due to contralateral carotid stenosis; 80 percent of these events were reported as transient; the remainder were described as strokes with minimal residual deficits. Two-thirds of the patients were asymptomatic with regard to both cerebral hemispheres. Medical exclusionary criteria included: previous cerebral infarction; previous carotid endarterectomy with restenosis; previous extracranial-to-intracranial bypass; high surgical risk due to associated medical illness, chronic anticoagulant therapy, aspirin intolerance or chronic higher dose aspirin therapy; life expectancy less than five years; surgically inaccessible lesions; and noncompliance or refusal to participate in the protocol.

All patients initially received aspirin at a dosage of 650 mg twice daily, but this was modified to a lower dose regimen (325 mg daily) for patients with aspirin intolerance during subsequent clinical follow-up.[17,18] Patients randomized to carotid endarterectomy underwent operation within 10 days of randomization. Patients who experienced clinically defined neurological outcome events were evaluated independently by the participating vascular surgeon and neurologist and their conclusions submitted to the End-points Committee for blinded review and adjudication. Enrollment of patients began April 1, 1983; patient acquisition was completed in

Table 17-2 Patient Characteristics at Entry[a]

Characteristics	Surgical group	Medical group
Number of patients	211	233
Mean age (SD)	64.1 (6.8)	64.7 (6.7)
Race (%)		
Caucasian	88	86
African American	6	8
Hispanic	1	3
Native American	2	3
Asian American	2	0
Previous contralateral symptoms (%)	32	33
Daily smoker (%)	52	49
Previous smoker (%)	43	42
History of (%)		
Diabetes	30	27
Myocardial infarct	28	25
Angina pectoris	30	25
Congestive heart failure	5	7
Hypertension	63	64
Arrhythmia	17	14
Peripheral vascular disease	61	59

[a]No significant differences between treatment groups

SOURCE: From Hobson RW et al.[8] Reproduced by permission.

Table 17-3 Incidence of Combined Neurological Endpoints for Ipsilateral and Contralateral Events

	Surgical group 211 patients		Medical group 233 patients	
Neurological endpoint	Number	%	Number	%
Transient ischemic attack	9	4.3	17	7.3
Transient monocular blindness	1	0.5	12	5.2
Stroke (nonfatal and fatal)	17	8.1	28	12.0
Total[a]	27	12.9	57	24.5

[a] $p<.002$ for the comparison between groups (relative risk, 0.51; 95% confidence interval, 0.32 to 0.81)
SOURCE: From Hobson RW et al.[8] Reproduced by permission.

October 1987; and clinical follow-up ended March 31, 1991. The mean duration of follow-up, as measured from time of entry to first neurological event, death, or loss to follow-up, was 47.9 months.

Morbidity and mortality data for the 211 patients treated by carotid endarterectomy have been reported previously.[8,19] The 30-day operative mortality was 1.9 percent (4 of 211). Three deaths resulted from myocardial infarction and one from myocardial infarction followed by stroke. There were five nonfatal postoperative strokes, for an incidence of 2.4 percent (5 of 211). Three nonfatal strokes (0.4 percent, 3 of 714) occurred as a result of arteriography: one was associated with significant hemiparesis, and two were associated with minimal neurological deficits. Assigning all complications of arteriography to the surgical group, the permanent stroke and death rate within 30 days after randomization was 4.7 percent for the patients randomized to carotid endarterectomy. In contrast, during the first 30 days after randomization of patients to the medical group one suicide (0.4 percent) and two neurological events (0.9 percent) occurred, including one stroke and one TIA.

Results for all neurological outcome events, contralateral and ipsilateral, are summarized in Table 17-3. Eighty-four events were observed, 27 (12.9 percent) in the surgical group and 57 (24.5 percent) in the medical group, representing an absolute risk reduction of 11.6 percent ($p<.002$) and a relative risk (surgical group vs. medical group) of 0.51 (95 percent confidence interval, 0.32 to 0.81). Results for ipsilateral neurological events only are presented in Table 17-4. There were 65 ipsilateral events, 17 (8.0 percent) in the surgical group and 48 (20.6 percent) in the medical group,

Table 17-4 Incidence of Combined Neurological Endpoints for Ipsilateral Events Only

	Surgical group 211 patients		Medical group 233 patients	
Neurological endpoint	Number	%	Number	%
Transient ischemic attack	6	2.8	15	6.4
Transient monocular blindness	1	0.5	11	4.7
Stroke (nonfatal and fatal)[a]	10	4.7	22	9.4
Total[b]	17	8.0	48	20.6

[a] $p=.056$
[b] $p<.001$ for the comparison between groups (relative risk, 0.38; 95% confidence interval, 0.22 to 0.67)
SOURCE: From Hobson RW et al.[8] Reproduced by permission.

giving an absolute risk reduction of 12.6 percent ($p < .001$) and a relative risk of 0.38 (95 percent confidence interval, 0.22 to 0.67). Analysis of the ipsilateral neurological events in the medical group for stenoses of 50 to 75 percent and 76 to 99 percent showed the following: 24 events in 19.2 percent of patients with 50 to 75 percent stenoses (12 strokes, 7 TIAs, 5 episodes of transient monocular blindness), and 24 events in 22.4 percent of patients with 76 to 99 percent stenoses (10 strokes, 8 TIAs, 6 episodes of transient monocular blindness). These differences were not statistically significant.

The temporal distribution of neurological outcome events over the duration of follow-up was determined by construction of Kaplan-Meier survival curves, where survival was defined as the time to the first neurological event. Data for ipsilateral events are summarized in Fig. 17-2. Comparisons of treatment groups by the log-rank test showed significant differences in favor of the surgical group ($p < .001$). The incidence of stroke and death for this high risk group of patients is presented in Table 17-5. No significant differences were observed between treatment groups for the endpoints of stroke and death.

Other Clinical Trials

Data from another clinical trial, the Asymptomatic Carotid Atherosclerosis Study (ACAS),[9] should be available within the next year or so. This randomized clinical trial, sponsored by the National Institutes of Health, is similar in design to the previously published Veterans Affairs cooperative study on asymptomatic carotid stenosis. The ACAS has two major advantages in that both male and female patients have been randomized and a large sample (approximately 1600 patients) was chosen. The randomization of patients was concluded November 1, 1993, and the final phases of clinical follow-up are in progress.

Although the end-point of TIA plus stroke, as utilized in the Veterans Affairs trial, was also selected for follow-up of patients in the ACAS, the investigators have now modified the ACAS protocol because of concerns about the combined neurological end-points used in the Veterans Affairs trial.[8] Consequently, significant differences will be evaluated for stroke alone, as well as stroke plus death, in patients from the medical and surgical groups of the ACAS. In addition, although the risk of neurological events did not appear to be directly related to the severity of carotid stenosis in the Veterans Affairs trial, these neurological events were recorded in patients whose stenoses were characterized at the point of randomization rather than during follow-up or at the time of the neurological event. Since prospective data from serially obtained duplex scans will be available in the ACAS, it should be possible to identify this important group of patients having progression of carotid disease, and presumably, an increased risk of neurological complications. Thus, although the Veterans Affairs trial has assisted by confirming that carotid endarterectomy can reduce neurological events (TIA plus stroke) when compared with optimal medical management, prospective confirmation that carotid endarterectomy reduces stroke alone, or possibly stroke and death, must await publication of the ACAS data.

Data acquired from the European Carotid Surgery Trialists will be of additional significance.[10] This trial, initiated during 1993, will also compare medical and surgical management for asymptomatic carotid stenosis. In addition to having serial duplex scan results available during the follow-up period, data on plaque morphology will be analyzed prospectively, and the incidence of silent cerebral infarctions will be documented with prerandomization CT scans and appropriate follow-up studies.

These latter two studies will become increasingly important as data on the end-points

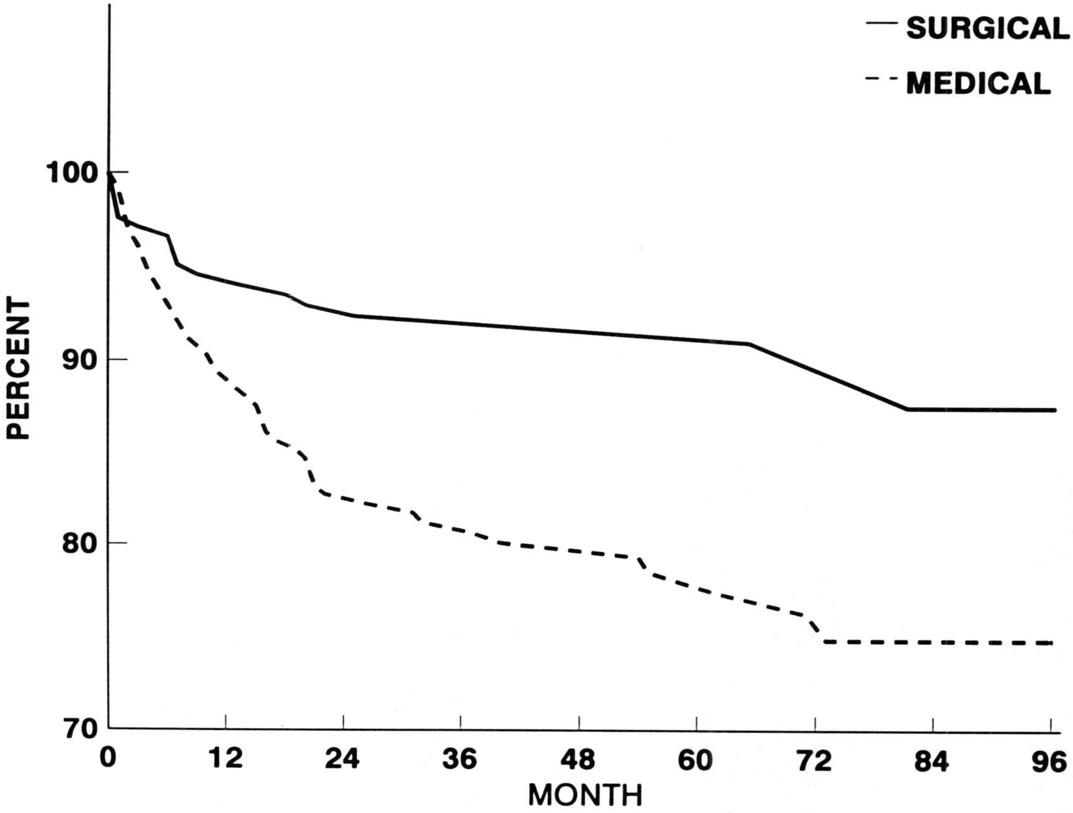

N = ———	211	181	163	150	122	88	45	18
N = — — —	233	194	166	148	121	85	58	32

Figure 17-2. Event-free rates for first ipsilateral stroke and transient ischemic attack including transient monocular blindness in the Veterans Affairs Cooperative Study. These are Kaplan-Meier curves for an analysis of time to the first event for the surgical and medical groups. The numbers (*n*) of patients remaining event-free and on study at the beginning of each 12-month period are provided under the graph. Treatment group comparisons by the log-rank test demonstrated significant differences in favor of the surgical group ($p<.001$). The relative risk (surgical group vs. medical group) was 0.38 (95% confidence interval, 0.22 to 0.67). (*From Hobson RW et al.*[8] *Reproduced by permission.*)

of stroke alone and stroke plus death are analyzed. An assumption that carotid endarterectomy will increase patient longevity probably is overly optimistic; however, a reduction in stroke alone will require confirmation before prophylactic carotid endarterectomy can be strongly recommended for all patients with asymptomatic carotid stenosis. Furthermore, important cost-effectiveness analyses will be needed once clinical efficacy has been established.

A further challenge for clinicians is to identify the subsets of patients with asymptomatic carotid disease who will clearly benefit from operation. Of significance is the fact that 20 percent of the patients in the Veterans Affairs cooperative study sustained all the neurological events, whereas 80 percent of the study

Table 17-5 Incidence of Stroke, Stroke Deaths, and All Other Deaths

	Surgical group 211 patients		Medical group 233 patients	
Endpoint	Number	%	Number	%
Nonfatal stroke	17	8.0	25	10.7
Stroke death	1	0.5	4	1.7
Other deaths				
MI, cardiac causes, sudden death[a]	44	20.9	47	20.2
Other medical causes	19	9.0	17	7.3
Unknown causes	6	2.8	10	4.3
Total[b]	87	41.2	103	44.2

[a]Includes 4 perioperative deaths; MI = Myocardial infarction
[b]No significant difference between groups (relative risk, 0.92; 95% confidence interval, 0.69 to 1.22)
SOURCE: From Hobson RW et al.[8] Reproduced by permission.

population passed through the four year mean period of observation without neurological complications.[8] This suggests that the percentage of stenosis is, at best, only an approximate predictor of the true neurological risk. Additional data on carotid plaque morphology, the influence of silent cerebral infarction on CT scan, measurements of cerebral collateral circulation, and the analysis of major risk factors such as coronary artery disease, diabetes mellitus, and symptomatic peripheral vascular disease, will also influence selection of patients. Once these factors have been thoroughly evaluated, the role of carotid endarterectomy for asymptomatic carotid artery disease will be more apparent, and the operation can be applied in a more cost-effective manner.

CURRENT CLINICAL RECOMMENDATIONS

Retrospective and prospective clinical analyses have demonstrated that carotid endarterectomy combined with optimal medical management can reduce the incidence of ipsilateral neurological outcome events in high-risk patients with arteriographically confirmed asymptomatic carotid stenosis. However, despite the increased risk of TIA and stroke in this population, most will die as a result of coronary atherosclerosis. Consequently, care must be exercised in the selection of patients for operation. Acceptably low perioperative complication rates (Table 17-6) should be confirmed by clinical audit at each institution before proceeding with a program of operative intervention for asymptomatic carotid disease.

Although the Veterans Affairs trial demonstrated a trend toward reduction in stroke alone for patients treated by carotid endarterectomy (Table 17-4), the more definitive analysis of stroke plus death must await publication of the ACAS results. For those patients randomized in the ACAS protocol, continued clinical follow-up is recommended. However, for those patients with asymptomatic carotid stenosis who are unwilling or unable to participate in the ACAS, carotid endarterectomy offers important advantages in selected individuals whose surgeons have demonstrated low complication rates.

Another clinically important group of patients are those identified as having asymptomatic carotid stenoses during preoperative evaluation for major general surgical or cardiovascular operative procedures. Intraoperative hypotension combined with carotid stenosis may predispose a patient to carotid artery occlusion and has been suggested as a

Table 17-6 Morbidity and Mortality Associated with Carotid Endarterectomy for Asymptomatic Carotid Disease in Different Studies

			Morbidity	
Authors	Operations	Mortality	Transient	Permanent
Thompson et al.[20]	167	0	2 (1.2%)	2 (1.2%)
Moore et al.[21]	78	0	2 (2.6%)	0
Hertzer et al.[22]	95	1 (1.1%)	—	4 (4.2%)
Whitney et al.[23]	279	3 (1.1%)	5 (1.8%)	6 (2.2%)
Javid et al.[24]	65	1 (1.5%)	1 (1.5%)	1 (1.5%)
Anderson et al.[25]	120	0	2 (1.7%)	0
VA Clinical Trial[8]	211	4 (1.9%)	2 (0.9%)	5 (2.4%)

mechanism for the development of stroke. Nevertheless, the overall risk of perioperative stroke is only 0.3 to 0.5 percent in patients undergoing general abdominal procedures, 1 to 2 percent in those undergoing vascular surgical procedures, and 2 to 5 percent in those undergoing coronary bypass grafting.[26] Although there is no well-documented relationship between the presence of a carotid bruit and the incidence of perioperative stroke, the perioperative risk of stroke in asymptomatic patients with carotid stenoses of 75 percent or greater has not been fully evaluated.

Barnes and coworkers used spectral analysis and cerebrovascular Doppler examinations to evaluate 449 patients undergoing coronary or peripheral vascular operations.[27] Fourteen percent of the patients had carotid stenoses that exceeded 50 percent of the arterial diameter; however, the range and distribution of these stenoses were not detailed. Nevertheless, no correlation between the presence of carotid stenosis and the incidence of perioperative stroke was reported. However, the incidence of postoperative death from myocardial infarction was significantly increased in the group of patients with asymptomatic carotid stenoses. Brener and coworkers used noninvasive techniques to study 2026 patients prior to coronary artery bypass, and 47 of these patients (2.3 percent) were identified as having hemodynamically significant carotid stenoses.[28] Although this prevalence of severe carotid disease was significantly less than the 12.3 percent reported by Barnes and colleagues[27] and the 11.8 percent reported by Turnipseed and coworkers[29] there was a 15 percent incidence of perioperative neurological deficits in patients with significant carotid occlusive disease undergoing coronary artery bypass compared with a 2 percent incidence in patients without significant carotid stenoses.[28] Nevertheless, Brener and coworkers recommended against prophylactic endarterectomy in this population because of the high incidence of perioperative complications for combined carotid endarterectomy and aortocoronary bypass procedures.

The decision to perform a prophylactic carotid endarterectomy prior to a major operative procedure must be based on the severity of carotid disease and the associated surgical risk. Although the overall incidence of stroke associated with aortic reconstruction or coronary artery bypass is low, patients with carotid stenoses of 75 percent or greater, or those with significant bilateral carotid disease, may constitute a group in which staged or combined operative intervention is appropriate. Currently, we recommend combined procedures only for asymptomatic patients with bilateral stenoses of more than 75 percent area-reduction or a comparable unilateral stenosis coupled with an asymptomatic contralateral occlusion. The subject of combined carotid and coronary artery disease is discussed in more detail in Chap. 20.

Whether concomitant carotid endarterectomy reduces the incidence of perioperative stroke in these patients remains controversial. However, subsequent or staged carotid endarterectomy once the patient has recovered from the cardiac or other surgical procedure may be indicated as part of a program of long-term stroke prevention. Furthermore, the ACAS group is studying this question in a prospective randomized fashion.[9] Until this information is available, no definitive conclusion regarding this group of patients is possible.

REFERENCES

1. Barnett HJM, Plum F, Walton JN: Carotid endarterectomy—an expression of concern. *Stroke* 15:941–943, 1984.
2. Easton JD, Sherman DG: Stroke and mortality rate in carotid endarterectomy: 228 consecutive operations. *Stroke* 8:565–568, 1977.
3. Brott T, Thalinger K: The practice of carotid endarterectomy in a large metropolitan area. *Stroke* 15:950–955, 1984.
4. NASCET Collaborators: Beneficial effect of carotid endarterectomy in symptomatic patients with high-grade carotid stenosis. *N Engl J Med* 325:445–453, 1991.
5. European Carotid Surgery Trialists' (ECST) Collaborative Group: MRC European Carotid Surgery interim results for symptomatic patients with severe (70–99%) or mild (0–29%) carotid stenosis. *Lancet* 337:1235–1243, 1991.
6. Mayberg MR, Wilson SE, Yatsu F, et al: Carotid endarterectomy and prevention of cerebral ischemia in symptomatic carotid stenosis. *JAMA* 266:3289–3294, 1991.
7. CASANOVA Study Group: Carotid surgery versus medical therapy in asymptomatic carotid stenosis. *Stroke* 22:1229–1235, 1991.
8. Hobson RW, Weiss DG, Fields WS, et al and the Veterans Affairs Cooperative Study Group: Efficacy of carotid endarterectomy for asymptomatic carotid stenosis. *N Engl J Med* 328: 221–227, 1993.
9. The Asymptomatic Carotid Atherosclerosis Study Group: Study design for randomized prospective trial of carotid endarterectomy for asymptomatic atherosclerosis. *Stroke* 20:844–849, 1989.
10. Nicolaides AN: European clinical trial on asymptomatic carotid stenosis, personal communication. 1993.
11. Wolf PA, Kannel WB, Sorlie P, McNamara P: Asymptomatic carotid bruit and the risk of stroke. *JAMA* 245:1442–1445, 1981.
12. Heyman W, Wilkinson WE, Heyden S, et al: Risk of stroke in asymptomatic persons with cervical arterial bruits: A population study in Evans County, Georgia. *N Engl J Med* 302: 838–841, 1980.
13. Norris JW, Zhu CZ, Bornstein NM, Chambers BR: Vascular risks of asymptomatic carotid stenosis. *Stroke* 22:1485–1490, 1991.
14. Gee W, Mehigan JT, Wylie EJ: Measurement of collateral cerebral hemispheric blood pressure by ocular pneumoplethysmography. *Am J Surg* 130:121–127, 1975.
15. Blackshear WM Jr, Phillips DJ, Thiele BL, et al: Detection of carotid occlusive disease by ultrasonic imaging and pulsed Doppler spectrum analysis. *Surgery* 86:698–706, 1979.
16. Hobson RW, Strandness DE: Carotid artery stenosis: What's in the measurement? (editorial) *J Vasc Surg* 18:1069, 1993.
17. Krupski WC, Weiss DG, Rapp JH, et al and the VA Cooperative Asymptomatic Carotid Artery Stenosis Study Group: Adverse effects of aspirin in the treatment of asymptomatic carotid artery stenosis. *J Vasc Surg* 16:588–600, 1992.
18. Hobson RW, Krupski WC, Weiss DG, and the VA Cooperative Study Group on Asymptomatic Carotid Stenosis: Influence of aspirin in the management of asymptomatic carotid artery stenosis. *J Vasc Surg* 17:257–265, 1993.
19. Towne JB, Weiss DG, Hobson RW: First phase report of Veterans Administration asymptomatic carotid stenosis study—operative morbidity and mortality. *J Vasc Surg* 11:252–259, 1990.
20. Thompson JE, Patman RD, Talkington CM: Asymptomatic carotid bruit: Long-term outcome in patients having endarterectomy compared with unoperated controls. *Ann Surg* 188: 308–316.

21. Moore WS, Boren C, Malone JM, Goldstone J: Asymptomatic carotid stenosis: Immediate and long-term results after prophylactic endarterectomy. *Am J Surg* 138:228–233, 1979.
22. Hertzer NR, Beven EG, Greenstreet RL, Humphries AW: Internal carotid back pressures, intraoperative shunting, ulcerated atheromata, and the incidence of stroke during carotid endarterectomy. *Surgery* 83:306–312, 1978.
23. Whitney DG, Kahn EM, Estes JW, Jones CE: Carotid artery surgery without a temporary indwelling shunt. *Arch Surg* 115:1393–1399, 1980.
24. Javid H, Ostermiller WE, Hengesh JW, et al: Carotid endarterectomy for asymptomatic patients. *Arch Surg* 102:389–391, 1971.
25. Anderson RJ, Hobson RW, Padberg FT, et al: Carotid endarterectomy for asymptomatic carotid stenosis: A ten year experience with 120 procedures in a fellowship training program. *Ann Vasc Surg* 5(2):111–115, 1991.
26. Long JB, Lynch TG, Hobson RW: Asymptomatic carotid stenosis, in Wilson SE, Veith FJ, Hobson RW, Williams RA (eds): *Vascular Surgery: Principles and Practice*. New York, McGraw-Hill, pp 581–591, 1987.
27. Barnes RW, Liebman PR, Marszalek PB, et al: The natural history of asymptomatic carotid disease in patients undergoing cardiovascular surgery. *Surgery* 90:1075–1083, 1981.
28. Brener BJ, Brief DK, Alpert J, et al: A four-year experience with preoperative noninvasive carotid evaluation of two thousand twenty-six patients undergoing cardiac surgery. *J Vasc Surg* 1:326–338, 1984.
29. Turnipseed WD, Berkoff HA, Belzer FO: Postoperative stroke in cardiac and peripheral vascular disease. *Ann Surg* 192:365–368, 1980.
30. Lynch TG, Hobson RW: Noninvasive cerebrovascular diagnostic techniques, in Wilson SE, Veith FJ, Hobson RW, Williams RA (eds). *Vascular Surgery: Principles and Practice*. New York: McGraw-Hill, 105–134, 1987.

18

Indications for Carotid Endarterectomy

R. Eugene Zierler

The purpose of this chapter is to summarize the currently accepted indications for carotid endarterectomy. Suggested algorithms are presented for the management of asymptomatic and symptomatic carotid artery disease. Whenever possible, recommendations are based on the results of randomized clinical trials, as discussed in Chaps. 16 and 17. In clinical situations for which prospective data are not yet available, the most applicable retrospective studies have been used. Since the conclusions of nonrandomized, uncontrolled studies are subject to a variety of interpretations, some of the specific indications for carotid endarterectomy will remain controversial.

In addition to the clinical presentation and the severity of extracranial carotid artery disease, a decision to proceed with carotid endarterectomy must take into account the general medical condition of the patient and, most important, the presence of cardiac risk factors. Cardiac complications are clearly the principal source of perioperative morbidity and mortality—and of decreased long-term survival—following carotid surgery. In a series of patients undergoing coronary arteriography prior to elective peripheral vascular reconstructions at the Cleveland Clinic, the prevalence of severe correctable coronary artery disease was 26 percent among the 295 patients under consideration for carotid endarterectomy.[1] Kazmers and coworkers evaluated the cardiac risks of carotid endarterectomy in 73 patients by measurement of left ventricular ejection fraction.[2] They observed that perioperative cardiac complications were more frequent in patients with ejection fractions of 35 percent or less (43 percent) compared to patients with ejection fractions greater than 35 percent (9 percent). Although there was no significant difference in operative mortality, overall survival was significantly lower in patients having an ejection fraction of 35 percent or less.

The many clinical factors that must be considered in the decision-making process leading up to carotid endarterectomy are covered elsewhere in this book. For example, the timing of carotid endarterectomy after an acute stroke is critical to a favorable clinical outcome, and the role of computed tomography (CT) in the timing of carotid surgery is described in Chap. 13. The problem of combined carotid and coronary artery disease is discussed in Chap. 20, including suggested management algorithms. Chap. 21 gives several algorithms related to the issue of performing carotid endarterectomy without preoperative arteriography. The preoperative details that are most important from the anesthesiologist's point of view are discussed in Chap. 22. Recurrent carotid stenosis and reoperative carotid surgery are unique problems that require individualized decision-making, as covered in Chaps. 27 and 28. Finally, as described in Chap. 29, the rare occurrence of significant occlusive lesions in the innominate and proximal common carotid arteries may require more than a routine carotid endarterectomy for effective treatment.

Minor differences between the management algorithms presented in this chapter and others elsewhere in this book should not be regarded as significant contradictions. There will continue to be differences of opinion regarding such aspects of carotid surgery as the minimum degree of stenosis that should qualify as a "surgical" lesion and the relative value of various preoperative tests. These algorithms obviously do not account for all possible clinical circumstances. They are intended to provide general guidelines that can serve as a constructive framework for clinical decision-making.

ASYMPTOMATIC CAROTID DISEASE

A key element in determining the clinical role of carotid endarterectomy is the safety of the operation. The primary rationale for operative treatment of asymptomatic carotid disease is the prevention of neurologic events. Since the risk of such events associated with asymptomatic high-grade carotid stenosis is relatively low, significant benefit can be achieved only if the risk of operation is also extremely small. In other words, if the surgical morbidity and mortality rates exceed those of medical therapy, any beneficial effects of operation will be lost.

In 1989, the Stroke Council of the American Heart Association proposed guidelines for acceptable complication rates associated with carotid endarterectomy.[3] The specified rates for combined operative morbidity and mortality varied according to the preoperative neurologic status of the patient as follows: less than 3 percent for asymptomatic patients; less than 5 percent for patients with transient ischemic attacks (TIAs); less than 7 percent for patients with ischemic stroke; and less than 10 percent for patients undergoing repair of recurrent carotid disease. The 30-day mortality rate following carotid endarterectomy should not exceed 2 percent. Complication rates within these ranges are clearly attainable by experienced surgeons.

As described in Chap. 11, natural history studies of asymptomatic high-grade carotid artery stenoses indicate that these lesions are not entirely benign.[4–6] A serial follow-up study based on duplex scanning strongly suggested that the finding of an 80 to 99 percent internal carotid stenosis identified a group of patients at high risk for TIA, stroke, or internal carotid occlusion.[4] Patients with asymptomatic stenoses in this range had a 46 percent incidence of one or more of these events within a 36-month period, while patients with less severe stenoses had only a 1.5 percent incidence. The mean interval between the finding of an 80 percent or greater stenosis and an event was 4.9 months. While no strokes occurred in patients with less than 80 percent stenoses, the incidence of stroke alone among patients in the high-risk group was 12.5 percent.

If an asymptomatic 80 to 99 percent internal carotid stenosis is associated with a high risk for neurologic symptoms or internal carotid occlusion, the clinically important question is whether this risk can be reduced by carotid endarterectomy. This issue was addressed in a retrospective review of 129 asymptomatic high-grade internal carotid stenoses, of which 56 were treated by carotid endarterectomy and 73 were followed without surgery.[7] Although the patients were not randomized to treatment groups, there were no significant differences between the operated and nonoperated patients for characteristics such as age, diabetes mellitus, hypertension, ischemic heart disease, and aspirin use. There was no operative mortality, but one perioperative stroke occurred. During 24 months of follow-up, neurologic symptoms and internal carotid occlusion were significantly more frequent in the nonoperated patients (48 percent) than in operated patients (9 percent). These results suggest that endarterectomy improves the natural history of high-grade asymptomatic internal carotid stenoses, provided the perioperative complication rate is low.

As discussed in Chap. 17, the Veterans Affairs Cooperative Study indicated that carotid endarterectomy can reduce the risk of ipsilateral neurologic events in patients with asymptomatic carotid stenosis.[8] Although this study was unable to show a benefit from carotid endarterectomy for the combined end-points of stroke and death, a modest effect could not be excluded because of the relatively small sample size. The exact severity of stenosis at which endarterectomy is justified for asymptomatic carotid disease was not resolved; however, this question should be addressed in the Asymptomatic Carotid Atherosclerosis Study.[9]

A management algorithm for patients with suspected asymptomatic carotid stenosis is shown in Fig. 18-1. It is assumed that patients will be selected for noninvasive carotid screening by the presence of a neck bruit or other risk factors for carotid artery disease. Recognizing that the neurologic risk associated with asymptomatic carotid disease appears to be most closely related to the severity of stenosis, the screening test of choice is duplex scanning. While the indirect noninvasive tests may continue to play a limited clinical role, duplex scanning is clearly the only acceptable screening test for extracranial carotid disease.[10] Serial follow-up studies suggest that it is safe to follow asymptomatic patients with 50 to 79 percent internal carotid stenoses by duplex scanning at approximately six-month intervals.[4] If neurologic symptoms or progression to 80 percent or greater stenosis are observed, the patient should be considered for carotid endarterectomy. The recommended follow-up intervals are considered optimal for the detection of progressive or recurrent disease. Whether such follow-up programs are practical or cost-effective remains to be determined.

The management of patients found to have asymptomatic carotid disease while being evaluated for major general or cardiovascular surgical procedures is discussed in Chaps. 17 and 20. In general, coexisting asymptomatic carotid disease should be approached as outlined above, and treatment of this problem may take precedence over other elective procedures.

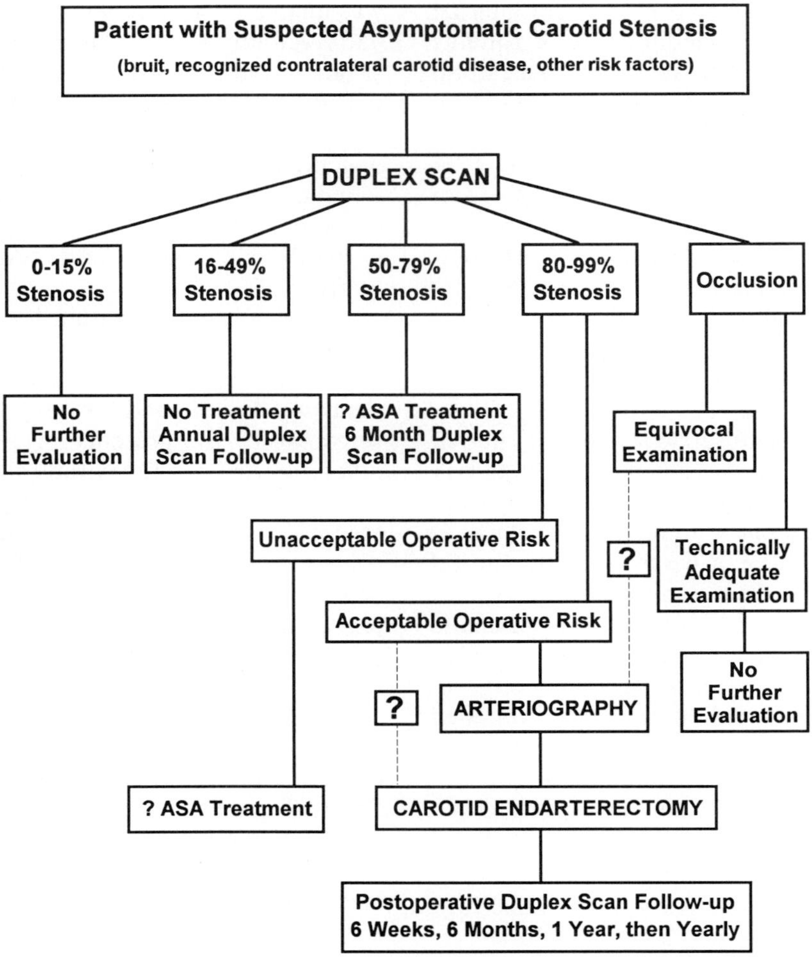

Figure 18-1. Management algorithm for patients with suspected asymptomatic carotid stenosis. Question marks signify optional or especially controversial aspects of management.

Prophylactic carotid endarterectomy or combined operations may be indicated in patients with bilateral high-grade carotid stenoses or unilateral high-grade stenosis with contralateral carotid occlusion.

SYMPTOMATIC CAROTID DISEASE

The three randomized clinical trials discussed in Chap. 16—the North American Symptomatic Carotid Endarterectomy Trial (NASCET), the European Carotid Surgery Trial (ECST), and the Veterans Affairs Trial—all clearly support a recommendation for carotid endarterectomy in symptomatic patients with 70 percent or greater stenosis of the appropriate internal carotid artery.[11–13] The circumstances surrounding the conclusions of the NASCET were particularly dramatic, since they were announced before the average patient follow-

A8 Seattle Post-Intelligencer, Saturday, February 23, 1991

Stroke surgery works so well, study is halted

The Associated Press

SAN FRANCISCO – A form of surgery to prevent strokes works so well that the government has called an emergency halt to further study and is scrambling to inform the nation's doctors of its effectiveness.

After an all-night meeting, researchers decided Thursday that a government study of the treatment should be stopped because the surgery was too effective to deny it to the study's control group of subjects, said Dr. Murray Goldstein, director of the National Institute of Neurological Disorders and Stroke.

The move was announced yesterday at the annual stroke meeting of the American Heart Association.

Figure 18-2. Headline from a Seattle newspaper dated February 23, 1991, announcing the results of the NASCET study.

up goal of five years specified in the original protocol had been attained.[11,14] On February 1, 1991, after an average follow-up of only 18 months, the preplanned rule for stopping randomization was applied because of statistically convincing evidence of treatment efficacy for patients with 70 to 99 percent stenoses undergoing carotid endarterectomy. The results of this study were promptly announced in the lay press (Fig. 18-2), and on February 25, 1991, a Clinical Alert was issued by the sponsoring agency, the National Institute of Neurological Disorders and Stroke, to rapidly transmit a summary of the NASCET results to physicians in North America (Fig. 18-3). A complete report of the interim NASCET results was published in the August 15, 1991 *New England Journal of Medicine*.[11]

It is important to emphasize that the NASCET results do not establish a 70 percent stenosis as the absolute threshold for benefit

National Institute of Neurological Disorders and Stroke

CLINICAL ALERT

BENEFIT OF CAROTID ENDARTERECTOMY FOR PATIENTS WITH HIGH-GRADE STENOSIS OF THE INTERNAL CAROTID ARTERY

Summary. The investigators of the North American Symptomatic Carotid Endarterectomy Trial (NASCET) are reporting the results of an interim analysis of the findings of a randomized controlled clinical trial of carotid endarterectomy for patients with a recent hemispheric, transient ischemic attack (TIA) or a mild (non-disabling) stroke and ipsilateral narrowing of the internal carotid artery. Two groups in the Trial received best medical care, including antiplatelet therapy; one of the two groups also had endarterectomy. For patients with high-grade stenosis (70-99% narrowing in the luminal diameter), surgery was highly beneficial. Consequently, patients with high-grade stenosis are no longer being entered into the Trial. Since the question of surgical benefit for patients with moderate stenosis (30-69%) has not yet been answered, that part of the Trial dealing with symptomatic patients with moderate stenosis will continue. Since it is also not yet known whether asymptomatic patients will benefit from carotid endarterectomy, other trials for those patients will also continue.

Figure 18-3. Clinical Alert issued by the National Institute of Neurological Disorders and Stroke, February 25, 1991. This summary of the NASCET results was distributed to physicians across North America.

from carotid endarterectomy. Rather, this degree of stenosis represents the current lower limit for which statistically valid conclusions can be reported. Because of continuing uncertainty about symptomatic patients with carotid stenoses in the range of 30 to 69 percent diameter reduction, randomization of such patients will continue.

Carotid endarterectomy is generally an elective procedure, and there is ample time to evaluate thoroughly both the carotid disease and other medical factors before proceeding with surgery. Although the role of emergency carotid endarterectomy is controversial, there are occasional circumstances in which it appears justified.[15,16] These situations arise in patients with acute neurologic symptoms that fall into the categories of stroke-in-evolution, waxing and waning neurologic deficit, and crescendo TIAs. When symptoms of this nature are associated with a 95 percent or greater stenosis or extensive thrombus in the ipsilateral carotid bifurcation, emergency carotid endarterectomy may be beneficial.[15] These preocclusive or thrombotic lesions are considered to be unstable because of their tendency to embolize or to progress to complete internal carotid occlusion. An algorithm for management of patients with acute neurologic deficits is presented in Fig. 18-4.

As discussed in Chap. 13, the timing of carotid endarterectomy after an acute completed stroke is determined by the degree of neurologic recovery and the findings on CT of the head. Patients with profound neurologic deficits and no evidence of recovery are not candidates for carotid endarterectomy; however, patients who show rapid resolution of their neurologic symptoms with minimal residual deficits may benefit from early operation. If a CT scan obtained during the acute stage of a stroke shows an ischemic infarct, the risk of perioperative stroke is increased, and these patients should be considered for carotid endarterectomy after an interval of four to six weeks.[17] In contrast, it appears that patients with negative CT scans, both on presentation and approximately five days following a stroke, can safely undergo carotid endarterectomy within two weeks of the neurologic event.[18]

A general algorithm for the management of patients with symptomatic carotid stenosis is given in Fig. 18-5. As in the preceding algorithms, duplex scanning is used as the primary noninvasive screening test. Although the NASCET recommendations for carotid endarterectomy in symptomatic patients require a 70 percent or greater stenosis by arteriography, virtually all lesions in the 80 to 99 percent stenosis category and many of the lesions in the 50 to 79 percent stenosis category by duplex scanning (Table 11-1 in Chap. 11) will fall into this group. The ratio of the peak systolic velocities in the internal and common carotid arteries (ICA/CCA ratio) also can be used to select patients for further evaluation and treatment according to the NASCET guidelines.[19]

A question that arises frequently in the clinical setting is how to manage asymptomatic or symptomatic patients with degrees of carotid stenosis near the thresholds that determine different approaches to treatment. Such borderline lesions will occur with any technique for grading the severity of carotid disease. For example, how should the patient with hemispheric TIAs and a 50 or 60 percent carotid stenosis be managed? While there are no simple answers, it is helpful to remember that there is some variability in the results of both carotid duplex scanning and arteriography.[20,21] Therefore, if a patient has a carotid stenosis close to 70 percent and is otherwise a candidate for carotid endarterectomy according to the NASCET criteria, it is reasonable to proceed with surgery. A similar rationale can be used in selecting patients with asymptomatic high-grade carotid stenoses for carotid endarterectomy.

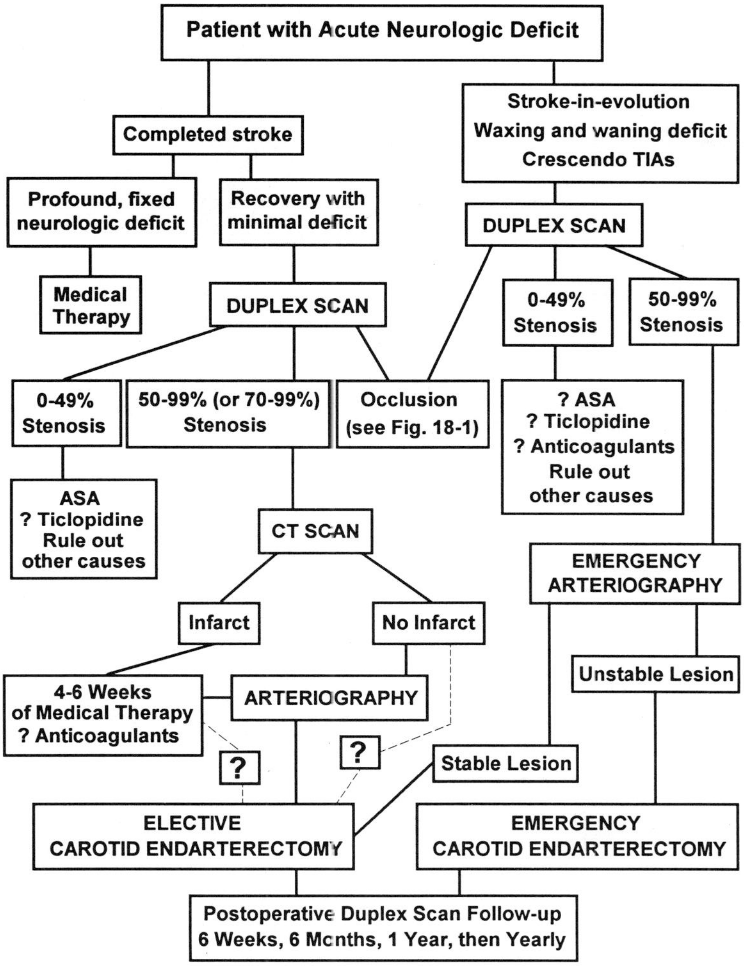

Figure 18-4. Algorithm for management of patients with an acute neurologic deficit associated with carotid artery disease. Question marks signify optional or controversial aspects of management. The 70 to 99 percent stenosis category represents the guidelines specified in the NASCET (see text).

NONHEMISPHERIC SYMPTOMS

Many surgeons approach the treatment of patients with nonhemispheric neurologic symptoms and carotid artery disease in much the same way they proceed with asymptomatic patients. In contrast to hemispheric symptoms, which produce distinct clinical manifestations in the distribution of a particular carotid artery, nonhemispheric or vertebrobasilar symptoms are relatively nonspecific and often do not implicate a unique vascular territory (Chap. 7). Therefore, in addition to screening for extracranial carotid artery disease, vascular evaluation in these patients should include an assessment of the proximal aortic arch vessels and the intracranial circulation. Other potential causes of vertebrobasilar symptoms also should be considered, including postural hypotension, cardiac arrhythmias, and vestibular or auditory disorders. Techniques such as CT scanning or mag-

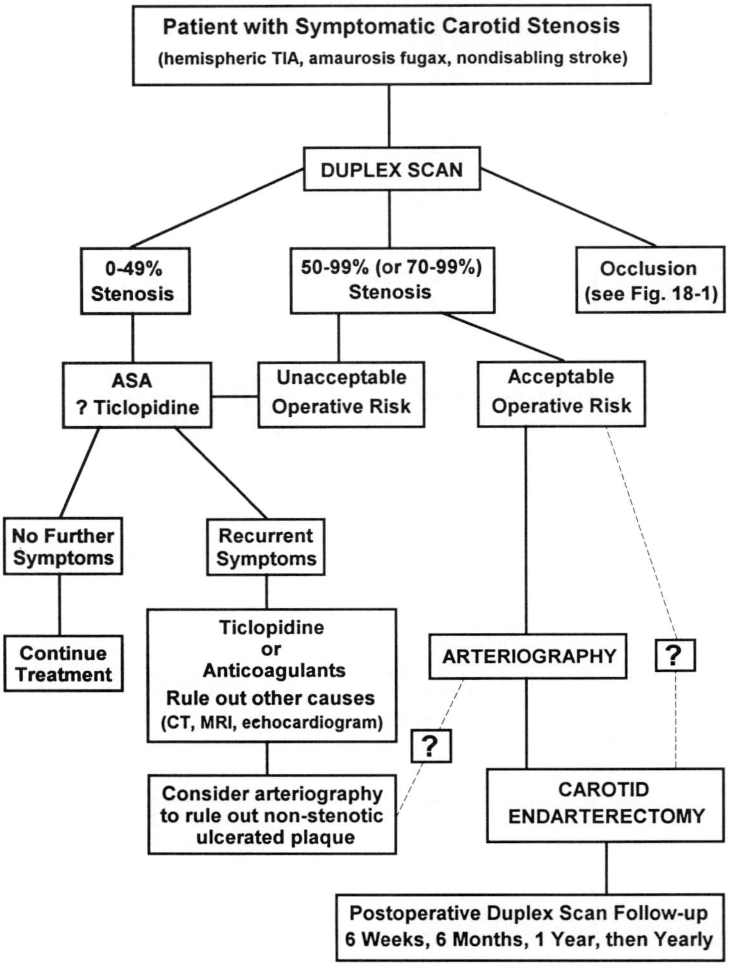

Figure 18-5. Management algorithm for patients with symptomatic carotid stenosis. Question marks signify optional or controversial aspects of management. The 70 to 99 percent stenosis category represents the guidelines specified in the NASCET (see text).

netic resonance imaging may be useful in selected cases (Chap. 13).

Unlike symptoms in the carotid artery distribution, which are more likely to result from small emboli, nonhemispheric symptoms are generally attributed to decreased blood flow in the posterior cerebral circulation (Chap. 4). Consequently, treatment is directed toward increasing cerebral perfusion. This can be achieved by direct vertebral artery repair when indicated (Chaps. 19 and 30), or by carotid revascularization. The latter approach relies on an intact circle of Willis, particularly the posterior communicating arteries, to increase blood flow to the vertebrobasilar circulation.[22]

The results of carotid endarterectomy for nonhemispheric symptoms have been variable. McNamara and coworkers reported that eight of 18 patients (44 percent) having carotid endarterectomy for nonhemispheric symptoms and followed for a mean of 40 months had recurrent symptoms identical to those noted preoperatively.[23] However, in the series of 50 carotid endarterectomies performed by Ford and coworkers[24] and 24 carotid endarterectomies performed by Rosenthal and colleagues.[25] for vertebrobasilar symptoms, postoperative improvement was noted in 95 and 88 percent of cases, respectively. Thus, carotid endarterectomy should be considered after nonvascular causes have been excluded in patients with nonhemispheric symptoms and severe occlusive disease involving multiple extracranial cerebral vessels.

CONCLUSIONS

With the successful completion of the first randomized clinical trials on the management of carotid artery disease, a major clinical milestone has been reached. While the most definitive conclusions have come from trials involving symptomatic patients, the results of these studies already have influenced the diagnosis and treatment of both symptomatic and asymptomatic carotid disease.

It is now clear that carotid endarterectomy is more effective than nonoperative therapy alone for symptomatic patients with 70 to 99 percent stenosis of the appropriate internal carotid artery. Whether lesser degrees of symptomatic carotid stenosis also will benefit from endarterectomy remains to be determined. For patients with asymptomatic high-grade carotid stenoses, it appears that endarterectomy can reduce the risk of ipsilateral neurologic events, but the minimum stenosis that justifies surgical treatment has not yet been established. Whenever possible, prospective data should serve as the basis for clinical decision-making; when such data are not available, satisfactory guidance is provided by retrospective studies.

REFERENCES

1. Hertzer NR, Beven EG, Young JR, et al: Coronary artery disease in peripheral vascular patients: A classification of 1000 coronary angiograms and results of surgical management. *Ann Surg* 199:223, 1984.
2. Kazmers A, Cerqueira MD, Zierler RE: The role of preoperative radionuclide left ventricular ejection fraction for risk assessment in carotid surgery. *Arch Surg* 123:416, 1988.
3. Beebe HG, Clagett GP, DeWeese JA, et al: Assessing the risk associated with carotid endarterectomy: A statement for health professionals by an ad hoc committee on carotid surgery standards of the stroke council, American Heart Association. *Stroke* 20:314, 1989.
4. Roederer GO, Langlois YE, Jager KA, et al: The natural history of carotid arterial disease in asymptomatic patients with cervical bruits. *Stroke* 15:605, 1984.
5. Chambers BR, Norris JW: Outcome in patients with asymptomatic neck bruits. *N Engl J Med* 315:860, 1986.
6. Bougousslavsky J, Despland PA, Regli F: Asymptomatic tight stenosis of the internal carotid artery: Long-term prognosis. *Neurology* 36:861, 1986.
7. Moneta GL, Taylor DC, Nicholls SC, et al: Operative versus nonoperative management of asymptomatic high-grade internal carotid artery stenosis: Improved results with endarterectomy. *Stroke* 18:1005, 1987.
8. Hobson RW, Weiss DG, Fields WS, et al. and the Veterans Affairs Cooperative Study Group: Efficacy of carotid endarterectomy for asymptomatic carotid stenosis. *N Engl J Med* 328:221, 1993.
9. The Asymptomatic Carotid Atherosclerosis Study Group: Study design for randomized prospective trial of carotid endarterectomy for asymptomatic atherosclerosis. *Stroke* 20:844, 1989.
10. Strandness DE Jr, Andros G, Baker JD, et al: Vascular laboratory utilization and payment: Report of the Ad Hoc Committee of the Western Vascular Society. *J Vasc Surg* 16:163, 1992.
11. North American Symptomatic Carotid Endarterectomy Trial Collaborators: Beneficial effect

of carotid endarterectomy in symptomatic patients with high-grade carotid stenosis. *N Engl J Med* 325:445, 1991.
12. European Carotid Surgery Trialists' Collaborative Group: MRC European carotid surgery trial. Interim results for symptomatic patients with severe (70–99%) or with mild (0–29%) stenosis. *Lancet* 337:1235, 1991.
13. Mayberg MR, Wilson SE, Yatsu R, et al: Carotid endarterectomy and prevention of cerebral ischemia in symptomatic carotid stenosis. *JAMA* 266:3289, 1991.
14. North American Symptomatic Carotid Endarterectomy Trial (NASCET) Steering Committee: North American Symptomatic Carotid Endarterectomy Trial: Methods, patient characteristics, and progress. *Stroke* 22:711, 1991.
15. Goldstone J, Moore WS: Emergency carotid artery surgery in neurologically unstable patients. *Arch Surg* 111:1284, 1976.
16. Mentzer RM, Finkelmeier BA, Crosby IK, et al: Emergency carotid endarterectomy for fluctuating neurologic deficits. *Surgery* 89:60, 1981.
17. Graber JN, Vollman RW, Johnson WC, et al: Stroke after carotid endarterectomy: Risk as predicted by preoperative computerized tomography. *Am J Surg* 147:492, 1984.
18. Pitrowski JJ, Bernhard VM, Rubin JR, et al: Timing of carotid endarterectomy after acute stroke. *J Vasc Surg* 11:45, 1990.
19. Moneta GL, Edwards JM, Chitwood RW, et al: Correlation of North American Symptomatic Carotid Endarterectomy Trial (NASCET) angiographic definition of 70% to 90% internal carotid artery stenosis with duplex scanning. *J Vasc Surg* 17:152, 1993.
20. Chikos PM, Fisher LD, Hirsch JH, et al: Observer variability in evaluating extracranial arterial stenosis. *Stroke* 14:885, 1983.
21. Kohler T, Langlois Y, Roederer GO, et al: Sources of variability in carotid duplex examination: A prospective study. *Ultrasound Med Biol* 4:571, 1985.
22. Harward TRS, Wickborn IG, Otis SM, et al: Posterior communicating artery visualization in predicting results of carotid endarterectomy for vertebrobasilar insufficiency. *Am J Surg* 148:43, 1984.
23. McNamara JO, Heyman A, Silver D, et al: The value of carotid endarterectomy in treating transient cerebral ischemia of the posterior circulation. *Neurology* 27:682, 1977.
24. Ford JJ, Baker WH, Ehrenhaft JL: Carotid endarterectomy for nonhemispheric transient ischemic attacks. *Arch Surg* 110:1314, 1975.
25. Rosenthal D, Cossman D, Ledig CB, et al: Results of carotid endarterectomy for vertebrobasilar insufficiency. *Arch Surg* 113:1361, 1978.

19

Indications for Vertebral Artery Surgery

Stephen C. Nicholls

Despite the observation by Astley Cooper in 1836 that, unlike ligation of the carotid arteries, vertebral artery ligation would not be tolerated because they supplied more vital centers, the clinical importance of the cervical portions of the vertebral arteries has been largely ignored until relatively recently. Furthermore, although Taylor described embolism involving the left vertebral artery in the *British Medical Journal* in 1871, at that time clinical symptoms were generally attributed to local factors, and extracranial causes were not considered.

In 1927 deKleyn and Nieuwenhuyser[1] demonstrated in cadavers that flow in the vertebral artery could be reduced or stopped with neck movement, and in 1946 Kubik and Adams[2] described occlusion of the basilar artery and its associated clinical syndrome. Biemond[3] reported in 1951 that nystagmus and dysarthria could be produced by neck rotation and extension in patients thought to be suffering from cerebral arteriosclerosis, and in 1956 Schwartz and coworkers[4] described a patient sustaining brain stem infarction following chiropractic manipulation. In 1957 Hutchinson and Yates observed that lesions of the carotid and vertebral arteries occurred with equal frequency and that with vertebral artery lesions infarcts were found in the cerebellum and brain stem, suggesting a causal relationship.[5] Castaigne and coworkers supported this theory in 1973 when, based on an autopsy study, they concluded that atheromatous lesions of the vertebral artery were the cause of basilar territory infarcts.[6]

Although the initial concept of vertebrobasilar insufficiency was formulated by Millikan and Siekert in 1955,[7] its clear distinction from carotid insufficiency has continued to evolve in the literature. Evidence that vertebral artery lesions are not rare was presented by the Joint Study of Extracranial Arterial Occlusion, in which 22 percent of 4748 patients had stenosis at the origin of the left vertebral artery and 18 percent had similar lesions of the right vertebral artery.[8] However, surgical treatment of these lesions has been performed infrequently. In describing his experience of 25 years, Rob reported 149 patients undergoing vertebral artery surgery, while during the same period 4362 patients underwent operations on the internal carotid artery.[9] As recently as 1981, Carney noted "the vertebral artery lies buried in a sea of generalities, prejudices, fear and ignorance."[10]

The anatomic location and course of the vertebral arteries has always hindered diagnostic evaluation, pathologic examination, and surgical exploration. In addition, the clinical presentation of posterior circulation insufficiency is often vague and, as a result, the management of vertebral artery disease has lagged far behind that of carotid disease. Recent recognition that embolization is far more common in the posterior circulation than previously believed,[11] and the increasing sophistication of diagnostic techniques such as transcranial Doppler (TCD) and magnetic resonance imaging (MRI), are enabling better delineation of pathophysiologic mechanisms in cerebral ischemia and infarction. This will permit more precise correlation of symptoms with anatomic lesions and improve selection of patients for surgical intervention.

ANATOMY OF THE VERTEBROBASILAR SYSTEM

By convention the arterial supply of the brain is divided into two major systems—the carotid and the vertebrobasilar—which are synonymous with the terms "anterior" and "posterior" cerebral circulations. However, such a distinction is somewhat arbitrary and at variance with the known functional interdependence of these two systems through an abundance of collateral pathways (Chap. 2).

The paired vertebral arteries arise at an acute angle from the subclavian arteries and constitute their largest and most proximal branches. Anomalies of the vertebral artery origins occur, the most frequent variation being a left vertebral artery originating directly from the arch of the aorta which is present in up to 8 percent of individuals. The vertebral artery is divided into four segments (Fig. 19-1). The first segment courses cephalad until it enters the transverse foramina of the cervical vertebrae. This occurs at the level of C6 in 88 percent of cases, although entry may occur higher at C5 (7 percent) or C4 (1 percent), or lower at C7 (4 percent).[12] Thus, the second segment of the vertebral artery typically is formed by the intraosseous course through the transverse foramina of the C2 through C6 vertebrae. The third segment begins as the artery exits the transverse foramen of C2 and terminates at the dura. The fourth segment is intracranial and terminates at the level of the pontomedullary junction, where the two vertebral arteries join to form the basilar artery (Fig. 19-2). The two most important branches of the intracranial segment are the

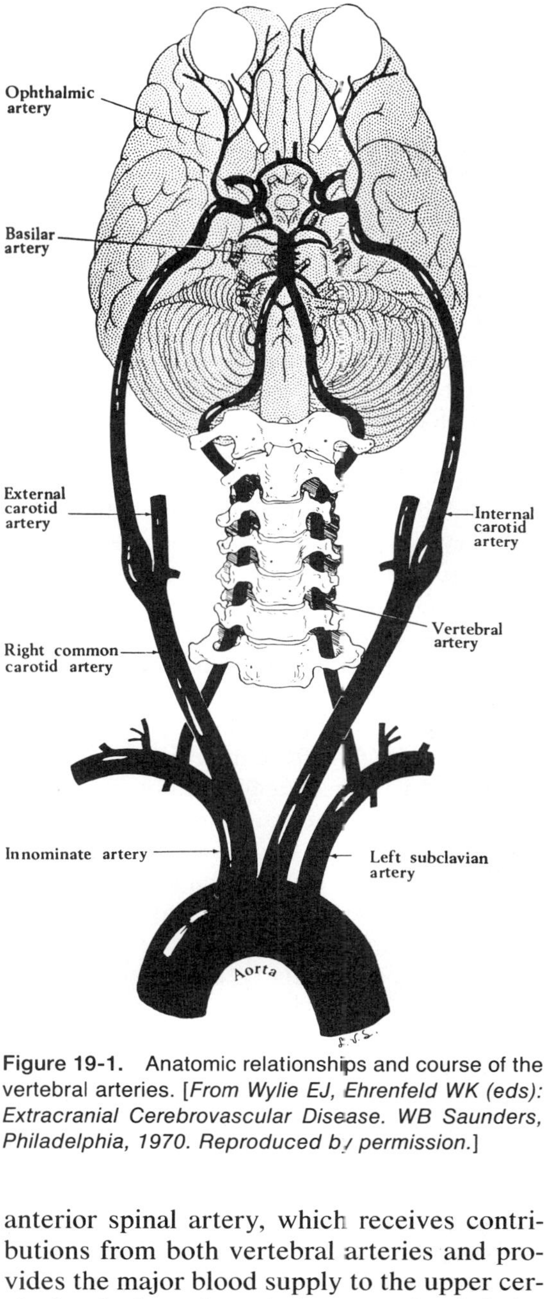

Figure 19-1. Anatomic relationships and course of the vertebral arteries. [*From Wylie EJ, Ehrenfeld WK (eds): Extracranial Cerebrovascular Disease. WB Saunders, Philadelphia, 1970. Reproduced by permission.*]

anterior spinal artery, which receives contributions from both vertebral arteries and provides the major blood supply to the upper cervical spinal cord, and the posterior inferior cerebellar artery (PICA).

The basilar artery runs along the base of the

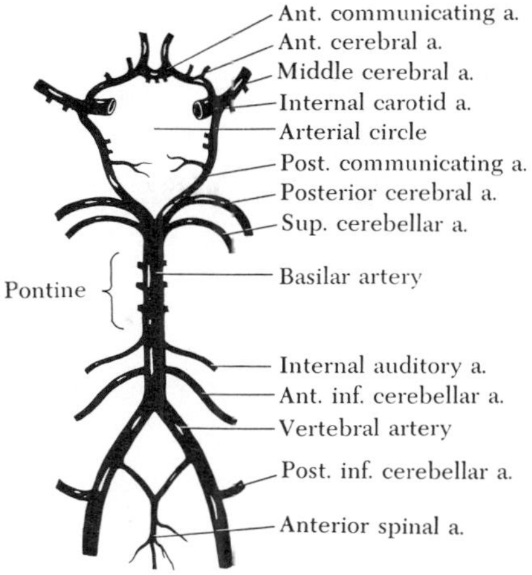

Figure 19-2. Normal configuration of the distal branches of the vertebrobasilar system and circle of Willis. [*From Wylie EJ, Ehrenfeld WK, (eds): Extracranial Cerebrovascular Disease. WB Saunders, Philadelphia, 1970. Reproduced by permission.*]

pons and at its termination gives off a pair of basilar communicating arteries, which form the initial portion of the posterior cerebral artery (PCA) on each side. These PCA segments receive the posterior communicating arteries from the internal carotid circulation, forming a potential collateral route between the anterior and posterior circulations and completing the posterior aspect of the circle of Willis (Fig. 19-2). Occasionally, the vertebral artery terminates in the PICA rather than the PCA. It should be emphasized that hypoplastic anterior or posterior communicating arteries are frequent, and the circle of Willis is functionally complete in less than 50 percent of individuals.[13]

CAUSES OF VERTEBROBASILAR INSUFFICIENCY

Atherosclerosis

Of all the causes of posterior circulation ischemia listed in Table 19-1, atherosclerosis is the

Table 19-1 Causes of Vertebrobasilar Insufficiency

Atherosclerosis
Nonatherosclerotic disease
Intrinsic disease
Fibromuscular disease
Takayasu's disease
Trauma
Spontaneous dissection
Aneurysms
Arteriovenous fistulas
Extrinsic disease (compression)
Cervical spondylosis
Fibrous bands
Craniocleidal dysostosis
Cervical spinal canal stenosis
Infantile atlanto-occipital instability
Atlanto-occipital subluxation in rheumatoid arthritis
Congenital cervical spine fusion
Thoracic outlet syndrome
Cervical spine tumors

most important. The underlying mechanisms include hypoperfusion secondary to vertebral artery stenosis or occlusion and embolization from a more proximal arterial lesion. The most common site of stenosis in the vertebral artery is its origin, but narrowing also can occur where the artery exits from the bony canal, possibly due to mechanical factors, and in the proximal portion of the basilar artery. Cardiogenic emboli affect the posterior circulation more frequently than previously suspected, and arterio-arterial emboli can originate from within a stenosed or occluded vertebral artery.

Subclavian Steal Although retrograde flow in a vertebral artery was first described by Harrison over 100 years ago,[14] the clinical relevance of this observation was not defined until 1961.[15] As discussed in Chaps. 4 and 7, the clinical manifestations associated with this pattern of flow are commonly referred to as the "subclavian steal syndrome." When there is a high-grade stenosis or occlusion in a proximal subclavian or innominate artery, the ipsilateral vertebral artery becomes a collateral vessel, diverting blood from the posterior circulation to supply the arm. Under certain circumstances, most commonly with a contralateral vertebral artery occlusion, flow in the basilar artery may be reversed and lead to a loss of adequate blood supply to the brain stem. This steal of blood from the posterior circulation classically is exacerbated by arm exercise, which increases the pressure gradient favoring blood flow to the arm. Thus, patients who are asymptomatic at rest may develop symptoms or signs of posterior circulation ischemia with exercise of the ipsilateral arm.

Most patients with a hemodynamic subclavian steal are asymptomatic, both at rest and with arm exercise, whereas some patients become symptomatic only during exercise. A small proportion of patients demonstrate vertebrobasilar insufficiency at rest, and some may even have oscillating flow at rest that completely reverses with arm exercise.[16]

In almost all cases, reversed flow in a vertebral artery is compensated for at the basilar artery level by flow from the contralateral vertebral artery. Consequently, although patients with reversed vertebral artery flow have a hemodynamic steal, they can only be considered to have brain stem ischemia if flow reversal is demonstrated in the basilar artery. This fact became appreciated recently with routine TCD insonation of this vessel.[17] Patients with a symptomatic subclavian steal also usually have a concomitant deficiency of the posterior communicating arteries that prevents adequate collateral flow from the anterior circulation. There is a particular group of patients who have adequate posterior communicating arteries but restriction of flow from bilateral high-grade carotid artery disease.[18] These patients may be cured or improved by carotid endarterectomy. The surgical management of subclavian steal syndrome is discussed in Chap. 29.

Embolization in the Posterior Circulation In the past, the incidence of embolization in the posterior circulation was thought to be extremely low. However, it now appears that emboli are the cause of posterior circulation ischemia in a significant proportion of cases. The evidence for this conclusion will be briefly reviewed.

The PCA is the most distal branch of the vertebrobasilar system and is therefore the most likely recipient vessel for emboli to the posterior circulation. Castaigne and coworkers[6] reported on an autopsy series of 30 vertebrobasilar occlusions in 22 patients with infarction in the PCA territory. Only two patients had thrombosis of the PCA related to areas of stenosis. In five patients basilar artery thrombus extended into the PCA and accounted for occlusion. All the other instances were embolic. In 11 patients (50 percent), emboli originated from occlusive lesions in the more proximal vertebrobasilar system, while one patient had a recognized cardiac source.

Caplan and coworkers reported 67 patients with vertebrobasilar insufficiency in whom cardiac emboli accounted for 21 percent of cases and arterial emboli for 13 percent.[11] Of the nine cases with emboli from lesions in the vertebral artery, there was an occlusion of the vertebral artery origin in three, dissection of the distal extracranial vertebral artery in three, and two patients who had posterior circulation events after surgery. These postoperative events presumably were related to neck positioning and occlusion of the vertebral artery during anesthesia with subsequent embolization. An additional patient had thrombus in the intracranial portion of the vertebral artery. Of the recipient territories, three involved the intracerebral vertebral artery-PICA territory, and three involved the distal basilar artery-superior cerebellar artery territory. Three patients were noted to have pontine infarcts due to basilar artery embolic material. How often platelet and platelet-fibrin emboli arise from ulcerative lesions within the extracranial vertebral arteries is unknown.

Rancurel and coworkers[19] studied 460 patients with a well-documented history of transient ischemic attack (TIA) in the vertebrobasilar distribution. Of the 460 cases, 136 had one or more brain stem infarcts in addition to TIA. The underlying etiology in the patients with infarcts was determined to be cardiac disease in 31, arterial emboli in 82, and unknown in 23. Mean follow-up was 64 months. Among the 460 patients, two main etiologic groups were distinguishable. There was a homogeneous group of 97 patients who had thromboembolic TIA and one or more infarcts demonstrated by computed tomography (CT) or MRI. These were related to an arterial or cardiac source. In most cases the TIA preceded infarction. A second group of 210 patients, also homogeneous, showed a stereotyped and repetitive pattern of TIA, often closely associated with postural changes or specific neck positions. Orthostatic hypotension and low cardiac output were ruled out in all patients before inclusion in the study. In the latter group with hemodynamic TIA related to postural or positional changes, there was no clinical, CT, or MRI evidence of infarction. A third group of 95 patients showed both thromboembolic and hemodynamic TIA with clinical features differing from one attack to the next. Finally, a fourth group of 58 patients had only vertebrobasilar TIA but did not fit into any of the preceding categories and remained unclassified.

More recently TCD has been used in the detection of cerebral emboli (Chap. 12).[20] Applications of this technique are now being extended to monitor the basilar artery and identify those patients with vertebrobasilar territory embolization (Fig. 19-3). Since the prognosis of embolic events in the vertebrobasilar territory is worse than that for simple

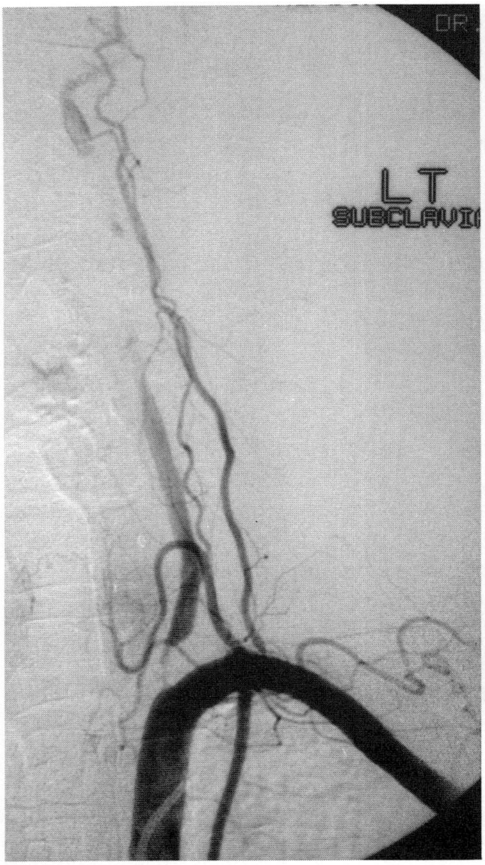

A

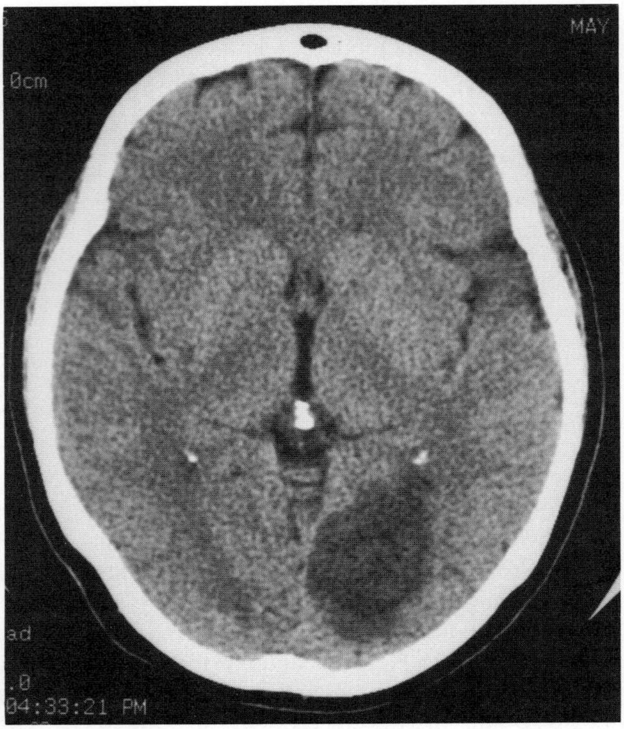

B

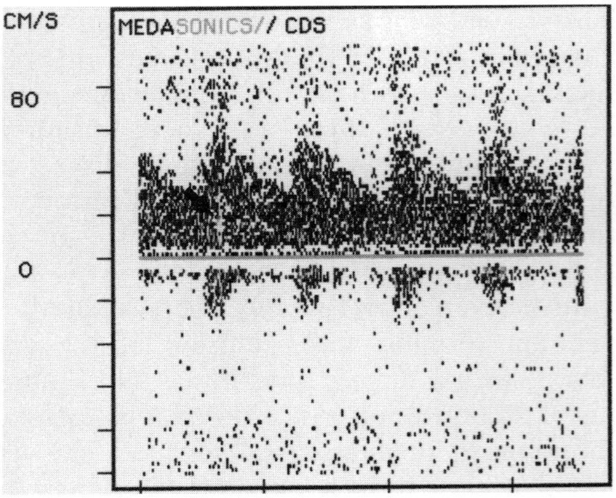

Figure 19-3. *A.* Angiogram of a 61-year-old woman presenting with aphasia and ataxia. Arch injection with a blood pressure cuff inflated on the left arm shows a very tight stenosis at the origin of the left vertebral artery. *B.* CT scan demonstrates a large infarct in the cerebellum. There were two other sites of infarction in the left brain stem territory. *C.* TCD monitoring of the basilar artery demonstrates evidence of ongoing embolization. Embolus signature is indicated by the arrow.

hemodynamic events, future efforts should be directed toward careful evaluation of these patients for embolic disease, including duplex scanning, TCD, and selective four-vessel angiography.

Nonatherosclerotic Disease

Intrinsic nonatherosclerotic disease of the vertebral artery is similar in nature to that of other arteries, whereas the mechanisms of extrinsic compression are unique to the vertebral artery (Table 19-1).

Intrinsic Disease Fibromuscular dysplasia usually affects the second and third segments of the vertebral arteries and commonly is associated with corresponding lesions in the internal carotids. It may present with thromboembolic symptoms, and aneurysm formation or dissection may also occur. Vertebral artery lesions in Takayasu's disease are typically at the origin from the subclavian where relative stenoses occur, especially when the vertebral artery enlarges to compensate for bilateral carotid involvement.

Penetrating trauma to the vertebral artery is rare. Blunt trauma may be associated with spinal fracture or dislocation. Most often injury occurs to the third segment when extreme neck rotation and hyperextension cause forceful stretching of the artery. Injury also may result from therapeutic manipulations. Arteriovenous fistulas involving the vertebral artery may be congenital or acquired secondary to trauma. Arterial dissection and aneurysm formation may be related to trauma as well as fibromuscular dysplasia. Secondary thromboembolic complications can occur after a variable interval following the initial injury, resulting in brain stem stroke.

Extrinsic Disease Compression of the vertebral artery tends to occur when there is rotation and hyperextension of the neck. The vertebral artery on the side opposite to the direction of neck rotation usually is affected (Fig. 19-4). Normally, this compression is not clinically significant, but it can assume importance if one vertebral artery is occluded or hypoplastic and collateral flow from the anterior circulation through the posterior communicating arteries is limited. While extrinsic compression of the vertebral arteries is much less common than occlusive disease from atherosclerosis, it should be considered in all patients presenting with vertebrobasilar symptoms, particularly those in the younger age group and when symptoms are provoked by changes in head position. While symptoms are typically transient, repetitive compression can lead to thrombosis or formation of emboli.

Underlying causes of extrinsic vertebral artery compression are cervical spondylosis, fibrous bands, craniocleidal dysostosis, cervical spinal canal stenosis, infantile atlanto-occipital instability, atlanto-occipital subluxation in rheumatoid arthritis, congenital cervical spine fusion, thoracic outlet syndrome, and cervical spine tumors (Fig. 19-5). All of these may result in an interruption of flow in the vertebral artery, either unilaterally or bilaterally, with specific head and neck positions (Fig. 19-6).

SYMPTOMS

While the indications for surgery in vertebral artery disease are based on the demonstration of significant anatomic lesions in the presence of posterior circulation insufficiency, it must be emphasized that vertebrobasilar symptoms more often are due to other causes. In addition, the symptoms of vertebrobasilar ischemia are highly variable, and the patterns are more complex than symptoms in the carotid territory. Many symptoms, such as loss of balance, dizziness, and bilateral visual blurring,

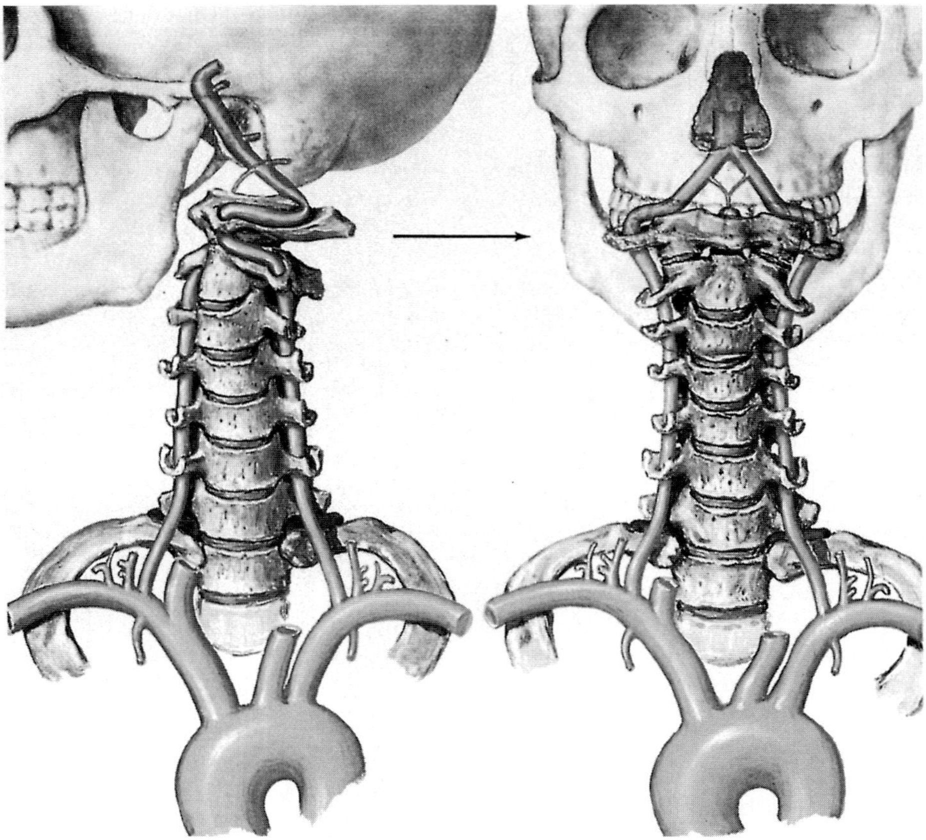

Figure 19-4. Physiologic compression of the left vertebral artery associated with head turning to the right. There is concomitant rotation of the atlas, which can lead to sharp angulation of the vertebral artery contralateral to the direction of head turning and a temporary obstruction of the lumen. [*From Clinical Symposia: Aortocranial Occlusive Vascular Disease, (Stroke) Volume 26, number 4. New Jersey: CIBA, 1974. Reproduced by permission.*]

are vague or nonspecific and difficult to interpret. Although dizziness is the most common presenting symptom in vertebrobasilar insufficiency,[21] syncope or presyncope are more frequently the result of nonvascular conditions.

Certain posterior circulation symptoms may be the result of global cerebral ischemia caused by severe carotid artery disease; however, objective signs are very important. Nystagmus, extraocular muscle palsies, and cerebellar signs cannot be mimicked by anterior circulation lesions. While certain symptoms are relatively specific for the posterior circulation, they also may be caused by disorders such as multiple sclerosis. Posterior fossa tumors can cause prominent cranial nerve and brain stem symptoms. A vascular cause is suggested by features such as advanced age, diabetes, hypertension, other manifestations of vascular disease, evidence of infarction in the vertebrobasilar territory on CT or MRI, and

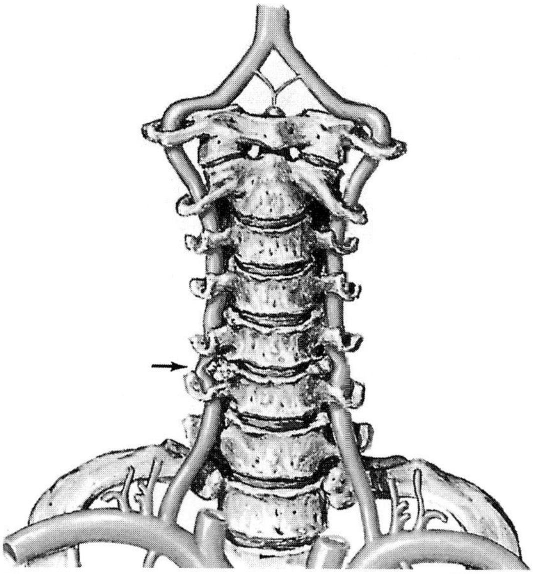

Figure 19-5. Mechanical compression of the right vertebral artery by an osteophyte at the C5-C6 level (*arrow*), which can result in complete cessation of flow in the affected vertebral artery. [*From Clinical Symposia: Aortocranial Occlusive Vascular Disease, (Stroke) Volume 26, number 4. New Jersey: CIBA, 1974. Reproduced by permission.*]

appropriate lesions on noninvasive or angiographic evaluation.

DIAGNOSTIC EVALUATION

The diagnosis of extrinsic compression of the vertebral arteries has traditionally depended on plain x-ray films, CT of the cervical spine, and a careful history verifying the onset of symptoms with specific head movements. However, the definitive diagnostic test has been angiography of the vertebrobasilar system with the head in the anteroposterior and rotated positions.

Noninvasive evaluation of the vertebrobasilar system remains less developed than that of the carotid circulation, and precise classification of stenosis severity is not possible. The standard duplex examination (Chap. 11) allows identification of the vertebral artery at its origin from the subclavian artery, and the stenoses that occur most commonly at that site can be assessed qualitatively. The vertebral artery can then be evaluated up into the bony canal. Determination of flow direction, with and without provocative testing (reactive hyperemia of the ipsilateral arm), can establish the diagnosis of a hemodynamic subclavian steal.

A study by Bendick and Glover suggests that cerebral artery flow can be assessed by duplex scanning, allowing comparisons among different patient groups.[22] Despite the lack of a gold standard and significant overlap among measurements, there is evidence that low-volume flow is associated with a higher incidence and severity of posterior circulation ischemic symptoms. More recently, success has been reported using TCD monitoring of the vertebral, basilar, posterior cerebral, and posterior communicating arteries to demonstrate the hemodynamic patterns and collateral pathways of the intracranial circulation.[23] The advantages of this approach are the avoidance of the associated morbidity and mortality of an invasive procedure and the ability to reproduce extreme neck movements and relate them to clinical symptoms without the constraints imposed by the angiography suite. TCD monitoring with neck maneuvers offers the potential to replace dynamic angiography in the future (Fig. 19-7). Detection of emboli with TCD monitoring of the basilar and posterior cerebral arteries has recently been developed. With the addition of carotid and middle cerebral artery monitoring, TCD may be helpful in identifying the embolic source.

MEDICAL MANAGEMENT

In the 1950s Millikan and coworkers treated a group of patients assumed to have vertebrobasilar insufficiency with systemic anticoagulation.[24] They reported a decline of mortality

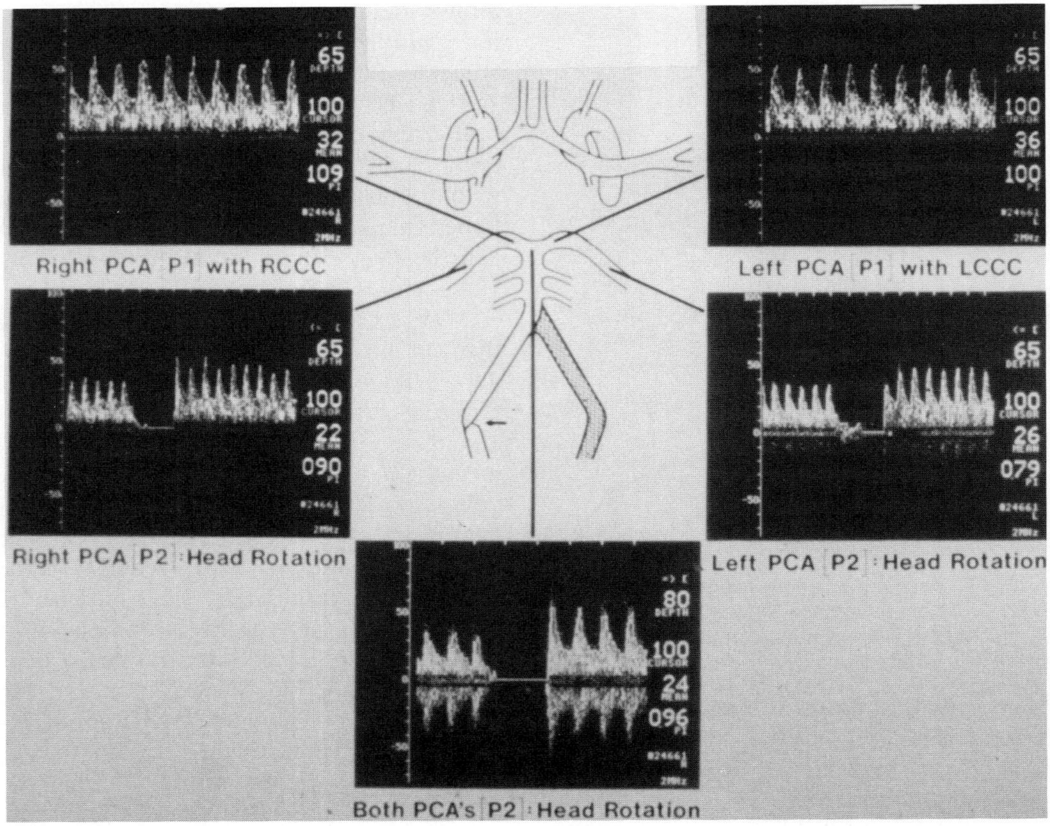

Figure 19-6. Patient presenting with loss of consciousness on neck turning. The status of the circle of Willis may be established by TCD monitoring during various maneuvers. No significant increases in flow velocities are noted in the P-1 segments of either posterior cerebral artery (PCA) with ipsilateral common carotid compressions (CCC), suggesting that neither posterior communicating artery is functional (*top row*). Complete cessation of flow is noted in the P-2 segments of both PCAs with head turning to the left. A hyperemic response occurs when the head is returned to the neutral position.

from 43 percent in an untreated group to 14 percent in the group treated with anticoagulants. Although this was a landmark study, angiography was not performed in any of the patients, nonvascular causes of symptoms were not ruled out, and patients were not assigned to the treatment group in a random fashion. All patients were assumed to have impending basilar artery occlusion.

Whisnant and coworkers in 1978 reported a population study including 15-year follow-up of patients with vertebrobasilar ischemic symptoms.[25] They reported a drop in stroke incidence from 35 to 15 percent within four years among patients receiving oral anticoagulants. Unfortunately, the treatment and control groups were chosen in a nonrandom fashion. Use of antiplatelet and other agents, including calcium channel blockers, has been reported, but there have been no controlled

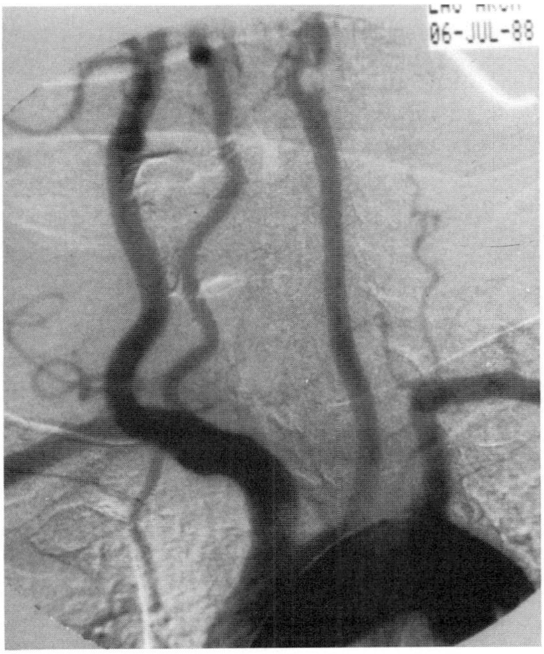

A

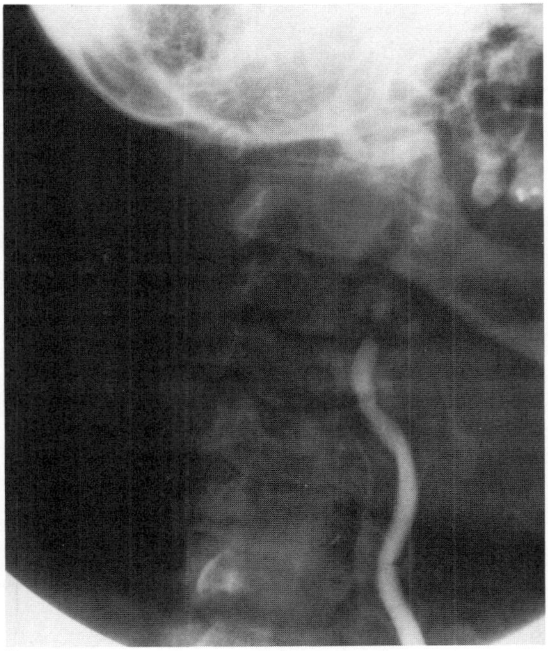

B

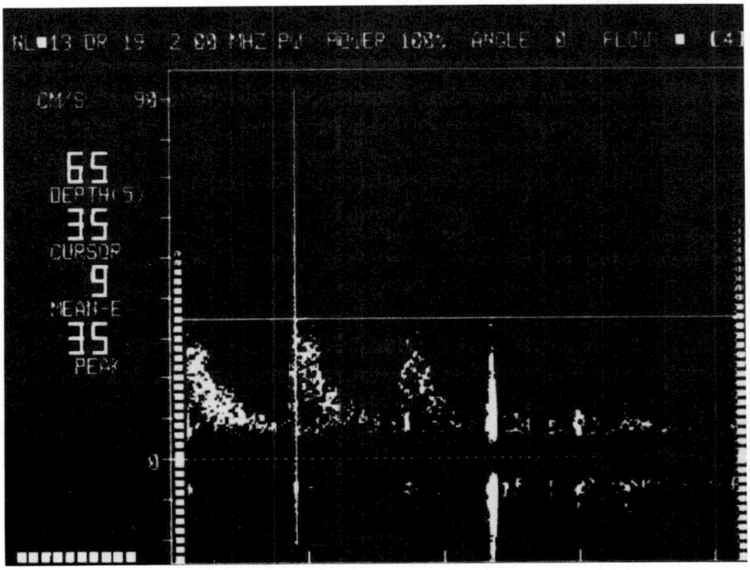

C

Figure 19-7. *A.* Angiogram of a normal right vertebral artery and hypoplastic or absent left vertebral artery in a patient presenting with light headedness and dizziness on neck rotation. *B.* Angiographic demonstration of a cut-off in the right vertebral artery with neck rotation associated with onset of symptoms. *C.* Demonstration by TCD monitoring of obliteration of right vertebral artery flow with neck rotation.

studies to assess their efficacy for treating vertebrobasilar insufficiency.[26] The use of intraarterial thrombolytic therapy has also been reported in patients with acute basilar artery thrombosis; however, the results have been inconclusive.[27]

Balloon angioplasty of basilar artery stenosis was reported by Sundt and coworkers in 1980, but multiple complications led them to conclude that the technique was inappropriate in these circumstances.[28] In 1987 George and colleagues reported initial success with balloon angioplasty for relieving stenosis and improving symptoms associated with proximal vertebral artery lesions, although long-term results were not available.[29]

PATIENT SELECTION

There are two basic objectives of vertebral artery reconstruction—relief of existing symptoms and prevention of future neurologic impairment or death from posterior circulation stroke. The decision to proceed with vertebral artery reconstruction rests on four main issues: (1) that the demonstrated arterial lesion or lesions are specifically responsible for the neurologic symptoms; (2) that repair of the lesions is likely to improve the symptoms; (3) that the lesions, if not treated, will eventually result in disabling neurologic deficit or death; and (4) that the operative risk is acceptable. A fundamental consideration in the assessment of patients prior to vertebral artery reconstruction is the delineation of causes other than vertebral artery disease for vertebrobasilar ischemic symptoms. Such causes include low cardiac output, cardiac arrhythmias, and Meniere's disease. Clearly, reconstruction of the vertebral artery is indicated only when the patient has an anatomic lesion appropriate to symptoms that cannot be ascribed to any other cause.

Although not always possible, an effort should be made to distinguish symptoms related to hypoperfusion from those due to thromboembolic phenomena. As previously discussed, symptoms of vertebrobasilar hypoperfusion may occur as the result of stenosis, occlusion, or diversion of flow. These usually are associated with atherosclerotic disease, but may also be secondary to dissection or extrinsic compression of the vertebral artery (Table 19-1). Under normal circumstances, complete absence of flow in one vertebral artery will be compensated for by a contralateral normal side. If the contralateral vertebral artery is hypoplastic or terminates in the PICA, lesser degrees of disease in the remaining vertebral artery may result in a reduction of basilar artery flow and ischemic brain stem symptoms. Generally, arterial lesions must produce at least a 50 percent diameter stenosis to cause significant reductions in distal pressure and flow. Intermittent vertebrobasilar symptoms may be related to neck and head movements when one vertebral artery is absent and the contralateral vertebral artery is stenotic. In patients with thromboembolic disease, flow-reducing lesions are not necessary for symptoms to occur.

Based on the above considerations, specific indications for vertebral artery reconstruction in patients with vertebrobasilar symptoms are: (1) severe stenosis of a dominant or single vertebral artery, including cases with intermittent compression; (2) bilateral severe vertebral artery stenoses; and (3) a demonstrated source of emboli to a vertebral artery in a patient with vertebrobasilar insufficiency or evidence of infarction on imaging studies.

SURGICAL MANAGEMENT

The role of carotid endarterectomy for the relief of nonhemispheric symptoms remains controversial. Some authors have reported success rates of up to 95 percent when the procedure is employed in patients presenting with vertebrobasilar insufficiency.[30–33] Others have noted that carotid endarterectomy is of limited benefit in patients with nonhemispheric transient ischemia, compared with patients presenting with hemispheric symptoms, and have suggested that this operation does not alter the natural history of vertebrobasilar ischemic disease.[34] The problem with such analyses has been a failure to correlate the clinical outcome with the status of the circle of Willis. This is crucial, since the circle of Willis is functionally intact in less than half the population.[13]

Recent work by von Reutern and von Büdingen[35] has demonstrated that flow velocity in the region of the vertebrobasilar junction, as determined by TCD, depends on the severity of disease in the internal carotid arteries. This flow velocity is lowest in patients with no stenosis or occlusion of the internal carotid arteries, increases in those patients with unilateral internal carotid artery occlusion, and is highest in patients with either bilateral internal carotid artery occlusion or unilateral occlusion and contralateral high-grade stenosis (Fig. 19-8). Such data support a selective role for carotid endarterectomy in relieving vertebrobasilar symptoms.

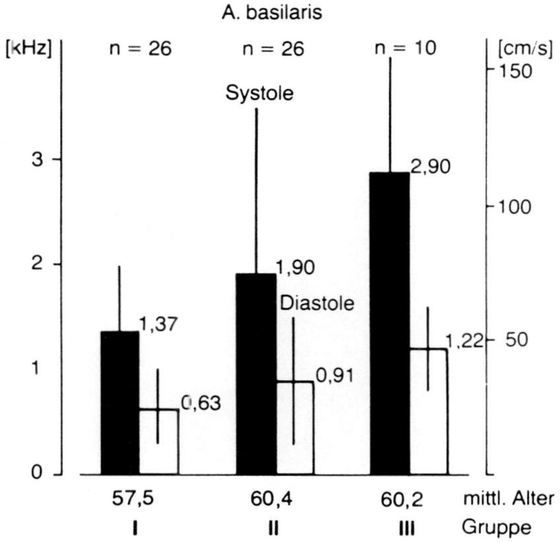

Figure 19-8. Flow velocity at the vertebrobasilar junction (suboccipital insonation) in three groups of patients. Group I: No stenosis or occlusion of the internal carotid arteries. Group II: Unilateral occlusion of the internal carotid artery. Group III: Bilateral occlusion of the internal carotid arteries or unilateral occlusion and contralateral high-grade stenosis. (*From von Reutern GM, von Büdingen HJ.[35] Reproduced by permission.*)

Therefore, selection of patients with vertebrobasilar symptoms for carotid endarterectomy is dependent on demonstrating the extent of communication between the anterior and posterior circulations through the posterior communicating arteries. At the present time, the results of carotid endarterectomy in patients for whom such data are known are limited. Dilley reported a series of 51 patients with classic symptoms of vertebrobasilar insufficiency and a flow-limiting lesion of the carotid bifurcation who underwent carotid endarterectomy.[36] Of the 24 patients who had a posterior communicating artery visualized on selective carotid angiography, 17 became asymptomatic and five were improved (91 percent); when the posterior communicating artery was not visualized, only 67 percent of the patients were improved. This difference was statistically significant ($p < .05$). It can be concluded that patients presenting with symptoms of vertebrobasilar insufficiency and carotid bifurcation disease should be carefully assessed with regard to the status of the posterior communicating arteries, preferably with both TCD and angiography, to select those patients who are most likely to benefit by improving flow from the anterior circulation to the basilar artery. Occasionally the vertebral artery ends in the PICA, and such arteries are considered functionally occluded and should not be revascularized (Fig. 19-9).

Certain uncommon conditions such as arteriovenous fistulas and false aneurysms of the vertebral artery should be corrected surgically irrespective of symptoms because of their potential for complications. Specific ap-

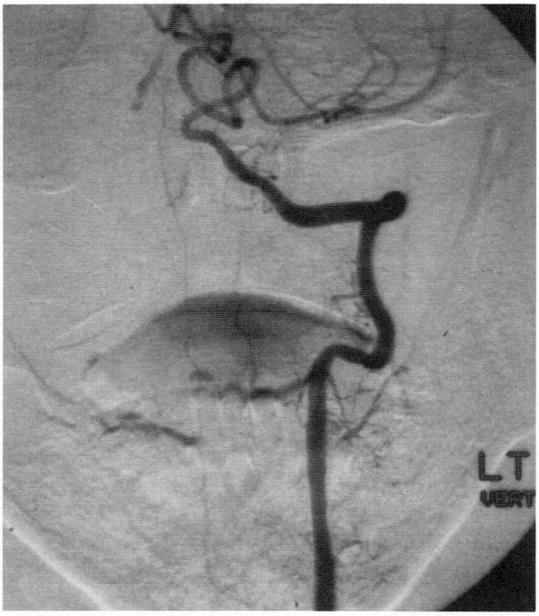

Figure 19-9. Angiogram of a left vertebral artery terminating in a posterior inferior cerebellar artery (PICA).

proaches to vertebral artery reconstruction and the details of their performance are discussed in Chap. 30.

REFERENCES

1. deKleyn A, Nieuwenhuyser P: Schwindelaufalle und nystagmus bei einer bestimmten stellung des kopfes. *Acta Otolaryngol* 11:155, 1927.
2. Kubik CS, Adams RD: Occlusion of the basilar artery—a clinical and pathological study. *Brain* 69:73, 1946.
3. Biemond A: Thrombosis of the basilar artery and vascularisation of the brainstem. *Brain* 74:300, 1951.
4. Schwartz GA, Gieger JK, Spano AW: Posterior inferior cerebellar artery syndrome of Wallenberg after chiropractic manipulation. *Arch Intern Med* 97:352, 1956.
5. Hutchinson EC, Yates PO: Carotid-vertebral stenosis. *Lancet* 1:2–8, 1957.
6. Castaigne P, Lhermitte K, et al: Arterial occlusions in the vertebrobasilar system. *Brain* 96: 133–154, 1973.
7. Millikan CH, Siekert RG: Studies in cerebrovascular disease I. The syndrome of intermittent insufficiency of the basilar arterial system. *Proc Staff Meet Mayo Clin* 30:61, 1955.
8. Hass WK, Fields WS, North RR, et al: Joint study of extracranial arterial occlusion. *JAMA* 203:961–968.
9. Rob C: Occlusive disease of the extracranial cerebral arteries. A review of the past 25 years. *J Cardiovasc Surg* 19:487–498, 1978.
10. Carney AW: Vertebral artery surgery: Historical development, basic concepts of brain hemodynamics, and clinical experience of 102 cases. *Adv Neurol,* 30:249–282, 1981.
11. Caplan LR, Tettenborn B: Embolism in the posterior circulation, in Berguer R, Caplan LR (eds): *Vertebrobasilar Arterial Disease.* St Louis, Quality Medical Publishing, chap 6, 1992.
12. Bell RH, Swigart LL, Anson BJ: The relation of the vertebral artery to the cervical vertebrae. *Q Bull Northwestern U Med* 24:184–185, 1950.
13. Fields WS, Bruetman ME, Weibel J: Collateral circulation of the brain. *Monogr Surg Sci* 2: 183–259, 1965.
14. Contorni L: The true story of the "subclavian steal syndrome" or "Harrison Smyth's Syndrome." *J Cardiovasc Surg* 14:408–417, 1973.
15. Reivich M, Holling HE, Roberts B, et al: Reversal of blood flow through the vertebral artery and its effect on cerebral circulation. *N Engl J Med* 265:878–885, 1961.
16. Nicholls SC, Koutlas TC, Strandness DE: Clinical significance of retrograde flow in the vertebral artery. *Ann Vasc Surg* 5:331–336, 1991.
17. von Büdingen HJ, Staudacher T: Evaluation of vertebrobasilar arterial disease, in Newell DW, Aaslid R (eds): *Transcranial Doppler.* New York, Raven Press, chap 16, 1992.
18. Bogousslavsky J: Vertebrobasilar transient ischemic attacks in internal carotid artery occlusion or tight stenosis. *Arch Neurol* 42:64–68, 1985.
19. Rancurel G, Kieffer E, Arzinanoglou A, et al:

Hemodynamic vertebrobasilar ischemia: Differentiation of hemodynamic and thromboembolic mechanisms, in Berguer R, Caplan LR (eds): *Vertebrobasilar Arterial Disease*. St. Louis, Quality Medical Publishing, chap 5, 1992.

20. Spencer MP, Thomas GI, Sauvage LR, Nicholls SC: Detection of middle cerebral artery emboli during carotid endarterectomy using transcranial Doppler. *Stroke* 21:415–423, 1990.
21. Kline RA, Berguer R: Vertebral artery reconstruction. Basic data underlying clinical decision making. *Ann Vasc Surg* 497–501, 1993.
22. Bendick PJ, Glover JL: Vertebrobasilar insufficiency: Evaluation by quantitative duplex flow measurements. *J Vasc Surg* 5(4):594–600, 1987.
23. Fujioka KA, Ernsberger AM, Nicholls SC, Spencer MP: Transcranial Doppler assessment of mechanical compression of the vertebral arteries. *J Vasc Tech* 15(5):254–259, 1991.
24. Millikan CH, Siekert RG, Shick RM: Studies in cerebrovascular disease III. The use of anticoagulant drugs in the treatment of insufficiency or thrombosis within the basilar arterial system. *Proc Staff Meet Mayo Clin* 30:116–126, 1955.
25. Whisnant TP, Cartlidge NEF, Elvebach LR: Carotid and vertebrobasilar transient ischemic attacks. Effects of anticoagulants, hypertension and cardiac disorders on survival and stroke occurrence. A population study. *Ann Neurol* 3:107–115, 1978.
26. Swedish Cooperative Study: High dose acetylsalicylic acid after cerebral infarction. *Stroke* 18:325–334, 1984.
27. Sloane MA: Thrombolysis and stroke. *Arch Neurol* 44:748–768, 1987.
28. Sundt TM, et al: Transluminal angioplasty for basilar artery stenosis. *Mayo Clinic Proc* 55: 673–680, 1980.
29. George B: Angioplasty, in George B, Lavrian C (eds): *The Vertebral Artery: Pathology and Surgery*. New York, Springer-Verlag, 1987.
30. Ouriel K, Ricotta JJ, Green RM, DeWeese JA: Carotid endarterectomy for nonhemispheric cerebral symptoms: Patient selection with ocular pneumoplethysmography. *J Vasc Surg* 4: 115–118, 1986.
31. Humphries AW, Young JR, Bevin EG, et al: Relief of vertebrobasilar symptoms by carotid endarterectomy. *Surgery* 57:48–52, 1965.
32. Rosenthal D, Cossman D, Ledig CB, Callow AD: Results of carotid endarterectomy for vertebrobasilar insufficiency. *Arch Surg* 113:1361–1364, 1978.
33. Ford JJ, Baker WH, Ehrenhaft JL: Carotid endarterectomy for nonhemispheric transient ischemic attacks. *Arch Surg* 110:1314–1317, 1975.
34. McNamara JO, Heyman A, Silver D, Mandel ME: The value of carotid endarterectomy in treating transient cerebral ischemia of the posterior circulation. *Neurology* 27:682–684, 1977.
35. von Reutern GM, von Büdingen HJ: *Ultrasound Techniques in Cerebrovascular Diagnosis*. Stuttgart/New York, Thieme, 1992.
36. Dilley RB: Discussion of Ouriel K, May AG, Ricotta JJ, Deweese JA, Green RM: Carotid endarterectomy for non hemispheric symptoms: Predictors of success. *J Vasc Surg* 1:339–345, 1984.

20

Combined Carotid and Coronary Artery Disease

Glenn E. Esses, Joseph L. Mills,
Dennis F. Bandyk

The management of concomitant extracranial carotid stenosis (CS) and coronary artery disease (CAD) persists as a clinical dilemma. The primary concern is whether an operation on one diseased arterial segment will precipitate an ischemic event in the distribution of the other. With the advent of carotid duplex scanning and transcranial Doppler, patients can be accurately screened for both extracranial and intracranial arterial disease based on abnormalities of local and regional blood flow patterns. Improved diagnostic techniques have increased the detection rate of severe carotid disease in asymptomatic patients undergoing major vascular and cardiac procedures and has resulted in a greater number of prophylactic carotid endarterectomies. This approach is controversial, since no appropriately designed clinical trial has been conducted to identify the cohort of patients who will benefit from simultaneous or staged coronary and carotid revascularizations. Because of this, clinicians have relied on either their personal experience or published retrospective clinical reports to make management decisions.

The published experience of institutions performing large numbers of vascular procedures has contributed to our understanding of the pathogenesis of perioperative and late stroke in patients undergoing coronary artery bypass grafting (CABG). Despite the limitations of such reports, these data provide the basis for the diagnostic and therapeutic algorithms proposed in this chapter. In general, intervention should be based on both presenting symptoms and signs, as well as the severity of extracranial CS as assessed by duplex scanning and arteriography. Guidelines for the management of three patient groups will be discussed: (1) symptomatic CAD with asymptomatic CS; (2) carotid territory symptoms with CAD evident by abnormal stress testing; and (3) symptomatic CAD with symptomatic CS.

MAGNITUDE OF THE PROBLEM

In 1991, 265,000 patients underwent CABG and 65,000 patients underwent carotid endarterectomy (CEA) in the United States, excluding Department of Veterans Affairs medical centers.[1] The reported incidence of stroke associated with open heart surgery varies widely (1 to 10 percent), but is relatively low (less than 2 percent) following CABG.[2,3] Perioperative neurologic syndromes following CABG span a clinical spectrum from focal cortical infarcts, to nonfocal or global deficits, to ill-defined personality disorders. Careful neurologic testing can identify deficits in up to 40 percent of postoperative cardiac patients. While the causes of nonfocal deficits or cognitive dysfunction can be difficult to establish with certainty, the etiology of focal neurologic deficits, which account for approximately 5 to 10 percent of all neurologic complications, often can be identified.

Table 20-1 Etiology of Stroke in 22 Coronary Artery Bypass Patients at the Cleveland Clinic

Identified etiology	No. patients (%)
Cardiac arrhythmia intra/periop	6 (27)
Internal carotid artery disease	5 (23)
Air embolism from left ventricle	2 (9)
Carotid trauma	1 (4.5)
Aortic disease/clamp injury	1 (4.5)
Prolonged hypotension	1 (4.5)
No cause identified	6 (27)

Table 20-1 lists the causes of stroke associated with CABG reported by one institution.[4] Only about 20 percent of the focal neurologic events were thought to be the direct result of carotid artery occlusive disease. Thus, based on the estimated prevalence of carotid disease in the patient population undergoing CABG, fewer than 1000 patients annually would potentially benefit from a prophylactic CEA performed as a simultaneous or staged procedure. It should be emphasized that this analysis considers only the risk of perioperative stroke and does not address the important problem of late stroke in this patient population.

RISK FACTORS FOR STROKE IN CARDIAC SURGERY PATIENTS

A number of patient and clinical risk factors have been associated with an increased risk for stroke (Table 20-2). The significance of a carotid bruit as a risk factor has varied.[2,3,5,6] This discrepancy may be due to the poor correlation between the physical sign of a carotid bruit and a significant stenosis of the internal carotid artery as documented by ultrasound studies or arteriography.[7] Reed and coworkers[2] found that the presence of a carotid bruit increased the risk of stroke or tran-

Table 20-2 Risk Factors for Stroke in Patients Undergoing Coronary Artery Bypass Grafting

Patient factors
Age >60 years
History of
Peripheral vascular disease
Transient ischemic attack/stroke
Clinical factors
Carotid bruit
Duplex identified internal carotid stenosis
Congestive heart failure
Concomitant valvular disease
Cardiopulmonary bypass time >2 h
Air embolism
Intraoperative hypotension (mean pressure <70 torr)

sient ischemic attack (TIA) by 3.9 times in CABG patients, but many of the strokes were not ipsilateral to the bruit. When a significant common or internal CS is defined as a lesion of 50 percent or greater diameter reduction, 5 to 11 percent of patients undergoing CABG will have concomitant carotid disease.[8–10] Demonstrable carotid disease has been correlated with an increased ipsilateral stroke rate after CABG. Faggioli and colleagues,[11] using duplex scanning, reported that 8.7 percent of patients undergoing CABG had 75 percent or greater internal CS, and this cohort experienced a 14.3 percent stroke rate with CABG, significantly higher than the 1 percent rate reported in patients with less severe stenoses ($p<.002$).

Other factors associated with stroke after CABG are age,[12,13] history of peripheral vascular disease,[3] history of TIA or stroke, congestive heart failure, mitral regurgitation,[2] and a pump time of greater than 2 h.[2,12] Age is a particularly important risk factor. The annual stroke mortality for all Americans over 65 years is 2.3 percent, but stroke rates of 8 to 10 percent have been reported after CABG in patients 70 years or older. The incidence and severity of carotid occlusive disease increase with age, but patients 70 or older appear to have an increased risk of stroke after CABG independent of carotid disease.[11,12]

Because the incidence of perioperative stroke in patients undergoing CABG is low, we recommend routine screening with carotid duplex scanning in patients over 65 years. The increased prevalence of carotid disease in recent screening studies reflects the current trend in coronary artery surgery toward operations on older patients as either primary or secondary bypass procedures. Noninvasive carotid testing is appropriate in all patients with a carotid bruit on physical examination or a history of a carotid artery territory ischemic event (TIA, stroke, amaurosis fugax) within the previous six months.

The majority of strokes associated with cardiac surgery occur intraoperatively, with less than one-third developing more than 24 h after surgery. Intraoperative strokes are most commonly attributed to technical problems with hypotension, aortic clamping or cannulation, or inadequate venting of air and debris from the heart or aorta at the conclusion of the procedure. The risk of perioperative stroke with valve replacement is two to three times greater than with CABG. There is no evidence that prior CEA reduces the risk of stroke in cardiac surgery patients.[13]

CLINICAL STUDIES

Two types of clinical studies—screening and intervention-based—have been conducted to help define appropriate treatment algorithms for patients with combined carotid and coronary artery disease. Screening studies have documented the prevalence of carotid disease and have focused on the outcome of asymptomatic patients undergoing CABG without treatment of identified carotid stenoses. In contrast, intervention-based studies have evaluated the use of CEA in patients undergoing cardiac surgery in relation to other patient groups undergoing CABG. Differences in operative mortality and morbidity, as well as the late occurrence of stroke, have been compared. While these clinical studies were not designed to determine the optimal management of patients with combined CS and CAD, the epidemiologic and treatment data are valuable, even though it is recognized that lack of patient randomization to treatment groups can result in both Type I and II statistical errors.

In general, all reports indicate that patients with combined CS and CAD represent a high-risk group for stroke compared with patients who have disease isolated to one of these areas. Table 20-3 lists data from four studies that reported operative mortality and stroke rates in patients undergoing CABG with documented asymptomatic CS of greater than 50 percent diameter reduction.[9,11,14,15] The overall mortality for this patient group was 7.1 percent, and the risk of a focal neurologic deficit was 6.2 percent. Operative morbidity in these patients with combined CS and CAD was higher than the mortality and stroke rates in patients undergoing CABG without significant carotid disease. Schultz and coworkers[16] matched risk factors of advanced age, sex, and associated illnesses in patients with and without known CS undergoing CABG and found that both patient groups exhibited high but similar perioperative and late morbidity. These data indicate that severe carotid disease does correlate with an increased risk of stroke associated with CABG, and patients with combined CS and CAD are older, have more associated medical problems, and exhibit a decreased life-expectancy.

Simultaneous carotid and coronary operations are associated with increased perioperative morbidity. Table 20-4 summarizes the results of simultaneous CEA and CABG procedures in 1556 patients compiled from 15 reports that each included at least 50 patients.[9,15–28] The operative mortality rates in these series ranged from 0 to 12 percent, with a mean of 5.1 percent. The incidence of postoperative neurologic events ranged from 1.6 to 15 percent, with an average of 7.0 percent. By comparison, studies of patients having CEA alone have consistently cited a mortality of less than 2 percent and a permanent stroke rate of less than 4 percent. The incidence of myocardial infarction with simultaneous procedures was not given in all the reports listed in Table 20-4, but when provided it ranged from 0 to 7.7 percent.

An important management question addressed by retrospective clinical reviews is whether patients with combined CS and CAD should be treated by simultaneous or staged procedures. In addition, if the operations are staged, should CEA be performed prior to or following CABG, and what should the time interval be between the operations? As a practical matter, should staged procedures be performed during the same hospitalization? Table 20-5 presents results for staged operations from three institutions.[11,15,20] Two of these series had the CABG performed initially. The

Table 20-3 Mortality and Stroke Rates of Patients with Significant Carotid Disease[a] Undergoing Coronary Artery Bypass Grafting

Author	Year	No. patients	Mortality (%)	Focal stroke (%)
Ivey	1984	16	0 (0)	0 (0)
Brener	1987	64	10 (15.6)	4 (6.3)
Hertzer	1989	58	2 (3.4)	4 (6.9)
Faggioli	1990	88	4 (4.5)	6 (6.8)
Total		226	16 (7.1)	14 (6.2)

[a]Defined as greater than 50% diameter reduction of the internal carotid artery.

Table 20-4 Stroke Rate and Mortality for Simultaneous Carotid Endarterectomy and Coronary Artery Bypass Grafting in Reports with More Than 50 Patients

Author	Year	No. patients	Mortality (%)	Neurologic events (%)	MI[a] (%)
Rice	1980	54	0 (0)	2 (3.7)	0 (0)
Jones	1984	132	4 (3.0)	2 (1.6)	— (<1.0)
Babu	1985	57	3 (5.2)	3 (5.2)	—
Reul	1986	143	6 (4)	5 (3.5)	—
Brener	1987	57	6 (10.5)	5 (8.8)	—
Schultz	1988	62	4 (6.5)	5 (8.0)	—
Perler	1988	63	7 (11)	3 (4.8)	2 (3.2)
Hertzer	1989	275	13 (4.7)	24 (8.9)	—
Cambria	1989	71	2 (2.8)	2 (4.2)	2 (2.8)
Duchateau	1989	82	6 (7.3)	12 (15)	3 (3.6)
Pomé	1991	52	0 (0)	3 (5.7)	4 (7.7)
Vermeulen	1992	230	8 (3.5)	22 (8.7)	4 (1.7)
Rizzo	1992	127	7 (5.5)	7 (5.5)	6 (4.7)
Carrel	1992	52	2 (3.8)	1 (1.9)	0 (0)
Bass	1992	99	12 (12)	12 (12)	6 (6)
Total		1556	80 (5.1)	109 (7.0)	

[a]MI = myocardial infarction

data appear to indicate that mortality (2.5 percent) and stroke (3.3 percent) rates are less with staged procedures than with simultaneous operations (mortality 5.1 percent, stroke rate 7.0 percent). However, such a comparison probably is not appropriate, since a significant number of patients who underwent simultaneous operations presented with symptomatic CS and were not considered candidates for a staged approach. This clinical experience suggests that when patients are stable from both cardiac and neurologic viewpoints, the mortality and neurologic morbidity may be lower with staged procedures.

Questions regarding the timing of staged procedures have been best addressed by Reul and coworkers[20] and Hertzer and colleagues.[15] Both reports recommended not performing the carotid surgery during the same hospitalization. Reul and colleagues[20] reported a mortality following staged CABG and CEA of 5 percent when performed during the same hospitalization, but only 0.5 percent when CEA was performed during a later hospitalization. Similarly, Hertzer and coworkers[15] demonstrated a decrease in stroke rate from 11 to 2.2 percent when the CEA was performed at a separate hospitalization. The time interval be-

Table 20-5 Mortality and Morbidity for Staged Operations (Combined Figures from Both Operations)

Author	Year	Staging	No. patients	Mortality (%)	Neurologic complications (%)
Reul	1986	CABG-CEA	350	9 (2.6)	8 (2.3)
Hertzer	1989	CABG-CEA	110	3 (2.7)	8 (7.3)
Faggioli	1990	CEA-CABG	19	0 (0)	0 (0)
Total			479	12 (2.5)	16 (3.3)

tween the hospitalizations has not been well defined, but four to six weeks appears appropriate in patients with an uncomplicated postoperative course following CABG.

Only one study attempted to randomize patients to either "staged" or "simultaneous" operations for combined CS and CAD. Hertzer and coworkers[15] randomized 129 patients with unilateral, asymptomatic CS and unstable CAD to receive either simultaneous CEA and CABG or CABG followed by CEA at a later date. In the 71 patients undergoing simultaneous operations, there were three (4.2 percent) deaths and two (2.8 percent) perioperative strokes. In the 58 patients assigned to staged operations, there was a combined mortality of 5.3 percent (CABG 3.4 percent, CEA 1.9 percent) and an overall 14 percent incidence of stroke. The risk of stroke (2.8 versus 14 percent) was significantly higher for the staged operations ($p = .042$). The variability of outcomes with simultaneous and staged CABG and CEA emphasizes the need for more definitive studies. An ad hoc committee of the Joint Vascular Societies (SVS and ISCVS) has recommended that a multicenter, randomized clinical trial of staged versus simultaneous CEA and CABG be conducted.[29]

Although not frequently reported, an alternative approach, termed the "reverse staged" method, is performance of the CEA prior to CABG. Riles and Pasternack[30] advocated CEA under regional block anesthesia prior to CABG based on a review of 26 patients with arteriographic evidence of triple-vessel CAD. Of note, 58 percent of these patients had a previous myocardial infarction, and 54 percent had angina at rest. This patient cohort experienced three myocardial infarctions in the course of 30 carotid operations, but no deaths or strokes occurred. These results are certainly acceptable, but the "protective" value of regional block anesthesia in this high risk patient group is questionable.

Patients with symptomatic carotid disease and unstable cardiac status should undergo carotid surgery with a "cardiac technique" of anesthesia that includes hemodynamic monitoring (arterial line, mixed venous saturation Swan-Ganz catheter), selective perioperative β-blocker administration, and careful, prolonged postoperative monitoring. The value of this approach was assessed by Mackey and colleagues[31] in a retrospective study of patients with and without overt CAD undergoing CEA. Mortality among 324 patients with CAD was 1.5 percent, with major morbidity rates of 2.8 percent for stroke and 4.3 percent for myocardial infarction—levels comparable to or less than those for simultaneous CEA and CABG. Both mortality and myocardial infarction rates were significantly higher than for patients undergoing CEA without overt CAD. The patients with CAD had a five-year actuarial survival rate of 69 percent, which was significantly less than patients without overt CAD. These survival statistics support the recommendation of offering CABG to patients with left main or triple vessel coronary disease and an ejection fraction of less than 50 percent.[32]

LONG-TERM RESULTS AFTER CABG WITH CAROTID DISEASE

The efficacy of CEA and CABG in patients with combined disease is linked to the natural history of atherosclerosis involving these arterial segments. Data from the Cleveland Clinic clearly indicate that patient survival is increased when severe carotid and coronary occlusive disease are successfully treated.[15] Three studies have addressed the natural history of CABG patients with unoperated, asymptomatic significant (greater than 50 percent diameter reduction) carotid stenoses (Table 20-6).[9,16,33] Barnes and associates reported only one stroke among 40 patients during a mean follow-up period of 35 months. Whether

Table 20-6 Patients Undergoing Coronary Artery Bypass Grafting with Significant Unoperated Carotid Stenoses[a]—Late Events (>1 month)

Author	Year	No. patients	Follow-up	Death (%)	Stroke (%)	Neurologic events (%)
Brener	1987	44	<3 yrs	2 (4.5)	2 (4.5)	3 (6.8)
Schultz	1988	50	41 mo	—	4 (8.0)	9 (18)
Barnes	1985	40	35 mo	4 (10)	1 (2.5)	7 (18)

[a]Defined as greater than 50% diameter reduction of the internal carotid artery.

the stroke occurred ipsilateral to the CS was not stated, but an additional six patients did develop ipsilateral TIAs as their initial neurologic event. Based on this experience, the authors did not recommend prophylactic CEA for patients with asymptomatic CS and symptomatic CAD about to undergo CABG.[33]

Recent randomized clinical trials of CEA in patients with and without neurologic symptoms have shown benefit in selected patients with high-grade carotid stenoses (Chaps. 16 and 17.)[34–36] Thus, natural history studies must stratify for high-grade CS to avoid the possibility of a Type II statistical error due to an inadequate number of study patients with this risk factor.

Long-term follow-up of patients after simultaneous CEA and CABG indicates a low stroke rate and prolonged survival (Table 20-7).[15,16,23,27] The duration of patient follow-up varied in each of the studies listed, but five-year actuarial survival ranged from 65 to 91 percent. These survival rates compare favorably with the results of the Coronary Artery Surgery Study, which reported an 83 percent five-year survival following CABG,[32] and another study reporting an 87 percent five-year survival following CABG for 1718 patients without CS.[37] Major risk factors adversely affecting long-term survival after CEA and CABG have been determined in a number of prospective studies and include cardiac ejection fraction less than 50 percent,[16,25–27] age greater than 70 years,[25,27] prior myocardial infarction,[25,16] and triple vessel CAD.[16]

PATHOGENESIS OF STROKE ASSOCIATED WITH CABG

An understanding of the mechanisms of stroke associated with CABG is necessary for the development of rational treatment protocols

Table 20-7 Long-Term Clinical Outcome in Patients after Simultaneous Carotid Endarterectomy and Coronary Artery Bypass Grafting

Author	Year	No. patients	Mean months follow-up	Death (%)	Stroke (%)	Total neurologic events (%)	MI[a] (%)	% 5-Year Survival
Schultz	1988	58	—	17 (29)	4 (6.9)	—	—	65
Hertzer	1989	257	26	38 (15)	6 (2.3)	1 (0.4)	—	81
Duchateau	1989	76	29	3 (4)	2 (2.6)	3 (4)	—	86
Pomé	1991	52	35	4 (7.6)	1 (1.9)	6 (11.5)	3 (6)	83
Rizzo	1992	127	46	3 (2.4)	5 (3.9)	7 (5.5)	6 (5)	70
Vermeulen	1992	129	180	66 (51)	9 (6.9)	27 (21)	9 (7)	74
Carrel	1992	52	42	5 (9.6)	0 (0)	0 (0)	—	91

[a]MI = myocardial infarction

for individual patients. Data from radiologic, pathologic, and physiologic monitoring of CABG patients with stroke, and cerebral blood flow studies during cardiopulmonary bypass, are helpful in defining possible mechanisms.

Radiologic Signs of Stroke in CABG Patients

At one institution, computed tomography (CT) of the brain in patients with stroke following CABG revealed lesions consistent with embolization in approximately one-third of patients.[37] Only a minority of patients (2/22) had evidence of watershed infarcts that would implicate hypoperfusion as a causative factor. Notably, most patients had normal CT scans, and there were no cases in which intracranial hemorrhage was seen.

Autopsy Findings in CABG Patients with Stroke

Cardiopulmonary bypass is clearly responsible for some of the neurologic events seen after CABG. A pathologic study of five patients and four dogs who came to autopsy after recent cardiopulmonary bypass described "dramatic and ubiquitous alterations consisting of small capillary and arteriolar dilatations or microaneurysms."[39] These vascular abnormalities were seen in terminal arterioles and capillaries measuring 10 to 40 microns in size. Some lesions had evidence of birefringence under polarized light, indicating particulate microemboli, and were located in the border zone regions of the anterior, middle, and posterior cerebral arteries. Using extrapolation from several sections of basal ganglia, one patient had evidence of 15×10^6 microemboli in his brain.[39] The majority were felt to represent fat or air emboli, although cholesterol emboli have also been documented on postmortem examination.

A recent autopsy study indicated that atherosclerotic disease of the aortic arch was an important source for embolic material. Ulcerated lesions were demonstrated in 26 percent of patients who died of stroke not directly related to CABG, compared to 5 percent of patients who died of nonfocal or diffuse central nervous system injury ($p<.001$).[40] Other investigators have also observed a significant ($p<.005$) correlation between the presence of severe calcific disease of the aorta and the occurrence of stroke with CABG.[12]

Cerebral Flow Physiology during Cardiopulmonary Bypass

Physiologic monitoring of cerebral blood flow also can provide insights into the mechanisms of stroke during cardiopulmonary bypass. Transcranial Doppler interrogation of middle cerebral artery flow velocity, electromagnetic flow monitoring, and radioactive xenon measurements of regional cerebral blood flow during cardiopulmonary bypass have provided useful information on blood flow alterations in patients undergoing CABG.

In 1985 Lundar and coworkers[41] used an electromagnetic flow probe in five patients to document the effect of cardiopulmonary bypass on internal carotid artery flow. Carotid flow changes were correlated with arterial blood pressure, intracranial pressure (measured with an epidural probe placed through a burrhole), and a three-lead EEG monitor. A rapid increase in carotid flow was observed upon initiation of cardiopulmonary bypass, corresponding to hemodilution from the pump primer fluid. A reduction in carotid flow was observed with decreases in arterial blood pressure, effectively decreasing the cerebral perfusion pressure. The response of internal carotid flow and cerebral perfusion pressure to changes in arterial pressure indicated a pressure-passive system, which was consistent with a disturbance in cerebral autoregulation. In two of three patients monitored for cerebral function there was a fall in electrical activity associated with the initial drop in blood pressure. The abnormal electrical pattern occurred in spite of increased carotid flow, which indicates that there was insufficient cerebral perfusion pressure to maintain normal neuronal activity. These events may be related to the markedly decreased hematocrit in the initial stages of cardiopulmonary bypass that prevents sufficient oxygen transport to the cells.[41]

The physiologic changes of cardiopulmonary bypass also have been confirmed using transcranial Doppler to monitor middle cerebral artery flow. Again, a decrease in cerebral activity was recorded in 10 of 11 patients at the initiation of cardiopulmonary bypass, despite measured increases in middle cerebral artery flow velocity of 140 to 260 percent. The pressure-dependent changes in cerebral perfusion indicated a disturbance of autoregulation during nonpulsatile cardiopulmonary bypass.[42] These data emphasize the need to avoid hypotension and severe anemia during CABG procedures to avoid inadequate cerebral perfusion. Also, increases in cerebral blood flow do not always correlate with EEG activity or neuronal oxygen requirements.

The effect of extracranial carotid occlusive disease on cerebral blood flow during CABG is unpredictable. Johnsson and coworkers[43] used xenon 133 imaging of regional cerebral blood flow in patients with CS undergoing CABG and concluded that flow was not significantly diminished ipsilateral to the stenosis. Intraoperative transcranial Doppler monitoring was used by von Reutern and colleagues[44] in 69 patients undergoing CABG of whom 18 had significant internal CS or occlusion. Reduction in middle cerebral artery blood flow was found not to be a factor in postoperative stroke; however, microemboli were identified by transcranial Doppler in two of the three patients who suffered a major stroke.

In summary, strokes associated with CABG are rarely caused by flow reduction. Inadequate venting of the heart and microemboli from diseased valves, cannulation sites, and the aortic arch are the major causes of focal neurologic deficits. In patients with identified CS the mechanisms of stroke are less clear but may be related to hypercoagulability in the early postoperative period which induces thrombus formation on a stenotic or ulcerated lesion of the extracranial carotid arteries or aortic arch. Perioperative alterations in blood rheology or the coagulation system, or specific acquired hypercoagulable conditions (heparin-induced platelet aggregation, antiphospholipid antibodies), also predispose postoperative patients to thrombotic complications.

TECHNIQUE OF SIMULTANEOUS CEA AND CABG

There is no standard technique for performing simultaneous carotid and coronary revascularization. At our institution, we favor two separate operating teams, a cardiac team for the CABG and a separate vascular team for the CEA. In patients who are clinically stable prior to and following induction of anesthesia, simultaneous CEA and harvesting of the saphenous vein for CABG are undertaken before the median sternotomy. In high-risk patients, such as those with left main CAD or depressed ejection fraction, median sternotomy and preparation for cardiopulmonary bypass cannulation are completed prior to exposure of the carotid bifurcation. Carotid endarterectomy is performed under general anesthesia with standard dose heparinization (approximately 100 units/kg). EEG monitoring has not been routinely employed. A shunt is used in all cases, and saphenous vein patch angioplasty of the endarterectomy site is generally performed. Intraoperative color duplex imaging is used to document the technical adequacy of the repair site. The neck wound is left open to be closed over a drain following reversal of systemic heparinization at the completion of the CABG.

Carotid endarterectomy during temporary hypothermic extracorporeal perfusion has been recommended by some authors for patients with difficult access to the carotid bifurcation.[25,45] Disadvantages of this approach include the added complexity of the procedure and the longer pump times required for simultaneous operations which have been associated with an increased frequency of neurologic events.[2,12]

RECOMMENDED TREATMENT ALGORITHMS

Based on the available data, we propose separate management algorithms for patients with asymptomatic or symptomatic CS in whom CABG is necessary, and patients with known or suspected CAD who are under consideration for CEA (Figs. 20-1 and 20-2). In most patients, either the carotid or the coronary disease is the primary vascular problem and should be treated according to standard clinical guidelines, taking into account the risks associated with concurrent medical problems. Patients with symptomatic CAD should be screened for CS prior to CABG with duplex scanning if any of the following characteristics are present: age over 65 years; audible neck bruit; or history of focal cerebral ischemia (Fig. 20-1). The goal in this situation is to identify patients with severe carotid lesions that in-

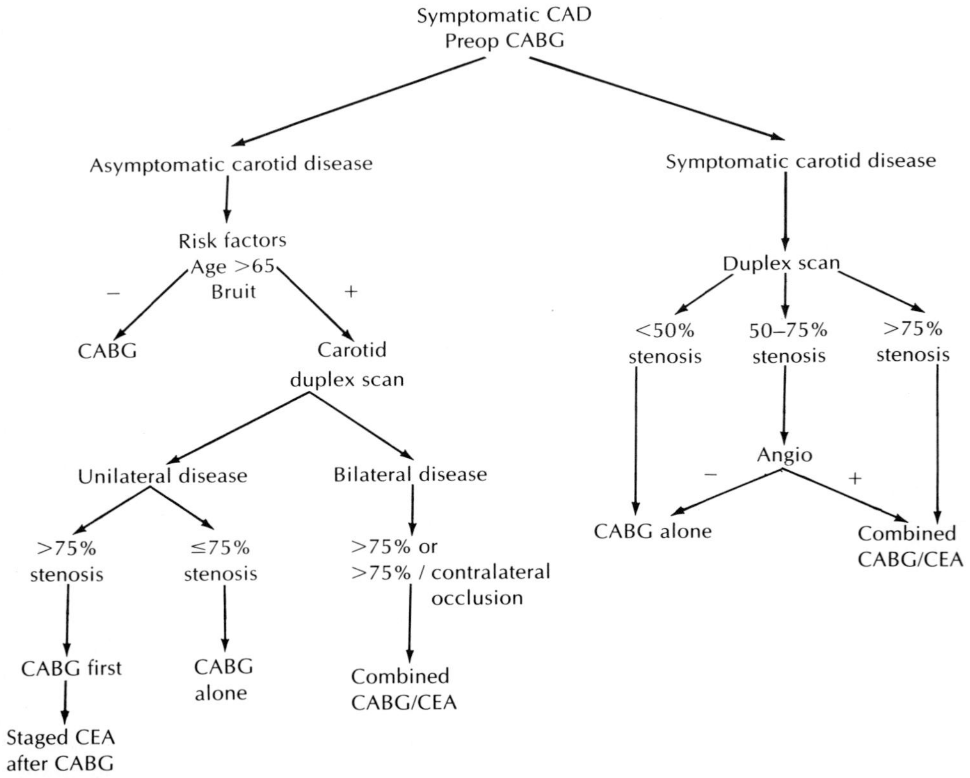

Figure 20-1. Screening and treatment algorithm for patients scheduled for CABG with suspected asymptomatic or symptomatic carotid disease. Symptomatic carotid disease refers to a history of a recent focal neurologic deficit. Angio (+) and (−) refers to the presence or absence of ulceration, thrombus, or high-grade stenosis seen on angiography in patients who have symptomatic carotid disease and a 50 to 75 percent stenosis by duplex scan.

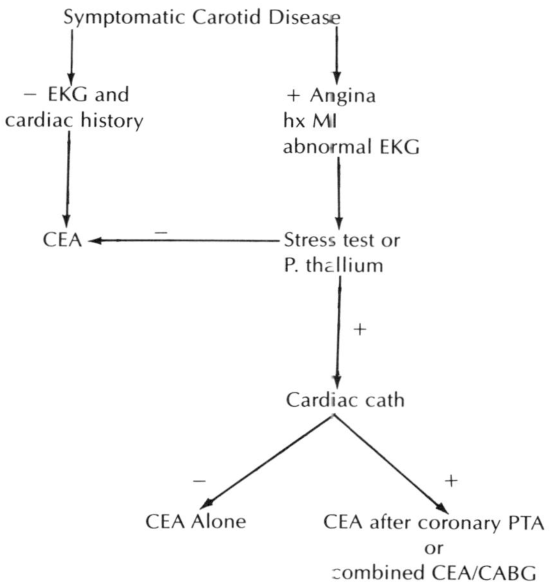

Figure 20-2. Screening and treatment algorithm for patients scheduled for CEA. *P. thallium* refers to Persantine thallium imaging. Patients with triple vessel or left main coronary artery disease by cardiac catheterization should be considered for combined CEA and CABG. Lesions amenable to coronary PTA may be treated before the CEA is performed. PTA = percutaneous transluminal angioplasty.

crease the risk of both perioperative and late stroke. In the absence of these risk factors, routine screening is not recommended. A patient with high-grade CS is subject to increased operative mortality and morbidity and decreased long-term survival.

The least controversial indication for simultaneous CEA and CABG is in patients with both symptomatic CS and severely symptomatic CAD with unstable angina. Although an uncommon clinical presentation, the occurrence of crescendo TIAs or stroke with recovery ipsilateral to a high-grade (greater than 70 percent diameter reduction) internal CS in a patient with unstable CAD is an indication for simultaneous CEA and CABG. Depending on the institutional accuracy of duplex scanning and the experience of the vascular team, CEA can be undertaken safely without preliminary diagnostic arteriography in most cases (Chap. 21).

The role for simultaneous CEA and CABG in patients with asymptomatic CS is controversial, since no study has confirmed that CS is a primary cause of stroke in CABG patients. Many cardiac surgery patients have extracranial carotid disease by duplex scanning, with greater than 50 percent diameter-reducing stenoses in approximately 10 percent of patients and greater than 75 percent stenoses in less than 5 percent of patients. In general, high-grade lesions should be treated for the same indications as carotid disease in other patients. Repair of an asymptomatic high-grade internal CS is appropriate if the vascular team has demonstrated a mortality and stroke rate of less than 3 percent following carotid surgery. The authors have recommended repair of high-grade internal carotid lesions when they are bilateral or when a contralateral internal carotid occlusion is present. Simultaneous CEA and CABG is preferred in managing patients with bilateral CS and evidence by arteriography, OPG-Gee, or transcranial Doppler of inadequate collateral pathways or a reduction in basal cerebral blood pressure or flow. The rationale for the simultaneous procedure rather than the "reverse staged" approach is that the stress of carotid surgery will precipitate myocardial ischemia.

Asymptomatic patients with greater than 75 percent internal CS and normal middle cerebral artery velocity should undergo staged CEA and CABG. Since there is controversy regarding the morbidity of simultaneous versus staged CEA and CABG procedures, a guiding principle should be repair of the "most" symptomatic lesion first, followed by correction of stable or asymptomatic lesions. Carotid endarterectomy prior to CABG is appropriate, but only in carefully selected patients and with realization of the potential cardiac morbidity of this approach. Use of local anesthesia and intensive cardiac monitoring, coupled with medical management of myocardial ischemia, may minimize the risk of myocardial infarction and life-threatening arrhythmias. If CABG is done first, CEA should be performed during a separate hospitalization after the patient has recovered from the cardiac procedure, typically four to six weeks later.

It is important to emphasize that prophylactic CEA will not result in a substantial decrease in the incidence of stroke following CABG. However, repair of symptomatic carotid stenoses of greater than 70 percent diameter reduction or high-grade asymptomatic lesions can be expected to reduce the likelihood of future ipsilateral stroke. Whether an individual patient benefits from treatment of combined CS and CAD is highly dependent on appropriate patient selection and the experience of the vascular and cardiac surgeons involved.

Since the majority of strokes associated with either CABG or CEA are related to technical problems, meticulous attention to technical details and intraoperative assessment of repair sites are essential. The frequency of concomitant carotid and coronary atherosclerotic disease is increasing as surgeons intervene in older patients to alleviate symptoms. Screening of patients based on risk factors and testing to assess the severity and extent of disease will identify the subset of patients likely to benefit from simultaneous or staged CEA and CABG.

REFERENCES

1. AHA statistics, 1991.
2. Reed G, Singer D, Picard E, DeSanctis R: Stroke following coronary-artery bypass surgery. *N Engl J Med* 319:1246, 1988.
3. Coffey C, Massey W, Roberts K, et al: Natural history of cerebral complications of coronary artery bypass graft surgery. *Neurology* 33: 1416, 1983.
4. Furlan A, Craciun A: Risk of stroke during coronary artery bypass graft surgery in patients with internal carotid artery disease documented by angiography. *Stroke* 16:797, 1985.
5. Turnipseed W, Berkoff H, Belzer F: Postoperative stroke in cardiac and peripheral vascular disease. *Ann Surg* 192:365, 1980.
6. Ropper A, Wechsler L, Wilson L: Carotid bruit and the risk of stroke in elective surgery. *N Engl J Med* 307:1388, 1982.
7. David T, Humphries A, Young F, et al: A correlation of neck bruits and arteriosclerotic carotid arteries. *Arch Surg* 107:729, 1973.
8. Barnes R, Liebman P, Marszalek P, et al: The natural history of asymptomatic carotid disease in patients undergoing cardiovascular surgery. *Surgery* 90:1075, 1981.
9. Brenner B, Brief D, Alpert J, et al: The risk of stroke in patients with asymptomatic carotid stenosis undergoing cardiac surgery: A follow-up study. *J Vasc Surg* 5:269, 1987.
10. Jausseran J, Bergeron P, Reggi M, et al: Single staged carotid and coronary arteries surgery. *J Cardiovasc Surg* 30:407, 1989.
11. Faggioli G, Curl R, Ricotta J: The role of carotid screening before coronary artery bypass. *J Vasc Surg* 12:724, 1990.
12. Gardner T, Horneffer P, Manolio T, et al: Stroke following coronary artery bypass grafting: A ten-year study. *Ann Thorac Surg* 40:574, 1985.
13. Weintraub W, Craver J, Cohen C, et al: Influence of age on results of coronary artery surgery. *Circulation* 84 (suppl III):226, 1991.
14. Ivey T, Strandness D, Williams D, et al: Management of patients with carotid bruit undergoing cardiopulmonary bypass. *J Thorac Cardiovasc Surg* 87:183, 1984.
15. Hertzer N, Loop F, Beven E, et al: Surgical staging for simultaneous coronary and carotid disease: A study including prospective randomizations. *J Vasc Surg* 9:455, 1989.
16. Schultz R, Sterpetti A, Feldhaus R: Early and late results in patients with carotid disease undergoing myocardial revascularization. *Ann Thorac Surg* 43:603, 1988.

17. Rice P, Pifarré R, Sullivan H, et al: Experience with simultaneous myocardial revascularization and carotid endarterectomy. *J Thorac Cardiovasc Surg* 79:922, 1980.
18. Jones E, Craver J, Michalik R, et al: Combined carotid and coronary operations: When are they necessary? *J Thorac Cardiovasc Surg* 87:7, 1984.
19. Babu S, Shah P, Singh B, et al: Coexisting carotid stenosis in patients undergoing cardiac surgery: Indications and guidelines for simultaneous operations. *Am J Surg* 150:207, 1985.
20. Reul G, Cooley D, Duncan J, et al: The effect of coronary bypass on the outcome of peripheral vascular operations in 1093 patients. *J Vasc Surg* 3:788, 1986.
21. Perler B, Burdick J, Minken S, Williams G: Should we perform carotid endarterectomy synchronously with cardiac surgical procedures? *J Vasc Surg* 8:402, 1988.
22. Cambria R, Ivarsson B, Akins C, et al: Simultaneous carotid and coronary disease: Safety of the combined approach. *J Vasc Surg* 9:56, 1989.
23. Duchateau J, Nevelsteen A, Sergeant P, et al: Combined myocardial and cerebral revascularization. *J Cardiovasc Surg* 30:715, 1989.
24. Pomè G, Passini L, Colucci V, et al: Combined surgical approach to coexistent carotid and coronary artery disease. *J Cardiovasc Surg* 32: 787, 1991.
25. Vermeulen F, Hamerlijnck R, Defauw J, Ernst S: Synchronous operation for ischemic cardiac and cerebrovascular disease: Early results and long-term follow-up. *Ann Thorac Surg* 53:381, 1992.
26. Rizzo R, Whittemore A, Couper G, et al: Combined carotid and coronary revascularization: The preferred approach to the severe vasculopath. *Ann Thorac Surg* 54:1099, 1992.
27. Carrel T, Stillhard G, Turina M: Combined carotid and coronary artery surgery: Early and late results. *Cardiology* 80:118, 1992.
28. Bass A, Krupski W, Dilley R, Bernstein E: Combined carotid endarterectomy and coronary artery revascularization: A sobering review. *Israel J Med Sci* 28:27, 1992.
29. Bernstein E: Staged versus simultaneous carotid endarterectomy in patients undergoing cardiac surgery. *J Vasc Surg* 15:870, 1992.
30. Riles T, Pasternack P: Management of concomitant carotid and coronary arterial occlusive disease, in Ernst C, Stanley J (eds): *Current Therapy in Vascular Surgery,* 2d ed., Philadelphia, BC Decker, 1991.
31. Mackey W, O'Donnell T, Callow A: Cardiac risk in patients undergoing carotid endarterectomy: Impact on perioperative and long-term mortality. *J Vasc Surg* 11:226, 1990.
32. CASS Principal Investigators: Myocardial infarction and mortality in the coronary artery surgery study (CASS) randomized trial. *N Engl J Med* 310:750, 1984.
33. Barnes R, Nix M, Sansonetti D, et al: Late outcome of untreated asymptomatic carotid disease following cardiovascular operations. *J Vasc Surg* 2:843, 1985.
34. NASCET Collaborators: Beneficial effect of carotid endarterectomy in symptomatic patients with high-grade carotid stenosis. *N Engl J Med* 325:445, 1991.
35. European Carotid Surgery Trialists' Collaborative Group: MRC European carotid surgery trial: Interim results for symptomatic patients with severe (70–99%) or with mild (0–29%) carotid stenosis. *Lancet* 337:1235, 1991.
36. Mayberg M, Wilson S, Yatsu F, et al: Carotid endarterectomy and prevention of cerebral ischemia in symptomatic carotid stenosis. *JAMA* 166:3289, 1991.
37. Hoffmann R, Blumiein S, Anderson A, et al: The probability of surviving coronary artery surgery. *JAMA* 243:1341, 1980.
38. Hise J, Nipper M, Schnitker J: Stroke associated with coronary artery bypass surgery. *AJNR* 12:811, 1991.
39. Moody D, Bell M, Challa V, et al: Brain microemboli during cardiac surgery or aortography. *Ann Neurol* 28:477, 1990.
40. Amarenco P, Cuyckaerts C, Tzourio C, et al: The prevalence of ulcerated plaques in the aortic arch in patients with stroke. *N Engl J Med* 326:221, 1992.
41. Lundar T, Frøysaker T, Lindegaard K, et al: Some observations on cerebral perfusion dur-

ing cardiopulmonary bypass. *Ann Thorac Surg* 39:318, 1985.
42. Lundar T, Lindegaard K, Frøysaker T, et al: Cerebral perfusion during nonpulsatile cardiopulmonary bypass. *Ann Thorac Surg* 40:144, 1985.
43. Johnsson P, Algotsson L, Ryding E, et al: Cardiopulmonary perfusion and cerebral blood flow in bilateral carotid artery disease. *Ann Thorac Surg* 51:579, 1991.
44. von Reutern G, Hetzel A, Birnbaum D, Schlosser V: Transcranial Doppler ultrasonography during cardiopulmonary bypass in patients with severe carotid stenosis or occlusion. *Stroke* 19:674, 1988.
45. Schwartz R, Garrett J, Karp R, Kouchoukos N: Simultaneous myocardial revascularization and carotid endarterectomy. *Circulation* 66 (suppl I):97, 1982.

21

Carotid Endarterectomy without Arteriography

David L. Dawson

Duplex scanning is now considered the noninvasive method of choice for the diagnosis of extracranial cerebrovascular disease.[1] Because of its sensitivity, low cost, and widespread availability, duplex scanning is a valuable screening test for patients with lateralizing neurologic symptoms. In addition, duplex scanning can be used to evaluate asymptomatic patients with bruits or other risk factors for carotid artery disease to identify those patients who warrant operation or close clinical follow-up.[2,3] The use of noninvasive cerebrovascular testing has largely eliminated the need for arteriography as a diagnostic screening method.[4] Generally, arteriography need not be performed for patients with minimal disease (less than 15 percent stenosis by duplex scanning), since these patients have a negligible risk of future stroke or transient neurologic events.[5]

Over the past decade there has been increasing interest in performing carotid endarterectomy (CEA) on the basis of noninvasive diagnostic studies without preoperative arteriography. This was first done for patients who had a clear contraindication to arteriography, but, with the increasing reliability of noninvasive testing, some surgeons have adopted this approach for the majority of CEAs they perform. For many surgeons, duplex scanning has progressed from the status of a screening test to a definitive diagnostic modality. There are two principal reasons to eliminate arteriography from the preoperative evaluation of patients being considered for CEA: (1) arteriography adds significantly to the cost of patient care; and (2) the risks associated with arteriography.

Routine preoperative arteriography would still be appropriate, despite these disadvantages, if it made the conduct of the operation safer or the outcome better. Those who advocate routine arteriography have asserted that the diagnostic information obtained with noninvasive tests is incomplete or not sufficiently reliable to serve as the basis for surgical decisions. However, clinical experience contradicts this view.

The initial sections of this chapter discuss the strengths and weaknesses of available diagnostic methods and the specific information required to plan CEA safely. This is followed by a review of the experience of performing carotid surgery without preoperative arteriography. More specifically, this chapter focuses on the adequacy of duplex scanning and clinical evaluation as sufficient preoperative assessment for CEA. The role of newer noninvasive diagnostic tests, such as magnetic resonance angiography and transcranial Doppler, is also briefly addressed.

INDICATIONS FOR OPERATION

The indications for CEA need to be considered before developing a logical algorithm for preoperative evaluation. Although there are individual and regional variations in surgical practice, there are some general indications for CEA on which most surgeons agree. For example, the North American Symptomatic Carotid Endarterectomy Trial (NASCET) clearly established the beneficial role of CEA for the treatment of 70 percent or greater internal carotid artery stenoses associated with transient ischemic attack (TIA), stroke, or amaurosis fugax (Chap. 16).[6] The management of moderately severe (30 to 69 percent diameter-reducing) carotid stenoses is not uniformly agreed on. While definitive information from randomized prospective clinical trials is still not available, there appears to be adequate data from nonrandomized series and natural history studies to suggest that CEA is beneficial for symptomatic carotid stenoses of 50 percent or greater, especially if the symptoms occur while the patient is receiving antiplatelet therapy.[7]

Asymptomatic patients also are candidates for CEA if: (1) they have a high-grade internal carotid artery stenosis; (2) the operation can be performed with less than a 3 percent incidence of stroke and death; and (3) there is no concomitant condition limiting life expectancy.[7,8] Data from the Veterans Affairs Cooperative Study, a randomized clinical trial of CEA for asymptomatic patients, suggested a beneficial role for CEA in selected cases (Chap. 17). However, the validity of this study may have been compromised by the inclusion of patients with only moderately severe internal carotid artery stenoses (50 percent diameter-reducing).[9] This limited the ability of the study to confirm the benefit of CEA for the group of asymptomatic patients at highest risk for neurologic events, that is, patients with stenoses of more than 75 to 80 percent diameter-reduction. It has been established that the risk of stroke, TIA, or progression of internal carotid stenosis to occlusion increases with the degree of luminal narrowing.[2,10] Nonrandomized but prospective evaluations of CEA and medical therapy for asymptomatic 80 percent or greater carotid stenoses have shown markedly better outcomes with surgery in this group.[11,12]

Noninvasive cerebrovascular tests, duplex scanning in particular, can identify operable carotid bifurcation disease in both symptomatic and asymptomatic patients. As discussed in Chap. 11, duplex scanning can accurately detect 50 percent or greater stenoses of the internal carotid artery and can distinguish lesions in the range of 80 to 99 percent stenosis. Furthermore, duplex scanning can provide the other information needed by the surgeon for preoperative planning and performing the operation.

REQUIREMENTS OF PREOPERATIVE STUDIES

Before selecting a diagnostic test or series of tests, it is appropriate to consider what specific information is needed from preoperative studies.

Establish the Diagnosis

The principal role of preoperative studies is to identify carotid artery disease that merits surgical intervention. The diagnostic tests used must be sufficiently sensitive to ensure that patients with operable lesions will not be missed. In addition, internal carotid arteries with high-grade stenoses need to be differentiated from those with mild stenoses or complete occlusions. Patients with minimally stenotic, nonulcerated plaques who will not benefit from operation should be distinguished from those with complicated, ulcerated plaques and more severe stenoses. The evaluation of symptomatic patients also should identify those who have neurologic symptoms from causes other than cerebrovascular disease.

Anatomic Definition and Localization

As discussed in Chap. 3, the location and distribution of atherosclerotic lesions of the extracranial carotid artery are remarkably constant (Fig. 21-1). Plaque is typically localized to the carotid bifurcation, and the lesion usually tapers off to normal intima within 3 cm of the internal carotid origin, a site easily reached with the standard cervical exposure for CEA.

Some technical aspects of carotid surgery make it important to recognize anatomic variants and atypical pathology prior to operation. Special maneuvers for exposure may be required if there is an unusually distal extent of disease or a particularly high carotid bifurcation. Tortuosity, kinks, or distal plaque in the internal carotid artery may interfere with placement of a shunt. Patients with innominate or proximal common carotid artery disease may require endarterectomy or bypass of these lesions. Such proximal disease can be flow-limiting or a source of atheroemboli and thus could compromise the success of a carotid bifurcation endarterectomy.

ARTERIOGRAPHY

Intraarterial contrast arteriography is the established "gold standard" for evaluation of cerebrovascular disease. Arteriographic techniques and interpretation are reviewed in

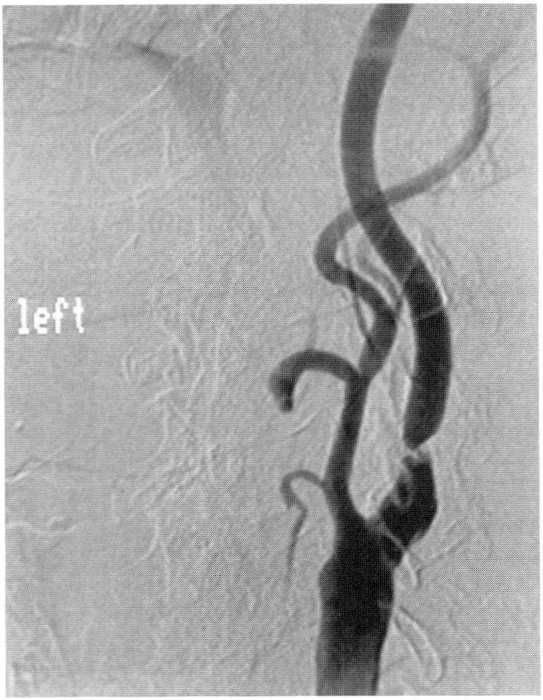

Figure 21-1. The typical atherosclerotic lesion of the internal carotid artery is focal and localized to within 3 cm of the internal carotid origin.

Chap. 14. Some aspects relevant to the clinician's choice of diagnostic methods prior to CEA will be discussed in this section.

Arteriography is a well-established imaging method, and vascular surgeons are accustomed to using the information it provides. It is also widely available, although the quality of an arteriogram depends greatly on the radiologist performing the study. In addition to evaluating the carotid bifurcation, arteriography gives information about the aortic arch, the other intrathoracic vessels, and the intracranial circulation.

The formal recommendations of vascular technology and vascular surgery societies include the use of arteriography before CEA.[7,13] Practice guidelines for CEA published by the Ad Hoc Committee of the Joint Council of the Society for Vascular Surgery and the North American Chapter of the International Society for Cardiovascular Surgery cite preoperative contrast arteriography as a "practice standard." In 1992 Moore and colleagues wrote: "The role of duplex scanning as an alternative to angiography is currently in evolution."[7] All major clinical trials examining the safety and efficacy of CEA have used arteriography to establish the presence and severity of carotid artery disease. Surgeons or referring physicians whose decision-making is based strictly on these study protocols are obliged to use arteriography. In some practice settings, the use of arteriography is required by third-party payers to provide "objective" and "definitive" proof that accepted indications for surgery are present.

However, it may be better to consider arteriography as a "reference standard" for validating other techniques, rather than to assume that the arteriogram is irrefutably correct. Measuring the percentage of stenosis from arteriograms does not yield an absolute numerical value. With carefully performed multiple measurements based on multiplanar arteriography, the interobserver variability for the estimation of internal carotid artery stenosis was 6.0 percent, and the standard deviation of the measurement was 8.1 percent.[14] Furthermore, studies that correlated findings at CEA with preoperative estimates of carotid disease severity based on arteriography and ultrasound found arteriography inferior to ultrasound for the evaluation of ulcerated lesions or plaques that were not associated with severe arterial narrowing.[15–17]

LIMITATIONS OF NONINVASIVE TESTS

Duplex Scanning

Duplex scanning is the combination of B-mode imaging and pulsed Doppler assessment of flow characteristics. This approach is generally accepted as the best noninvasive method for detecting and characterizing lesions of the extracranial carotid arteries.[1] The details of the technique and interpretation of carotid duplex scanning are discussed in Chap. 11.

One problem with duplex scanning is that it is highly dependent on the examiner's skill. Accurate studies require well-trained and experienced technologists. Developing a "true picture" of the patient's disease depends on acquiring many images and the interpretation of physiologic information. In addition, there are specific technical limitations of carotid ultrasound imposed by the equipment or particular clinical circumstances (Table 21-1). However, with an understanding of the limitations of carotid duplex scanning, the pathology or other factors that interfere with accurate characterization of carotid disease can be recognized.

In some cases, additional diagnostic maneuvers or adjustments in diagnostic criteria can compensate for the technical limitations of duplex scanning. For example, categorization of stenosis severity can be inaccurate if there is severe contralateral disease. There is often a compensatory increase in flow through a carotid artery if there is an occlusion or high-grade stenosis of the contralateral internal carotid.[18–21] This can lead to overestimating the degree of stenosis if standard diagnostic criteria are used. Thus, as discussed in Chap. 11, modified criteria have been proposed for use in cases of contralateral carotid occlusion.[22]

Although experience in the vascular labo-

Table 21-1 Sources of Error With Carotid Duplex Scanning

	Sources of error	Examples
General	Operator inexperience	ECA[a] mistaken for ICA[b] Atypical pathology unrecognized
	Incorrect instrument set-up or operation	
B-mode imaging	Calcified plaque	Acoustic shadowing obscures imaging and Doppler
	Eccentric plaque	Appearance of lumen narrowing and plaque thickness varies in different scan planes
	Image appearance changes with transmitting power, receiver gain, TGC[c], dynamic range, pre- and postprocessing settings	Hypoechoic plaque or thrombus may be unrecognized
Pulsed Doppler	Angle error	Operator error in sample volume positioning or angle of ultrasound insonation Flow disturbances and nonaxial flow jets with carotid artery kinks, coils, and dilatations
	ICA stenosis misclassified (severity underestimated) because of diminished inflow	Severe stenosis or occlusion of innominate artery (evaluating right ICA) Severe stenosis of ipsilateral proximal CCA[d]
	ICA stenosis misclassified (severity overestimated) because of increased flow	Contralateral ICA occlusion
	High-grade ICA stenosis mistakenly classified as ICA occlusion	Low velocity ICA flow undetected by Doppler
	ICA occlusion unrecognized	ECA mistaken for ICA

[a]ECA: external carotid artery
[b]ICA: internal carotid artery
[c]TGC: time-gain compensation (depth-gain compensation)
[d]CCA: common carotid artery

ratory has improved the accuracy of diagnosing internal carotid artery occlusion by duplex scanning, discriminating a very tight stenosis from a complete occlusion still can be difficult. Absence of a detectable flow signal in the imaged internal carotid lumen is the principal Doppler finding with internal carotid occlusion, but diagnostic errors occur if the very narrow flow channel through a preocclusive stenosis is missed (Fig. 21-2). Furthermore, extensive plaque calcification associated with

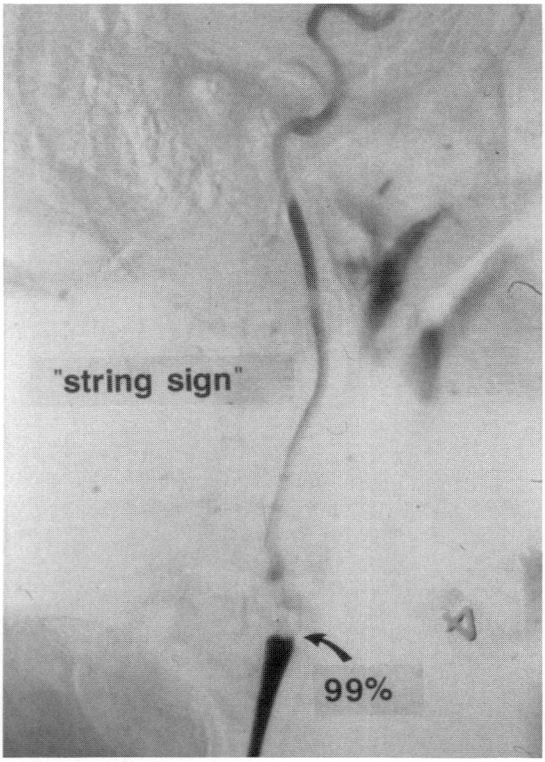

Figure 21-2. The arteriographic "string sign" is produced distal to a very high-grade stenosis (approximately 99 percent) by the slow flow of contrast. Flow is inadequate to show complete filling of the arterial lumen distal to the stenosis. A tight stenosis such as this can be mistaken for an occlusion by either duplex scanning (if the flow is too slow to be detected by Doppler) or by arteriography (without selective carotid injection or if delayed films are not obtained).

some severe stenoses can interfere with ultrasound imaging and Doppler flow detection. Thus, several factors can lead to the misclassification of a very high-grade internal carotid artery stenosis as an occlusion.[21,23–25]

Other duplex scan criteria can help with the accurate diagnosis of internal carotid artery occlusion (Table 21-2). There are changes in the ipsilateral common carotid artery flow pattern that characterize an internal carotid artery as occluded.[26] The absence of diastolic forward flow in the common carotid artery is 93 percent accurate in detecting internal carotid artery occlusion.[27] It should be noted that this loss of diastolic forward flow is a nonspecific marker for increased outflow resistance. This high-resistance type of common carotid flow pattern also has been observed with intracranial internal carotid artery occlusion (or near occlusion) when the internal carotid at the level of the bifurcation is not significantly diseased (Figs. 21-3 and 21-4) and with severe intracranial hypertension.[28]

When a technically satisfactory duplex scan demonstrates internal carotid artery occlusion in an asymptomatic patient, no further evaluation should be necessary. When the examination is limited or difficult, or if the patient presents with acute ipsilateral neurologic symptoms (especially crescendo TIAs or recurrent episodes of amaurosis fugax), arteriography is appropriate to ensure that a surgically treatable lesion is not missed. However, in some instances even arteriography fails to differentiate a high-grade stenosis from an occlusion.[29] Newer ultrasound systems, including the use of color-flow imaging, have been reported to be more sensitive than digital subtraction arteriography in identifying "trickle flow" distal to a very high-grade internal carotid artery stenosis.[30]

Some disagreements between duplex scanning and subsequent arteriography regarding internal carotid occlusion may not represent diagnostic errors at all. If there is a delay be-

Table 21-2 Duplex Scan Criteria for Diagnosis of Internal Carotid Artery Occlusion

Criteria	Specific ultrasound findings
No detected ICA flow	No detectable Doppler flow in adequately visualized ICA segment[a]
	No color-flow signal in adequately visualized ICA segment[b]
Loss of low resistance CCA outflow	Absent or very low velocity flow in diastole in ipsilateral CCA
	"Thump" at location of suspected occlusion
	Asymmetric contralateral CCA waveform
CCA collateral outflow through ECA	Increased flow velocities in ipsilateral ECA
Correct carotid branch identification	ECA identification confirmed by:
	percussion of superficial temporal artery
	visualization of branches
	high-resistance outflow pattern

[a]Minimal wall filter, low Doppler pulse repetition frequency, large Doppler sample volume, high Doppler gain.

[b]Minimal color wall filter, low color pulse repetition frequency, high color write priority, high color gain, optimal color Doppler angle.

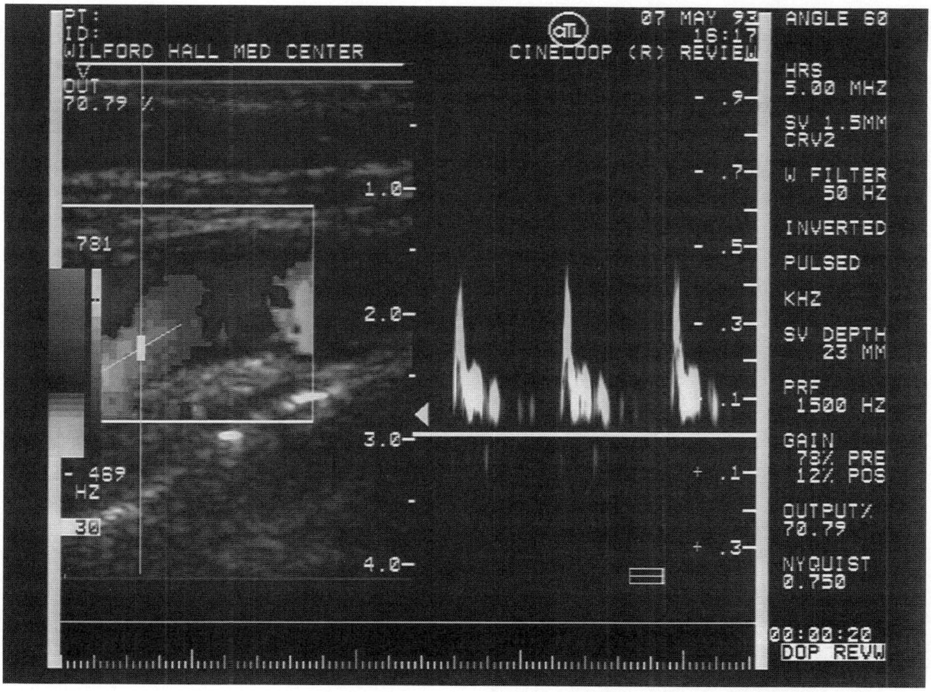

Figure 21-3. Carotid duplex scanning did not show any significant carotid bifurcation disease in this patient, who presented with a mild stroke low peak systolic velocities and the absence of diastolic forward flow in the internal carotid artery suggested abnormal outflow resistance.

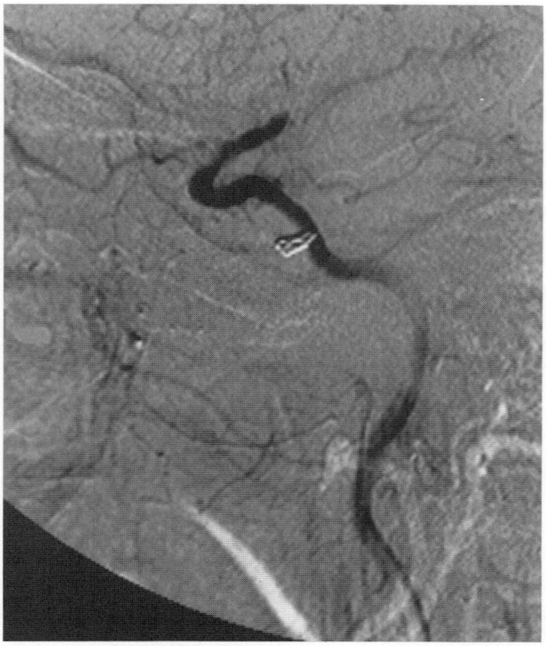

Figure 21-4. Lateral projection from a selective carotid arteriogram on the same patient as in Fig. 21-3 demonstrates occlusion of the intracranial portion of the internal carotid artery just distal to the origin of the ophthalmic artery.

tween a duplex scan that shows a high-grade carotid stenosis and a later arteriogram or operation, the stenosis may progress to occlusion. This reflects the natural history of high-grade carotid stenoses, and these cases should not be counted as duplex scan errors. Internal carotid artery end-diastolic frequencies greater than 6.0 kHz are associated with the greatest risk of progression to occlusion.[12] While internal carotid artery thrombosis may be accompanied by a transient or permanent neurologic deficit, it may also occur without symptoms.[2,31] If a patient with a documented high-grade internal carotid stenosis must wait more than a few days to undergo CEA, the duplex scan should be repeated to ensure that the diseased vessel has not progressed to occlusion.

While duplex scanning is an excellent method for evaluating the carotid arteries in the neck, it gives limited information about the proximal or distal vessels. The aortic arch and its proximal branches cannot be directly examined in most cases, and there are no established criteria for grading lesions of these vessels if they are detected. In general, duplex scanning is also insensitive to the presence of stenoses in the carotid siphon or intracranial vessels. Finally, duplex scanning cannot detect other intracranial lesions, such as tumors or arteriovenous malformations.

Ocular Pneumoplethysmography

The use of ocular pneumoplethysmography (OPG-Gee)[32–34] in the vascular laboratory continues, but its clinical applications have diminished with the increasing availability of duplex scanning (Chap. 10). This method was widely used, and many studies of carotid artery disease that were published before the mid-1980s were based on the OPG-Gee.[35]

The OPG-Gee can accurately detect a pressure-reducing lesion (approximately 60 percent or greater diameter reduction) in the ipsilateral internal carotid artery.[33,34] However, as for the indirect tests in general, the OPG-Gee cannot further classify the severity of the lesion. Thus, the OPG-Gee cannot distinguish a high-grade stenosis from a complete occlusion. Furthermore, it provides no information on the exact location of any pressure-reducing arterial lesions. The accuracy of the OPG-Gee also may be reduced in the presence of bilateral high-grade carotid artery disease.

Transcranial Doppler and Transcranial Duplex Scanning

Transcranial Doppler (TCD) and transcranial duplex scanning use low frequency (2 MHz) ultrasound to penetrate through thin areas of the skull or other imaging windows to detect flow in the intracranial vessels. These methods are useful for detection and monitoring of cerebral vasospasm and several other clinical applications, but their role in the evaluation of patients with extracranial carotid artery disease is less well defined (Chap. 12).

Transcranial Doppler has been used for intraoperative monitoring of patients undergoing CEA.[36,37] It is one means of assessing cerebral blood flow with carotid clamping, and may help to determine the need for shunting or the adequacy of shunt function. However, the utility of TCD in the preoperative evaluation of patients with carotid artery disease is largely speculative. It has been suggested that TCD-derived information about intracranial vascular disease or the adequacy of transhemispheric collateral pathways may be helpful in selecting patients for CEA,[38] but there are no objective data to support this assertion.

REASONS TO ELIMINATE ARTERIOGRAPHY

Arteriography is relatively unpleasant for the patient and adds significantly to the costs associated with the management of cerebrovascular disease. There are also risks associated with cerebral arteriography, including contrast toxicity, arterial complications at the puncture site, transient neurologic complications, and stroke. Since arteriography is regarded as a preoperative investigation, it has been pointed out that the morbidity of arteriography should be added to the operative complication rate when considering the overall morbidity and mortality of the surgical treatment of cerebrovascular disease.[6,39–41]

Risks Associated with Arteriography

Death, stroke, renal failure, and local arterial injury are the most significant potential complications associated with cerebral arteriography. Obtaining a preoperative arteriogram usually delays surgery by at least a day, and this delay may be detrimental to patients with crescendo TIAs and a high-grade internal carotid artery stenosis. Complication rates vary markedly between studies, and it is important to consider that the mortality and morbidity rates reported in older studies may not accurately reflect the risk to patients evaluated by more up-to-date techniques.[42] The mortality associated with cerebral arteriography in the Joint Study of Extracranial Arterial Occlusion reported in 1968 was 0.5 percent[43]; more modern series report mortality rates of 0 to 0.6 percent.[39] Elderly patients with cerebrovascular disease are at highest risk for complications of cerebral arteriography. A retrospective analysis of 5000 cerebral arteriograms by Mani and Eisenberg found a neurologic complication rate of 1.9 percent for patients with vascular occlusive disease, a figure significantly higher than the 0.2 to 0.5 percent complication rate for patients with tumor, seizures, or headache undergoing cerebral arteriography.[44,45]

The incidence of neurologic complications associated with arteriography can exceed the typical neurologic complication rate associated with CEA. In a prospectively evaluated series of cerebrovascular arteriograms in 147 patients who presented with stroke or TIA, Faught and coworkers observed a 6.8 percent rate of temporary neurologic deficits and a 5.4 percent rate of permanent neurologic complications.[46] Hankey and colleagues reviewed eight prospective studies with a total of 2227 cerebral arteriograms and concluded that the average neurologic complication rate for conventional cerebral arteriography was 4.1 percent.[39] Most of these events were TIAs, and the permanent neurologic complication rate was 1.0 percent. These high complication rates may be avoidable. In a prospective study of 1095 patients published in 1990, Gryzska and coworkers found that, with careful technique, the use of small catheters, nonionic contrast media, and a digital imaging system, the rate of permanent neurologic complications was only 0.09 percent.[42]

Radiographic contrast media cause severe anaphylactoid reactions in less than 2 percent of cases.[47] A prior reaction to contrast does not mean that a patient will have a similar episode with subsequent exposure to a contrast agent, but the risk is increased, even after premedication with histamine blockers and steroids.[48] Contrast nephrotoxicity is another potential problem. Patients with preexisting renal disease, diabetes mellitus, heart failure, and those over 70 years of age have the highest risk for acute renal dysfunction following contrast administration.[49,50] A review by Berkseth and Kjellstrand found that the reported incidence of contrast-induced nephropathy varied from 0.5 percent or less in an unselected population to 92 percent in a group of patients with diabetes and renal insufficiency.[51] Acute renal dysfunction also occurs with the nonionic contrast agents in up to 5.5 percent of high-risk patients.[50]

Femoral artery puncture is the safest route for aortic and brachiocephalic vessel catheterization,[52] but it still carries a risk of complications related to arterial access. Puncture site complications include hematoma formation, pseudoaneurysm, arteriovenous fistula, hemorrhage, arterial thrombosis, and femoral neuralgia. The reported incidence of local complications varies widely, partly due to differences in how small hematomas are reported or classified. Clinically significant local arterial complications occur in 0.1 to 5 percent of cases.[39,44,52–54]

Cost Containment

Approximately 80,000 to 100,000 carotid operations are performed each year in the United States, with associated costs of nearly 1 billion dollars.[55] With current concerns about the rising costs of health care, cost containment with CEA has become an important issue. Several means by which savings can be achieved have been identified, including the use of local or regional anesthesia,[56,57] elimination of routine intensive care unit monitoring,[56–58] shortened postoperative hospital stays,[57] and the selective use of preoperative arteriography.[57] In a 1992 cost analysis by Kraiss and coworkers, a therapeutic approach that combined these cost-saving measures resulted in a decrease in hospital charges for CEA from $10,429 to $6927 per patient—a 34 percent savings.[57] Notably, the cost of arteriography was the most significant avoidable expense associated with hospitalization for CEA.

Arteriography is undeniably expensive, and the true cost of the procedure is difficult to establish. An average cost of about $2500 was reported in two articles from 1987 that included cost estimates for arteriography.[59,60] The effects of inflation and other associated hospital charges may make the true figure significantly higher (Table 21-3).[61] In addition, the costs associated with the complications of arteriography should be considered. Based on an estimated 80,000 CEAs, a cost of $2000 per arteriogram, and the use of arteriography in one-third of cases, it is likely that more selective use of arteriography could reduce health care expenses in the United States by more than $50 million annually.

Table 21-3 Cost of Carotid Arteriography[a]

Cervicocerebral arteriography, 3–4 vessel, room charge (first 60 min)	$2354.75
Additional room time, each block of 30 min	194.75
Additional film runs, each	158.75
Miscellaneous and other supplies	
ISOVUE, 200 ml at $150.00/100ml	300.00
Professional fee, neuroradiologist	736.00
Short-stay admission	475.00
TOTAL	$4219.25

[a]Based on patient charges at the University Medical Center, Seattle, Washington. Data from: University of Washington Physicians, University of Washington Department of Radiology, and University of Washington Medical Center Financial Services Office, January 1992.

Is Routine Arteriography Necessary for Clinical Decision-Making?

Atherosclerotic lesions tend to be localized to the carotid bifurcation (Fig. 21-1), and duplex scanning frequently provides a complete assessment of this arterial segment. The most critical diagnostic information concerns the presence of atherosclerotic disease and the severity of any stenotic lesions. Duplex scanning has an overall accuracy of 93 percent for distinguishing between less than and greater than 50 percent diameter-reducing lesions.[62,63] It can further stratify the clinically significant lesions of more than 50 percent diameter reduction into categories of very high-grade stenosis (80 to 99 percent) or less severe stenosis (50 to 79 percent) with an accuracy of 87 percent (sensitivity 83 percent, specificity 86 percent).[64] Therefore, the use of arteriography simply to confirm the presence of carotid bifurcation disease is unnecessary if a technically adequate duplex scan has been performed. Unsuspected diagnostic errors are rare, and most of the inconsistencies in interpretation, when comparing carotid duplex scanning and arteriography, come from attempting to differentiate normal and mildly diseased vessels. However, this is not an issue when screening patients for significant disease.[65]

Aortic Arch Vessel Disease Complete evaluation of the aortic arch, innominate artery, and the origins of the common carotid arteries requires arteriography. However, arterial lesions of these proximal vessels are far less common than carotid bifurcation disease. Intrathoracic abnormalities were found in only 1.8 percent of 1000 studies reviewed by Akers and coworkers.[66] In addition, significant disease of the proximal arch vessels often is evident from a careful clinical examination.[66,67] In the study by Akers and coworkers significant proximal disease was suspected prior to arteriography on the basis of unequal brachial artery blood pressures in two-thirds of cases.

Duplex scanning can identify these proximal lesions in many cases, either by direct examination or by indirect findings. When it is not possible to position the Doppler sample volume proximal enough to identify the high velocity jet of a stenosis near the common carotid artery origin, the presence of a proximal stenosis may be indicated by poststenotic turbulence in the more distal common carotid artery. The velocity waveform in the distal common carotid may also be damped with reduced peak systolic velocities (Fig. 21-5). Ackerstaff and colleagues found that duplex scanning could detect significant (50 percent or greater diameter-reducing) stenoses of the vertebral artery origins with a sensitivity of 80 percent and a specificity of 83 percent.[68] They also obtained good results with duplex scanning for evaluating subclavian artery disease, with a 73 percent sensitivity and 91 percent specificity.

Intracranial Arterial Disease Intracranial arterial disease is not directly evaluated by the standard cervical duplex scan. Potential intracranial vascular lesions include atherosclerosis, aneurysms, tumors, and arteriovenous malformations. In terms of pathophysiology, intracranial carotid artery atherosclerosis appears to be far less important than disease of the carotid bifurcation. Arteriography commonly demonstrates atherosclerotic changes of the intracranial portions of the internal carotid artery. Intracranial atherosclerosis most frequently involves the cavernous portion of the internal carotid artery, a segment also referred to as the carotid siphon. The reported prevalence of carotid siphon atherosclerosis in patients with carotid bifurcation disease ranges from 6 to 84 percent.[69–77] If only more severe stenoses are considered (50 percent or greater diameter reduction), the prevalence is in the range of 0 to 9 percent. When these tandem lesions occur, the more severe stenosis usually is at the bifurcation. Only 8 to 20 percent of tandem lesions have the more severe lesion distally.[76,77] Isolated siphon disease can

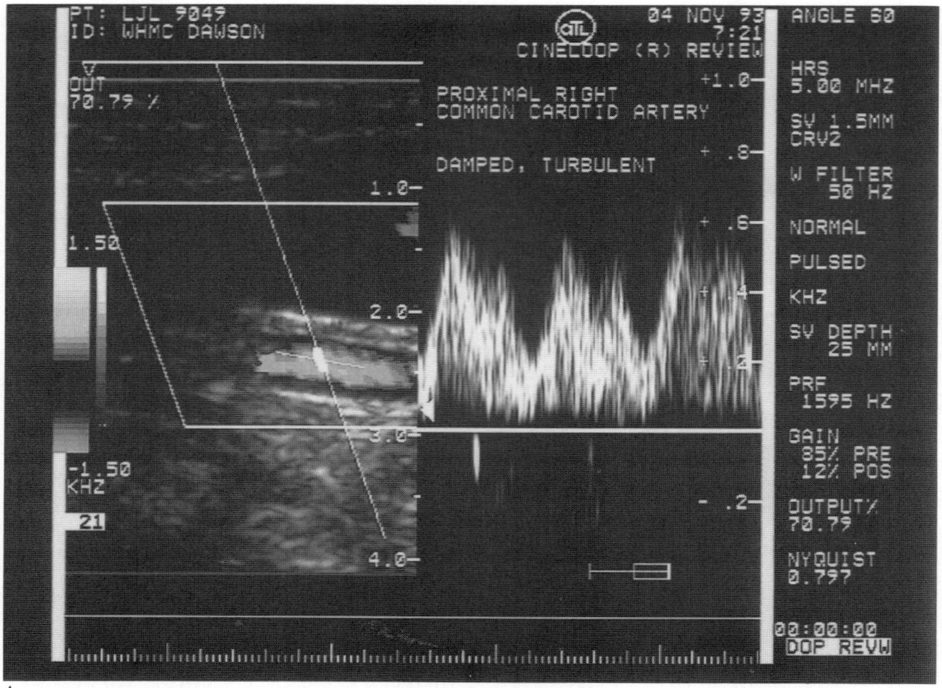

A

Figure 21-5. This 63-year-old woman was asymptomatic, but the right brachial artery pressure was 50 mmHg less than the pressure on the left. Duplex scanning of the right common carotid artery showed very low velocity turbulent flow, although no proximal lesion could be directly identified (*A*). Arch aortography demonstrated innominate artery occlusion (*B*). Late imaging after selective left subclavian artery injection showed subclavian steal and collateral filling of the right common carotid artery (*C*). Because of the low concentration of contrast filling the right carotid artery, the duplex scan was better than arteriography at demonstrating the high-grade (≥80 percent diameter-reducing) recurrent stenosis at the right carotid bifurcation (*D*).

be implicated in only 5 percent of patients presenting with stroke or TIA.[43,72,78] Currently, the identification of this small subset of patients has limited therapeutic value since these lesions are not accessible surgically.

In earlier publications, some authors suggested that the presence of tandem lesions should be considered a contraindication to CEA. Specific concerns included an increased risk of perioperative stroke,[71,79,80] recurrence of symptoms,[81–84] and shortened long-term stroke-free survival[71,85,86] due to the untreated distal lesion. However, clinical experience has not supported these concerns, and intracranial atherosclerosis appears to have a much more benign natural history than does disease of the carotid bifurcation. It has been hypothesized that morphologic differences between atherosclerosis of the carotid bifurcation and siphon result in a lower risk of plaque ulceration and embolization from the intracranial lesions.[87–89] Whatever the reason, intracranial atherosclerosis does not seem to have a major effect on either the short-term or long-term success of CEA.

Schuler and coworkers followed 79 patients undergoing 91 CEAs and compared the outcome of patients with isolated carotid bifur-

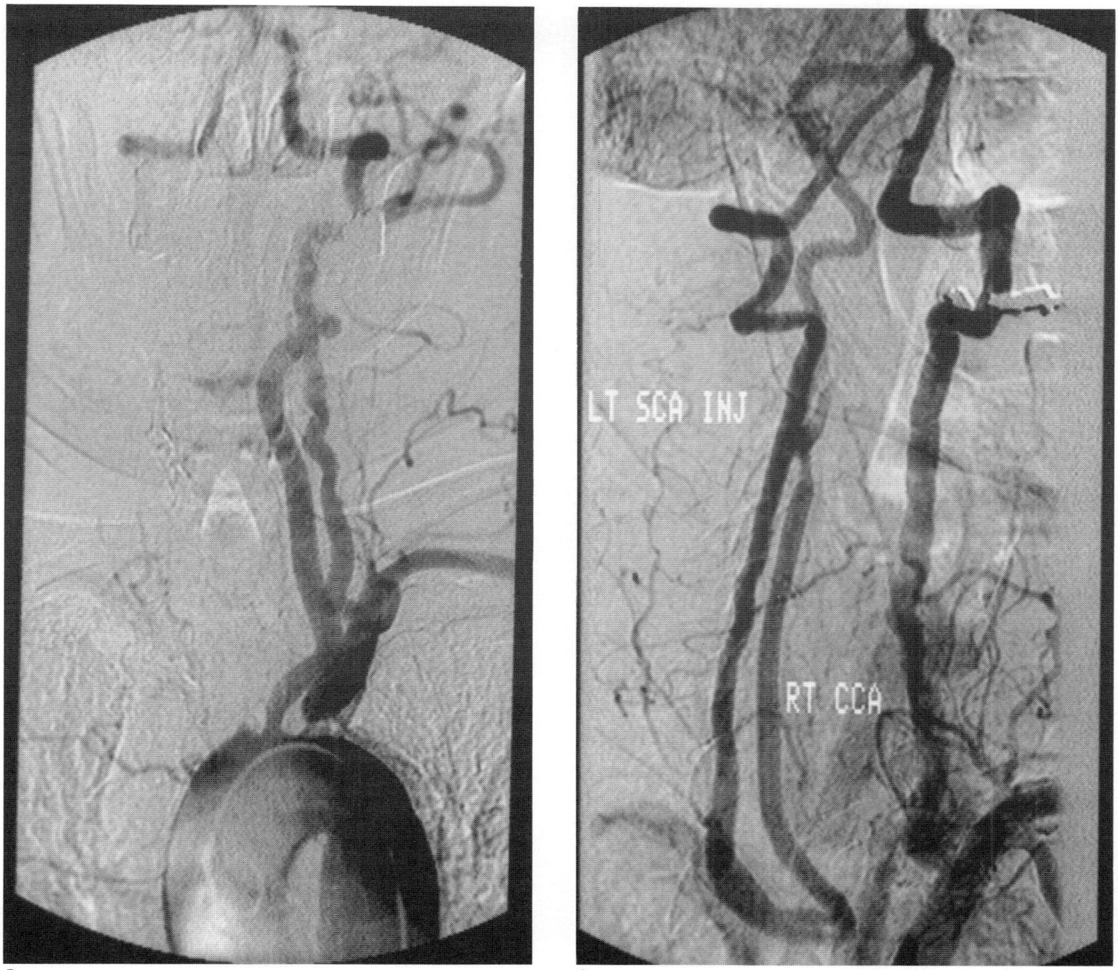

B *C*

Figure 21-5. (*Continued*)

cation stenoses ($n=44$) to the outcome of those with tandem lesions ($n=35$).[77] They found that CEA provided effective and immediate relief of symptoms in both groups, and there were no statistically significant differences in perioperative stroke and death rates. Furthermore, when the patients with severe (50 percent or greater) siphon stenoses were compared to patients with less severe lesions or normal carotid siphons, the early and late complication rates were nearly identical.

In an effort to study the effect of siphon disease on the clinical outcome of CEA, Roederer and colleagues followed 125 patients having 133 operations for a mean of 22 months.[76] Mild to moderate (1 to 49 percent) siphon stenoses were found in 63 percent of the sides examined. Severe siphon stenosis (50

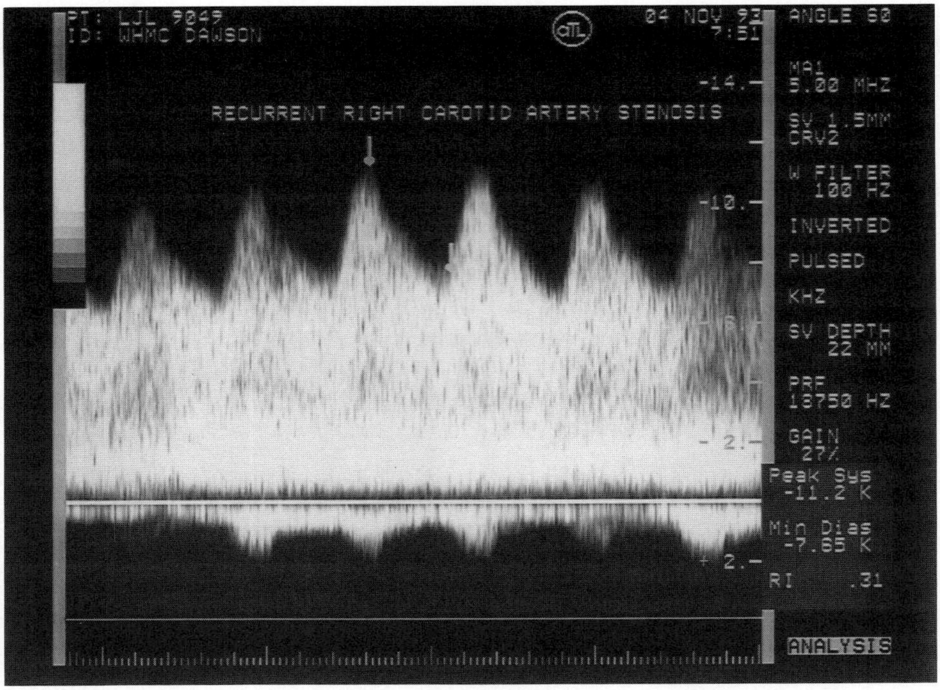

D

Figure 21-5. (*Continued*)

to 99 percent) was present in 9 percent, and 10 percent had intracranial carotid artery occlusions. They found no correlation between the severity of siphon disease and the success of CEA, nor did the severity of siphon disease predict the recurrence of focal neurologic symptoms on either the operated or contralateral side. The severity of the carotid bifurcation stenosis had no relationship to the severity of the intracranial lesion. In symptomatic patients, the severity of siphon disease was equal on the symptomatic and asymptomatic sides. Siphon disease was found in only 6 percent of 784 arteriograms reviewed by Akers and coworkers.[69] In their series, the long-term outcome (4 to 20 months) was unaffected by the presence or absence of a siphon stenosis. Mattos and colleagues reported ipsilateral siphon stenosis in 21 percent of 354 patients having 393 carotid operations and also found no difference in perioperative outcome or late stroke risk.[75] However, the presence of carotid siphon disease was associated with a higher late cardiac death rate.

One criticism of studies on the significance of intracranial arterial disease is that they consider only the outcome of patients having CEA. It is possible that patients with the most severe intracranial disease were not offered operation, thus biasing the data. However, recognizing the generally aggressive approach to the treatment of carotid bifurcation disease, it is likely that the reported experience reflects the true impact of intracranial disease on clinical outcome after CEA. The evidence summarized above suggests that carotid bifurcation lesions should be considered independently of any more distal carotid disease. Consequently, routine arteriography to detect intracranial atherosclerotic disease becomes unnecessary. This rationale also obviates any need for routine TCD or transcranial duplex scanning, which have been advocated as noninvasive methods to identify intracranial vascular disease.

Intracranial Aneurysm The combination of carotid bifurcation disease and an intracranial berry aneurysm has been cited as another potential contraindication to CEA.[90] The major concern is the hypothetical risk of aneurysm rupture related to perioperative hypertension, anticoagulation, and the hemodynamic effects of relieving the proximal stenosis. However, clinical experience does not support these theoretical concerns. Ladowski and colleagues performed 20 CEAs in 19 patients with concurrent intracranial berry aneurysms without perioperative complications.[91] The largest aneurysm in their series was 25 mm in diameter. They also reviewed the literature on the prior experience with this problem.[90,92–96] Of 20 previously reported cases, they found only one instance of a ruptured intracranial aneurysm within 30 days of CEA.[96] Orecchia and coworkers added to this experience, reporting the successful operative management of symptomatic carotid bifurcation disease in 10 patients with concomitant asymptomatic intracranial aneurysms ranging from 2 mm to 13 mm.[97] Six of the 10 patients required nitroglycerin or nitroprusside postoperatively, and transient severe hypertension was noted in two cases. All the intracranial aneurysms remained intact.

Specific indications for prophylactic repair of berry aneurysms have not been clearly defined.[98,99] The risk of rupture for small asymptomatic intracranial aneurysms is low. Weibers and colleagues observed 65 patients with 81 aneurysms for a mean of 98.5 months.[98] None of the 44 aneurysms less than 10 mm in diameter ruptured, although 28 percent of the aneurysms larger than 10 mm ruptured during the period of follow-up. The prevalence of intracranial aneurysms is in the range of 2 to 5 percent in both autopsy series[100,101] and in a review of 784 arteriograms performed for the evaluation of patients with suspected carotid artery disease.[69] It is not known exactly how often the combination of significant carotid artery disease and an intracranial aneurysm of more than 10 mm occurs. However, it is exceedingly rare, and certainly not common enough to justify routine arteriography as a screening method for asymptomatic intracranial aneurysms. Magnetic resonance imaging is the best screening test when intracranial aneurysm is suspected, followed by arteriography for definitive vascular evaluation.[102]

Tumors and Other Intracranial Pathology Patients with brain tumors, arteriovenous malformations, or other uncommon intracranial lesions can present with a variety of neurologic symptoms (Chap. 9). These include seizures, headaches, cranial nerve palsies, and other findings usually distinct from the symptoms of carotid artery disease. Thromboemboli from carotid disease cause hemispheric TIAs, cerebral infarcts in the distribution of the anterior or middle cerebral arteries, or retinal embolization with symptoms of amaurosis fugax and the finding of Hollenhorst plaques. Arteriography performed for the evaluation of patients with carotid disease has been reported to demonstrate tumors in only 0.1 percent of cases.[69] However, arteriography is inferior to computed tomography (CT) or magnetic resonance imaging for the detection of such lesions. Martin and coworkers prospectively examined the utility of routine CT scanning before CEA in 469 consecutive patients over a five-year period.[103] This was accomplished at a cost of approximately $500,000. Infarcts, already suspected clinically, were common, but no tumors were found. In no instance did the CT scan findings alter patient management.

CLINICAL EXPERIENCE

Need for Preoperative Arteriography Critically Examined

By the early 1980s noninvasive tests for cerebrovascular disease had become well established, and some groups had accumulated enough experience with the techniques to suggest that arteriography was no longer necessary in screening for cerebrovascular disease.[104] It was becoming apparent that arteriography usually confirmed the results of the noninvasive tests and that it rarely added information that influenced patient management. In a retrospective study using a combination of oculoplethysmography (OPG-Gee) and ultrasonic arteriography, Ricotta and colleagues found that two-thirds of their patients with hemispheric cerebral symptoms or asymptomatic bruits would have been adequately evaluated for surgery without a subsequent arteriogram.[67] These findings are especially significant when one considers the relatively limited diagnostic capabilities of OPG-Gee and ultrasonic arteriography compared with modern color-flow duplex scanners.

Amaurosis fugax is a distinctive symptom of carotid disease. Walsh and coworkers retrospectively reviewed the evaluation of 28 patients who presented with transient monocular blindness.[105] No significant information was added by arteriography after a thorough noninvasive evaluation that combined bidirectional Doppler analysis, oculoplethysmography, and carotid artery B-mode imaging. They concluded that arteriography was unnecessary in patients with amaurosis fugax if noninvasive studies showed that significant carotid bifurcation disease was present.

The preoperative decision-making process was further evaluated by clinical researchers at the University of Illinois. Flanigan and colleagues presented duplex scan information and arteriograms separately to two vascular surgeons, who were asked to make decisions regarding therapy based on the clinical findings and the diagnostic study results.[106] The surgeons made similar decisions on the need for carotid surgery based on duplex scanning or arteriography in 89 and 91 percent of the cases. Most of the disagreements involved operative indications in patients with symptomatic but nonstenotic carotid lesions. From this experience they developed an algorithm for patient management and estimated that 99.4 percent of cases could be appropriately treated with selective use of arteriography (Fig. 21-6). The same group subsequently evaluated their algorithm in a series of patients with focal hemispheric or retinal embolic symptoms and found it to be highly accurate for the identification of patients who should have CEA.[60] Duplex scanning was equal to arteriography for identifying significant (50 percent or greater) carotid stenoses. Comparing the preoperative diagnostic studies to operative specimens from 72 patients who underwent 78 CEAs, they found that all operative specimens had been correctly characterized by duplex scanning. They concluded that for patients with hemispheric neurologic symptoms, CEA could be safely performed on the basis of duplex scan findings.

Moore and coworkers confirmed the findings of earlier retrospective studies with a prospective analysis of noninvasive testing for the selection of patients for CEA.[107] They assembled a panel of eight surgical and medical specialists and asked them to assess 85 patients. Each clinician was provided with duplex scan and OPG-Gee data and asked to classify the anatomic or pathologic status of the 170 carotid bifurcations. When compared to arteriography, the noninvasive tests were 100 percent accurate for the diagnosis of carotid

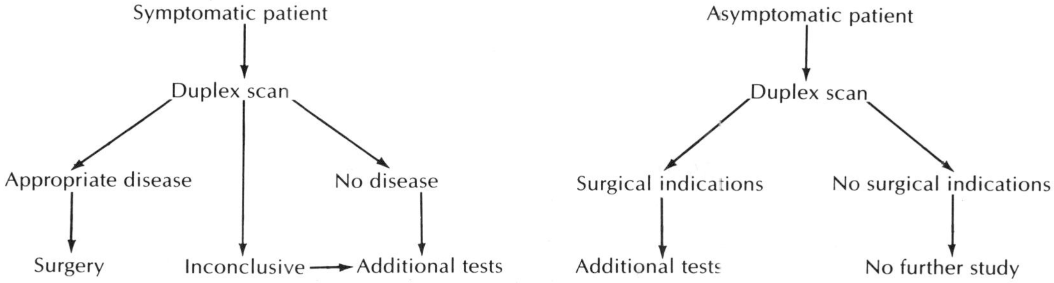

Figure 21-6. Management algorithm developed by Flanigan et al.[106]

occlusion, 100 percent accurate for the diagnosis of a hemodynamically significant lesion, and 93.5 percent accurate overall. This experience prompted them to start performing CEA without preoperative arteriography in selected cases. While retrospective studies have documented the accuracy of duplex scanning in the selection of patients for CEA, they have also suggested that the diagnosis of carotid occlusion, at least in symptomatic patients, probably should be confirmed with arteriography.[108–110]

Not all vascular surgeons share this willingness to give up routine arteriography. Geuder and colleagues performed a retrospective comparison of duplex scanning and arteriography for preoperative decision-making.[111] They found that arteriography altered their clinical management in eight of 100 consecutive cases and concluded that arteriography was a necessary complement to duplex scanning. However, their conclusions were challenged in the discussion of the paper because the management changes cited by the authors involved such controversial situations as tandem lesions, patients with symptoms of vertebrobasilar insufficiency, and errors in duplex scan interpretation. Two patients in this series had strokes as a complication of arteriography, and one stroke resulted in death.

Walters and coworkers also examined the feasibility of eliminating arteriography before CEA, and on the basis of this experience they continued to prefer routine arteriography.[21] In their series of 51 patients, five (9.8 percent) had a clinically significant change in management based on the arteriographic findings. In each case the patient was symptomatic and the duplex scan identified carotid bifurcation disease. In three of the five patients, high-grade carotid stenoses were mistaken for occlusions, thus emphasizing the need for confirmatory arteriography when noninvasive tests suggest internal carotid occlusion in an acutely symptomatic patient. In one patient who presented with a stroke, an internal carotid artery occlusion was missed when the patent but diseased external carotid artery was mistakenly identified as a diseased internal carotid artery. The authors discussed this error, pointing out that the simple maneuver of tapping on the superficial temporal artery while performing the duplex scan readily identifies the external carotid artery, enabling the technician to recognize this situation. In the remaining case, the duplex scan underestimated the severity of a symptomatic lesion. Examining this series, it appears that the cases in which clinically useful information was provided by arteriography could have been identified by the clinical circumstances or a carefully performed duplex scan.

Initial Reports of CEA without Arteriography (1979 to 1985)

The first reports of CEA without preoperative arteriography came from Europe. By the late 1970s, von Reutern and colleagues in Germany had started to perform CEAs on the basis of noninvasive studies in selected cases.[112] In 1982 Blackshear and Connar published the first English-language report of CEA without preoperative arteriography.[113] They had four patients with documented severe contrast media allergies who presented with symptoms of carotid territory TIAs. Their patients were studied with a combination of ultrasonic arteriography and pulsed Doppler spectral waveform analysis. A significant stenosis at the level of the carotid bifurcation was identified ipsilateral to the symptomatic hemisphere in each case. Five carotid endarterectomies were performed without complications, and in each case the operative findings and pathologic specimens confirmed the preoperative diagnosis.

Reports by Gonzalez and coworkers and Crew and colleagues were the first to describe the use of duplex scanning without confirmatory arteriography as a means for evaluating patients prior to CEA. Gonzalez mentioned several CEAs performed without preoperative arteriography in a report on their use of oculoplethysmography and duplex scanning for postoperative follow-up.[114] They proceeded directly to operation in six patients with contrast allergy, two who refused arteriography, and six more who had prior arteriograms and later developed new neurologic symptoms. Crew and colleagues presented data from a four-year period during which they performed 65 CEAs without arteriography.[115,116] This approach was used electively, not just for patients who had contrast allergies or refused arteriography. They had no deaths and a 3 percent perioperative stroke rate. Pathologic evaluation confirmed the preoperative diagnosis in each case.

Changes in Practice Patterns (1986 to Present)

The practice of CEA without preoperative arteriography was used initially for patients who had specific contraindications to arteriography. Relative contraindications that have prompted CEA without arteriography include contrast allergy, progression of previously documented carotid disease, patient fear of arteriography, and severe peripheral vascular disease that interferes with femoral artery catheterization.[59,113,115] In addition, arteriography is not always feasible in patients who require an urgent operation, such as those with evolving strokes[59] and patients with concomitant carotid and coronary artery disease requiring urgent coronary bypass.[115,117] This experience led to a gradual change in practice patterns and a greater reliance on the information obtained by duplex scanning.

Recognizing the advantages of avoiding preoperative arteriography, some surgeons adopted this approach as routine, reserving arteriography for specific indications.[57,59,107,118–120] In the largest prospective series, Hill and coworkers reported 130 consecutive CEAs without arteriography, all in symptomatic patients.[118] During this period they obtained only one arteriogram that confirmed the duplex scan finding of a distal internal carotid artery occlusion. Operative findings confirmed the preoperative diagnoses. There was no operative mortality, one stroke, two TIAs, and one asymptomatic carotid occlusion.

While there are no prospective case-control series that compare the outcome of CEA with and without arteriography, there are large series that offer historical controls. In 1984 Wagner and coworkers reported that they obtained arteriograms prior to CEA in 95 percent of cases.[121] By the two-year period 1988 to 1989 this proportion had decreased to only 32 percent. Patients having operations after preoperative arteriography ($n = 484$) had the same perioperative stroke and death rates as those who had operations on the basis of duplex scanning alone ($n = 255$). During the same period, Ranaboldo and colleagues reported a similar shift in their practice patterns and also found no change in perioperative outcomes.[119]

How Frequently Is It Practical?

The initial reports[57,59,107,112,113,115–121] and subsequent clinical reviews[122–125] all indicate that CEA without preoperative arteriography is effective and safe, but they stress that it is not appropriate for every case. How often can patients with suspected significant carotid artery disease be completely evaluated without arteriography?

This question was examined in a step-wise fashion at the University of Washington. Since essentially all patients at that institution with known or suspected carotid artery disease have a duplex scan, the first step was to determine retrospectively how often arteriography added useful or important information to the clinical evaluation and duplex scan findings. Based on a review of hospital records, it appeared that no important information was added by the arteriogram in 83 percent of cases. In the minority of cases in which arteriography yielded clinically valuable data, the need for arteriography was evident from the patient's circumstances or duplex scan findings.[109]

This was followed by a prospective study of decision-making by vascular surgeons performing CEA.[126] For each case, the surgeon's management plan was recorded after a clinical evaluation and review of the duplex scan findings, but before arteriography. This plan was later compared to the patient's ultimate clinical management. There were 94 carotid arteries considered for endarterectomy in this study. Carotid duplex scans were diagnostic in 87 of the 94 cases (93 percent). The carotid lesion was incompletely assessed by duplex scanning in seven patients for the following reasons: the disease was not limited to the distal common or proximal internal carotid artery ($n = 4$); anatomic or pathologic features of the carotid artery interfered with imaging or accurate Doppler assessment ($n = 1$); and an internal carotid artery occlusion could not be distinguished from a high-grade stenosis ($n = 2$). When a technically adequate duplex scan showed significant carotid bifurcation disease, arteriography contributed information that affected the clinical management in only a single case (1 percent). This patient had a middle cerebral artery occlusion distal to a high-grade carotid bifurcation stenosis and went on to have a fatal stroke without operation (Fig. 21-7). Clinical assessment and duplex scanning were sufficient for the preoperative evaluation of 93 percent of the candidates for CEA.

Acceptability of the Approach

Available data suggest that vascular surgeons consider CEA without preoperative arteriography to be within acceptable standards of surgical practice. In 1985 Baker surveyed 494 practicing vascular surgeons across the United States to determine how noninvasive tests were being used.[35] For cerebrovascular testing, oculoplethysmography and periorbital Doppler testing were still widely used; however, acceptance of newer ultrasound technology was confirmed by the finding that 71 percent used some imaging modality. At that time, 19 percent of the survey respondents had performed CEA on the basis of duplex scanning, direct Doppler examination, or Doppler imaging, but most still reserved CEA without arteriography for exceptional circumstances.

Seven years later, in 1992, the members of the Pacific Northwest Vascular Society were surveyed about their approach to CEA and how they used preoperative tests.[127] Each of the 80 respondents had an average of 16 years in practice and had performed an average of 26 CEAs the previous year. In this survey, the proportion reporting performance of CEA

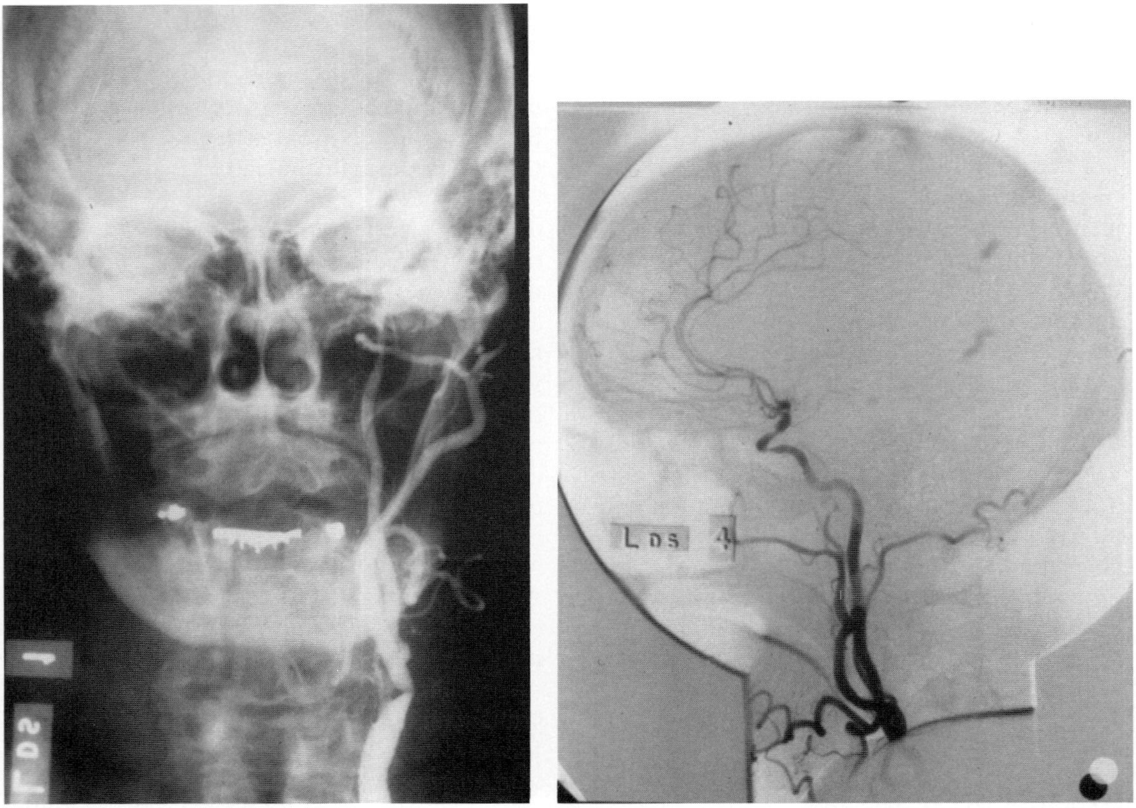

A *B*

Figure 21-7. Arteriography after good functional recovery in this patient who presented with a left hemispheric stroke demonstrated both a tight stenosis at the origin of the left internal carotid artery (*A*) and occlusion of the left middle cerebral artery at its origin (*B*). This is an extreme example of a "tandem lesion." Because of these findings the patient was not offered CEA. Four months later the internal carotid artery occluded, resulting in a fatal stroke, as documented by CT scan (*C*).

without arteriography was 63 percent. Most surgeons used this approach only when there were specific contraindications to arteriography, but several stated that duplex scanning alone had become their routine preoperative evaluation.

FUTURE DIRECTIONS: MAGNETIC RESONANCE ANGIOGRAPHY

Magnetic resonance angiography (MRA) has been proposed as another noninvasive means to select patients for CEA (Chap. 13).[61,128–130] MRA usually is obtained with a magnetic resonance image study of the brain; thus, a single examination can provide both structural and vascular information. Flowing blood causes a localized signal loss, and these areas of attenuation are computer-reconstructed in either two or three dimensions to yield images of both the extracranial and intracranial vessels. Magnetic resonance techniques may be superior to high-resolution B-mode imaging for plaque characterization.[131] Since its first clini-

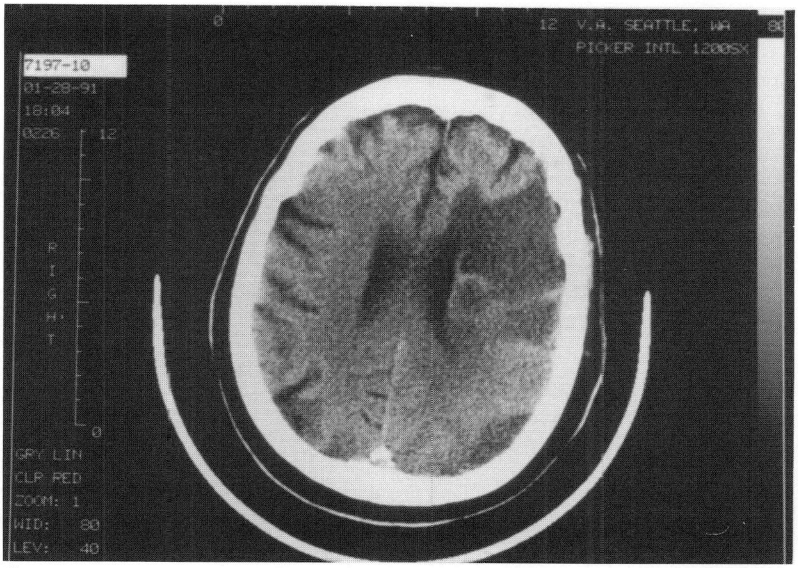

C

Figure 21-7. *(Continued)*.

cal applications in 1985, the hardware and imaging software have dramatically improved, but MRA remains subject to a variety of artifacts that can exaggerate or mimic the appearance of stenoses.[132] These limitations may be overcome by future technologic advances.

MRA can increase the costs of diagnosis. Because charges for a complete magnetic resonance study can be three to four times the cost of a carotid duplex scan,[61] MRA is not an appropriate screening examination. Thus, patients typically get referred for an MRA after a duplex scan demonstrates disease of the carotid bifurcation, adding to the total cost of the diagnostic evaluation. However, if MRA obviates the need for an otherwise indicated arteriogram, there will be a net cost savings.

Studies evaluating the accuracy of MRA for assessing carotid bifurcation disease have not found it to be more accurate than duplex scanning. In a prospective study of 128 patients, Wesbey and coworkers showed that duplex scanning and MRA were equal in their correlation with contrast arteriography.[129] Adequate images were not always obtained with MRA, and nondiagnostic tests occurred in 10 of the 128 patients. Riles and coworkers found duplex scanning to be slightly more accurate than MRA.[128] A total of 25 carotid arteries were evaluated in 42 patients by conventional cerebral arteriography, duplex scanning, and MRA. They found that MRA correlated exactly with conventional arteriography in 52 percent, while duplex scanning correlated with conventional arteriography in 65 percent. Compared with conventional arteriography, both of the noninvasive methods tended to overestimate the degree of stenosis. The tendency of MRA to overestimate the degree of internal carotid stenosis and problems distinguishing high-grade stenosis from occlusion have been observed in several other studies.[61,128,132,133] However, while Turnipseed and colleagues found that MRA tended to overestimate moderate stenoses, in another smaller study they obtained excellent correlations between MRA and arteriography for lesions of 70 percent or greater internal carotid artery stenosis.[61] Edelman and coworkers found that MRA correctly identified 17 internal carotid occlusions in 202 carotid bifurcations.[132]

The additional information about the intracranial circulation that MRA provides is probably of limited value. There has not been any validation of the accuracy of MRA for the diagnosis of intracranial atherosclerotic occlusive disease. It is still difficult to separate flow-related artifacts from true stenotic lesions, although new technology may solve this problem in the near future.[134] However, even if MRA information about the intracranial circulation is shown to be valid, studies using arteriography indicate that the presence of intracranial disease does not affect the perioperative or late outcome after CEA.[74–77] While magnetic resonance imaging and MRA are techniques that may be valuable in the evaluation of patients with carotid artery disease, the appropriate clinical role of these methods has not been established, and their routine use is limited by the relatively high cost.[135]

GUIDELINES FOR CEA WITHOUT ARTERIOGRAPHY

It should be emphasized that the selective use of arteriography before CEA requires that the surgeon consider the specific duplex scan findings, the technical quality of the study, and the clinical status of the patient. Algorithms for the preoperative evaluation of patients with carotid artery disease based on selective use of arteriography are given in Figs. 21-8 and 21-9.

No surgeon would consider operating solely on the basis of a radiologist's report of the arteriographic findings. Before planning and performing an operation, the responsible surgeon needs to review personally whatever diagnostic studies have been obtained. When arteriography has been omitted from the preoperative evaluation, the surgeon should review the

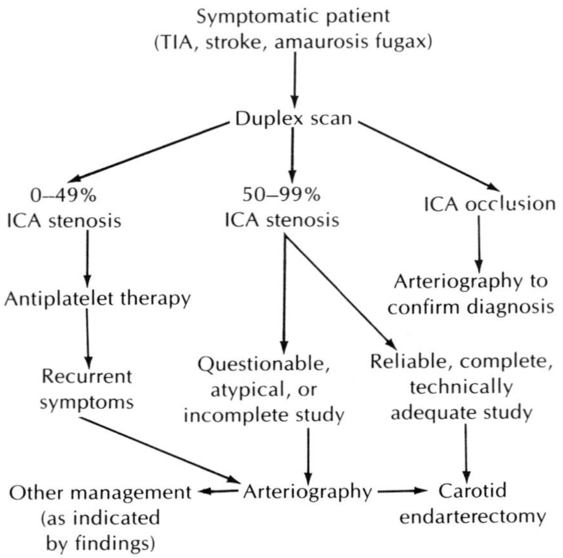

Figure 21-8. Management algorithm for patients with symptomatic carotid artery disease.

duplex scan findings, confirm the interpretation, and make a judgment about the adequacy of the diagnostic information before proceeding with surgery. If information from the initial diagnostic studies incompletely explains the clinical findings, further evaluation is required.

Indications for Selective Use of Arteriography

Even with the best noninvasive vascular laboratory there will be some cases that are insufficiently evaluated without arteriography. In general, these cases can be identified by clinical criteria or duplex scan findings. The conditions that usually require arteriography are listed below. The designation of indications for arteriography as absolute or relative admittedly is subjective.

Absolute Indications for Preoperative Arteriography There are a number of situations that would generally be considered as absolute indications for contrast arteriography before CEA. These include the following:

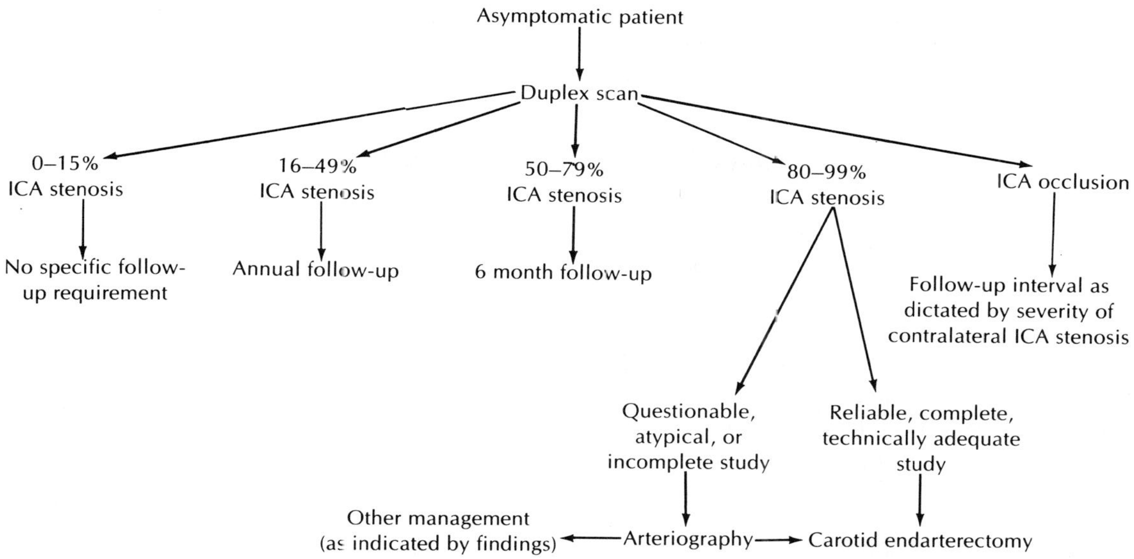

Figure 21-9. Management algorithm for patients with asymptomatic carotid artery disease.

1. Undocumented accuracy or uncertain reliability of the vascular laboratory performing the duplex scan.
2. The duplex scan is technically inadequate or incomplete.
3. The duplex scan suggests significant proximal common or distal internal carotid artery disease (either by imaging or spectral waveform analysis).
4. The duplex scan indicates unusual carotid anatomy that would affect the operation performed or the accuracy of the duplex scan (carotid coil or kink).
5. Nonhemispheric neurologic symptoms.
6. Clinically significant posterior circulation disease is suspected.
7. Nonatherosclerotic cerebrovascular disease is suspected (fibromuscular dysplasia, dissection).

High-quality noninvasive vascular studies are not universally available. Critics of CEA without preoperative arteriography can cite reports of several recent clinical trials that examined the role of CEA for symptomatic and asymptomatic carotid disease. Significant variability in the results of carotid duplex scanning between centers remains a major problem.[40] The NASCET,[6] the Asymptomatic Carotid Atherosclerosis Study,[136] and the Veterans Affairs Cooperative Trial[137] all found relatively poor correlations between noninvasive vascular laboratory findings and arteriography. However, the instrumentation and techniques for noninvasive carotid testing were not standardized in these studies.

Arteriography is also required if the surgical procedure may be something other than a routine CEA, or when the duplex scan has provided insufficient information to establish that appropriate indications for surgical intervention are present. Clinical examples include patients requiring median sternotomy for innominate artery disease, subclavian-carotid bypass for proximal common carotid artery disease, or the use of special maneuvers to expose the distal cervical internal carotid artery.

It is practical to eliminate routine preoperative arteriography because atherosclerosis of the carotid artery has a characteristic clinical presentation and the pathologic process is frequently limited to the carotid bifurcation. Arteriography remains appropriate when evaluating other types of cerebrovascular disease. Examples include determining the extent of a spontaneous carotid dissection, evaluation of patients with suspected fibromuscular dysplasia or other nonatherosclerotic arterial disease (Chap. 5), and the assessment of posterior circulation symptoms.

Relative Indications for Preoperative Arteriography Other situations in which arteriography may be indicated include: (1) recurrent carotid stenosis; (2) a fixed neurologic deficit; and (3) CEA for other than standard indications (TIAs associated with an ulcerated but nonstenotic plaque).

The relative indications are not universally agreed upon. Recurrent carotid stenosis due to intimal hyperplasia has a distribution and natural history different from atherosclerosis, but it can usually be fully evaluated by duplex scanning (Chap. 27).[59,114] Fixed neurologic deficits have been associated with more severe intracranial disease,[126] but the importance of such lesions in patients requiring CEA for significant carotid bifurcation disease is uncertain. Some surgeons obtain an arteriogram to evaluate patients without significant carotid stenosis who have recurrent TIAs despite antiplatelet therapy (Fig. 21-10). Others point out that ultrasound may be more sensitive than arteriography for detecting nonstenotic ulcerated atheromatous lesions.[60]

CONCLUSIONS

The costs and associated morbidity of arteriography can be reduced markedly by more selective use of this diagnostic modality. If omitting arteriography were to result in higher complication rates, the inappropriate selection of patients for operation, or the inappropriate exclusion of patients from indicated surgery, the total costs of patient care could increase.

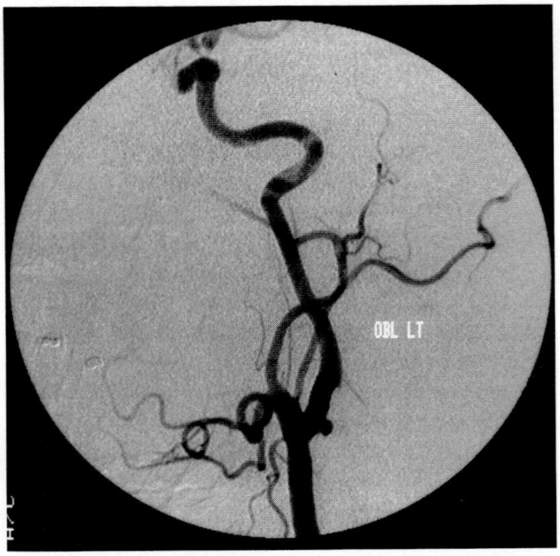

Figure 21-10. Although duplex scanning showed only mild spectral broadening consistent with 1 to 15 percent diameter reduction, arteriography demonstrated a deeply ulcerated lesion. This patient had recurring episodes of amaurosis fugax, despite aspirin therapy. CEA eliminated the symptoms.

However, several studies have demonstrated that arteriography does not change patient selection for CEA, and there are no data to suggest that outcomes after CEA are better if arteriography is routinely obtained.

Duplex scanning is safe and reliable, and several series suggest that it is sufficient to accurately characterize carotid artery disease in the majority of patients. However, it is not adequate in all cases. With experience, the unusual situations that impair duplex scan accuracy are recognizable, and further diagnostic testing can be obtained. While the role of ultrasonic methods to assess intracranial disease is being explored, experience with arteriography suggests that this may not be important.

Selective use of preoperative arteriography is not a revolutionary approach to carotid artery surgery. Surgeons who now perform CEA on the basis of noninvasive studies have not made sudden changes in their practice patterns, nor have they completely abandoned contrast arteriography. As the indications for CEA are better defined, and as the capabilities and limitations of different imaging modalities are better understood, diagnostic algorithms will be developed to meet the clinical requirements. The informed surgeon will adopt an approach that considers the scope, quality, and costs of locally available diagnostic services. The selective use of arteriography before CEA is an acceptable approach when the costs and potential morbidity of diagnostic studies are considered and when the diagnostic evaluation is tailored to the individual patient's situation.

REFERENCES

1. Kempczinski RF, Thiele BL, Strandness DE Jr, Bandyk DF: Accreditation of vascular laboratories. *J Vasc Surg* 12:629, 1990.
2. Roederer G, Langlois Y, Jäger K, et al: The natural history of carotid artery disease in asymptomatic patients with cervical bruits. *Stroke* 15:605, 1984.
3. Moore WS: Diagnosis and management of patients with asymptomatic carotid artery bruit. *Compr Ther* 16:46, 1990.
4. Hill SL: The positive effect of accurate noninvasive studies in decreasing the number of normal radiographic studies. *Am Surg* 55:543, 1989.
5. Zierler RE, Kohler TR, Strandness DE Jr: Duplex scanning of normal or minimally diseased carotid arteries: Correlation with arteriography and clinical outcome. *J Vasc Surg* 12:447, 1990.
6. NASCET collaborators: Beneficial effect of carotid endarterectomy in symptomatic patients with high-grade carotid stenosis. *N Engl J Med* 325:445, 1991.
7. Moore WS, Mohr JP, Najafi H, et al: Carotid endarterectomy: Practice guidelines. Report of the Society for Vascular Surgery and the North American Chapter of the International Society for Cardiovascular Surgery. *J Vasc Surg* 15:469, 1992.
8. Beebe HG, Clagett GP, DeWeese JA, et al: Assessing risk associated with carotid endarterectomy. *Stroke* 20:314, 1989.
9. Hobson RW II, Weiss DG, Fields WS, et al: Efficacy of carotid endarterectomy for asymptomatic carotid stenosis. *N Engl J Med* 328: 221, 1993.
10. Chambers BR, Norris JW: Outcome in patients with asymptomatic neck bruits. *N Engl J Med* 315:860, 1986.
11. Moneta G, Taylor D, Nicholls S, et al: Operative versus nonoperative management of asymptomatic high-grade carotid artery stenosis: Improved results with endarterectomy. *Stroke* 18:1005, 1987.
12. Moneta G, Taylor D, Zierler R, et al: Asymptomatic high-grade internal carotid artery stenosis: Is stratification according to risk factors or duplex spectral analysis possible? *J Vasc Surg* 10:475, 1989.
13. Thiele BL: Standards in noninvasive cerebrovascular testing, in Bernstein EF (ed): *Recent Advances in Noninvasive Diagnostic Techniques in Vascular Disease*. St. Louis, CV Mosby, p 15, 1990.
14. Chikos P, Fisher L, Hirsch J, et al: Observer variability in evaluating extracranial carotid artery stenosis. *Stroke* 14:885, 1983.
15. Ricotta JJ, Schenk EA, Ekholm SE, DeWeese JA: Angiographic and pathologic correlates in carotid artery disease. *Surgery* 99:284, 1986.
16. Ricotta JJ, Bryan FA, Bond MG, et al: Multicenter validation study of real-time (B-mode) ultrasound, arteriography, and pathologic examination. *J Vasc Surg* 6:512, 1987.
17. Dawson DL, Strandness DE Jr: Arterial wall thickness with high-resolution B-mode imaging, in Bernstein EF (ed): *Vascular Diagnosis*, 4th ed. Chicago, Mosby-Year Book, p 420, 1993.
18. Cato FR, Bandyk DF, Livigni D, et al: Carotid collateral circulation decreases the diagnostic accuracy of duplex scanning. *Bruit* 10:68, 1986.
19. Hayes AC, Johnston KW, Baker WH, et al: The effect of contralateral disease on the carotid Doppler frequency. *Surgery* 103:19, 1988.

20. Spadone DP, Barkmeier LD, Hodgson KJ, et al: Contralateral internal carotid artery stenosis or occlusion: Pitfall of correct ipsilateral classification—a study performed with color-flow imaging. *J Vasc Surg* 11:642, 1990.
21. Walters GK, Jones CE, Meyd CJ, et al: The role of carotid duplex ultrasonography in the therapeutic algorithm of extracranial carotid artery disease. *J Vasc Tech* 17:177, 1993.
22. Fujitani RM, Mills JL, Wang LM, Taylor SM: The effect of unilateral internal carotid arterial occlusion upon contralateral duplex study: Criteria for accurate interpretation. *J Vasc Surg* 16:459, 1992.
23. O'Connor TJ, Coble RV, Embry BM, Isobe JH, Gaskin TA: Pseudo-occlusion of the internal carotid artery: How not to miss it. *South Med J* 79:588, 1986.
24. Bornstein N, Beloev Z, Norris J: The limitations of diagnosis of carotid occlusion by Doppler ultrasound. *Ann Surg* 207:315, 1988.
25. Maiuri F, Gallicchio B, Cinalli G: Diagnosis of carotid artery occlusion by duplex scanning. *Neurol Res* 12:75, 1990.
26. Bodily KC, Phillips DJ, Thiele BL, Strandness DE Jr: Noninvasive detection of internal carotid artery occlusion. *Angiology* 32:517, 1981.
27. Breslau PJ, Fell G, Phillips DJ, et al: Evaluation of carotid bifurcation disease: The role of common carotid artery velocity patterns. *Arch Surg* 117:58, 1982.
28. Rosendahl T, Muller C, Foran R: Internal carotid and vertebral duplex scanning for the determination of brain death (abstr). *J Vasc Tech* 17:195, 1993.
29. Archie JP Jr: Carotid endarterectomy for string sign internal carotid arteries. Presented at the 1993 meeting of the North American Chapter, International Society for Cardiovascular Surgery. Washington, DC.
30. Bryant PS, Comeaux ME, Harkrider WW Jr: Color Doppler imaging versus angiography in near-total occlusion of the internal carotid artery (abstr). *J Vasc Tech* 17:199, 1993.
31. Perler BA, Burdick JF, Williams GM: Progression to total occlusion is an underrecognized complication of the medical management of carotid disease. *J Vasc Surg* 14:821, 1991.
32. Gee W: Carotid physiology with ocular pneumoplethysmography. *Stroke* 13:666, 1982.
33. Gee W: Physiologic principles of ocular pneumoplethysmography, in Bernstein EF (ed): *Noninvasive Diagnostic Techniques in Vascular Disease,* 2d ed. St. Louis, CV Mosby, p 57, 1982.
34. Gee W, Reed JF: Ocular pneumoplethysmographic evaluation of carotid lesions: Gee method, in: *Current Therapy in Vascular Surgery,* 2d ed. Toronto, BC Decker, p 20, 1992.
35. Baker JD: How vascular surgeons use noninvasive testing. *J Vasc Surg* 4:272, 1986.
36. Bergeron P, Benichou H, Rudondy P, et al: Stroke prevention during carotid surgery in high risk patients (value of transcranial Doppler and local anesthesia). *J Cardiovasc Surg* 32:713, 1991.
37. Jorgensen LG, Schroeder TV: Transcranial Doppler for detection of cerebral ischaemia during carotid endarterectomy. *Eur J Vasc Surg* 6:142, 1992.
38. Bernstein EF: Role of transcranial Doppler in carotid surgery. *Surg Clin North Am* 70:225, 1990.
39. Hankey GJ, Warlow CP, Molyneux AJ: Complications of cerebral angiography for patients with mild carotid territory ischaemia being considered for carotid endarterectomy. *J Neurol Neurosurg Psychiatry* 53:542, 1990.
40. Masaryk TJ, Obuchowski NA: Noninvasive carotid imaging: Caveat emptor. *Radiology* 186:325, 1993.
41. Vitek JJ: Femoro-cerebral angiography: Analysis of 2,000 consecutive examinations, special emphasis on carotid arteries catheterization in older patients. *AJR* 118:633, 1973.
42. Grzyska V, Freitag J, Zeumer H: Selective intraarterial DSA: Complication rate and control of risk factors. *Neuroradiology* 32:296, 1990.
43. Hass WK, Fields WS, North RR, et al: Joint study of extracranial arterial occlusion. II. Arteriography, techniques, sites, and complications. *JAMA* 203:159, 1968.
44. Mani RL, Eisenberg RL: Complications of catheter cerebral arteriography: Analysis of 5000 procedures. II. Relation of complication rates to clinical and arteriographic diagnoses. *AJR* 131:867, 1978.

45. McIvor J, Steiner TJ, Perkin GD, et al: Neurological morbidity of arch and carotid arteriography in cerebrovascular disease. The influence of contrast medium and radiologist. *Br J Radiol* 60:117, 1987.
46. Faught E, Trader SD, Hanna GR: Cerebral complications of angiography for transient ischemia and stroke: Prediction of risk. *Neurology* 29:4, 1979.
47. Mani RL, Eisenberg RL, McDonald EJ, et al: Complications of catheter cerebral arteriography: Analysis of 5,000 procedures. I. Criteria and incidence. *AJR* 131:861, 1978.
48. Madowitz JS, Schweiger MJ: Severe anaphylactoid reaction to contrast media. Recurrence despite premedication with diphenhydramine and prednisone. *JAMA* 241:2813, 1979.
49. Martin-Paredero V, Dixon SM, Baker JD, et al: Risk of renal failure after major angiography. *Arch Surg* 118:1417, 1983.
50. Gomes A, Lois J, Baker J, et al: Acute renal dysfunction in high-risk patients after angiography. Comparison of ionic and nonionic contrast media. *Radiology* 170:65, 1989.
51. Berkseth RO, Kjellstrand CM: Radiologic contrast-induced nephropathy. *Med Clin North Am* 68:351, 1984.
52. Hessel S, Adams D, Abrams H: Complications of angiography. *Radiology* 138:273, 1981.
53. Earnest F, Forbes G, Sandok B, et al: Complications of cerebral angiography: Prospective assessment of risk. *AJR* 142:247, 1984.
54. Dion J, Gates P, Fox A, et al: Clinical events following neuroangiography: A prospective study. *Stroke* 18:997, 1987.
55. Pokras R, Dyken ML: Dramatic changes in the performance of endarterectomy for diseases of the extracranial arteries of the head. *Stroke* 19:1289, 1988.
56. Corson JD, Chang BB, Shah DM, et al: The influence of anesthetic choice on carotid endarterectomy outcome. *Arch Surg* 122:807, 1987.
57. Kraiss LW, Kilberg L, Critch S, Johanson KH: Cost-effective carotid endarterectomy. Presented at the 1993 meeting of the Washington State Chapter, American College of Surgeons, Sunriver, OR.
58. O'Brien MS, Ricotta JJ: Conserving resources after carotid endarterectomy: Selective use of the intensive care unit. *J Vasc Surg* 14:796, 1991.
59. Thomas GI, Jones TW, Stavney LS, et al: Carotid endarterectomy after Doppler ultrasonographic examination without angiography. *Am J Surg* 151:616, 1986.
60. Goodson S, Flanigan D, Bishara R, et al: Can carotid duplex scanning supplant arteriography in patients with focal carotid territory symptoms? *J Vasc Surg* 5:551, 1987.
61. Turnipseed WD, Kennell TW, Turski PA, et al: Combined use of duplex imaging and magnetic resonance angiography for evaluation of patients with symptomatic ipsilateral high-grade stenosis. *J Vasc Surg* 17:832, 1993.
62. Taylor DC, Strandness DE Jr: Carotid artery duplex scanning. *J Clin Ultrasound* 15:635, 1987.
63. Zierler RE: Carotid artery evaluation by duplex scanning. *Semin Vasc Surg* 1:9, 1988.
64. Roederer G, Langlois Y, Jäger K, et al: A simple spectral parameter for accurate classification of severe carotid disease. *Bruit* 8:174, 1984.
65. Kohler T, Langlois Y, Roederer G, et al: Sources of variability in carotid duplex examination: A prospective study. *Ultrasound Med Biol* 11:571, 1985.
66. Akers DL, Markowitz IA, Kerstien MD: The value of aortic arch study in the evaluation of cerebrovascular disease. *Am J Surg* 154:230, 1987.
67. Ricotta JJ, Holen J, Schenk E, et al: Is routine angiography necessary prior to carotid endarterectomy? *J Vasc Surg* 1:96, 1984.
68. Ackerstaff R, Hoeneveld H, Slowikowski J, et al: Ultrasonic duplex scanning in atherosclerotic disease of the innominate, subclavian, and vertebral arteries: A comparative study with angiography. *Ultrasound Med Biol* 10:409, 1984.
69. Akers DL, Bell WH III, Kerstein MD: Does intracranial dye study contribute to evaluation of carotid artery disease? *Am J Surg* 156:87, 1988.
70. Angel F, Cross JN, Tedeschi GM, et al: Ischaemic carotid strokes. Angiographic investigation of 523 patients. *Scott Med J* 17:1, 1972.
71. Bauer RB, Sheehan S, Weschler N, Meyer JS:

Arteriographic study of sites, incidence, and treatment of arteriosclerotic cerebrovascular lesions. *Neurology (Minneap)* 12:698, 1962.
72. Borozan PG, Schuler JJ, LaRosa MP, et al: The natural history of isolated carotid siphon stenosis. *J Vasc Surg* 1:744, 1984.
73. Harrison MJG, Marshall J: Angiographic appearance of carotid bifurcation in patients with completed stroke, transient ischemic attacks, and cerebral tumour. *Br Med J* 1:205, 1976.
74. Mackey WC, O'Donnell TF Jr, Callow AD: Carotid endarterectomy in patients with intracranial vascular disease: Short-term risk and long-term outcome. *J Vasc Surg* 10:432, 1989.
75. Mattos MA, van Bemmelen PS, Hodgson KJ, et al: The influence of carotid siphon stenosis on short- and long-term outcome after carotid endarterectomy. *J Vasc Surg* 17:902, 1993.
76. Roederer GO, Langlois YE, Chan ARW, et al: Is siphon disease important in predicting outcome of carotid endarterectomy? *Arch Surg* 118:1177, 1983.
77. Schuler JJ, Flanigan DP, Lim LT, et al: The effect of carotid siphon stenosis on stroke rate, death, and relief of symptoms following elective carotid endarterectomy. *Surgery* 92: 1058, 1982.
78. Eisenberg RL, Nemzek WR, Moore WS, Mani RL: Relationship of transient ischemic attacks and angiographically demonstrable lesions of the carotid artery. *Stroke* 8:483, 1977.
79. Sundt TM, Sandok BA, Whisnant JP: Carotid endarterectomy. Complications and preoperative assessment of risk. *Mayo Clin Proc* 50:301, 1975.
80. Day AL, Rhoton AL, Quisling RG: Resolving siphon stenosis after carotid endarterectomy. *Stroke* 11:278, 1980.
81. Blaisdell WF, Clauss RH, Galbraith JG, et al: Joint study of extracranial arterial occlusion. IV. A review of surgical considerations. *JAMA* 209:1889, 1969.
82. Wylie EJ, Ehrnfeld WK: *Extracranial Occlusive Cerebrovascular Disease: Diagnosis and Management*. Philadelphia, WB Saunders, 1970.
83. Fields WS: Selection of stroke patients for arterial reconstructive surgery. *Am J Surg* 125: 527, 1973.
84. Fields WS: Selection of patients with ischemic cerebrovascular disease for surgery. *World J Surg* 3:147, 1979.
85. Craig DR, Meguro K, Watridge C, et al: Intracranial internal carotid artery stenosis. *Stroke* 13:825, 1982.
86. Marzewski DJ, Furlan AJ, St. Louis P, et al: Intracranial internal carotid artery stenosis: Long-term prognosis. *Stroke* 13:821, 1982.
87. Ratinov G: Extradural intracranial portion of carotid artery: A clinicopathologic study. *Arch Neurol* 10:66, 1964.
88. Fisher CM, Gore I, Okabe N, et al: Calcification of the carotid siphon. *Circulation* 32:538, 1965.
89. Scotti G, Degrandi C: Intimal and medial calcifications of the carotid siphon and cerebrovascular disease. *Radiology* 116:667, 1975.
90. Adams HP Jr: Carotid stenosis and coexisting ipsilateral intracranial aneurysm. A problem in management. *Arch Neurol* 34:515, 1977.
91. Ladowski J, Webster M, Yonas H, et al: Carotid endarterectomy in patients with asymptomatic intracranial aneurysm. *Ann Surg* 200: 70, 1984.
92. Fields WS, Weibel J: Coincidental internal carotid artery stenosis and intracranial saccular aneurysm. *Trans Am Neurol Assoc* 95:237, 1970.
93. Portnoy HD, Avellanosa A: Carotid aneurysm and contralateral carotid stenosis with successful surgical treatment of both lesions. Case report. *J Neurosurg* 32:476, 1970.
94. Denton IC Jr, Gutmann L: Surgical treatment of symptomatic carotid stenosis and asymptomatic ipsilateral intracranial aneurysm. *J Neurosurg* 38:662, 1973.
95. Shoumaker RD, Avant WS, Cohen GH: Coincidental multiple asymptomatic intracranial aneurysms and symptomatic carotid stenosis. *Stroke* 7:504, 1976.
96. Stern J, Whelan M, Brisman R, Correll JW: Management of extracranial carotid stenosis and intracranial saccular aneurysm. *J Neurosurg* 51:147, 1979.
97. Orecchia PM, Clagett GP, Youkey JR, et al: Management of patients with symptomatic extracranial carotid artery disease and incidental

intracranial berry aneurysm. *J Vasc Surg* 2: 158, 1985.

98. Weibers DO, Whisnant JP, O'Fallon WM: The natural history of unruptured intracranial aneurysm. *N Engl J Med* 304:696, 1981.
99. Dell S: Asymptomatic cerebral aneurysm: Assessment of its risk of rupture. *Neurosurgery* 10:162, 1982.
100. Silverstein A: Arteriography of stroke. I. Incidence of mass lesions in patients with clinical diagnosis of occlusive cerebrovascular disease. *Arch Neurol* 12:387, 1965.
101. Weisberg L, Nice C, Katz M, et al: Rapid onset of neurological deficit (stroke syndrome): aneurysmal subarachnoid hemorrhage, in *Cerebral Computed Tomography: A Text-Atlas*. Philadelphia, WB Saunders, p 135, 1984.
102. Atkinson DP, Jacobs LA, Weaver AW: Elective carotid resection for squamous cell carcinoma of the head and neck. *Am J Surg* 148:483, 1984.
103. Martin JD, Valentine RJ, Myers SI, et al: Is routine CT scanning necessary in the preoperative evaluation of patients undergoing carotid endarterectomy? *J Vasc Surg* 14:267, 1991.
104. Sumner D, Russell J, Miles R: Are noninvasive tests sufficiently accurate to identify patients in need of carotid arteriography? *Surgery* 91:700, 1982.
105. Walsh J, Markowitz I, Kerstein MD: Carotid endarterectomy for amaurosis fugax without angiography. *Am J Surg* 142:172, 1986.
106. Flanigan DP, Schuler JJ, Vogel M, et al: The role of carotid duplex scanning in surgical decision making. *J Vasc Surg* 2:15, 1985.
107. Moore WS, Ziomek S, Quiñones-Baldrich WJ, et al: Can clinical evaluation and noninvasive testing substitute for arteriography in the evaluation of carotid artery disease? *Ann Surg* 208:91, 1988.
108. Farmilo RW, Scott DJ, Cole SE, et al: Role of duplex scanning in the selection of patients for carotid endarterectomy. *Br J Surg* 77:388, 1990.
109. Dawson DL, Zierler RE, Kohler TR: Role of arteriography in the preoperative evaluation of carotid artery disease. *Am J Surg* 161:619, 1991.
110. Gertler JP, Cambria RP, Kistler JP, et al: Carotid surgery without arteriography: Noninvasive selection of patients. *Ann Vasc Surg* 5:253, 1991.
111. Geuder JW, Lamparello PJ, Riles TS, et al: Is duplex scanning sufficient evaluation before carotid endarterectomy? *J Vasc Surg* 9:193, 1989.
112. von Reutern GM, Ortega-Schrkamp E, Spillner S: Is noninvasive Doppler sonography alone sufficient to indicate carotid surgery? Proceedings of the 9th Salzburg Conference, Salzburg, Austria, p 46, 1979.
113. Blackshear W, Connar R: Carotid endarterectomy without angiography. *J Cardiovasc Surg* 23:477, 1982.
114. Gonzalez LL, Partusch L, Wirth P: Noninvasive carotid artery evaluation following endarterectomy. *J Vasc Surg* 1:403, 1984.
115. Crew JR, Dean M, Johnson JM, et al: Carotid surgery without arteriography. *Am J Surg* 148:217, 1984.
116. Crew JR, Dean M, Johnson JJ: Carotid surgery without angiography. *Surgical Rounds* Sept: 18, 1985.
117. Marshall WG Jr, Kouchoukos NT, Murphy SF, Pelate C: Carotid endarterectomy based on duplex scanning without preoperative arteriography. *Circulation* 78(suppl I):I-1, 1988.
118. Hill JC, Carbonneau K, Baliga PK, et al: Safe extracranial vascular evaluation and surgery without preoperative arteriography. *Ann Vasc Surg* 4:34, 1990.
119. Ranaboldo C, Davies J, Chant A: Duplex scanning alone before carotid endarterectomy: A 5-year experience. *Eur J Vasc Surg* 5:415, 1991.
120. Balas P, Pagratis N, Massouridou E, Ioannou N: Is cerebral arteriography necessary for decision making in carotid endarterectomy? *Int Angiol* 10:213, 1991.
121. Wagner WH, Treiman RL, Cossman DV, et al: The diminishing role of diagnostic arteriography in carotid artery disease: Duplex scanning as definitive preoperative study. *Ann Vasc Surg* 5:105, 1991.
122. Sanders R: Duplex scanning for carotid artery disease: Is angiographic confirmation required? *Am J Surg* 156:2, 1988.

123. Gelabert HA, Moore WS: Carotid endarterectomy without angiography. *Surg Clin North Am* 70:213, 1990.
124. Balas P: Are the ultrasonic imaging technics (duplex or triplex) alone sufficient for decision-making in carotid endarterectomy? Pros and cons (editorial). *Int Angiol* 11:91, 1992.
125. Polak JF: Noninvasive carotid evaluation: Carpe diem. *Radiology* 186:329, 1993.
126. Dawson DL, Zierler RE, Strandness DE Jr, et al: The role of duplex scanning and arteriography before carotid endarterectomy: A prospective study. *J Vasc Surg* 18:73, 1993.
127. Dawson DL, Kohler TR: Results of a survey of PNWVS members: Role of duplex scanning prior to carotid endarterectomy. Annual Meeting of the Pacific Northwest Vascular Society. Tacoma, WA, 1992.
128. Riles TS, Eidelman EM, Litt AM, et al: Comparison of magnetic resonance angiography, conventional angiography, and duplex scanning. *Stroke* 23:341, 1992.
129. Wesbey GE, Bergan JJ, Moreland SI, et al: Cerebrovascular magnetic resonance angiography: A critical verification. *J Vasc Surg* 16: 619, 1992.
130. Polak JF, Kalina P, Donaldson MC, et al: Carotid endarterectomy: Preoperative evaluation of candidates with combined Doppler sonography and MR angiography. Work in progress. *Radiology* 186:333, 1993.
131. Vinitski S, Consigny PM, Shapiro MJ, et al: Magnetic resonance chemical shift and spectroscopy of atherosclerotic plaque. *Invest Radiol* 26:703, 1991.
132. Edelman RR: MR angiography, present and future. *AJR* 161:1, 1993.
133. Klop RB, Eikelboom BC, Mali WP, et al: Carotid bifurcation imaging: Magnetic resonance angiography compared to conventional angiography and Doppler ultrasound. *Eur J Vasc Surg* 7:245, 1993.
134. Urchuk SN, Plewes DB: Mechanism of flow-induced signal loss in MR angiography. *JMRI* 2:453, 1992.
135. Litt AW: MR angiography: Reaching adolescence. *AJR* 158:389, 1992.
136. Howard G, Chambless LE, Baker WH, et al: A multicenter validation study of Doppler ultrasound versus angiography. *J Stroke Cerebrovasc Dis* 1:166, 1991.
137. Mayberg MR, Wilson SE, Yatsu F, et al: Carotid endarterectomy and prevention of cerebral ischemia in symptomatic carotid stenosis. *JAMA* 266:3289, 1991.

Part Five

Surgical Management

22

Anesthesia for Carotid Surgery

Basil F. Matta
Arthur M. Lam

In symptomatic patients with severe carotid stenosis (70 to 99 percent diameter reduction), carotid endarterectomy confers a significant benefit.[1–3] There is no demonstrable benefit in patients with mild stenosis (0 to 29 percent),[2] but in moderate stenosis (30 to 69 percent) the situation is less clear, and clinical trials are still ongoing to establish its efficacy in preventing stroke. In asymptomatic patients, the effectiveness of carotid endarterectomy in preventing stroke remains controversial, despite a recent study that has shown some benefit.[4]

The major indications for carotid endarterectomy are transient ischemic attack (TIA) and reversible ischemic neurologic deficit (RIND). The prevalence of TIA increases with age from 16/100,000 between 45 and 54 years, to 69/100,000 between 55 and 64 years, and

220/100,000 in the 65 to 74 year group.[5] As the prevalence of coronary artery disease also increases with age, it is not surprising that the major cause of mortality and morbidity from carotid endarterectomy is myocardial infarction (MI). Irrespective of anesthetic and surgical technique, recent surveys indicate that the procedure is associated with a perioperative mortality of about 2 percent and a stroke rate of about 4 percent.[6] To realize the potential benefits of carotid surgery, it is essential to provide the optimal physiologic environment during the operation, and this necessitates a thorough understanding of the pathophysiology of carotid artery disease and the anesthetic implications.

PREOPERATIVE CONSIDERATIONS

The Mayo Clinic classification system is a well-accepted method for grading operative risk according to neurologic, medical, and angiographic findings (Table 22-1).[7] The primary complications of carotid surgery are MI and mild to severe neurologic deficits. Preoperative assessment must therefore include a thorough evaluation of cardiovascular and neurologic status, in addition to studies of the carotid lesions. The usefulness of this classification was recently reaffirmed.[8]

Neurologic System

Evaluation of the cerebrovascular system should document carefully the presence of transient or permanent neurologic deficits. This is essential as a baseline for assessing both postoperative progress and perioperative risk. Frequent daily TIAs, multiple neurologic deficits secondary to cerebral infarctions, or a progressive neurologic deficit increase the risk of new postoperative neurologic events.[7] Results of tests assessing the cerebrovascular system such as duplex scanning and cerebral angiography should be available.

Cardiovascular System

The occurrence of TIAs is a marker for generalized atherosclerosis, and many patients will have concomitant coronary artery disease. Among patients with TIAs, up to 18 percent have had previous MIs.[9] The annual long-term mortality rate from cardiac disease in these patients is 5 percent, similar to the 6 percent rate among patients with symptomatic triple-vessel coronary artery disease, and far

Table 22-1 The Mayo Clinic Classification System for Predicting Morbidity and Mortality of Carotid Endarterectomy[a]

Grade	Neurologic status[b]	Medical status[c]	Angiographic findings[d]	Risk of MI or stroke (%)
1	Stable	− risk factors	− lesions	1
2	Stable	− risk factors	+ lesions	2
3	Stable	+ risk factors	+ or − lesions	7
4	Unstable	+ or − risk factors	+ or − lesions	10

[a] +, presence of major medical risk factors or significant angiographic lesions; −, absence of major medical risk factors or significant angiographic lesions; MI, myocardial infarction.

[b] Neurologic factors contributing to unstable status: A progressing neurologic deficit; a deficit of less than 24 h duration; frequent daily TIAs, or neurologic deficits due to multiple cerebral infarctions.

[c] Medical risk factors: Angina pectoris or MI within 6 months of operation; congestive heart failure; severe hypertension (>180/110 mmHg); chronic obstructive pulmonary disease; age over 70 years; and severe obesity.

[d] Angiographic lesions considered significant: Occlusion of the contralateral internal carotid artery; stenosis involving the carotid siphon; extension of plaque proximal or distal to the carotid bulb; a high carotid bifurcation; and thrombus associated with an ulcerative lesion.

SOURCE: Adapted from Sundt TM Jr, Sandok BA, Whisnant JP: Carotid endarterectomy: Complications and preoperative assessment of risk. Mayo Clin Proc 50: 301, 1975.

exceeding the mortality rate from stroke.[9] The cardiac risk is further increased by other associated medical conditions, such as hypertension and obesity.

In evaluating the cardiovascular system, it should be kept in mind that coronary artery disease is present in over 55 percent of these patients.[10] Patients with coronary artery disease as determined by history, electrocardiography, or cardiac catheterization have an increased risk of postoperative MI (5 percent) compared to patients without coronary artery disease (0.5 percent).[11] Evidence of cardiac disease should be sought by careful history and thorough examination, noting the presence of angina and its severity, any previously documented MI, and symptoms or signs of cardiac failure. The electrocardiogram (ECG) should be examined for abnormalities of rhythm and evidence of previous infarction or ischemia. When indicated, a chest radiograph is obtained for evidence of cardiac failure. Further cardiac work-up, including an exercise ECG, radionuclide studies, or coronary angiography, may be necessary and such studies are best coordinated with a cardiologist.

Hypertension is also frequently present and must be well controlled, as postoperative hypertension and transient neurologic deficits are more frequent in patients with poor preoperative blood pressure control (blood pressure greater than 170/95 mmHg) than in those with adequate control or normotension.[11] In patients who remain hypertensive, abrupt normalization of blood pressure should be avoided in order to prevent cerebral ischemia and stroke.

Elective surgery should be postponed in patients with uncontrolled hypertension, unstable angina, congestive heart failure, or MI in the previous six months, since the perioperative cardiac risk is greatly increased. In some unstable patients, combined coronary artery bypass and carotid endarterectomy may be necessary, as discussed in Chap. 20.

Other Systems

Other medical conditions such as diabetes mellitus and chronic obstructive pulmonary disease are often present in patients requiring carotid surgery. Patients with chronic obstructive pulmonary disease need optimal medical treatment preoperatively, which may include bronchodilators, corticosteroids, physiotherapy, and incentive spirometry. Whenever possible, cigarette smoking should be stopped for six to eight weeks preoperatively. Diabetes mellitus has been shown to exist in about 20 percent of patients presenting for carotid endarterectomy, and most of these patients are insulin-dependent.[12] Adequate blood glucose control and absence of ketoacidosis must be confirmed preoperatively. In experimental studies, even modest elevations in brain glucose have been shown to augment postischemic cerebral injury.[13] Such manifestations of diabetes mellitus as renal failure, silent myocardial ischemia, autonomic and sensory neuropathy, and ophthalmic complications also must be looked for.

Last but not least, the patient's preoperative medications should be reviewed. These patients are often receiving cardiac and antihypertensive drugs, antiplatelet agents, antacids, steroids, insulin, and anticoagulants. Most of these medications should be continued, except for anticoagulants.

ANESTHETIC MANAGEMENT

The goal of intraoperative anesthetic management is to minimize the risk of the two major complications: stroke and MI. Causes of stroke can be hemodynamic or embolic. No uniformly accepted anesthetic technique has emerged, and many aspects remain controversial.

Premedication

Premedication should be used to alleviate anxiety, especially in patients having regional anesthesia. We use a benzodiazepine (midazolam) with or without a short-acting opioid (fentanyl). Regional anesthesia allows neurologic assessment during and immediately following the procedure, but necessitates judicious use of preoperative sedation.

Regional or Local vs. General Anesthesia

No clear advantages have been demonstrated with either of these techniques. Local anesthesia or cervical plexus block allows evaluation of neurologic status during carotid cross-clamping to assess the need for shunting, and theoretically would facilitate prevention of stroke from hypoperfusion. However, perioperative strokes are more likely to be embolic than low-flow in origin.[13–15] Another potential advantage of regional or local anesthesia may be a lower incidence of postoperative hypertension—hence less need for vasoactive drugs and a shorter stay in the intensive care unit.[16] When this approach is used, constant communication with the patient is necessary throughout the operation because, even though neurologic function may appear normal at the time of carotid cross-clamping, signs of cerebral ischemia may develop later.[12]

Regional or local anesthesia has many potential disadvantages. It requires a high level of patient cooperation and the ability to remain still while supine for the duration of the procedure. Many patients will not be able to lie flat and refrain from coughing. The operation may be uncomfortable for the awake patient, and many would prefer to be unaware during such surgery. Anxiety, especially with the proximity of the surgical drapes, may result in hyperventilation and hypocapnia, leading to a reduction in cerebral blood flow and greater risk of cerebral ischemia. Autonomic responses to surgical manipulation of the carotid bulb may be excessive, resulting in hypotension or hypertension. There is also an ever-present risk of airway obstruction, as well as the occurrence of nausea and vomiting. Uncontrolled hemorrhage or sudden neurologic deterioration may require general anesthesia with rapid tracheal intubation.

Although regional anesthesia is still preferred by some surgeons, it is not widely practiced. Nevertheless, when used properly in carefully selected patients by experienced surgeons, regional anesthesia has a good safety record and is not associated with any increase in the rate of perioperative MI.[17]

Regional or Local Anesthesia

The patient is attached to all the standard monitors used for general anesthesia. An appropriate dose of sedation is given. Regional anesthesia is achieved with a deep cervical plexus block. This may be performed by a single injection or a multiple injection technique. For the single injection technique,[18] the patient is placed supine, with the head turned to the opposite side. The area is prepped and draped. The lateral margin of the clavicular head of the sternocleidomastoid muscle is identified at the level of C4, as indicated by the superior margin of thyroid cartilage. The middle and index fingers are rolled laterally over the anterior scalene muscle until the interscalene groove, between the anterior and middle scalene muscles, is palpated. This groove may be further enhanced by asking the patient to lift their head slowly off the table. After raising a skin wheal with 1% lidocaine, a short-bevel needle is inserted between the palpating fingers, perpendicular to all levels and slightly caudad, until paresthesia is elicited. After careful aspiration, 5 to 6 ml of local anesthetic suitable for the duration of surgery are injected (1% lidocaine or 0.5% bupivacaine with 1:200,000 epinephrine).

The local anesthetic should spread in the fascial sheath that extends from the cervical transverse processes to beyond the axilla and invests the cervical plexus between the middle and anterior scalene muscles. The slight caudad direction of the needle is important, because if the nerve is not encountered, advancing the needle in this direction is less likely to result in epidural or subarachnoid puncture, this complication being prevented by the transverse processes of the cervical vertebrae. There is no need to perform a superficial cervical plexus block with this technique, as the nerve roots are already anesthetized. It may be more comfortable for the patient, whose head will be turned laterally during the operation, if 5 ml of local anesthetic is deposited below the upper attachment of the sternocleidomastoid muscle, thus anesthetizing the accessory nerve. Local infiltration by the surgeon may be required if the upper end of the incision is in the trigeminal nerve area or if the midline is crossed. Judicious administration of intravenous midazolam or propofol can provide sedation without compromising the ability to evaluate the patient's neurologic function.

Possible complications of interscalene cervical plexus block include epidural, subarachnoid, and vertebral artery injection, all of which can be minimized by the caudad direction of the needle and by repeated aspiration before injecting the local anesthetic. Hoarseness may occur if the recurrent laryngeal nerve is blocked, and Horner's syndrome results if the cervical sympathetic chain is blocked. The lower roots of the brachial plexus also may be blocked by spread of local anesthetic. Local infiltration with or without superficial cervical plexus block has been used. A large volume of local anesthetic is required, and the results are not as satisfactory as with deep cervical plexus block.

General Anesthesia

Patients undergoing carotid endarterectomy exhibit a propensity to extreme blood pressure lability under general anesthesia. However, general anesthesia reduces cerebral metabolic demand and may offer some degree of cerebral protection.[19] It also allows for the precise control and manipulation of systemic blood pressure and arterial carbon dioxide tension to optimize cerebral blood flow. Several techniques are available, and the one used depends on the experience and preference of the anesthesiologist. "Light" general anesthesia that maintains the blood pressure at the preoperative level is preferred to "deep" general anesthesia that may necessitate the use of vasopressors to maintain blood pressure, since the risk of myocardial ischemia may be significantly increased by the latter.[11,20]

Induction The aim during induction is to maintain cerebral and myocardial perfusion with as little deviation from preoperative values as possible. Anesthesia can be induced in several ways. After preoxygenation, fentanyl and thiopental or etomidate are given in incremental doses, titrated against the patient's hemodynamic responses. Intravenous lidocaine, 1.5 mg/kg is given 2 to 3 min prior to laryngoscopy. Muscle relaxation is achieved using a nondepolarizing agent such as vecuronium, and a peripheral nerve stimulator is used to monitor the neuromuscular junction. When muscle relaxation is complete, laryngoscopy and intubation are performed. After confirmation of tracheal tube placement by breath sounds and end-tidal capnometry, the tube is secured away from the operative side. Some surgeons may prefer nasotracheal placement of the tube to allow maximum extension of the neck and better exposure. The lungs are ventilated to maintain adequate arterial oxygen saturation and normocarbia.

Maintenance

Choice of Anesthetic Agents Anesthesia can be maintained in many ways. The goal is to provide stable cerebral perfusion while minimizing stress to the myocardium. We use "light" general anesthesia with fentanyl (1 to 5 μg/kg), nitrous oxide (50 to 60%), isoflurane (0.5 to 1.0%), and muscle relaxants. The use of isoflurane is associated with a lower critical cerebral blood flow needed to maintain a normal electroencephalogram (EEG),[21] as well as a lower incidence of ischemic EEG changes as compared to halothane and enflurane, and therefore is the agent of choice if general anesthesia is employed.[22] Isoflurane has also been shown to be associated with a lower incidence of fatal MI (0.25 percent) than either enflurane (0.5 percent) or halothane (1.0 percent).[23] Total intravenous anesthesia with propofol and fentanyl, sufentanil, or alfentanil also may be used, but systemic hypotension is more likely with these combinations. Regardless of the anesthetic agents used, the regimen should be one compatible with early awakening, so that neurologic function can be assessed at the conclusion of the procedure.

Blood Pressure and Pa_{CO_2} Management Blood pressure should be maintained at the patient's normal preoperative level. Cerebral autoregulation may be impaired, and the autoregulation curve is shifted to the right in uncontrolled or poorly controlled hypertensive patients. As autoregulation may be completely lost in ischemic areas, maintaining an adequate blood pressure is a critical factor in the maintenance of cerebral blood flow. Should the blood pressure fall, "lightening" anesthesia by reducing isoflurane concentration is usually sufficient to raise it. Use of vasopressors to elevate the blood pressure during cross-clamping may be necessary, but it has been shown to induce ventricular dysfunction,[20] and in one early series was associated with a fourfold increase in the incidence of MI.[24] If necessary, a phenylephrine infusion (0.1 to 0.5 μg/kg per min) can be administered judiciously. On the other hand, patients who remain hypertensive during anesthesia may require an intravenous nitroglycerin infusion (1 to 5 μg/kg per min) for control. Surgical manipulation of the carotid sinus may cause marked alterations in heart rate and blood pressure. These reflexes can be minimized by prior local infiltration of the carotid bulb with lidocaine.[25] Should EEG changes occur shortly after infiltration, one must be aware that the injection may have been into the carotid artery, resulting in transient central nervous system lidocaine toxicity.[26]

Arterial blood gases are checked after tracheal intubation and regularly during the surgical procedure to ensure adequate oxygenation and normocapnia. Hypercapnia should be avoided, as it will only dilate blood vessels supplying the normal brain without affecting those supplying the ischemic regions that presumably are already maximally vasodilated. The result would be a diversion of blood away from the ischemic areas to the normal areas (intracranial steal), which further aggravates the ischemia. Hypocapnia, on the other hand, may increase flow to the ischemic tissues by constricting the blood vessels in the normal areas (Robin Hood effect). However, hypocapnia also causes a global reduction in cerebral blood flow. It is now generally accepted that the changes in regional cerebral blood flow associated with changes in Pa_{CO_2} in these individuals are unpredictable. Therefore, normocapnia is preferred.

Monitoring Basic monitoring should include intraarterial blood pressure, ECG (lead V_5), capnometry, pulse oximetry, and neuromuscular junction. A pulmonary artery catheter is indicated in patients with symptomatic cardiac disease or recent MI. No special cerebral monitoring is required in awake patients operated on under regional anesthesia. When general anesthesia is employed, physiologic considerations suggest that it is prudent to monitor brain function during cross-clamping of the carotid artery, although no difference in stroke rate has been convincingly demonstrated between patients treated with routine carotid shunting, selective shunting, and without shunting.[27–30]

Electroencephalogram Electrophysiologic monitoring with the 16-channel conventional

EEG remains the gold standard as a sensitive indicator of inadequate cerebral perfusion.[30] The unprocessed EEG displays voltage as a function of time. Proper use of this technique is tedious and time-consuming and requires the presence of an experienced electroencephalographer in the operating room to interpret the results. Nevertheless, intraoperative neurologic complications have been shown to correlate well with EEG signs of ischemia.[31,32] Ipsilateral or bilateral attenuation of high frequency amplitude or development of low frequency activity during carotid cross-clamping is indicative of inadequate cerebral perfusion.

The computer-processed EEG[33–35] and somatosensory evoked potentials (SSEPs)[36–40] also have been found to be useful. The processed EEG generally compresses the raw EEG data recorded from two hemispheric channels and displays them either as average power or voltage. This allows less experienced observers to concentrate on how the parameters are changing with respect to time instead of trying to analyze them directly. These devices range from the simple cerebral function monitor (CFM) to compressed spectral array, density spectral array, and aperiodic analysis. With the exception of the CFM, which displays average power, the rest perform a frequency analysis over a defined time and display the voltage according to frequency domain. Although computer-processed EEGs are easier to interpret, they have been shown not to be as accurate as the 16-channel EEG.[41] Despite extensive studies on the use of EEG to detect hemodynamic insufficiency during carotid cross-clamping, and reported success in individual series, review of the literature fails to establish a definite and conclusive role for EEG monitoring in reducing the incidence of perioperative stroke (Table 22-2).

Somatosensory Evoked Potentials SSEPs (median nerve stimulation) have been shown to be useful during carotid endarterectomy.[36–40] Early studies indicated that intraoperative loss of late cortical components was associated with a worsening of neuropsychologic abilities, and in some instances with subsequent stroke.[42] With the exception of one study,[43] recent reports suggest that SSEPs are useful for monitoring cerebral perfusion during carotid cross-clamping and have similar sensitivity and specificity to conventional EEG.[35–39] Because of the need for computer averaging, SSEPs do not provide continuous real-time monitoring. Stable anesthesia must also be maintained to minimize the influence of anesthetic agents on the amplitude. In general, more than 50 percent reduction or complete loss of amplitude of the cortical component is considered to be a significant indicator of inadequate cerebral perfusion. The SSEPs monitor the cortex as well as the subcortical pathways in the internal capsule, an area not reflected in the cortical EEG.[44]

Stump Pressure (Internal Carotid Artery Back Pressure) Since one important determinant of cerebral blood flow (CBF) is perfusion pressure, it seems reasonable to assume that the distal arterial pressure in the ipsilateral hemisphere during carotid occlusion should provide some indication of collateral flow to the brain. Stump pressure measurement was first described by Michal and colleagues in 1966.[45] This involves direct measurement of the retrograde internal carotid artery pressure during occlusion of the external and proximal common carotid arteries. This is achieved by placement of a 20-gauge needle, connected by fluid-filled tubing to a pressure transducer, in the common carotid artery. Early reports of stump pressure measurements concluded that a stump pressure of less than 50 mmHg indicated the need for placement of a shunt to avoid postoperative neurologic complications.[46,47]

Unfortunately, subsequent experience has shown that stump pressures are not always reliable. When stump pressure was compared to EEG monitoring by Kelly and coworkers,

Table 22-2 Techniques for Central Nervous System Monitoring

Monitor	Advantages	Disadvantages
Awake patient	Continuous neurologic assessment Avoids the risks of general anesthesia Lower incidence of postoperative hypertension Shorter ICU stay	Requires patient cooperation and ability to lie flat Anxiety leading to hyperventilation with potential risk of cerebral ischemia Risk of autonomic disturbances (nausea, vomiting) and airway obstruction
EEG (16-channel)	Gold standard	Cumbersome Difficult to interpret without electroencephalographer in the operating room
EEG (computer processed) CFM, DSA, etc.	Easier to use Less cumbersome set-up	Not as accurate as standard EEG More than one channel needed for accurate detection of ischemia
SSEPs	May detect subcortical ischemia	Intermittent monitor, cumbersome Affected by anesthetic agents
Stump pressure	Measures perfusion pressure Easy to perform Inexpensive	Unreliable except at extremes of values Does not reflect regional blood flow
rCBF	Measures actual cerebral blood flow	Invasive Time consuming, expensive
TCD	Continuous, easy to use Noninvasive, can be used pre-, intra-, and postoperatively Detects emboli	Not fully investigated Satisfactory flow signals cannot be obtained in all patients

6 percent of patients had ischemic EEG changes despite stump pressures in excess of 50 mmHg.[48] Several other studies have demonstrated the unreliability of stump pressures based on measurements of regional CBF (rCBF), EEG, and stump pressure in the same patients.[49] In 8 percent of the patients studied, stump pressures exceeded 50 mmHg, yet rCBF was less than 18 ml/min per 100 g, which is the commonly accepted lower limit of rCBF that allows a normal EEG and consciousness. Furthermore, in 28 percent of cases, stump pressures less than 50 mmHg were observed despite a rCBF above 24 ml/min per 100 g. Moreover, stump pressures lack specificity and are influenced by the anesthetic agent used.[49] On balance, extreme values (<25 mmHg or >50 mmHg) are probably useful indicators of the state of the cerebral circulation, but not the intermediate values.[50,51]

Intraoperative Measurement of CBF Intraoperative CBF measurement has also been used to determine the need for placement of shunts, but the associated cost makes this approach unsuitable for general use.[31] Measurement of CBF involves the intraarterial injection of 20 mCi of the inert radioactive gas Xenon 133 and measuring the wash-out of beta emissions by an extracranial collimated sodium iodide scintillation counter focused on the parietal cortex. The initial slope or fast component of the wash-out curve relates directly to regional blood flow. Newer measurement techniques involve single-photon emission computed tomography of inhaled xenon. Both techniques are useful as research tools but are unlikely to gain wide acceptance because of the equipment and expertise required to produce accurate results.

Transcranial Doppler Recently, transcranial Doppler (TCD) ultrasonography has been evaluated as a monitoring technique for measuring blood flow velocity in the middle cerebral artery during carotid endarterectomy.[52–57] The blood flow velocity is measured by placing an ultrasound probe on the temporal area just above the zygomatic arch.[58] TCD fulfills most of the requirements of an ideal monitoring technique, since it permits continuous noninvasive assessment of the changes in cerebral hemodynamics that take place during surgical occlusion of the carotid artery. In addition, it can be performed quickly without cumbersome equipment and is compatible with other monitoring techniques such as EEG. Ischemia is considered severe if the mean velocity after clamping is 0 to 15 percent of the preclamping value, mild if 16 to 40 percent, and absent if over 40 percent. TCD has been shown to be beneficial not only for detection of intraoperative cerebral ischemia following cross-clamping,[53] but also in detecting malfunctioning shunts due to kinking,[54] identifying high velocity flow states associated with hyperperfusion syndromes,[55] and detecting cerebral emboli both intra- and postoperatively (Chap. 12).[59,60] The different modalities available for intraoperative central nervous system monitoring are summarized in Table 22-2.

Intraoperative Cerebral Protection A detailed discussion of this topic can be found in Chap. 24. We would only comment briefly on cerebral protection from the anesthesiologist's viewpoint. The approach depends largely on the surgeon's decision regarding the placement of shunts. Where a carotid shunt is never used, it is reasonable to administer a bolus of thiopental (5 mg/kg) prior to cross-clamping of the carotid artery. With selective shunting according to EEG, thiopental should not be given, since it will interfere with monitoring; however, it can be used with SSEP monitoring. If routine carotid shunting is used, thiopental is not necessary as long as the shunt is functioning adequately, but it may still be given if additional pharmacologic protection is desired. Administration of thiopental is associated with systemic cardiovascular depression, and therefore the drug always should be used with caution.

The decision regarding whether to shunt is made by the surgeon. There are those who use shunts routinely, some who never use shunts, and others who shunt selectively according to signs of cerebral ischemia as detected by the various monitoring techniques discussed earlier in this chapter. Gummerlock and coworkers reviewed the literature and found no difference in the stroke or mortality rates associated with these approaches, although their own study favors the routine use of shunts.[61] The results from these studies are summarized in Table 22-3.

POSTOPERATIVE MANAGEMENT AND COMPLICATIONS

The goal at the end of carotid surgery is to allow smooth emergence and prompt assessment of neurologic function with stable systemic and cerebral hemodynamics. Our usual management is to taper the concentration of inhaled anesthetic toward the end of surgery and to discontinue it after wound closure. Lidocaine (1.5 mg/kg) is given intravenously to minimize coughing during emergence. Neuromuscular blockade is reversed, and the patient is allowed to breathe 100% oxygen spontaneously. When the patient is responsive and awake, the trachea is extubated. The patient

Table 22-3 Combined Results of Carotid Endarterectomy According to Use of Intraoperative Shunts for Cerebral Protection

		Neurologic deficit			Death		
Shunt use	Patients	No.	%	(range)	No.	%	(range)
Without shunt	4253	165	3.8	(1.1–8.0)	59	1.4	(0–2.0)
Routine shunt	4303	163	3.8	(2.1–7.1)	71	1.7	(0.5–3.5)
Selective shunt	4287	197	4.6	(1.4–6.2)	46	1.1	(0.5–1.5)

SOURCE: Data compiled from the literature based on: Halsey JH: Risks and benefits of shunting in carotid endarterectomy. Stroke 23:1583, 1992.

is carefully observed in the recovery room for cardiac, respiratory, and neurologic complications, the most important of which are mentioned below. The complications of carotid endarterectomy are discussed in more detail in Chap. 26.

Blood Pressure Abnormalities

Carotid endarterectomy is often complicated by postoperative hypertension or hypotension. Significant blood pressure elevation (greater than 40 mmHg above the preoperative value) is found in about 20 percent of patients, and the risk of hypertension is greatest in the first three postoperative hours.[62] The risk of postoperative hypertension is further increased in patients with poorly controlled preoperative hypertension. Patients who become hypertensive in the postoperative period (defined as systolic BP >200 mmHg) are at a much higher risk of developing neurologic deficits (10.2 percent) than are patients who remain normotensive (3.4 percent).[63] Hypertension may cause excessive cerebral perfusion in a circulation unable to autoregulate, resulting in the hyperperfusion syndrome and intracerebral hemorrhage.[64,65] Although rare, this syndrome is typically seen in patients with high-grade carotid stenosis who develop at least a 100 percent increase in CBF after endarterectomy.[64,66] Hypertension also may increase the incidence of wound hematoma with possible airway obstruction.

On the other extreme, hypotension may lead to hypoperfusion and ischemic infarction of the brain. Similarly, myocardial ischemia and infarction may occur as a result of either complication. Therefore, the blood pressure must be closely monitored and controlled in the immediate postoperative period. Regional anesthesia appears to be associated with a higher incidence of postoperative hypotension, whereas general anesthesia is more often associated with postoperative hypertension.[67]

Myocardial Ischemia and Infarction

Perioperative MI is the most frequent cause of mortality following carotid endarterectomy.[11] All causes of increased cardiac work must be minimized in order to avoid myocardial ischemia. The patient should be warm, pain-free, well-oxygenated, and normotensive with no tachycardia. Any signs of myocardial ischemia should be treated immediately.

Airway Obstruction

An expanding hematoma in the neck may cause compression of the trachea, resulting in airway obstruction. Damage to the recurrent laryngeal nerve may contribute to airway obstruction in addition to reducing the upper airway protective reflexes and placing the patient at risk for aspiration.

Hemorrhage

Persistent oozing from deep tissues, insecure ligation of vessels, and disruption of suture lines all may lead to bleeding into the operative site. This can be further aggravated by compromised coagulation due to use of anticoagulants or antiplatelet agents. An expanding hematoma may cause airway compression and necessitate exploration of the wound.

Neurologic Complications

Neurologic deficits following carotid endarterectomy are multifactorial. They may be related to embolization or thrombosis originating at the endarterectomy site or, less commonly, can be the result of intracerebral hemorrhage. The manifestations include both transient deficits and ischemic strokes. All potentially treatable causes, including technical problems such as intimal flaps or suture line stenoses, must be sought, and surgical exploration may be necessary. Evacuation of a wound hematoma requires meticulous airway management, and awake laryngoscopy or flexible fiberoptic laryngoscopy may be necessary. Cranial nerve injuries also have been reported, most commonly the hypoglossal and recurrent laryngeal nerves, and can lead to problems with upper airway control.[68]

Carotid Chemoreceptor and Baroreceptor Dysfunction

Carotid endarterectomy may result in loss of carotid body function with reduced ventilatory response to hypoxemia and hypercapnia.[69] This effect is further exaggerated in patients with coexisting pulmonary disease, especially in the presence of respiratory depressant drugs.

Much of the blood pressure lability observed after carotid surgery has been attributed to baroreceptor dysfunction. It is thought that atheromatous plaques dampen the pressure wave reaching the carotid sinus baroreceptors, and after the removal of these plaques increased stimulation of the baroreceptors results in bradycardia and hypotension.[70] On the other hand, hypertension may occur as a result of damage to the carotid sinus itself or the carotid sinus nerve which sends signals to the medulla. Interruption of these signals leads to tachycardia and hypertension.[71]

CONCLUSIONS

Although carotid endarterectomy reduces the incidence of stroke in selected patients with carotid artery stenosis, this benefit is only seen if the perioperative complications, mainly stroke and MI, are kept to a minimum. Therefore, to realize the potential benefits of this procedure, it is essential to provide the optimal physiologic environment during surgery, and this requires a thorough understanding of the pathophysiology of carotid artery disease and careful anesthetic management.

REFERENCES

1. North American Symptomatic Carotid Endarterectomy Trial Collaborators: Beneficial effect of carotid endarterectomy in symptomatic patients with high grade carotid stenosis. *N Engl J Med* 325:445, 1991.
2. European Carotid Surgery Trialists Collaborative Group. MRC European Carotid Surgery Trial. Interim results for symptomatic patients with severe (70–90%) stenosis or with mild (0–29%) stenosis. *Lancet* 337:1235, 1991.
3. Mayberg MR, Wilson SE, Yatsu F, et al: Carotid endarterectomy and prevention of cerebral ischemia in symptomatic carotid stenosis. Veterans Affairs Cooperative Studies Program 309 trialist group. *JAMA* 266:3289, 1991.
4. Hobson RW, Weiss DG, Fields WS, et al, and the Veterans Affairs Cooperative Study Group. Efficacy of carotid endarterectomy for asymptomatic carotid stenosis. *N Engl J Med* 328: 4:221, 1993.
5. Whisnant JP, Matsumoto N, Elveback LR: Transient cerebral ischemic attacks in a community: Rochester, Minnesota, 1955 through 1969. *Mayo Clin Proc* 48:844, 1973.
6. Fode NC, Sundt TM Jr, Robertson JT, et al: Multicenter retrospective review of results and complications of carotid endarterectomy in 1981. *Stroke* 17:370, 1986.
7. Sundt TM Jr, Sandok BA, Whisnant JP: Carotid endarterectomy: Complications and preoperative assessment of risk. *Mayo Clin Proc* 50:301, 1975.

8. Sieber FE, Toung TJ, Diringer MN, Long DM: Preoperative risks predict neurological outcome of carotid endarterectomy related stroke. *Neurosurgery* 30:847, 1992.
9. Adam HP Jr, Kassell NJ, Mazuz H: The patient with transient ischemic attacks—Is this the time for a new therapeutic approach? *Stroke* 15:371, 1984.
10. Asiddao CB, Donegan JH, Whitesell RC, Kalbfleisch JH: Factors associated with perioperative complications during carotid endarterectomy. *Anesth Analg* 61:631, 1982.
11. Riles TJ, Kopelman I, Imparato AM: Myocardial infarction following carotid endarterectomy: A review of 683 operations. *Surgery* 85:249, 1979.
12. Frost EAM: Some inquiries in neuroanesthesia and neurological supportive care. *J Neurosurg* 60:673, 1984.
13. Lanier WL, Stangland KJ, Scheithauer BW, et al: The effects of dextrose infusion and head position on neurologic outcome after complete ischemia in primates: examination of a model. *Anesthesiology* 66:39, 1987.
14. Toronto Cerebrovascular Study Group: Risks of carotid endarterectomy. *Stroke* 17:848, 1986.
15. Krul JMJ, van Gijn J, Ackerstaff RGA, et al: Site and pathogenesis of infarcts associated with carotid endarterectomy. *Stroke* 20:324, 1989.
16. Corson JD, Chang BB, Shah DM, et al: The influence of anesthetic choice on carotid endarterectomy outcome. *Arch Surg* 122:807, 1987.
17. Prough DS, Scuderi PE, Stullken E, Davis CH Jr: Myocardial infarction following regional anaesthesia for carotid endarterectomy. *Can Anaesth Soc J* 31:192, 1984.
18. Winnie AP, Ramamurthy S, Durrani Z, Radonjic R: Interscalene cervical plexus block: A single injection technique. *Anesth Analg* 54:370, 1975.
19. Wells BA, Keats AS, Cooley DA: Increased tolerance to cerebral ischaemia produced by general anesthesia during temporary carotid occlusion. *Surgery* 54:216, 1963.
20. Smith JL, Roizen MF, Cahalan MK, et al: Does anesthetic technique make a difference? Augmentation of systolic blood pressure during carotid endarterectomy: Effects of phenylephrine versus light general anesthesia and of isoflurane versus halothane on the incidence of myocardial ischemia. *Anesthesiology* 69:846, 1988.
21. Messick JM Jr, Casement B, Sharborough FW, et al: Correlation of regional cerebral blood flow (rCBF) with EEG changes during isoflurane anesthesia for carotid endarterectomy: Critical rCBF. *Anesthesiology* 66:344, 1987.
22. Michenfelder JD, Sundt TM, Fode N, Sharbrough FW: Isoflurane when compared to enflurane and halothane decreases the frequency of cerebral ischemia during carotid endarterectomy. *Anesthesiology* 67:336, 1987.
23. Cucchira RF, Sundt TM, Michenfelder JD: Myocardial infarction in carotid endarterectomy patients anesthetized with halothane, enflurane or isoflurane. *Anesthesiology* 69:783, 1988.
24. Riles TS, Kopelman I, Unoarati AM: Myocardial infarction following carotid endarterectomy: A review of 683 operations. *Surgery* 85:249, 1979.
25. Welch M, Tait WF, Durrans D, et al: Role of topical lignocaine during carotid endarterectomy. *Br J Surg* 79:1035, 1992.
26. Perkins WJ, Lanier WL, Sharbrough FW: Cerebral and haemodynamic effects of lidocaine accidentally injected into the arteries of patients having carotid endarterectomy. *Anesthesiology* 69:787, 1988.
27. Ferguson GG: Intra-operative monitoring and internal shunts: Are they necessary in carotid endarterectomy? *Stroke* 13:287, 1982.
28. Green RM, Messick WJ, Ricotta JJ, et al: Benefits, shortcomings, and costs of EEG monitoring. *Ann Surg* 201:785, 1985.
29. Van Alphen HAM, Polman CH: The value of continuous intra-operative EEG monitoring during carotid endarterectomy. *Acta Neurochir (Wien)* 91:95, 1988.
30. Reddy K, West M, Anderson B: Carotid endarterectomy without indwelling shunts and intraoperative electrophysiologic monitoring. *Can J Neurol Sci* 14:131, 1987.
31. Sundt TM, Sharborough FW, Piepgras DG: Correlation of cerebral blood flow and electroencephalographic changes during carotid en-

darterectomy with results of surgery and hemodynamics of cerebral ischemia. *Mayo Clin Proc* 56:533, 1981.

32. McFarland HR, Pinkerton JA, Fryre D: Continuous electroencephalographic monitoring during carotid endarterectomy. *J Cardiovasc Surg* 29:12, 1988.
33. Rampil IJ, Holzer JA, Quest DO, et al: Prognostic value of computerized EEG analysis during carotid endarterectomy. *Anesth Analg* 62:186, 1983.
34. Spackman TN, Faust RJ, Cucchiara RF, Sharbrough FW: A comparison of aperiodic analysis of the EEG with standard EEG and cerebral blood flow for detection of ischemia. *Anesthesiology* 66:229, 1987.
35. Tempelhoff R, Modica PA, Grubb RL Jr, et al: Selective shunting during carotid endarterectomy based on two channel computerized electroencephalographic compressed spectral array analysis. *Neurosurgery* 24:339, 1989.
36. Lam AM, Manninen PH, Ferguson GG, Nantau W: Monitoring electrophysiologic function during carotid endarterectomy: A comparison of somatosensory evoked potential and conventional electroencephalogram. *Anesthesiology* 75:15, 1991.
37. Dinkel M, Schweiger H, Goerlitz P: Monitoring during carotid surgery: somatosensory evoked potentials vs. carotid stump pressure. *J Neurosurg Anesth* 4:167, 1992.
38. Fava E, Bortolani E, Ducati A, Schieppati M: Role of SEP in identifying patients requiring temporary shunt during carotid endarterectomy. *Electroenceph Clin Neurophysiol* 84:426, 1992.
39. Tiberio G, Floriani M, Giulini SM, et al: Monitoring of somatosensory evoked potentials during carotid endarterectomy: Relationship with different haemodynamic parameters and clinical outcome. *Eur J Vasc Surg* 5:647, 1991.
40. Haupt WF, Horsch S: Evoked potential monitoring in carotid surgery: A review of 994 cases. *Neurology* 42:835, 1992.
41. Young WL, Moberg RS, Ornstein E, et al: Electroencephalographic monitoring for ischemia during carotid endarterectomy: Visual versus computer analysis. *J Clin Monit* 4:78, 1988.
42. Brinkman SD, Braun P, Gangi S, et al: Neuropsychological performance one week after carotid endarterectomy reflects intraoperative ischemia. *Stroke* 15:497, 1984.
43. Kearse LA Jr, Brown EW, McPeck K: Somatosensory evoked potentials sensitivity relative to electroencephalography for cerebral ischemia during carotid endarterectomy. *Stroke* 23: 498, 1992.
44. Gerwetz BL, McCaffrey M: Intraoperative monitoring during carotid endarterectomy. *Curr Probl Surg* 24:478, 1987.
45. Michal VV, Heighal L, First P: Zeitweilige shunts in der vaskularen chirurgir. *Thoraxchirurgie* 14:35, 1966.
46. Hays RJ, Levinson SA, Wylie EJ: Intraoperative measurement of carotid back pressure as a guide to operative management of carotid endarterectomy. *Surgery* 72:953, 1972.
47. Ricotta JJ, Charlton MH, Deweese JA: Determining criteria for shunt placement during carotid endarterectomy: EEG versus back pressure. *Ann Surg* 198:642, 1983.
48. Kelly JJ, Callow AD, O'Donnell TF, et al: Failure of carotid stump pressures: Its incidence as a predictor for a temporary shunt during carotid endarterectomy. *Arch Surg* 114:1361, 1979.
49. McKay RD, Sundt TM, Michenfelder JD, et al: Internal carotid artery stump pressure and cerebral blood flow during carotid endarterectomy. *Anesthesiology* 45:390, 1976.
50. Modica PA, Tempelhoff R: A comparison of computerized EEG with internal carotid artery stump pressure for detection of ischemia during carotid endarterectomy. *J Neurosurg Anesth* 1:211, 1989.
51. Cherry KJ Jr, Roland CF, Hallett JW Jr, et al: Stump pressure, the contralateral carotid artery, and electroencephalographic changes. *Am J Surg* 162:185, 1991.
52. Halsey JH, McDowell HA, Gelman S, Morawetz RB: Blood velocity in the middle cerebral artery and regional cerebral blood flow during carotid endarterectomy. *Stroke* 20:53, 1989.

53. Jorgensen LG, Schroeder TV: Transcranial doppler for detection of cerebral ischemia during carotid endarterectomy. *Eur J Vasc Surg* 6:142, 1992.
54. Padayachee TS, Bishop CCR, Gosling RG, Browse NL: Monitoring cerebral perfusion during carotid endarterectomy. Case report. *J Cardiovasc Surg* 31:112, 1990.
55. Powers AD, Smith RR, Graeber MC: Transcranial doppler monitoring of cerebral flow velocities during surgical occlusion of the carotid artery. *Neurosurgery* 25:383, 1989.
56. Spencer MP, Thomas GI, Moehring MA: Relationship between middle cerebral artery blood flow velocity and stump pressure during carotid endarterectomy. *Stroke* 23:1439, 1992.
57. Steiger HJ, Schaffler L, Boll J, Leichti S: Results of microsurgical carotid endarterectomy: A prospective study with transcranial Doppler sonography and EEG monitoring and elective shunting. *Acta Neurochir (Wien)* 100:31, 1989.
58. Aaslid R, Markwalder TM, Nornes H: Noninvasive transcranial Doppler ultrasound recording of flow velocity in basal cerebral arteries. *J Neurosurg* 57:769, 1982.
59. Spencer PM, Thomas GI, Nicholls SC, Savage LR: Detection of middle cerebral artery emboli during carotid endarterectomy using transcranial Doppler ultrasonography. *Stroke* 21:415, 1990.
60. Halsey JH: Risks and benefits of shunting in carotid endarterectomy. *Stroke* 23:1583, 1992.
61. Gummerlock MK, Neuwelt EA: Carotid endarterectomy: To shunt or not to shunt. *Stroke* 19:1485, 1988.
62. Bove EL, Fry WJ, Gross WS, Stanley JC: Hypotension and hypertension as consequences of baroreceptor dysfunction following carotid endarterectomy. *Surgery* 85:633, 1979.
63. Towne JB, Bernhard VM: The relationship of postoperative hypertension to complications following carotid endarterectomy. *Surgery* 88: 575, 1980.
64. Schroeder T, Sillesen H, Sorensen O, Engell HC: Cerebral hyperperfusion following carotid endarterectomy. *J Neurosurg* 66:824, 1987.
65. Piepgras DG, Morgan MK, Sundt TM Jr: Intracerebral hemorrhage after carotid endarterectomy. *J Neurosurg* 68:532, 1988.
66. Powers AD, Smith RR: Hyperperfusion syndrome following carotid endarterectomy: A transcranial Doppler evaluation. *Neurosurgery* 26:56, 1990.
67. Prough DS, Scuderi PE, McWhorter JM: Hemodynamic status following regional and general anesthesia for carotid endarterectomy. *J Neurosurg Anesth* 1:35, 1989.
68. Rogers W, Root HD: Cranial nerve injuries after carotid endarterectomy. *South Med J* 81: 1006, 1988.
69. Wade JG, Larson CP, Hickey RF, et al: Effect of carotid endarterectomy on carotid chemoreceptors and baroreceptors in man. *N Engl J Med* 282:823, 1970.
70. Taylor E, Schmidek H, Scott RM, et al: Reflex hypotension following carotid endarterectomy: Mechanisms and management. *J Neurosurg* 39:323, 1973.
71. Bore EL, Fry WL, Gross WS, Stanley JC: Hypotension and hypertension as consequences of baroreceptor dysfunction following carotid endarterectomy. *Surgery* 85:633, 1979.

23

Technique of Carotid Endarterectomy

Brian L. Thiele

Carotid endarterectomy has become one of the signature procedures performed by vascular surgeons today. Much of the debate regarding its appropriate place in the management of patients with carotid bifurcation atherosclerosis has been precipitated not only by the question of whether endarterectomy is effective, but also by the wide variation in technical skill with which it has been performed. In some circumstances, the results of this operation have been less than satisfactory.[1]

It is arguably true that the technical expertise of any vascular surgeon can best be assessed by observing the performance of carotid endarterectomy and evaluating postoperative results in large numbers of patients. This chapter provides a detailed description of the procedure, with emphasis on the technical factors that the author considers to be fundamentally important.

HISTORICAL NOTES

The classic operation for carotid bifurcation atherosclerosis—carotid endarterectomy—has evolved over the past 40 years. The technical aspects of this operation, which are the subject of this chapter, have undergone numerous changes. Early surgical procedures on the carotid arteries were performed while techniques of vascular surgery developed and the application of arteriography became common (Chap. 1), but the first successful carotid endarterectomy as we now know it was performed by DeBakey on August 7, 1953.[2,3] This patient, a 53-year-old male suffering from transient cerebral ischemia in the left carotid territory, had clinical evidence of left internal carotid artery disease. He underwent surgery without prior arteriography because, as DeBakey noted, "published reports had indicated that such lesions may be well localized at the bifurcation of the common carotid artery." A left carotid endarterectomy was performed, and at the time of surgery a partly organized fresh clot filling the lumen of the internal carotid artery was removed, along with an atheromatous plaque involving the carotid bifurcation. The report of this procedure was not published until 1959.[2]

The operation recognized by many vascular surgeons as the landmark carotid procedure was reported in the *Lancet* in November 1954 by Eastcott, Pickering, and Rob.[4] This patient was presented preoperatively at a sectional meeting of the American College of Surgeons held in London, England. Dr. Edwin J. Wiley suggested that a thromboendarterectomy should be performed, and at the subsequent surgery a very short, localized lesion was identified at the origin of the internal carotid artery. This lesion was resected, and the artery was reconstructed with an end-to-end anastomosis between the common and internal carotid arteries. To facilitate the end-to-end reconstruction, the external carotid artery was divided. The patient recovered and was symptom-free.

Since that time numerous technical features have been emphasized by various authors,[5–7] each of whom has had a substantial impact on the technique of carotid endarterectomy.

POSITIONING AND PREPARATION OF THE PATIENT

Although specific details of anesthetic technique vary considerably,[8,9] carotid endarterectomy generally is performed either under local anesthesia with regional block or general anesthesia. These approaches are discussed in Chap. 22, and anesthetic technique is mentioned here only insofar as it influences positioning of the patient.

In the patient who is undergoing general anesthesia, an optimal head position for exposing the carotid triangle structures can be obtained. This involves extension of the head on the neck, with rotation of the head to the contralateral side. Undue extension of the head may cause postoperative neck pain and headache owing to greater occipital nerve irritation. A satisfactory head position usually can be maintained while also supporting the neck with a circular, firm headrest and a rolled-up towel placed between the shoulder blades (Fig. 23-1).

Skin preparation of the operative field should be carried out in the shaded area

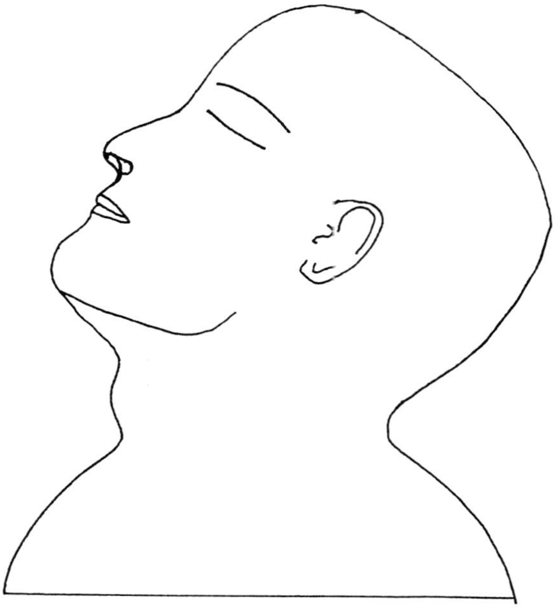

Figure 23-1. Positioning of the patient for optimal exposure of the carotid triangle anatomy.

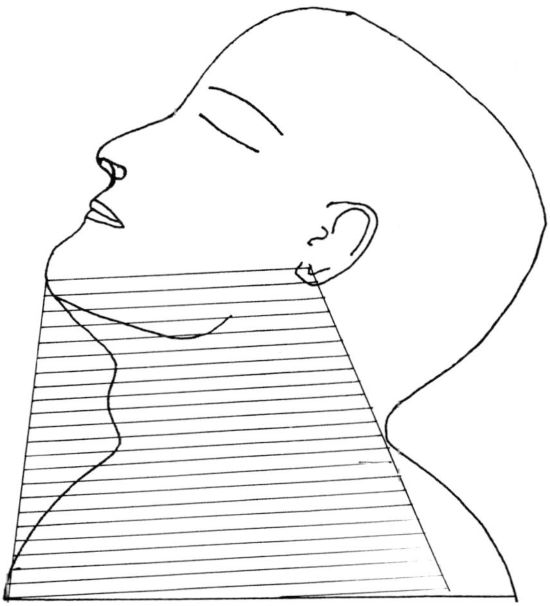

Figure 23-2. Operative field to be prepared and draped.

shown in Fig. 23-2. The simple technique of painting the skin with povidone-iodine or alcohol-chlorhexidine is adequate because the incidence of wound infections in the neck is extremely low and probably unrelated to the skin preparation method used. Vigorous scrubbing of the area is avoided because of the possibility that mechanical manipulation in the region of the carotid bifurcation could dislodge atheromatous or thrombotic debris from an arterial lesion.

The operative area should then be draped with towels, as shown in Fig. 23-3. Anteriorly, the drape extends from the symphysis menti to the suprasternal notch; superiorly, the drape extends from the symphysis menti to the lower portion of the earlobe. The posterior drape extends from the posterior earlobe to the acromioclavicular joint; the inferior drape extends from the suprasternal notch horizontally to the acromioclavicular joint. It is important that the earlobe and the angle of the mandible be included in the operative field, since both serve as surface markings for incision placement.

The author prefers that the patient be in slight reverse Trendelenburg position to reduce intracranial venous pressure and thereby facilitate cerebral perfusion. This also helps to minimize venous bleeding during the operation.

THE INCISION

The primary requirement for any incision in surgery is that it provide adequate exposure for the performance of the procedure. A variety of incisions has been described for carotid endarterectomy, but the most commonly used is the vertical incision along the anterior border of the sternocleidomastoid muscle (Fig. 23-4). The next most common is the modified

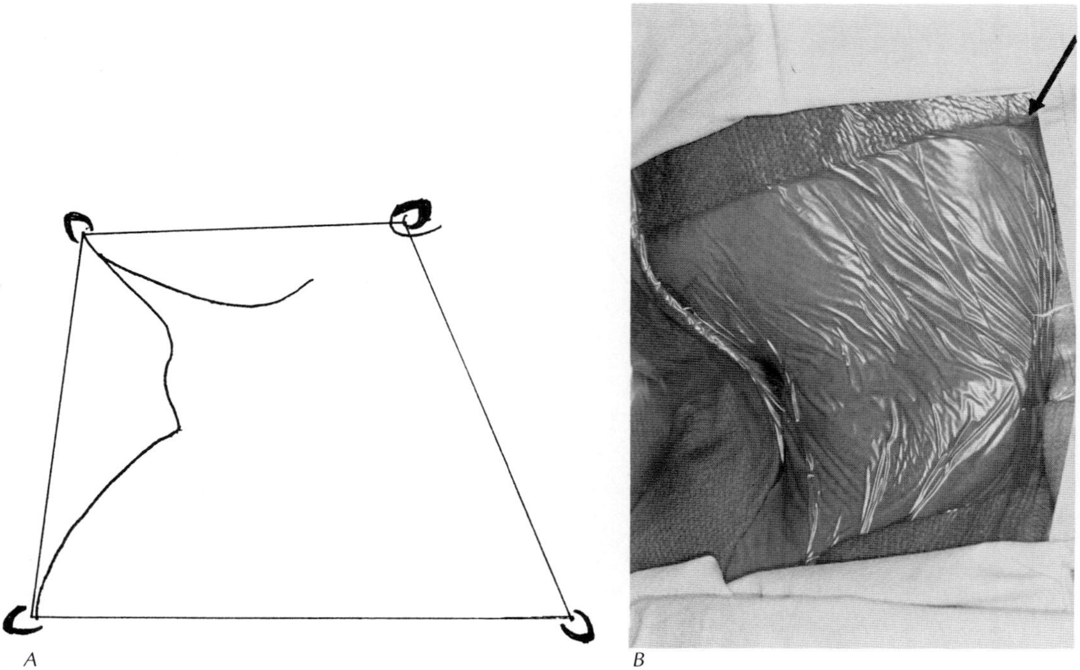

Figure 23-3. Operative field at completion of draping. Note earlobe exposed (arrow) as a point of reference.

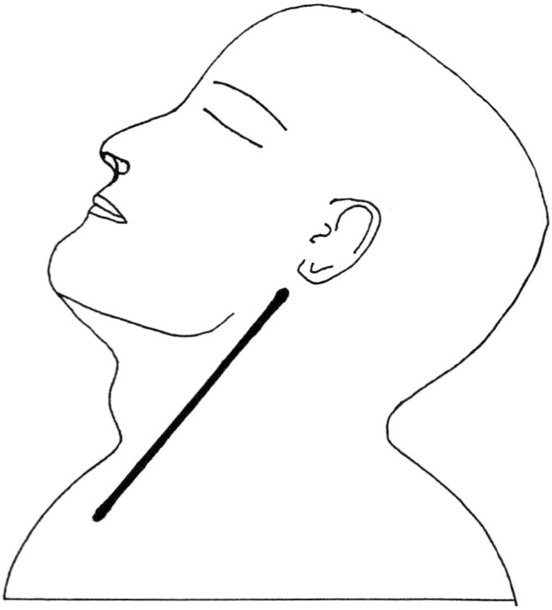

Figure 23-4. Placement of vertical skin incision along the anterior border of the sternocleidomastoid muscle.

transverse incision at the level of the upper border of the thyroid cartilage (Fig. 23-5). The author prefers the latter incision because it gives a more pleasing cosmetic result, avoids the tail of the parotid gland, and provides excellent exposure. A key point related to placement of this incision is identification of the level of the carotid bifurcation, either with preoperative arteriography or by duplex ultrasound. When a transverse incision is used, it is important that it cross the anterior border of the sternocleidomastoid muscle at the level of the carotid bifurcation. This transverse or oblique incision (Fig. 23-5) commences inferior to the earlobe and curves inferiorly to cross the anterior border of the sternocleidomastoid muscle, terminating at the greater cornu of the thyroid cartilage.

The frequent use of preoperative antiplatelet therapy, with its associated tendency to in-

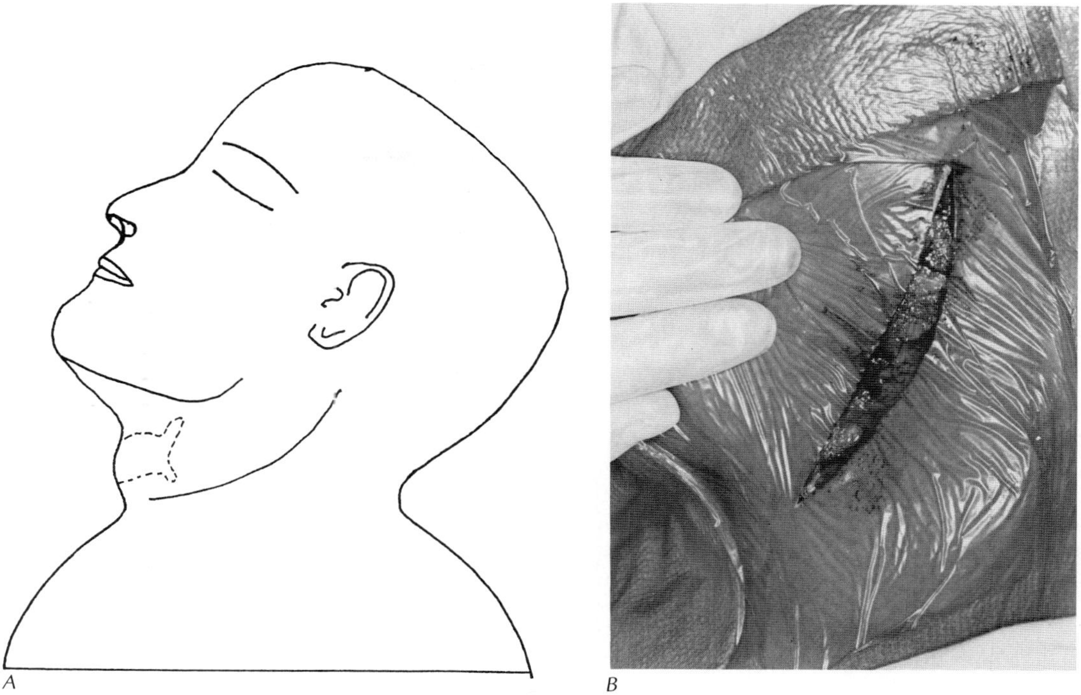

A B

Figure 23-5. Placement of oblique skin incision. The relationship of the thyroid cartilage is shown in the drawing.

crease perioperative bleeding, has prompted the use of electrocautery during the next phase of the operation. Cutting electrocautery is used to incise the platysma muscle in the line of the incision, and hemostasis is achieved with coagulation electrocautery. Care is taken to identify the external jugular vein, which is located in the roof of the carotid triangle. This structure is exposed by sharp dissection and divided between ligatures. During this part of the operation, it is common to encounter branches of the cervical plexus—particularly the great auricular nerve, which should be spared if at all possible. If this nerve must be sacrificed, it should be sharply divided with a scalpel, not with electrocautery.

After division of the platysma muscle, the surgeon has entered the carotid triangle bounded by the anterior border of the sternocleidomastoid muscle, the posterior belly of the digastric muscle, and the superior belly of the omohyoid muscle (Fig. 23-6).

MOBILIZATION OF THE STERNOCLEIDOMASTOID

The next stage of the operation involves mobilization of the sternocleidomastoid muscle, which is to be retracted laterally in the operative field. Electrocautery generally is used to separate the soft tissues from the anterior border of the sternocleidomastoid, extending from the region of the earlobe to the superior belly of the omohyoid muscle. During this maneuver, small muscular arterial branches to the sternocleidomastoid are encountered and can be controlled with electrocautery. These vessels may be enlarged in the presence of severe carotid artery disease.

At this point, it usually is appropriate to

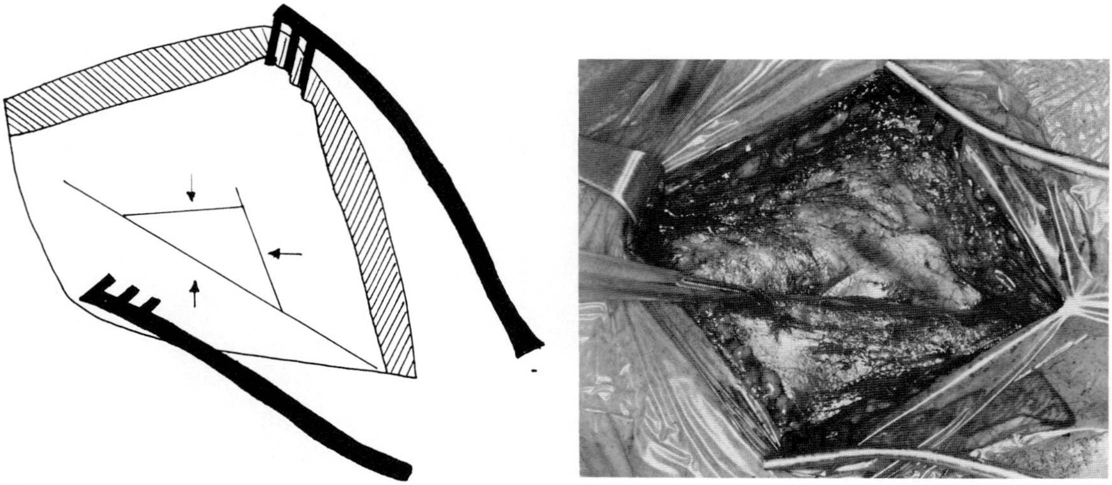

A B

Figure 23-6. Exposure of the carotid triangle bounded by the sternocleidomastoid muscle (posterior), the digastric muscle (superior), and the omohyoid muscle (inferior). The forceps indicate the anterior border of the sternocleidomastoid at the inferior boundary of the incision.

insert a self-retaining retractor in the lower portion of the incision, with the hooks of the lateral jaw placed into the deep surface of the mobilized sternocleidomastoid muscle in preparation for exposure of the carotid sheath.

MOBILIZATION OF THE INTERNAL JUGULAR VEIN

The subsequent dissection maneuvers are designed to mobilize the internal jugular vein and retract it laterally along with the sternocleidomastoid muscle. Sharp dissection is used throughout this part of the procedure to expose the superficial surface of the vein. Having identified the internal jugular vein, sharp dissection is then continued along the anterior border to identify any branches. The major branch is the common facial vein, which usually is a single large vessel (Fig. 23-7), but in some patients may be replaced by a number of smaller venous channels draining into the anterior aspect of the internal jugular vein. These small veins should be carefully identified, ligated with fine ligature material, and divided. The common facial vein, if it is large, should be both transfixed with a suture and ligated when it is divided.

As with the sternocleidomastoid muscle, it usually is necessary to dissect the deep surface of the internal jugular vein slightly to enable the vein to be retracted. If the internal jugular vein is mobilized completely, it tends to lie over the carotid bifurcation, making it more difficult to retract; however, leaving the internal jugular vein partly attached to the deep surface of the sternocleidomastoid muscle facilitates retraction of the vein. The sharp dissection along the anterior border of the internal jugular vein should extend from the omohyoid muscle inferiorly to the superior region of the carotid triangle.

After mobilization of the internal jugular vein, it usually is necessary to reposition the self-retaining retractor, with the blades somewhat deeper in the middle portion of the operative field.

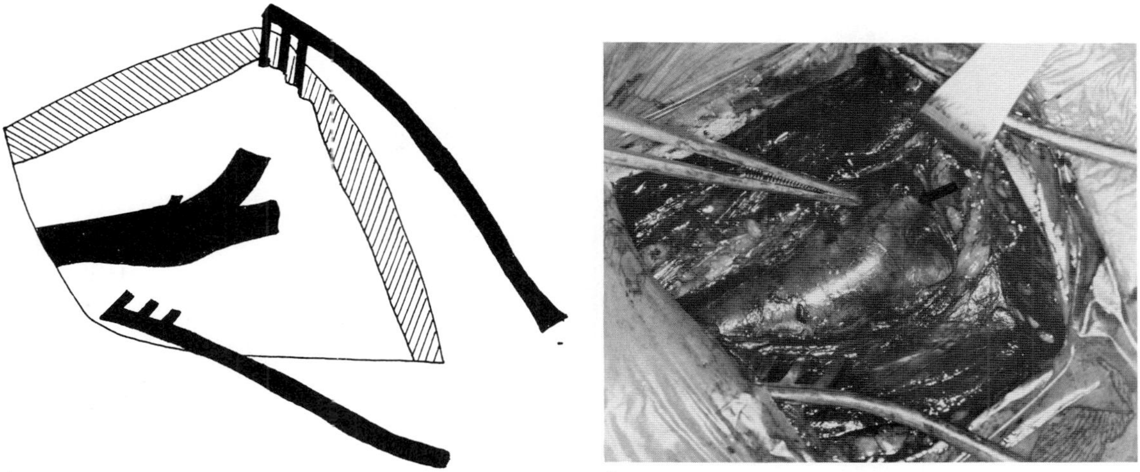

A B

Figure 23-7. Identification of the common facial vein (arrow). Ligation and division of this vein facilitates lateral retraction of the internal jugular vein to expose the carotid artery.

EXPOSURE OF THE CAROTID ARTERIES

The next phase of the procedure involves exposure of the common, internal, and external carotid arteries. This dissection should be started at the inferior portion of the operative field, with sharp dissection used to identify the common carotid artery at the level of the upper border of the omohyoid muscle (Fig. 23-8). It may be necessary to divide a small artery and vein to the omohyoid muscle belly at this location to fully expose the common carotid. The ansa hypoglossi (ansa cervicalis) usually is visualized as it enters the superior belly of the omohyoid muscle. While this nerve may be divided without deleterious effects, it is better to preserve all nerve structures in the operative field.

The second nerve identified at this point in the dissection should be the vagus nerve. This nerve usually courses vertically in the groove between the common carotid artery and internal jugular vein, but in some patients it may be located more anteriorly, where it can be mistaken for the ansa hypoglossi. This is an additional reason why all nerve structures should be carefully preserved until the identity of each is clear. If the vagus nerve does lie anteriorly, it may be gently encircled with a vessel loop and retracted. This nerve is also at risk for injury when the common carotid artery is being encircled for vascular control. Thus, when a right-angle clamp is passed circumferentially around the common carotid artery, care should be taken to ensure that the blades are closely applied to the arterial wall, thereby excluding the vagus nerve.

Throughout this part of the procedure, it is essential that the carotid artery be manipulated as little as possible. Retraction of the surrounding tissues to facilitate dissection may be accomplished by traction on these tissues without handling the carotid itself. Once the proximal common carotid artery has been completely exposed, the next step is to expose the distal portion of the common carotid and the internal carotid.

The author prefers that the initial sharp dissection be carried along the posterior border

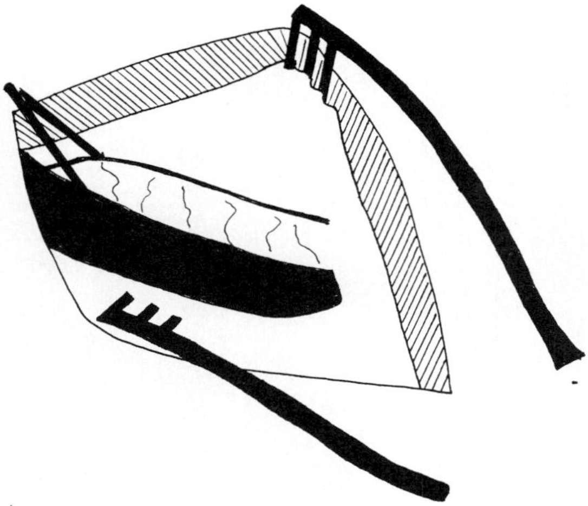

A

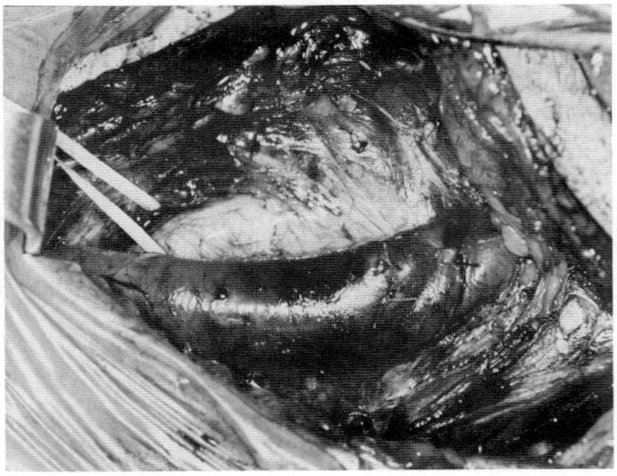

B

Figure 23-8. Exposure of the common carotid artery, encircled by an umbilical tape, at the inferior boundary of the carotid triangle.

of the common carotid artery such that the anterior and lateral surfaces are gradually exposed. Gentle traction is applied to the periarterial tissues to facilitate this dissection, and particular care is taken to minimize manipulation in the region of the carotid bifurcation and the bulb of the internal carotid. The vagus nerve is usually visualized during this part of the procedure and should not be disturbed. The plane between the carotid artery and the internal jugular vein is opened up as the dissection proceeds cephalad along the posterior surface of the internal carotid. The correct plane is directly adjacent to the internal jugular vein, which is gently retracted laterally. It is usually advantageous at this stage to place a second retractor in the superior margins of the operative field to facilitate identification of the tissue planes (Fig. 23-9).

At this point in the procedure the major goals are: (1) to expose the distal internal carotid artery at a location where there is no disease; (2) to avoid damage to the hypoglossal nerve; (3) to avoid damage to the vagus nerve; and (4) to minimize manipulation of the carotid bifurcation. The disease-free segment of internal carotid artery usually can be identified by a bluish tinge due to the relatively thin normal vessel wall. When this is apparent on the anterior surface of the internal carotid artery, sharp dissection can be used to encircle the vessel (Fig. 23-10). It is essential during placement of a right-angle clamp for the passage of a vessel loop or umbilical tape that the internal carotid artery not be disturbed from its bed. This normal segment of the internal carotid artery is commonly found without having visualized the hypoglossal nerve.

Dissection along the anterior border of the internal jugular vein is advised because there is usually a small venous branch draining into the internal jugular (Fig. 23-11) with the hypoglossal nerve deep to it (Fig. 23-12). If the internal carotid artery can be identified at an appropriate disease-free level without encountering this venous branch, the hypoglossal nerve is not at risk. The technique of "separate-and-cut" should be used in this area to ensure that this small vein can be readily identified, ligated, and divided to allow visualiza-

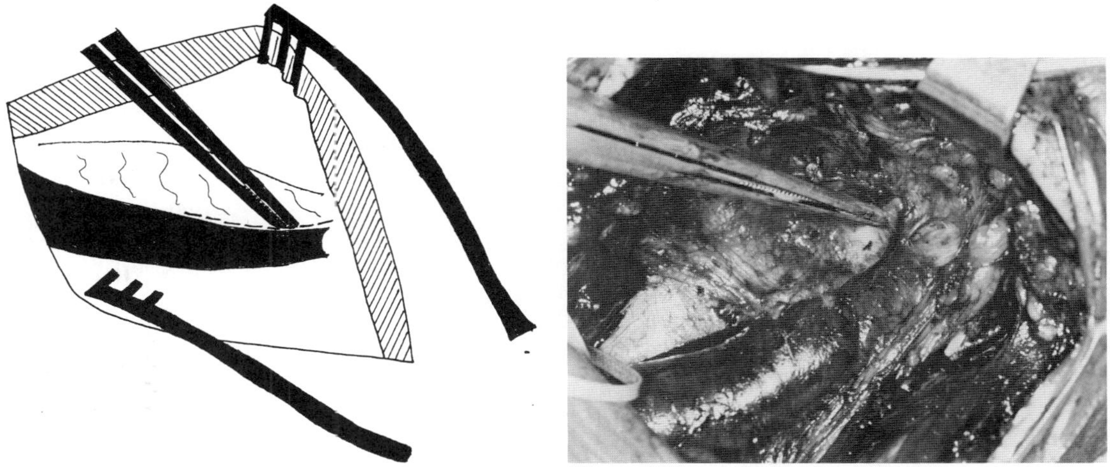

A *B*

Figure 23-9. Dissection plane between the internal carotid artery and internal jugular vein indicated by the forceps.

tion of the hypoglossal nerve. The plane of dissection with this approach is parallel to the hypoglossal nerve, minimizing the possibility of nerve damage. A second landmark that facilitates identification of the hypoglossal nerve is the ansa hypoglossi, which runs in the groove between the internal carotid artery and the internal jugular vein. The ansa hypoglossi can be followed superiorly to its junction with the hypoglossal nerve. If it is necessary to dissect above the level of the hypoglossal nerve, encircling this nerve with a vessel loop en-

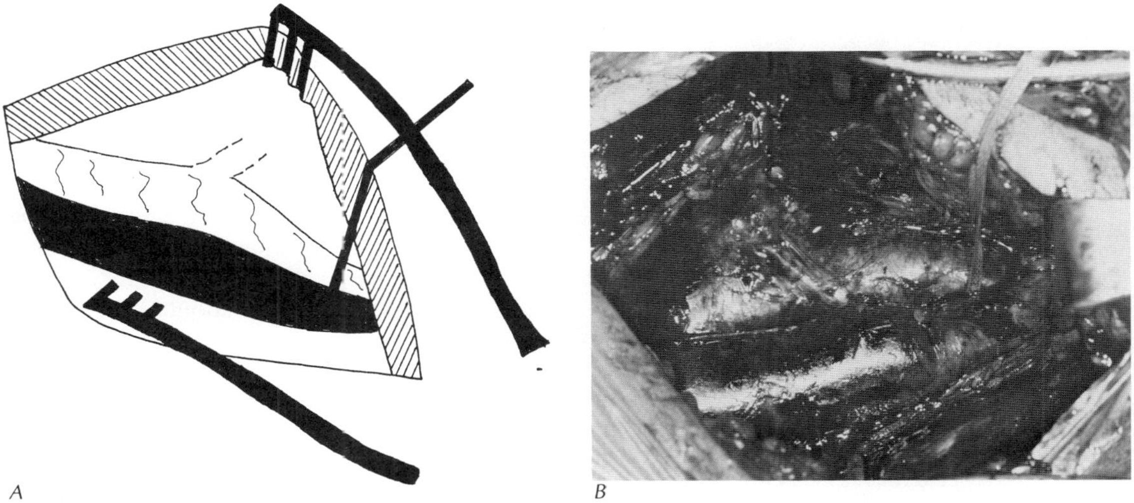

A *B*

Figure 23-10. Vascular control of the internal carotid artery obtained at a nondiseased level (umbilical tape).

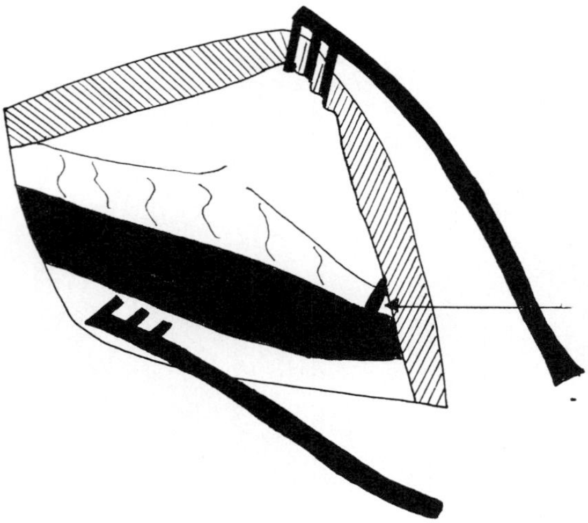

Figure 23-11. Venous tributary entering the internal jugular vein at the superior boundary of the dissection.

ables gentle retraction. Once the common and internal carotid arteries have been exposed and encircled with vessel loops, the surgeon's attention is directed toward gaining control of the superior thyroid artery and the external carotid.

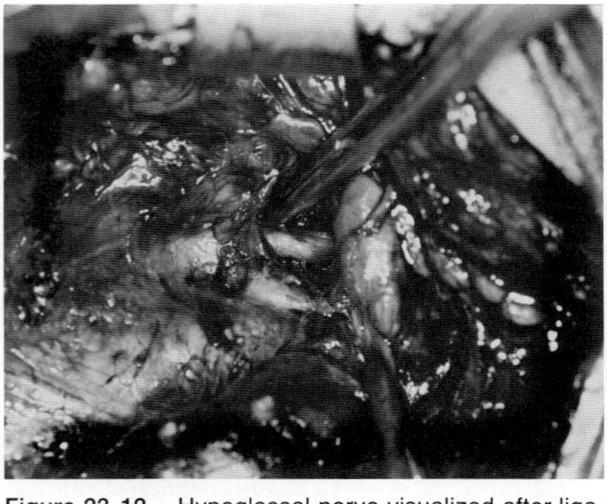

Figure 23-12. Hypoglossal nerve visualized after ligation and division of the venous tributary indicated in Fig. 23-11. The nerve is located under the tip of the forceps in the center of the photograph.

The superior thyroid artery is the first branch of the external carotid and can be identified by sharp dissection along the anterior border of the most proximal portion of the external carotid artery. This small branch should be encircled with a vessel loop for control adjacent to its origin to ensure that the laryngeal branch of the vagus nerve is not damaged. The external carotid artery is best controlled approximately 1 cm distal to its origin, where the periarterial tissues can be dissected relatively easily. If control of the external carotid is attempted directly at its origin, the fibrous tissue associated with the carotid body is difficult to remove and may be associated with annoying hemorrhage from small arterioles. Because the anatomy of the external carotid artery is variable, it may be simpler to identify and control branches of the external carotid rather than the main trunk of the vessel.

Reflex bradycardia may occur in some patients when dissection is performed in the region of the carotid bulb. If this becomes a problem, the effects can be minimized by injection of approximately 1 ml of 0.5% lidocaine into the connective tissue around the carotid body and carotid sinus nerve, which are deep to the common carotid bifurcation.

After completion of the dissection described above, intravenous heparin should be administered in a dose of 75 to 100 units/kg. If a shunt is to be used, it is appropriate at this time to make a selection based on the size of the undisturbed internal carotid artery. The technical details of shunt placement will be discussed later in this chapter.

A basic principle of vascular surgery is that complete vascular control should be obtained before opening the vessels so that the procedure can be performed in a bloodless field. Occlusion of the vessels is readily achieved with small, soft clamps, which should be applied sequentially to the distal internal carotid artery at the nondiseased level, the common carotid artery above the level of the omohyoid muscle, and the external carotid. Control of the superior thyroid artery usually can be obtained with a small vascular clamp or by traction on the encircling vessel loop. Placement of the clamps, in the order described above, is performed to avoid potential embolization from initial clamping of the common or external carotid.

EXPOSURE OF THE HIGH INTERNAL CAROTID ARTERY

On rare occasions, it may be necessary to expose the most distal portion of the cervical internal carotid artery immediately adjacent to where the internal carotid enters the skull. Circumstances that require this type of distal exposure include the high carotid bifurcation, trauma to the distal extracranial internal carotid, diffuse disease extending distally in the internal carotid, and fibromuscular dysplasia of the internal carotid artery.

Two approaches may be used to obtain control of the carotid artery at this level. The first involves controlled subluxation of the temporomandibular joint with displacement of the mandible anteriorly, thus enabling dissection between the internal jugular vein and the internal carotid artery toward the base of the skull. When this is done, it is also necessary to displace the hypoglossal nerve and to exercise caution regarding identification of the accessory nerve. Both of these nerves can be encircled with a vessel loop and gently retracted to facilitate the distal dissection and exposure.

A second approach is to change the plane of dissection from anterior to the internal jugular vein to posterior to the internal jugular. When this approach is used, the contents of the carotid sheath are displaced anteriorly, and the vagus nerve is visualized posteriorly. The accessory nerve needs to be identified high in the neck as it exits from the base of the skull and moved out of the way to expose the posterolateral aspect of the internal carotid artery. This approach provides excellent access to the distal internal carotid from the level of the bifurcation to the base of the skull. Furthermore, the dissection is usually simpler and faster because this is an avascular plane and the hypoglossal nerve is not at risk.

THE ARTERIOTOMY

After placement of the vascular clamps, the common carotid artery should be incised longitudinally, using a No. 11 scalpel blade. With the point of the scalpel, a sufficiently large incision should be made to ensure easy insertion of the deep blade of the Potts scissors into the arterial lumen. Care must be taken during this maneuver not to injure the opposite wall of the vessel. The arteriotomy should then be extended with the Potts scissors along the anterior surface of the common carotid artery, the carotid bulb, and the distal internal carotid to the point at which 4 to 5 mm of nondiseased internal carotid are visualized (Fig. 23-13). Difficulties may be encountered in cutting through heavily calcified plaques with fine scissors, and it may be safer simply to cut through the adventitia and outer layers of the media at the level of the plaque and enter the lumen at a point proximal or distal to the calcified area.

Careful placement of the arteriotomy is important to ensure that the subsequent closure is technically adequate. In particular, the arteriotomy should not curve anteriorly toward the origin of the external carotid artery; rather, it should pass through a point midway between the anterior and posterior surfaces of the bulb. This is facilitated if the surgeon and assistant grasp the cut edges of the arteriotomy in the common carotid artery and retract in a caudad direction to straighten out any minor curves or kinks in the internal carotid. Gentle suctioning within the vessel removes any blood trapped in the lumen and allows

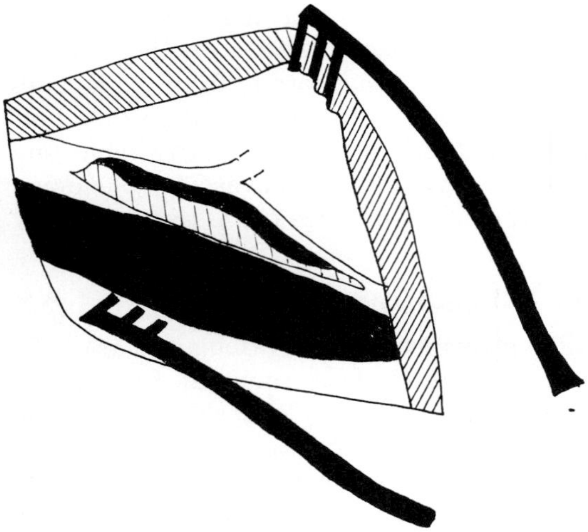

Figure 23-13. Arteriotomy placement in the common and internal carotid arteries. Note the extension of the arteriotomy into the distal nondiseased internal carotid artery.

performance of the arteriotomy under direct vision.

If a shunt is to be used, this is the point at which insertion should be carried out.

THE ENDARTERECTOMY

The next step in the operation is to perform an adequate endarterectomy of the common, internal, and external carotid arteries. The depth of the endarterectomy plane to be developed depends on the severity of the atherosclerotic process. In patients who have extensive atherosclerotic disease, endarterectomy typically requires removal of virtually all of the media out to the level of the adventitia. However, in patients with relatively mild disease, the proper cleavage plane is more difficult to identify, and care must be taken not to remove the nondiseased residual media along with the plaque. Therefore, the plane of the endarterectomy is not uniform in all patients, but is determined by the severity of their disease.

The author prefers to begin the endarterectomy at the region of the bifurcation where the disease is most severe. Gentle manipulation of the cut edge of the arterial wall enables the natural plane of separation in the arterial media to be identified. The adventitia of the carotid artery is then grasped with fine dissecting forceps, and a Freer elevator, Penfield, or a similar instrument is inserted into this cleavage plane. The endarterectomy then proceeds along the posterior surface of the carotid artery, and the Freer elevator is passed in a caudad direction toward the clamp on the common carotid. This is usually best accomplished by having the assistant grasp the residual adventitia, while the operating surgeon manipulates the plaque.

The plaque is mobilized circumferentially within the common carotid artery at the proximal apex of the arteriotomy using a series of distraction maneuvers with the Freer elevator. A small right-angle clamp may be inserted into the cleavage plane and gently passed circumferentially around the wall of the vessel to emerge from the opposite cut edge in the same plane. The right-angle clamp is then opened and the plaque sharply cut with Potts scissors to leave a beveled edge directed as shown in Fig. 23-14. This mobilizes the most proximal extent of the atherosclerotic plaque which can then be grasped and separated from the more cephalad portion of the common carotid artery by simply elevating the plaque and pushing the arterial wall away.

The next phase of the procedure is the external carotid endarterectomy. Careful separation of the adventitia from the atherosclerotic plaque at the origin of the external carotid artery is necessary to ensure adequate removal. This is the only portion of the endarterectomy not performed under direct vision. Obtaining a satisfactory end-point is facilitated by briefly releasing the clamp on the

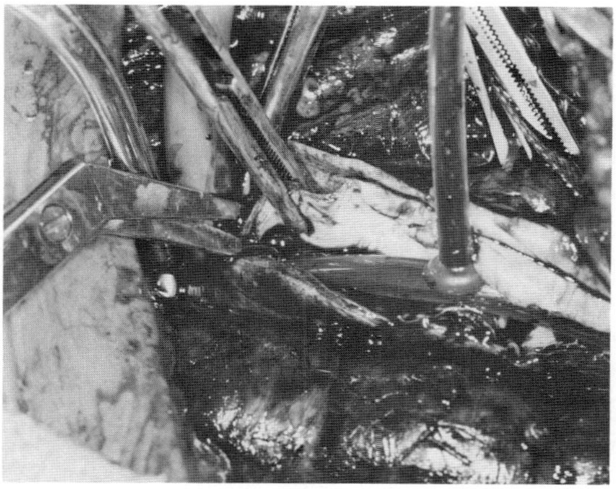

Figure 23-14. Definitive termination of the endarterectomy in the common carotid artery using sharp transection with Potts scissors. The sidearm of the T-shaped shunt is seen on the right of the photograph.

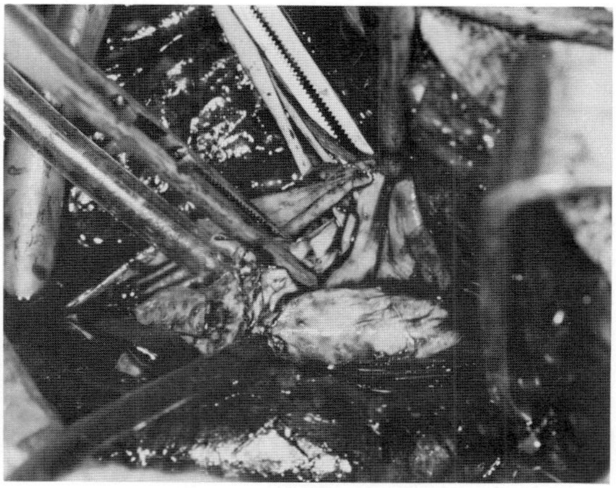

Figure 23-15. Endarterectomy of the external carotid artery facilitated by invagination into the lumen.

external carotid artery and invaginating the proximal segment of the external carotid into the lumen of the bifurcation while applying gentle traction to the plaque (Fig. 23-15).

The surgeon is now left with the most crucial part of the procedure—removal of the plaque from the bulb and the internal carotid artery. A common error at this point is simply to elevate the distal segment of the plaque in an attempt to complete the endarterectomy. Separation of the internal carotid plaque is best achieved by steady traction on the common carotid portion of the plaque in a caudad direction while gently separating the arterial wall from the plaque in the plane of cleavage. At the same time, gentle rotation of the plaque should be used to promote separation of the distal tongue of plaque from the relatively normal internal carotid (Fig. 23-16). Excessive elevation of the plaque during this maneuver often results in extension of the endarterectomy plane into the normal distal wall of the internal carotid. When this occurs, sharp division of the plaque is required to establish a satisfactory end-point, and tacking sutures may be necessary to avoid an intimal flap. Whether a smooth tapered end-point is obtained or tacking sutures are used, it is important to establish the internal carotid end-point under direct vision to avoid creating technical problems beyond the distal extent of the arteriotomy.

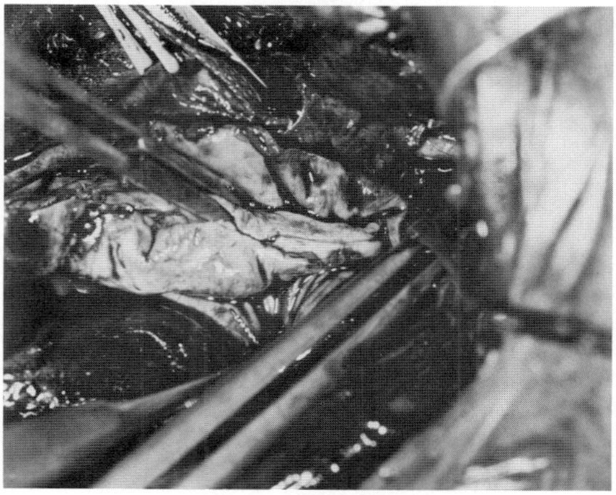

Figure 23-16. Spontaneous separation of the plaque in the distal internal carotid artery using traction and rotation.

After complete removal of the plaque, the surface of the arterial lumen should be irrigated copiously with heparinized saline solution, and gentle debridement should be performed with a miniature cotton swab (Fig. 23-17). This facilitates removal of any loosely adherent medial fibers not included with the endarterectomy specimen. Care should be taken not to traumatize the adventitia with forceps during this phase of the procedure.

The entire surface remaining after removal of the plaque must be inspected, particularly the critical distal end-point of the endarterectomy in the internal carotid artery. A syringe filled with heparinized saline solution and an 18-gauge blunt needle can be used to irrigate this area forcefully and to determine whether there are any small flaps that could be raised when blood flow is restored. These are readily identified in the pool of clear solution and removed with fine forceps.

When the surgeon is satisfied with the end-point in the internal carotid, the external carotid artery should be examined. At this stage, the author prefers a transient release of the clamp on the external carotid artery so that some back-bleeding occurs into the bulb. This can be suctioned out and the lumen of the proximal segment of the external carotid artery visualized directly. A small mosquito hemostat can then be inserted into the external carotid orifice to remove any residual loose atherosclerotic debris. It is frequently necessary to open the vascular occluding clamp during this maneuver. Complete removal of any atherosclerotic plaque at the origin of the external carotid artery is essential to avoid an intimal flap or the possibility of platelet-fibrin aggregates occurring at that site and embolizing after restoration of flow.

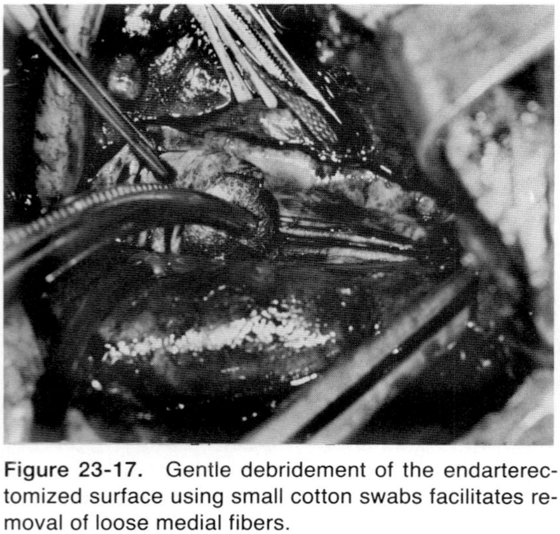

Figure 23-17. Gentle debridement of the endarterectomized surface using small cotton swabs facilitates removal of loose medial fibers.

Finally, the surface of the common carotid artery should be inspected to ensure that there is a relatively smooth transition from the non-endarterectomized vessel to the endarterectomized segment. This frequently requires some fashioning of the edge of the atherosclerotic plaque with Potts scissors. Once all these areas have been carefully inspected for any loose debris or flaps, the arteriotomy may be closed.

ARTERIOTOMY CLOSURE

The arteriotomy in the common and internal carotid arteries may be closed either primarily or by patch angioplasty. The technique of primary closure is considered first, followed by the author's technique for patch angioplasty closure.

Primary Closure

Closure of the internal carotid portion of the arteriotomy is best accomplished with 7-0 monofilament polypropylene suture material and a fine cardiovascular needle of the BV-1 type. A small through-and-through suture is placed above the apex of the arteriotomy and secured with six single throws. The excess short end of the suture is then cut, and the assistant applies traction to the long end of the suture that elevates the arterial edges at the apex of the arteriotomy (Fig. 23-18). Since the arteriotomy should extend to the nondiseased distal internal carotid artery, the vessel has not been endarterectomized at this location, and it is important not to manipulate the edges with forceps, as this frequently leads to fragmentation of the soft arterial wall. The edges can be positioned for suturing by grasping the adjacent endarterectomized segment. Extremely fine running sutures are placed along the internal carotid portion of the arteriotomy, with the size of bites increasing gradually as the closure moves caudad. Care should be taken to ensure that the carotid artery is reconstructed in an anatomic fashion without leaving too large a bulb. This part of the closure is carried to the level of the distal common carotid artery.

A 6-0 monofilament polypropylene suture is then used to insert a similar apical stitch at the proximal end of the arteriotomy in the common carotid artery. The common carotid is then closed with a running suture, using bites placed approximately 1 mm from the arterial edge and a travel of 1 mm between bites. This suture is carried cephalad to join the first suture from the internal carotid artery. As the closure proceeds, the endarterectomized surface is intermittently flushed with heparinized saline solution to remove small bits of thrombotic debris. Prior to completing the closure of the arteriotomy, all vessels are flushed by sequential removal of the vascular clamps.

Once the arteriotomy has been closed (Figs. 23-19 and 23-20), the clamp on the external carotid artery is removed, followed by the common carotid clamp, and finally the internal carotid clamp. Initial release of the external carotid artery clamp exposes the suture line to a low pressure head. If there are major defects, these can be identified and repaired. Subsequent restoration of flow by removal of the clamp on the common carotid artery ensures that any residual debris enters the external carotid rather than the internal carotid circulation.

Patch Angioplasty Closure

The author's preference for patch material is the distal greater saphenous vein obtained at the level of the ankle. The general indications

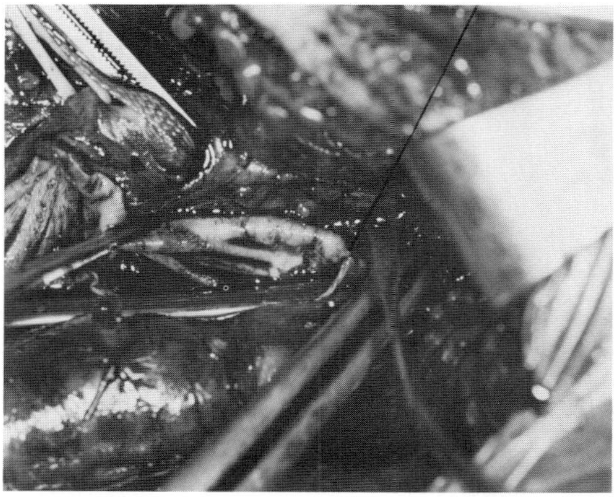

Figure 23-18. Placement of an apical stitch in the internal carotid artery with traction applied to facilitate presentation of the arterial edges for suturing.

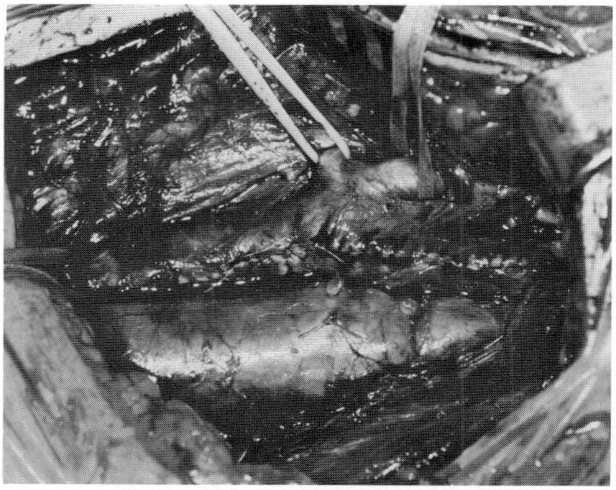

Figure 23-19. Primary closure of the arteriotomy, showing restoration of the normal anatomic contour. Umbilical tapes encircle the common and external carotid arteries; a vessel loop encircles the superior thyroid artery.

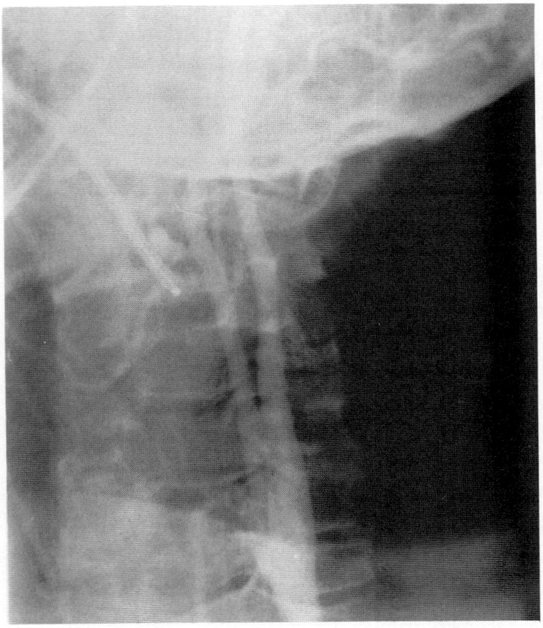

Figure 23-20. Operative arteriogram after primary closure, showing normal intraluminal architecture.

for use of patch angioplasty are: (1) technical factors related to the arteriotomy, such as lateral tears at the apex; (2) internal carotid arteries less than 3 mm in diameter; (3) to ensure that shunt removal can be performed without damage to the arteriotomy suture line; (4) operation for recurrent carotid stenosis; and (5) closure of kinked or tortuous carotid arteries.

A potential problem associated with patch angioplasty is inserting a patch that is so wide that the proximal portion of the internal carotid artery becomes aneurysmal. This can be avoided by splitting the saphenous vein segment approximately in half longitudinally. The author prefers to patch only the internal carotid artery and the bulb, not to extend the patch for the full length of the arteriotomy closure (Figs. 23-21 and 23-22). After an adequate length of saphenous vein has been harvested, opened with Potts scissors, and appropriately fashioned, a stay suture of 6-0 monofilament polypropylene is placed at one end of the patch (Figs. 23-21 and 23-22). A 7-0 monofilament polypropylene suture with BV-1 needles is then used to place a stitch between the opposite end of the vein patch and the apex of the arteriotomy in the distal internal carotid artery. This suture is secured with three throws, and each end is used to complete one side of the patch closure. After three or four running stitches have been placed with double passes, it usually is possible to proceed along the arteriotomy with single-needle passes. When performing patch angioplasty, the author closes the arteriotomy in the common carotid artery up to the region of the bulb primarily with a running 6-0 monofilament polypropylene suture prior to insertion of the patch. The suture along one edge of the patch is then carried down to this point, and the two sutures are tied.

Closure of the arteriotomy along the remaining edge of the patch proceeds with mod-

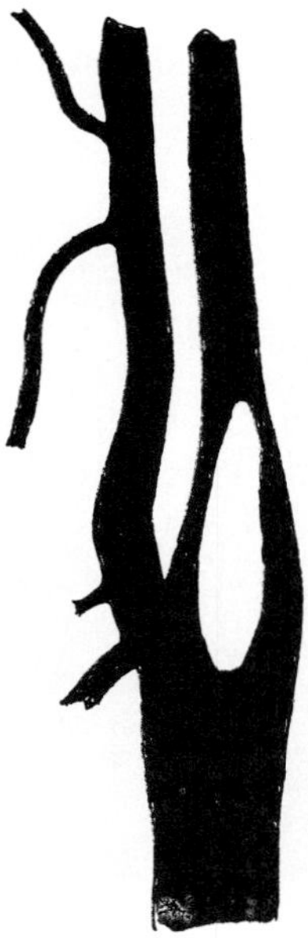

Figure 23-21. Diagram of a vein patch closure confined to the carotid bulb and internal carotid artery.

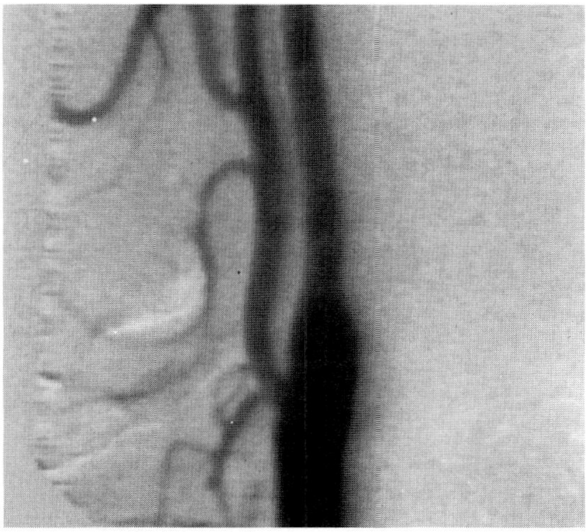

Figure 23-22. Operative arteriogram showing normal intraluminal architecture after vein patch closure.

erately large bites to ensure that this area is not excessively dilated. This suture is continued proximally to about 1 cm from the previously tied sutures, and one of these latter sutures is then run distally to complete the patch closure. The irrigation and flushing maneuvers utilized during patch closure are identical to those described for primary arteriotomy closure. A similar technique can be used, regardless of whether autologous or prosthetic material is chosen for the patch.

SHUNT PLACEMENT

A wide variety of shunts is available for use during carotid endarterectomy. The author believes that technical facility with a shunt is gained from repeated use. When selective shunting leads to infrequent shunt use, technical difficulties are more likely. Whichever type of shunt is used, there are a number of factors that the surgeon should consider:

1. The shunt should be of adequate size to deliver sufficient flow to maintain cerebral perfusion during clamping.

2. The shunt should fit snugly in the internal carotid artery without the possibility of trauma to the vessel.

3. The ends of the shunt should be smooth to ensure that dissection does not occur during placement.

4. The shunt should be inserted into the internal carotid artery first so that back-bleeding can be visualized, indicating that dissection or impingement of the shunt on the vessel wall has not occurred.

5. Care should be taken during insertion of the shunt into the common carotid to ensure that loose atherosclerotic debris does not enter the shunt.

6. Shunt function should be confirmed with a sterile Doppler instrument.

The author's preference is to use a tapered T-shaped shunt with a side-arm (Fig. 23-14), as discussed in Chap. 24. The advantages of this particular shunt are: (1) the tapered configuration fits the internal and common carotid arteries well; (2) the side-arm enables visualization of back-bleeding from the internal carotid artery and flushing from the common carotid prior to initiation of flow; (3) shunt flow can be assessed visually by removing the clamp from the side-arm; and (4) the shunt acts as a stent and facilitates primary closure of the internal carotid artery without narrowing.

Prior to insertion, the shunt should be flushed with heparinized saline solution and an atraumatic clamp applied on the common carotid end. Once the arteriotomy has been made and blood suctioned from within the lumen, the internal carotid end of the shunt is inserted into the lumen under direct vision, and the clamp on the internal carotid artery is removed. The shunt is then gently advanced, with the surgeon observing the back flow occurring from the side-arm. If this back-bleeding ceases, the shunt may have become lodged against the arterial wall. In this situation, the shunt should be withdrawn slightly to the point at which back-bleeding occurs again. The internal carotid end of the shunt is secured in place with a Rummel tourniquet (umbilical tape and red rubber tubing) or a double vessel loop, and the clamp on the common carotid end of the shunt is transferred to the internal carotid end just distal to the side-arm. The common carotid end of the shunt is then inserted into the common carotid artery under direct vision and advanced proximally. The flow from the common carotid artery initially emerges through the side-arm of the shunt, and once the common carotid end has been secured in place with a Rummel tourniquet, the clamp on the shunt is removed and applied to the side-arm, establishing flow to the internal carotid artery. The operative field is then filled with saline solution and a continuous-wave Doppler probe applied to the shunt to confirm the presence of flow.

Occasionally it may be difficult to secure the shunt in the internal carotid with a Rummel tourniquet or vessel loop, and a medium-sized Javid clamp may be necessary. This also facilitates exposure of high portions of the internal carotid artery.

Shunt removal is best accomplished by: (1) ensuring that there is an adequate gap in the arteriotomy suture line to remove the shunt without disrupting the arteriotomy closure; (2) removing the internal carotid end of the shunt first and observing the back-bleeding before clamping; and (3) removing the common carotid end and performing antegrade flushing to remove any residual debris.

ASSESSMENT OF TECHNICAL ADEQUACY

Evaluation of the technical adequacy of carotid endarterectomy is discussed in more detail in Chap. 25. The author's preference is to use either operative arteriography or duplex ultrasound.

The technique of operative arteriography involves inserting an 18- or 19-gauge needle into the common carotid and rapidly injecting approximately 15 cc of 60% methylglucamine iothalamate (Conray-60) prior to exposure of the x-ray film. This gives excellent visualization of the endarterectomized area, and the film should also include the intracranial portion of the internal carotid artery. After confirmation of the technical adequacy of the procedure, the arteriogram needle is removed and bleeding controlled with the placement of a 6-0 monofilament suture at the insertion site.

When technical problems occur, they typically involve the arteriotomy closure or the distal endarterectomy end-points in the internal or external carotid arteries. If the operative arteriogram shows a defect considered to be significant, such as an occlusion, greater than approximately 30 percent diameter stenosis, or intimal flap, immediate repair is indicated. This usually requires opening all or part of the arteriotomy and reinserting a shunt if one was used during the initial procedure. The specific repair depends on the nature of the defect and may require tacking an intimal flap, further endarterectomy, or addition of a patch angioplasty. If the problem is confined to the external carotid artery, the defect can often be repaired through a separate arteriotomy in the external carotid, and only the origin of this vessel needs to be clamped. Repeat operative arteriography should be performed to document the technical adequacy of the repair.

WOUND CLOSURE

After hemostasis has been secured along the arteriotomy closure and throughout the operative field, the anterior border of the sternocleidomastoid muscle is approximated to the fascia lying anterior to the carotid artery. This usually requires two or three interrupted sutures of 3-0 absorbable material (Fig. 23-23).

The platysma muscle is then meticulously closed, using a running 3-0 absorbable suture

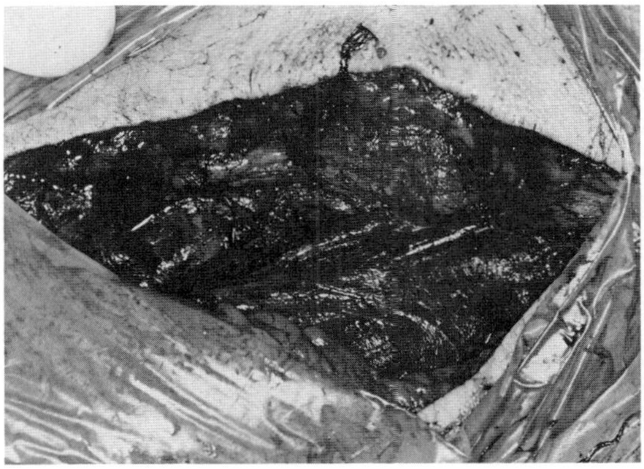

Figure 23-23. Approximation of the anterior border of the sternocleidomastoid muscle superficial to the exposed carotid arteries is the first step in wound closure.

to promote hemostasis and facilitate accurate apposition of the skin edges (Fig. 23-24). The skin is then closed with an absorbable running 4-0 subcuticular suture (Fig. 23-25). Steristrips are applied to the incision, and a small dry dressing is applied to the neck.

DRAINS

The author does not use drainage of the incision as a routine part of the procedure. If it is

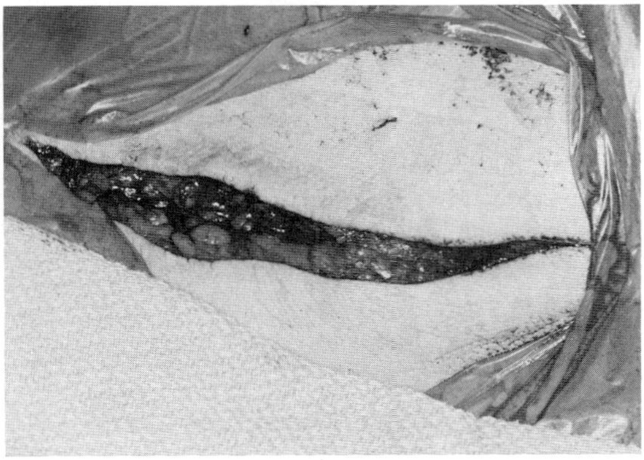

Figure 23-24. Closure of the platysma muscle with a running hemostatic suture, showing close apposition of the skin edges.

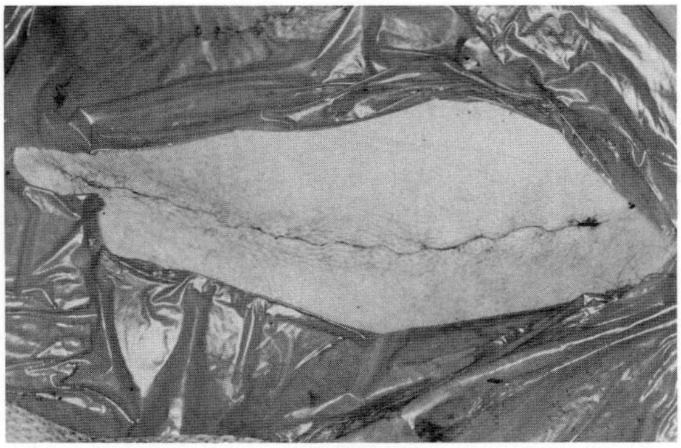

Figure 23-25. Accurate apposition of the skin edges with a running subcuticular suture provides an ideal skin closure.

required, a small (No. 7 French) flat drain is inserted deep to the sternocleidomastoid muscle, exiting through a separate stab-incision low in the neck. The drain usually needs to be cut short to fit within the wound and should be tethered to the skin at the exit site with nonabsorbable suture material.

EXTERNAL CAROTID ENDARTERECTOMY

In a small proportion of patients, atherosclerotic disease at the origin of the external carotid artery may serve as a source for emboli to the intracranial circulation through periorbital collaterals, particularly when the internal carotid is occluded.[10] These emboli also may originate from the occluded stump of the internal carotid artery, producing either visual or hemispheric symptoms.[11] In these circumstances, external carotid endarterectomy or remodeling of the bifurcation may be indicated.

Operative Technique

The incision and exposure for external carotid endarterectomy are similar to those described previously for carotid bifurcation endarterectomy. The major differences relate to the placement of the arteriotomy and the routine use of patch angioplasty for arteriotomy closure. When the internal carotid artery is occluded, it may be necessary to modify the configuration of the internal carotid stump to remove a potential source for emboli.

After satisfactory exposure and control of the common, internal, and external carotid arteries, the patient is heparinized and clamps are applied to the appropriate vessels. A definitive external carotid endarterectomy requires mobilization of a longer external carotid segment than that usually obtained for carotid bifurcation endarterectomy, and this often involves individual control of the first two or three external carotid branches. The arteriotomy is started in the common carotid artery with a No. 11 scalpel blade and extended through the distal common and the proximal external carotid arteries with Potts scissors. A nondiseased segment of the external carotid artery should be exposed at the most distal extent of the arteriotomy.

Endarterectomy of the common carotid artery is performed in a manner similar to that described in the preceding paragraphs, but the external carotid endarterectomy is now done under direct vision. The technique for separation of the distal portion of the plaque is analogous to that described for the internal carotid artery. After the endarterectomy specimen has been removed, gentle debridement and irrigation with heparinized saline solution are carried out, and the arteriotomy is routinely closed by vein patch angioplasty. In this situation, the patch extends along the entire arteriotomy from the apex of the distal portion in the external carotid to the proximal end in the common carotid.

In circumstances where "carotid stump syndrome" is considered to be the cause of symptoms, it is necessary to fashion the occluded origin of the internal carotid artery to obliterate the blind cul-de-sac at the stump. The author's preference for achieving this has been to transect obliquely the origin of the internal carotid artery and close the remaining arterial wall with a running 6-0 monofilament polypropylene suture. If oblique transection of the internal carotid artery and bulb is performed at this site, a smooth tapered transition from the common carotid to the origin of the external carotid artery can be obtained (Fig. 23-26).

The technical adequacy of the procedure should be assessed by operative arteriography as described previously, and wound closure is also performed in an identical manner. Shunting is rarely necessary during external carotid endarterectomy, and often is technically difficult owing to the small size of the distal branches of the external carotid artery.

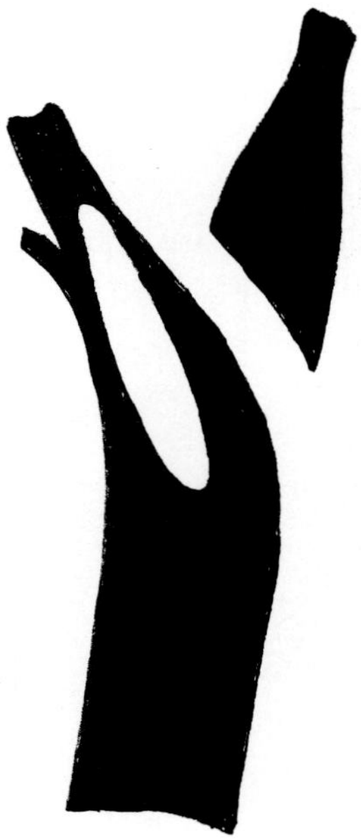

Figure 23-26. Diagram illustrating the technique of patch angioplasty of the external carotid artery and fashioning of the bulb for suspected "carotid stump syndrome."

REFERENCES

1. Kempczinski RF, Brott TG, Labutta RJ: The influence of surgical specialty and case load on the results of carotid endarterectomy. *J Vasc Surg* 3:911, 1986.
2. DeBakey ME, Crawford ES, Gooley DA, Morris GC Jr: Surgical considerations of occlusive disease of innominate, carotid subclavian, and vertebral arteries. *Ann Surg* 149:690–710, 1959.
3. DeBakey ME: Successful carotid endarterectomy for cerebrovascular insufficiency: Nineteen-year follow-up. *JAMA* 233:1083–1085, 1975.
4. Eastcott HHG, Pickering GW, Rob CG: Reconstruction of internal carotid artery in a patient with intermittent attacks of hemiplegia. *Lancet* 267(2):994–996, 1954.
5. Bahnson HT, Spencer FC, Ovattlebaum JK Jr: Surgical treatment of occlusive disease of the carotid artery. *Ann Surg* 149:74–720, 1959.
6. Thompson JE: The development of carotid artery surgery. *Arch Surg* 107:643–648, 1975.
7. Wylie EJ, Ehrenfeld WK: *Extracranial Occlusive Cerebrovascular Disease: Diagnosis and Management*. Philadelphia, WB Saunders, 1970.
8. Connelly JE: Carotid endarterectomy in the awake patient. *Am J Surg* 150:159–165, 1985.
9. Gillette MT: Anesthetic considerations in carotid artery surgery, in Robicsek F (ed): *Extracranial Cerebrovascular Disease—Diagnosis and Management*. New York, Macmillan, chap. 12, 1986.
10. Countee RW, Visayanathan T: Intracranial embolization via external carotid artery: Report of a case with angiographic documentation. *Stroke* 11:465–570, 1980.
11. Barnett JHM, Peerless SJ, Kaufmann JCE: "Stump" of internal carotid artery—A source for further cerebral embolic ischemia. *Stroke* 9:448–452, 1978.

24

Cerebral Protection during Carotid Surgery

Joseph A. Wasselle
Dennis F. Bandyk

Stroke or aggravation of a prior neurologic deficit is a grave complication of carotid artery surgery. Intraoperative cerebral ischemia can result from a variety of mechanisms, including embolization of atherosclerotic or thrombotic material, inadequate cerebral blood flow during carotid-clamping, intracerebral hemorrhage, and thrombotic occlusion of the operated internal carotid artery (ICA). To avoid these problems, technical precision in the conduct of the procedure is paramount. The spectrum of patient, anatomic, and disease variables involved in surgery for carotid bifurcation atherosclerosis mandates that surgeons employ an operative technique that ensures adequate cerebral blood flow throughout the procedure. Thus, cerebral protection is assured by maintaining adequate cerebral blood flow during and after carotid endarterectomy.

Cerebral protection can be achieved during carotid endarterectomy by three general approaches: (1) performing the operation in an awake patient using local anesthesia and shunt insertion if neurologic symptoms develop; (2) routine use of a shunt to maintain ICA blood flow during cross-clamping; or (3) intraoperative monitoring of cerebral function or blood flow to identify patients with clamp-induced cerebral ischemia for selective shunt insertion. Regardless of the approach used, careful monitoring of hemodynamic and coagulation parameters is vital to ensure a safe carotid repair.

The clinical efficacy of carotid endarterectomy depends on patient selection criteria and completing the procedure with an extremely low perioperative stroke and death rate. Results of randomized clinical trials conducted on both symptomatic and asymptomatic patients in North America (NASCET, VA Cooperative Trial 167, Mayo Clinic) and Europe (ECST) indicated a significant reduction in adverse events (stroke, death, transient ischemic attack) with carotid endarterectomy compared with medical treatment alone for severe atherosclerotic stenosis of the carotid artery (Chaps. 16 and 17).[1–4] In the NASCET, the perioperative stroke and death rate was 2.1 percent; in the ECST, the rate was 7.5 percent. Surgical intervention in asymptomatic patients enrolled in VA Cooperative Trial 167 was associated with a 4.3 percent rate of stroke or death.

The perioperative stroke and death rates recorded in these clinical trials significantly delayed the point at which patients realized a clear benefit from surgical intervention. In symptomatic patients the interval was approximately six months, but in asymptomatic patients the interval was prolonged to 18 months, during which time a number of patients sustained cardiac events. Thus, it is vital that surgeons employ appropriate intraoperative monitoring and surgical techniques to ensure cerebral protection and avoid both neurologic and cardiac complications. Only when perioperative morbidity and mortality are avoided can patients realize maximum benefits from carotid endarterectomy.

Stroke associated with carotid endarterectomy has been reported in 1 to 12 percent of patients, depending on the indication for surgery and the center where the operations were performed.[4–8] This chapter will emphasize techniques that are important for intraoperative cerebral protection to avoid neurologic deficits related to temporary carotid occlusion, as well as thromboembolism of plaque or clot during vessel exposure, shunt insertion, or after flow is restored.

PATHOPHYSIOLOGY OF PERIOPERATIVE STROKE

Strokes associated with carotid endarterectomy can occur during or following the procedure, with approximately 80 percent developing within hours to several days of surgery. Thrombotic occlusion of the ICA was the most common cause of neurologic deficit in patients randomized to surgical therapy in the clinical trials.[1–4] In descending order of frequency, perioperative strokes are the result of ICA thrombosis, intracerebral hemorrhage, clamp-induced cerebral ischemia, or thromboembolism from the endarterectomized arterial segment.

Carotid endarterectomy on awake patients has shown that when this technique is used most intraoperative strokes are the result of embolization during vessel manipulation. Surprisingly, inadequate collateral cerebral blood flow during cross-clamping of the ICA is an uncommon cause of intraoperative stroke. In a recent large retrospective review of 3062 carotid endarterectomies, ischemia during carotid artery clamping accounted for only 10 (15 percent) of 66 perioperative strokes.[9] The mechanisms responsible for cerebral ischemia included difficulty in placing a shunt, hypotension, and inadequate collateral flow due to contralateral ICA occlusion. In patients having carotid endarterectomy under local anesthesia, placement of a shunt to restore ICA blood flow has been required in between 8 and

16 percent of patients.[9–12] When operations are performed under general anesthesia, ascribing a time of onset or a cause to an intraoperative stroke is more difficult unless continuous electroencephalographic (EEG) monitoring has been utilized. Typically, the stroke is not recognized until the patient emerges from anesthesia.

Of the strokes that occur during carotid endarterectomy, approximately two-thirds appear to be the result of emboli, which vary in composition and site of origin (Table 24-1). Air embolization has been documented in up to 90 percent of patients undergoing carotid endarterectomy, particularly during shunt insertion and removal, and platelet emboli have been detected in approximately one-third of patients by continuous transcranial Doppler (TCD) monitoring of middle cerebral artery blood flow.[13] However, the significance of these air or platelet emboli is unclear, given their relatively high frequency during otherwise uncomplicated carotid procedures and the absence of neurologic sequelae. Emboli consisting of atherosclerotic debris, thrombus, or platelet-fibrin aggregates may occur during dissection of the carotid vessels, as a result of improper shunt placement, or after the endarterectomy has been completed and flow restored. In most studies, surface debris dislodged from the atherosclerotic plaque into the ipsilateral cerebral circulation accounts for the highest proportion of intraoperative strokes.

In clinical series that did not utilize shunts for cerebral protection, approximately 20 percent of operative strokes were the result of clamp-related cerebral ischemia.[10,15–17] The critical flow rate needed to maintain a normal EEG pattern is in the range of 15 to 20 ml/100g per min, but the ischemic tolerance of neural tissue also depends on the duration and severity of blood flow reduction. In some patients, hemispheric blood flow falls to near zero with carotid cross-clamping; in this situation, both clinical and laboratory data suggest that irreparable brain damage begins to occur within four to nine minutes.[18]

Insufficient collateral cerebral flow for maintaining neuron function occurs more frequently in symptomatic patients undergoing carotid endarterectomy than in asymptomatic patients with contralateral ICA occlusion.[15–17] While the reasons for this apparent discrepancy are unknown, symptomatic patients with severe carotid bifurcation atherosclerosis may have areas in the brain that are particularly sensitive to hypoperfusion; these are termed "watershed zones." Watershed zones are located at the boundaries of the territories supplied by the major cerebral arteries, e.g., between the anterior and middle cerebral

Table 24-1 Etiology and Origin of Intraoperative Strokes Associated with Carotid Endarterectomy

	Origin		
Etiology	ICA/CCA plaque	Shunt placement/removal	Repair site
Embolism			
Atherosclerotic debris	X	X	
Thrombus	X		X
Platelet aggregates			X
Air		X	X
Thrombosis		X	X
Inadequate cerebral blood flow			

NOTE: ICA: internal carotid artery; CCA: common carotid artery.

arteries, the anterior and posterior cerebral arteries, or the middle and posterior cerebral circulation.

Based on intraoperative monitoring of cerebral function during carotid endarterectomy, patients with a prior stroke or contralateral ICA or vertebral artery occlusion are at highest risk for clamp-related cerebral ischemia.[16,17] If the cerebral collateral circulation is adequate, no neurologic sequelae should result from the reduction in cerebral perfusion associated with carotid cross-clamping. Inadequate cerebral blood flow may occur regardless of collateral perfusion because of hypotension, intracranial arterial occlusive disease, cerebral vasospasm, or complications related to shunt placement (embolization of debris) or function (kinking, thrombosis). Both retrospective and prospective clinical studies have shown that patients with preexisting neurologic deficits are prone to aggravation of the deficit following carotid surgery unless cerebral protection is maintained by use of a shunt.[15–18]

As previously noted, thrombosis of the repaired ICA is the most common cause of perioperative stroke. This condition rarely develops during the procedure, but rather is manifest in the postanesthesia care unit as an acute neurologic deficit involving the cerebral hemisphere ipsilateral to the operated carotid artery. Asymptomatic ICA thrombosis has been reported in 0.5 to 1 percent of patients undergoing carotid endarterectomy. A variety of anatomic factors have been associated with early postoperative ICA thrombosis, including residual atherosclerotic plaque, intimal corrugation or flap formation, suture stricture following arteriotomy closure, stenosis produced by adventitial bands, and kinking of the ICA. Systemic factors that may also be associated with ICA thrombosis and stroke are inadequate anticoagulation, perioperative hypotension, and heparin-induced thrombocytopenia with its associated hypercoagulable state.

An additional but fortunately uncommon cause of perioperative stroke is intracerebral hemorrhage. This is a recognized complication of restoring blood flow to an area of recently infarcted brain and serves as the rationale for avoiding revascularization in patients with acute strokes. Carotid endarterectomy has a variable effect on cerebral hemodynamics.[18] Restoration of normal perfusion pressure to an area of brain with severely deranged autoregulation can result in a "hyperperfusion syndrome" with subsequent infarct extension or overt intracerebral hemorrhage (Chap. 26). This usually occurs several days after surgery, presenting with sudden onset of headache or migraine variants and paroxysmal lateralizing epileptiform discharges. Patients with severe hypertension, poor collateral reserve, clamp-induced cerebral ischemia, low baseline cerebral blood flow as documented by a low stump pressure, or severe contralateral carotid disease appear to be at highest risk for intracerebral hemorrhage. Monitoring by TCD during carotid endarterectomy may also identify patients with a hyperemic middle cerebral artery response to revascularization.

TO SHUNT OR NOT TO SHUNT

Although the circle of Willis is a critical determinant of collateral blood supply in the human brain, a completely intact circle of Willis has been demonstrated in only 21 percent of individuals.[14] Other potential collateral pathways include external carotid to ipsilateral internal carotid connections and leptomeningeal arterial connections (Chap. 2), but these collateral vessels may not contribute significantly to cerebral blood flow during carotid cross-clamping, even if the patient's blood pressure is elevated. Preoperative four-vessel, selective cerebral arteriography can identify the patient cohort at increased risk for cerebral ischemia during carotid surgery by demonstrating absence of anterior and middle cerebral artery cross-filling via the circle of Willis.[16] However, arteriographic confirmation of a patent circle of Willis does not completely ensure adequate cerebral collateral flow during carotid surgery.

The experience of the pioneers of carotid surgery led them to conclude that routine shunting or some form of monitoring (awake patient, stump pressure measurement, EEG) with selective shunting was advisable. Use of an intraluminal shunt to augment cerebral perfusion during carotid cross-clamping provides reliable cerebral protection in patients with inadequate collateral blood flow, and avoids the need to monitor cerebral function when carotid endarterectomy is performed under general anesthesia. Despite the documented safety of this approach, some surgeons advocate "selective" shunting based on the results of intraoperative monitoring. The arguments against routine shunt use have focused primarily on the technical difficulty added to the procedure when a shunt is in place, vessel trauma related to the shunt, and concern for either air or atheromatous embolization during shunt insertion.[17] In addition, the presence of a high carotid bifurcation, diffuse atherosclerotic disease extending to the base of skull, or a tortuous ICA further complicates the use and safety of temporary intraluminal shunts.

The controversy over routine shunt use has resulted in attempts to identify those patients who would benefit most from shunt placement. Monitoring the neurologic status of an awake patient is the most accurate method for determining the need for shunting during carotid endarterectomy. Other criteria used as a basis for selective shunt placement include assessment for pulsatile internal carotid backflow, measurement of ICA stump pressure, and changes in the EEG or somatosensory-evoked potentials (SSEPs) with carotid occlusion.

One of the earliest criteria used by surgeons to determine the need for a shunt was the quality of back-bleeding from the ICA. Pulsatile backflow was considered as reliable evidence of adequate cerebral collateral flow, while flow that merely seeped from the distal internal carotid was not. Since it was difficult to quantify back-bleeding, measurements of ICA stump pressure were proposed as a more quantitative index of collateral circulation from the vertebrobasilar and contralateral carotid systems. In 1969, Moore and Hall reported that if the mean ICA stump pressure was greater than 25 mmHg, carotid surgery could be performed safely without an intraluminal shunt; those patients with a lower stump pressure were at increased risk for intraoperative stroke if a shunt was not used.[20] Several years later, Hays and coworkers concluded that a systolic ICA stump pressure of 50 mmHg was safer, and this has become the threshold value most frequently used by surgeons who employ selective shunting based on stump pressure measurements.[21]

While stump pressure measurement and clinical assessment of carotid back-bleeding are the simplest methods for assessing collateral flow, subsequent changes in cerebral perfusion during the procedure will not be detected, and this initial assessment has been associated with a false-negative rate in the range of 6 to 15 percent.[16,22,23] Neurologic deficits after carotid endarterectomy and ischemic EEG changes during carotid cross-clamping have been reported with ICA stump pressures greater than 50 mmHg. Stump pressure measurements may be unreliable when compared with monitoring the awake patient, cerebral perfusion measurements, or EEG monitoring, particularly in patients with a prior stroke.

Neurologic Monitoring of the Awake Patient

It is generally accepted that continuous neurologic assessment of the awake patient is the most sensitive monitor of cerebral perfusion and function. Following carotid cross-clamping, up to one-quarter of patients will develop loss of consciousness, aphasia, contralateral paresis or paresthesias, confusion, or slowing of mentation. While the majority of these symptoms occur within one to three minutes after clamping, delayed onset of up to 20 minutes or more has been observed. When a trial of carotid occlusion confirms inadequate collateral circulation, insertion of a shunt will promptly correct the neurologic deficit; if the neurologic deficit is the result of embolization due to clamp placement, the deficit will not change even with a patent, functioning shunt. Monitoring the neurologic status of the awake patient is more sensitive than EEG monitoring, possibly because ischemic changes within the deeper structures of the brain can be detected.

Despite these advantages, most surgeons prefer that the patient not be awake during carotid endarterectomy. The perioperative morbidity and mortality of carotid surgery are comparable when either regional or general anesthesia is used, and some patients are not appropriate candidates for regional anesthesia because of anxiety, prior stroke, or concomitant medical problems. With skilled general anesthesia, the patient's airway is protected, and in cases of extensive atherosclerotic disease, exposure of the distal ICA is facilitated. Lastly, a significant problem when operating on the awake patient is hypertension, which increases myocardial oxygen demand and the risk of myocardial infarction. This is particularly important in patients with preexisting coronary artery disease, who account for over one-half of those undergoing carotid endarterectomy.

Electroencephalography and Somatosensory-Evoked Potentials

The EEG represents electrical activity arising from the superficial layers of the cerebral cortex and correlates with the level of cerebral perfusion. When blood flow falls below 18 ml/100 g per min, the neuronal electrical activity changes from high to low frequency, and the amplitude of the waves decreases.[22] The EEG becomes isoelectric when blood flow falls below 15 ml/100g per min, a level of perfusion that carries a high risk of neuron injury and cerebral infarction. Abnormalities in the EEG have been documented in 10 to 29 percent of patients following carotid cross-clamping. When an EEG abnormality is identified during carotid endarterectomy, the appropriate intervention is to place a shunt immediately, document its patency, and confirm that the patient's blood pressure and oxygenation are normal.

Unfortunately, the occurrence of EEG changes does not always correlate with the subsequent development of a neurologic deficit. Patients may sustain a perioperative stroke without EEG changes, and abnormalities of the EEG may be observed without a change in neurologic status. In a series of 458 consecutive carotid endarterectomies performed with general anesthesia and EEG monitoring, Kresowick and colleagues found that five of ten patients with immediate strokes—and all five patients with immediate transient neurologic deficits—had no ischemic EEG changes during the procedure.[23] There has also been a poor correlation between the severity of a neurologic deficit and the degree of intraoperative EEG change. These observations can be explained, in part, by the fact that the EEG monitors only the superficial layers of the cerebral cortex. Thus, cerebral infarcts occurring in subcortical or internal capsular areas will not result in significant EEG abnormalities.

Small emboli may cause very focal cerebral ischemia not detected by EEG monitoring. Similarly, if carotid cross-clamping produces critical ischemia in a small region secondary to intracerebral arterial disease or a prior cerebral infarct, the EEG may not be affected. When awake patients had concomitant EEG monitoring during carotid endarterectomy, up to one-quarter showed no EEG changes with carotid cross-clamping despite dramatic mental status changes that reversed promptly after shunt placement.[12] The inconsistent correlation between EEG changes and neurologic symptoms will most likely result in more patients being identified as candidates for shunt placement when EEG monitoring is used during general anesthesia, compared with patients undergoing carotid endarterectomy awake. When EEG monitoring is used as the primary criterion for shunt placement, failure of the EEG to return to baseline after shunt insertion should alert the surgeon to the possibility of an occluded or improperly positioned shunt.

An important disadvantage of EEG monitoring is the interpretation of the complex tracings. This has been particularly difficult in patients with preexisting EEG abnormalities, in whom subtle changes may be missed. Newer EEG instruments use a two-channel computerized system that processes the electrical signals by power spectral analysis. This permits a more objective assessment and demonstrates trends more clearly. A global power reduction of 50 percent or greater in three of six preselected frequency bands is an accepted threshold for shunt placement. In general, any EEG changes in patients with either a recent stroke (less than six weeks) or stroke-in-evolution should prompt shunt placement.

The SSEPs reflect the integrity of afferent pathways from peripheral nerves to the somatosensory cortex, as well as deep structures such as the internal capsule, and thus are more representative of overall brain function than the EEG. Measurements of SSEPs are obtained by stimulating the median nerve at the wrist and recording from the somatosensory cortex with scalp electrodes. Calculations of central conduction time and the amplitude of the primary cortical potential are then made. A 50 percent reduction in the amplitude of the primary cortical potential or prolongation of the central conduction time indicate impending cerebral ischemia and may be used as criteria for shunt placement. Use of SSEPs can decrease the frequency of shunt usage by up to 20 percent compared with shunting on the basis of ICA stump pressures.[16,12]

The principal advantage of monitoring the SSEPs is the ability to evaluate deeper structures of the brain. The major limitations are the time required to obtain meaningful data, operator dependence, and artifacts. As with EEG monitoring, amplitudes of SSEPs can be altered by anesthetic agents, sedative drugs, and hypotension. Schweiger and coworkers documented the efficacy of SSEPs in a prospective study of 400 carotid operations.[24] In 17 cases (4 percent), complete loss of amplitude occurred during the period of ICA clamping. Of these, seven patients underwent surgery without a shunt (clamp time 9 to 24 min); five developed a new contralateral hemiparesis that was transient in four and permanent in one. The 10 remaining patients had a shunt placed, and one sustained a permanent neurologic deficit due to inadequate shunt flow. Complete loss of amplitude on monitoring of SSEPs was observed in 25 percent of patients with a prior stroke and contralateral ICA occlusion.

Transcranial Doppler Ultrasonography

Low frequency ultrasound can be transmitted through the relatively thin temporal bone to assess the blood flow velocities in the basal cerebral arteries (Chap. 12). The intraoperative TCD instrument uses a probe fixed to the skull that continuously monitors the velocity in the middle cerebral artery (MCA). Predictable changes in MCA velocity appear to be associated with carotid cross-clamping and the need for shunt insertion. In addition, there is also good correlation between the velocities in the MCA and carotid stump pressures. A systolic carotid stump pressure of 50 mmHg corresponds to a peak MCA velocity of 42 cm/sec and a mean velocity of 30 cm/sec.[25] The major advantage of this approach over use of stump pressure alone is that a stump pressure is an isolated measurement, whereas TCD is a continuous monitoring technique. Since intracerebral flow increases during the first few minutes after carotid clamping, many patients may have a low stump pressure immediately after cross-clamping but subsequently develop adequate flow in the MCA as determined by TCD. Monitoring with TCD also can be helpful in assessing the adequacy of shunt function, diagnosis of ICA thrombosis in the immediate postoperative period, and differentiating between intraoperative hemodynamic or embolic neurologic events.

^{133}Xenon Clearance

The xenon washout or clearance technique provides a measurement of cerebral perfusion. This test is performed by injecting saline saturated with ^{133}Xe into the common carotid artery. An initial injection is made early in the operation to obtain a baseline blood flow determination. A second injection is then made immediately before cross-clamping, and monitoring is continued throughout the period of carotid occlusion. Comparison of the ^{133}Xe clearance between the first and second injections provides a determination of the change in cerebral perfusion during cross-clamping. A perfusion of 18 ml/100g per min is considered critical, and shunt placement is advised below this level.

This method has proved to be impractical for most institutions. In addition, it appears to be most sensitive to flow changes in the superficial layers of the cerebral cortex to the exclusion of the deeper regions of the brain, and can fail to detect ischemia in deep structures when the overlying areas are normally perfused. Furthermore, cerebral perfusion analysis with inert gas washout has not accurately correlated with intraoperative TCD recordings, EEG abnormalities, or neurologic outcome.

SAFE INTRALUMINAL SHUNTING

Since approximately 10 to 20 percent of patients undergoing carotid endarterectomy require the cerebral protection afforded by an intraluminal shunt (Table 24-2), surgeons must be familiar with a technique of shunt selection, placement, and monitoring that minimizes complications. A variety of shunts is commercially available, and the specific technical details of their use vary considerably. The senior author (D.F.B.) prefers a short, flexible shunt with a sidearm attachment (Brener carotid bypass tube, C.R. Bard, Inc., Billerica, MA). The T-shaped configuration of this shunt allows it to lie in the lumen of the exposed carotid bifurcation, and the presence of a sidearm in the middle of the shunt permits flushing of both limbs at the time of placement and verification of patency at any time during the procedure (Fig. 24-1).[27]

Shunt Placement

Following exposure of the carotid bifurcation and its branches, Rummel tourniquets are placed around the distal ICA and proximal common carotid artery (CCA). A shunt with the appropriate diameter (7 or 8 Fr) based on the size of the distal ICA is selected and

Table 24-2 Percentages of Patients with Signs of Clamp-Induced Cerebral Ischemia During Carotid Endarterectomy Relative to Monitoring Technique

	%
Awake patient under local anesthesia	8–16
EEG monitoring under general anesthesia	10–15
—with contralateral ICA occlusion	20–40
SSEPs monitoring under general anesthesia	6
Stump pressure < 50 mmHg	40–50

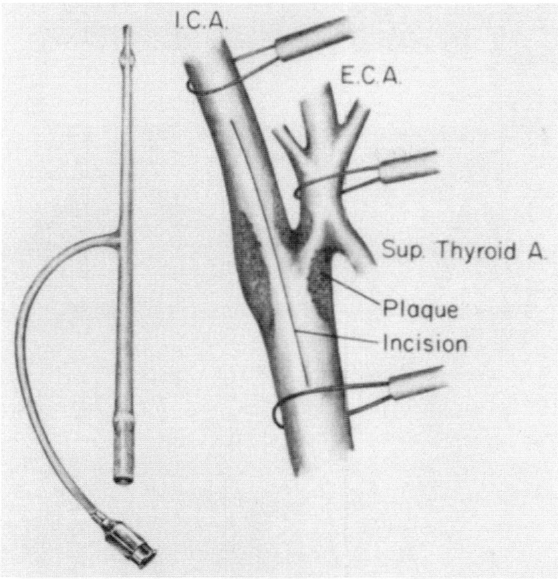

Figure 24-1. T-shaped Brener carotid bypass tube with sidearm and dissected carotid bifurcation with planned incision. Rummel tourniquets or Javid clamps are used to hold the shunt in place.

flushed with heparinized saline solution (1000 U of heparin/100 ml of normal saline). With the patient systemically heparinized, vascular clamps are applied sequentially to the distal ICA, CCA, and external carotid artery. Through a longitudinal arteriotomy extending from the CCA through the carotid bulb into the ICA beyond the obstructing plaque, the smaller end of the T-shaped shunt is introduced into the ICA with a hemostat placed on the shunt, as shown in Fig. 24-2*A*, observing the presence of retrograde ICA flow from the sidearm. This maneuver ensures that the end of the shunt does not impinge against the ICA wall and that a dissection will not be produced as the shunt tip is advanced. The distal end of the shunt is secured in place with either a Rummel tourniquet or a Javid clamp. The hemostat is then moved to the position shown in Fig. 24-2*B*, which halts retrograde flow through the sidearm. The larger end of the shunt is then inserted into the CCA and secured with a Rummel tourniquet. Flow through the proximal shunt limb exits initially from the sidearm, thus avoiding the embolization of air or atheromatous debris into the ICA circulation. When the surgeon is satisfied that flushing has been adequate and that flow through the sidearm is of good volume, the hemostat is transferred to the shunt sidearm to restore cerebral perfusion (Fig. 24-2*C*).

Immediate assessment of shunt function is carried out using a sterile continuous-wave Doppler probe. With the probe positioned over the shunt, a pulsatile flow signal with a continuous diastolic component should be heard. If the shunt is repositioned during the endarterectomy, repeat documentation of pulsatile flow should be obtained by either the Doppler instrument or unclamping the sidearm and assessing the patency of both proximal and distal shunt limbs. Prior to completion of the arteriotomy closure, the shunt is removed and the endarterectomized segment irrigated with heparinized saline solution. Usually, only an additional three or four sutures are required to complete vessel closure after removal of the shunt. The technique of shunt placement is also discussed in Chap. 23.

In the past 10 years, this technique of shunting has been used in approximately 500 patients undergoing carotid endarterectomy. There have been no instances of shunt thrombosis or vessel wall dissection with shunt placement. In four patients, atheromatous debris was observed exiting from the sidearm during shunt placement prior to establishing flow into the ICA (Fig. 24-3). Shunt placement and removal were consistently accomplished within two to three minutes and were associated with minimal blood loss.

The advantages of shunting during carotid endarterectomy include maintenance of normal regional cerebral blood flow during cross-clamping, elimination of the need for moni-

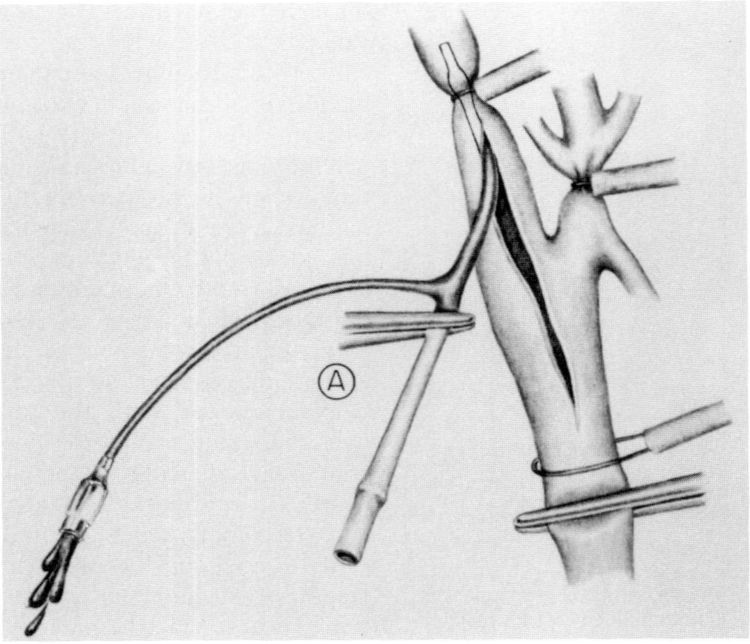

Figure 24-2. Technique of shunt placement. *A.* Shunt is introduced into the internal carotid artery with the proximal limb occluded by a hemostat to allow back-bleeding through the sidearm. *B.* Hemostat is moved to the position shown and the proximal limb placed in the common carotid artery, allowing the proximal limb to be flushed through the sidearm of the shunt prior to restoring flow to the brain. *C.* Shunt flow is established by transferring the hemostat to the sidearm. Flow is confirmed using a continuous-wave Doppler probe.

toring cerebral perfusion or function, and removal of the sense of urgency during the procedure, which allows time for carrying out a technically precise repair. Maintaining that a shunt is never necessary is not defensible based on reported experience with carotid endarterectomy. A safe technique for intraluminal shunting enables the surgeon to choose the security of routine shunting when the procedure is performed under general anesthesia.

ANESTHETIC CONSIDERATIONS

Cerebral blood flow is regulated by a multitude of factors. Anesthetic agents and manipulations may alter cerebral blood flow and offer varying degrees of cerebral protection. Vasopressors have been used to augment cerebral collateral blood flow by artificially elevating the systemic blood pressure to above 180 mmHg. However, this method is dangerous and can lead to myocardial ischemia and increased rates of myocardial infarction. Artificially-induced hypercarbia was tried in the past to reduce intracerebral vascular resistance. This can be achieved by inhalation of carbon dioxide, hypoventilation during general anesthesia, or administration of carbonic anhydrase inhibitors. The high number of intracerebral hemorrhages seen in association with induced hypercarbia has led to abandonment of this technique.

High-dose barbiturate anesthesia suppresses neuronal activity and reduces cerebral meta-

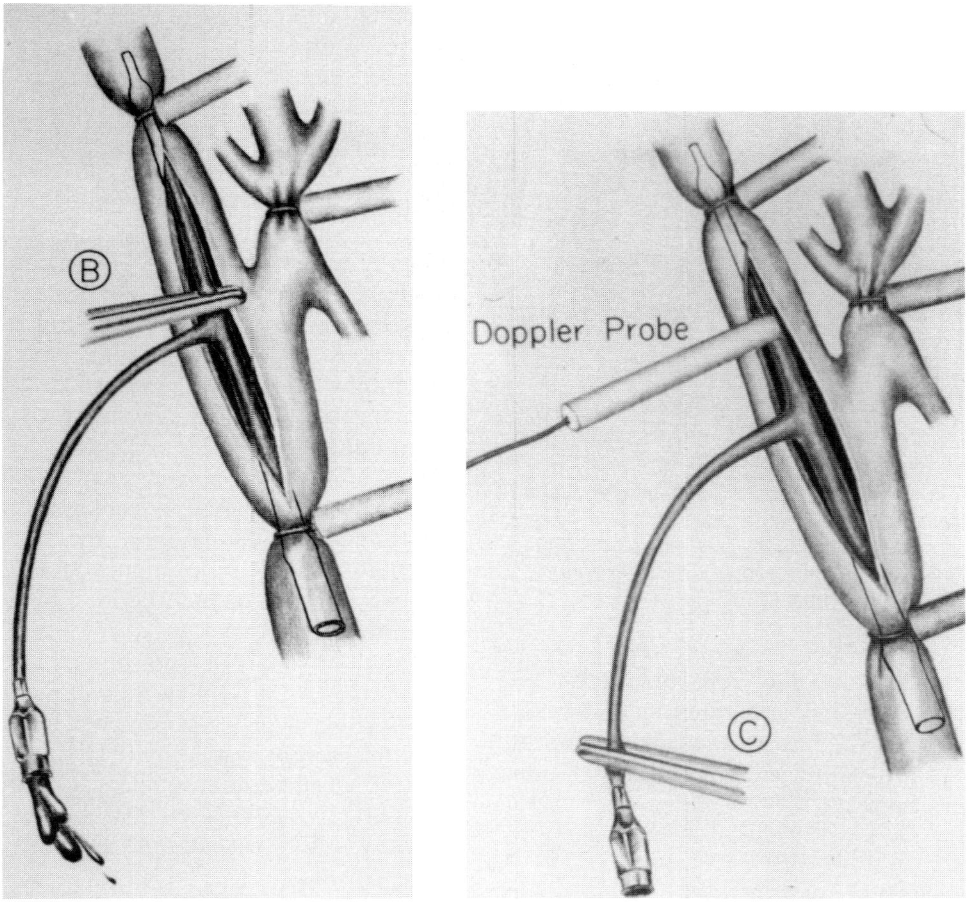

Figure 24-2. *(Continued)*

bolic demand, thereby increasing the tolerance of the brain to ischemia.[24] In large doses, barbiturates provide protection against focal ischemic cerebral injury, particularly when administered before the ischemic insult, and in some instances they may actually divert flow to areas of ischemia. Careful patient monitoring is mandatory when this approach is used, since high doses of barbiturates can lead to cardiovascular instability or delayed reversal of anesthesia. The use of barbiturates is probably most effective in patients undergoing simultaneous cardiac procedures, such as valve replacement, that require opening of the ventricle.

Isoflurane inhalation anesthetics offer cerebral protection by a mechanism similar to that of the barbiturates.[27] Isoflurane produces a dose-related decrease in cerebral oxygen consumption through a depression of synaptic transmission. Clinical studies have shown that the level of cerebral blood flow associated with ischemic EEG changes is lower for patients receiving isoflurane compared with halo-

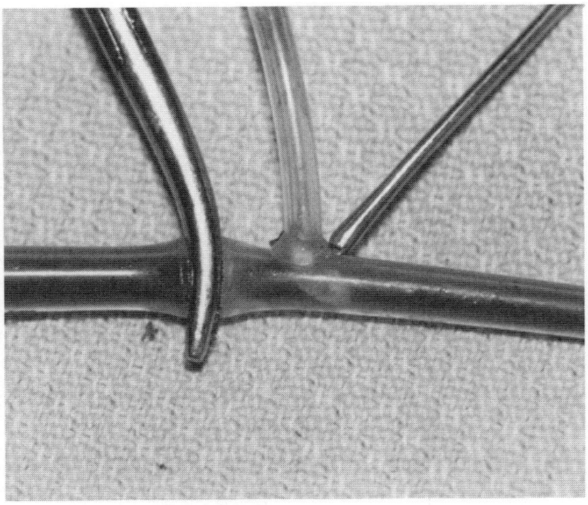

Figure 24-3. Close-up view of a T-shaped carotid shunt showing a clump of atheromatous debris lodged at the entrance to the sidearm. The hemostat is on the proximal (common carotid) limb, and the probe tip indicates the site of the debris.

thane anesthetics. Sundt reported decreased shunt usage in patients operated on under isoflurane anesthesia.[18] A detailed discussion of anesthesia for carotid endarterectomy is presented in Chap. 22.

INTRAOPERATIVE ASSESSMENT

Since the goal of carotid endarterectomy is to remove the obstructing lesion and provide an arterial segment free of anatomic and hemodynamic abnormalities, assessment of the repair prior to wound closure is strongly recommended (Chap. 25). Undetected defects (intimal flaps, luminal thrombus or platelet aggregates, suture stenoses, adventitial bands) can result in stroke by embolization or progression to occlusion. As previously mentioned, thrombosis of the repair accounts for most perioperative strokes, with a reported rate of approximately 2 percent.[9] Technical errors can be found at reexploration in most cases, and thus it is the responsibility of the surgeon to detect these problems before a neurologic event occurs.

Routine completion arteriography, performed by Blaisdell and colleagues in 1967, provided compelling early data on the fallibility of clinical assessment.[29] Significant abnormalities of the repair site, not evident by either palpation or inspection, were identified in 25 percent of cases. A variety of noninvasive methods, including angioscopy, continuous-wave Doppler assessment, pulsed Doppler spectral analysis, real-time B-mode imaging, and duplex ultrasonography have been used successfully to evaluate the technical adequacy of carotid endarterectomy sites.

Each intraoperative assessment method has unique advantages and disadvantages, increases operating time, and requires the surgeon to make an immediate decision concerning the adequacy of the reconstruction. Since decisions are best made on quantitative rather than qualitative information, the authors favor the routine use of duplex ultrasonography to evaluate the endarterectomy site for residual anatomic or flow abnormalities.[30] The advantages of intraoperative duplex scanning over arteriography include comparable or higher accuracy, safety, ease of repeated use, and relatively low cost.

In a series of 410 consecutive carotid endarterectomies, a normal intraoperative assessment ($n = 336$) was associated with a perioperative stroke rate of 1 percent, and the incidence of late ICA stenosis or occlusion was 8 percent at four years.[7] In contrast, when a residual flow abnormality in the ICA or CCA was accepted ($n = 74$), the perioperative stroke rate was 2.7 percent ($p = .55$), acute thrombosis of the repair occurred in one patient, and the incidence of late ICA stenosis or occlusion increased to 20 percent at four years ($p < .01$). This experience supports the view that objective intraoperative assessment is indicated following arteriotomy closure. Although confirming a technically adequate repair contributes only indirectly to the overall goal of cerebral protection, intraoperative assessment permits the surgeon to recognize correctable technical errors in approximately 5 percent of patients, resulting in improved operative technique and a reduction in procedure-related morbidity.

CONCLUSIONS

The elimination of neurologic events caused by inadequate or failed attempts at cerebral protection during carotid cross-clamping can decrease perioperative morbidity by 10 to 25 percent, depending on the characteristics of the patient population. Patients with prior strokes and multiple vessel cerebrovascular disease (carotid, vertebral, intracranial) are at highest risk for clamp-induced cerebral ischemia. In this subset of patients, recommended operative approaches are carotid endarterectomy with the patient awake, or if general anesthesia is used, routine shunt placement. When shunt function is inadequate, or anatomic considerations preclude the use of a shunt, barbiturate anesthesia can provide a measure of cerebral protection.

REFERENCES

1. North American Symptomatic Carotid Endarterectomy Trial Collaborators: Beneficial effect of carotid endarterectomy in symptomatic patients with high-grade carotid stenosis. *N Engl J Med* 325:445–453, 1991.
2. European Carotid Surgery Trialist's Collaborative Group: MRC European carotid surgery trial: Interim results for symptomatic patients with severe (70–99%) or mild (0–29%) carotid stenosis. *Lancet* 337:1235–1243, 1991.
3. Mayo Asymptomatic Carotid Endarterectomy Study Group: Results of a randomized controlled trial of carotid endarterectomy for asymptomatic carotid stenosis. *Mayo Clin Proc* 67:513–518, 1992.
4. Hobson RW, Weiss DG, and the Veterans Affairs Cooperative Study Group: Efficacy of carotid endarterectomy for asymptomatic carotid stenosis. *N Engl J Med* 221–227, 1993.
5. Easton JD, Sherman DG: Stroke and mortality rate in carotid endarterectomy. 228 consecutive operations. *Stroke* 8:565–568, 1977.
6. Roon AJ, Hoogerwerf D: Intraoperative arteriography and carotid surgery. *J Vasc Surg* 16:239–243, 1992.
7. Kinney EV, Seabrook GR, Kinney LY, et al: The importance of intraoperative detection of residual flow abnormalities after carotid endarterectomy. *J Vasc Surg* 17:912–913, 1993.
8. Moore WS, Mohr JP, Najafi H, et al: Carotid endarterectomy: Practice guidelines. *J Vasc Surg* 15:469–479, 1992.
9. Riles TS, Imparato AM, Jacobowitz GR, et al: The cause of perioperative stroke after carotid endarterectomy. *J Vasc Surg* 19:206–216, 1994.
10. Hafner CD, Evans WE: Carotid endarterectomy with local anesthesia: Results and advantages. *J Vasc Surg* 7:232–239, 1988.
11. Imparato AM, Ramirez A, Riles T, Minzer R: Cerebral protection in carotid surgery. *Arch Surg* 117:1073–1078, 1982.
12. Benjamin ME, Siva MB Jr, Watt C, et al: Awake patient monitoring to determine the need for shunting during carotid endarterectomy. *Surgery* 114:673–681, 1993.
13. Spencer MP, Thomas GI, Nicholls SC, Sauvage LR: Detection of middle cerebral artery emboli during carotid endarterectomy using transcranial Doppler ultrasonography. *Stroke* 21:415–423, 1990.
14. Schneider PA, Ringlestein EB, Rossman ME, et al: Importance of cerebral collateral pathways during carotid endarterectomy. *Stroke* 19:1328–1330, 1988.
15. Sundt TM Jr, Sharbrough FW, Marsh WR, et al: The risk-benefit ratio of intraoperative shunting during carotid endarterectomy: Relevancy to operative and postoperative results and complications. *Ann Surg* 203:196–204, 1986.
16. Sbarigia E, Speziale F, Colonna M, et al: The selection for shunting in patients with severe bilateral carotid lesions. *Eur J Vasc Surg* 7(suppl A):3–7, 1993.
17. Baker WH, Littooy FN, Hayes AC, et al: Carotid endarterectomy without a shunt: The control series. *J Vasc Surg* 1:50–56, 1984.

18. Sundt TM Jr: Cerebral blood flow measurements during carotid endarterectomy, in Bernstein EF (ed): *Vascular Diagnosis,* 4th ed. St. Louis, Mosby, pp 389–397, 1993.
19. Thompson JE: Complications of carotid endarterectomy and their prevention. *World J Surgery* 3:155–159, 1979.
20. Moore WS, Hall AD: Carotid artery back pressure. *Arch Surg* 69:702–710, 1969.
21. Hays RJ, Levison SA, Wylie EJ: Intraoperative measurement of carotid back pressure as a guide to operative management of carotid endarterectomy. *Surgery* 72:593–596, 1972.
22. Sundt TM Jr: Cerebral blood flow measurements and electroencephalograms during carotid endarterectomy. *J Neurosurg* 41:310–315, 1974.
23. Kresowik TF, Worsey MJ, Khoury MD, et al: Limitations of electrocephalographic monitoring in the detection of cerebral ischemia accompanying carotid endarterectomy. *J Vasc Surg* 13:439–434, 1991.
24. Schweiger H, Hans-Dieter K, Dinkel M: Somatosensory-evoked potentials during carotid artery surgery: Experience in 400 operations. *Surgery* 109:602–609, 1991.
25. Schneider PA, Rossman ME, Schlomo Torem RVT, et al: Transcranial Doppler in the management of extracranial cerebrovascular disease: Implications and monitoring. *J Vasc Surg* 7:223–231, 1988.
26. Frawley JE, Hicks RG, Horton DA, et al: Thiopental sodium cerebral protection during carotid endarterectomy: Perioperative disease and death. *J Vasc Surg* 19:732–738, 1994.
27. Michenfielder JD et al: Isoflurane when compared to enflurane and halothane decreased the frequency of cerebral ischemia during carotid endarterectomy. *Anesthesiology* 67:336–340, 1987.
28. Bandyk DF, Thiele BL: Safe intraluminal shunting during carotid endarterectomy. *Surgery* 93:260–263, 1983.
29. Blaisdell FW, Lim R, Hall AD: Technical result of carotid endarterectomy: Arteriographic assessment. *Am J Surg* 114:239–246, 1967.
30. Bandyk DF, Kaebnick HW, Adams MB, et al: Turbulence occurring after carotid bifurcation endarterectomy. A harbinger of residual and recurrent carotid stenosis. *J Vasc Surg* 7:261–274, 1988.

25

Intraoperative Assessment of Carotid Endarterectomy

Mark Wengrovitz
Dean A. Healy

The goal of carotid endarterectomy is stroke prevention in patients with extracranial carotid atherosclerosis. Factors that influence the outcome after surgical intervention include patient selection, timing of operation, perioperative morbidity and mortality, durability of the reconstruction, and the inherent reduction in stroke rate associated with removal of an internal carotid lesion. The anatomic and hemodynamic results of operation are directly related to surgical technique, and therefore it is the surgeon's responsibility to achieve the best technical result possible. Intraoperative assessment of the surgical site should be a routine component of carotid endarterectomy, and a variety of methods is available for this purpose.

The presence of a large intimal flap, residual atherosclerotic plaque, suture line stenosis, platelet-fibrin aggregation, or adventitial web is an unacceptable technical result which can be safely repaired as long as it is identified before the neck incision is closed. Many of these lesions will not cause immediate neurologic deficits, but since a postoperative neurologic deficit may be permanent even when a technical error is later identified and corrected, it is not justifiable to wait until the patient is awake to assess the surgical result. The detection of technical errors that have the potential to cause immediate or long-term neurologic sequelae requires the use of intraoperative methods to assess and assure the technical adequacy of the carotid reconstruction. These intraoperative methods are based on either anatomic imaging or assessment of the hemodynamic flow patterns in the area of the reconstruction.

IMAGING TECHNIQUES

Intraoperative Arteriography

Intraoperative arteriography is considered the standard for identifying technical errors after carotid endarterectomy[1–3] and other peripheral vascular reconstructions.[4,5] Completion arteriography is commonly performed to assess infrainguinal bypass grafts, but this approach has not become widely accepted as standard practice following carotid endarterectomy. Many surgeons are reluctant to perform intraoperative arteriography because they were not trained to use it in this setting, are unfamiliar with the technique and equipment, or feel concern over potential complications. The risk of complications is a valid consideration, but the technical aspects of this procedure can be readily learned, and every operating room should have the capability of performing arteriography after carotid endarterectomy.

The patient should be positioned on an operating room table that will allow placement of an x-ray cassette directly below the neck incision. A scout film can be taken to assure proper placement and exposure of the film so that time will not be wasted with multiple injections after the artery has been reconstructed. Once the endarterectomy has been completed, the arteriotomy closed, and flow reestablished, all retractors, vessel loops, and clamps must be removed from the incision to allow the artery to assume its natural configuration. A 19-gauge "butterfly" type needle is attached to one end of a length of intravenous infusion tubing, and the other end is connected to a syringe filled with heparinized Ringer's lactate or saline solution. All air must be carefully removed from the system. The needle is then inserted into the common carotid artery proximal to the arteriotomy suture line. The end of the needle can point either proximally or distally, but the contrast column will be less opaque and less likely to obscure a technical problem if it is pointed proximally so that more adequate mixing of contrast material and blood can occur. The needle is retained in the artery by the flanges at its base, clamping a nearby drape around the tubing, and by bending the needle slightly upward approximately 1.5 cm from the tip. Again, any air bubbles must be removed from the system before the injection is performed to avoid air embolism.

To ensure proper positioning of the needle, arterial blood should be easily aspirated. Once this is confirmed, the tubing is clamped and a syringe filled with 60% methylglucamine iothalamate (Conray 60) is attached in place of the syringe of heparinized fluid. The methylglucamine compounds have been advocated as the contrast media of choice for cerebral angiography as they are felt to be less toxic than the sodium-containing compounds.[6] The entire operative field is then covered with a sterile towel, the x-ray cassette is placed under the patient's head and neck, and the x-ray machine is moved into position. While standing behind a lead shield draped with a sterile sheet, the surgeon injects the contrast material as rapidly as possible, and the film is exposed after a volume of 15 to 20 ml has been infused. The infusion should continue while the film is being exposed to ensure the best image. Rarely is it necessary to clamp the common carotid artery proximal to the infusion needle to produce a satisfactory image. A 6-0 polypropylene suture is placed in the adventitia around the needle and is tied down as the needle is removed. The film is then developed and can be available for review by the surgeon within minutes (Fig. 25-1).

Surgeons usually interpret intraoperative carotid arteriograms themselves, but a radiologist's interpretation may be necessary. If the image is not of good quality, a second x-ray must be taken. In general, the technical result should be considered unacceptable if the operative arteriogram shows complete occlusion or greater than 30 percent diameter stenosis of any carotid bifurcation vessel, intraluminal thrombus, residual atherosclerotic plaque, or an intimal flap (Fig. 25-2*A* and *B*). These problems are most likely to occur at the distal extent of the endarterectomy in the internal and external carotid arteries. Even if a technical defect is found, immediate repair is not always considered necessary. Zierler and coworkers reported 150 intraoperative carotid arteriograms, of which 23 (15 percent) were considered to contain a technical abnormality; however, only 10 of these 23 abnormalities were surgically repaired.[7] More recently, Roon and Hoogerwerf reported their experience with 535 consecutive carotid endarterectomies which were assessed with intraoperative arteriography. Eleven abnormal arteriograms were felt to represent major defects, and all of these carotid arteries were reopened and repaired. Compared to 157 earlier procedures with no completion arteriograms, the group with intraoperative assessment had both sig-

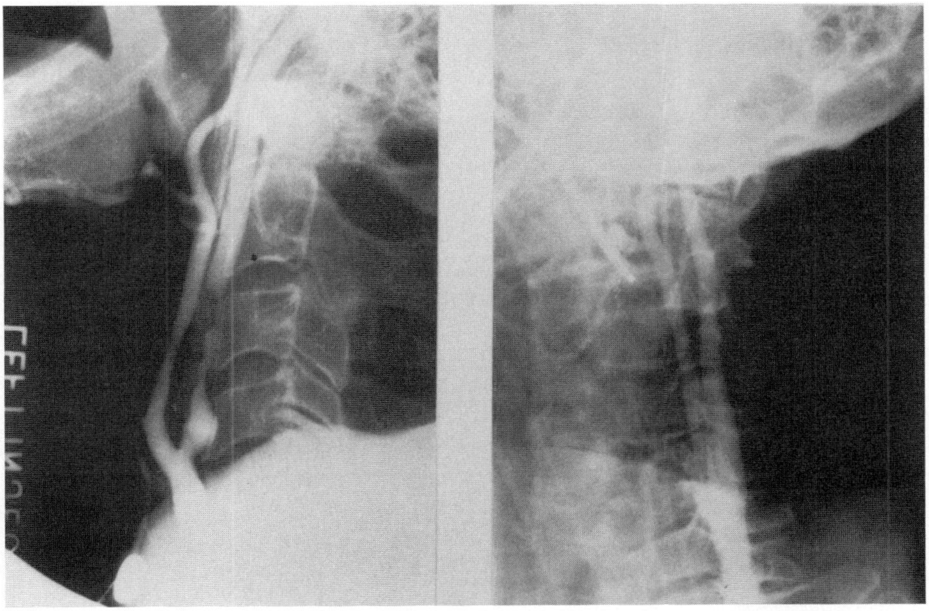

Figure 25-1. Preoperative arteriogram (*left*) of a high-grade internal carotid artery stenosis. Intraoperative arteriogram (*right*) taken after endarterectomy of this lesion showed a widely patent internal carotid artery with a smooth luminal surface.

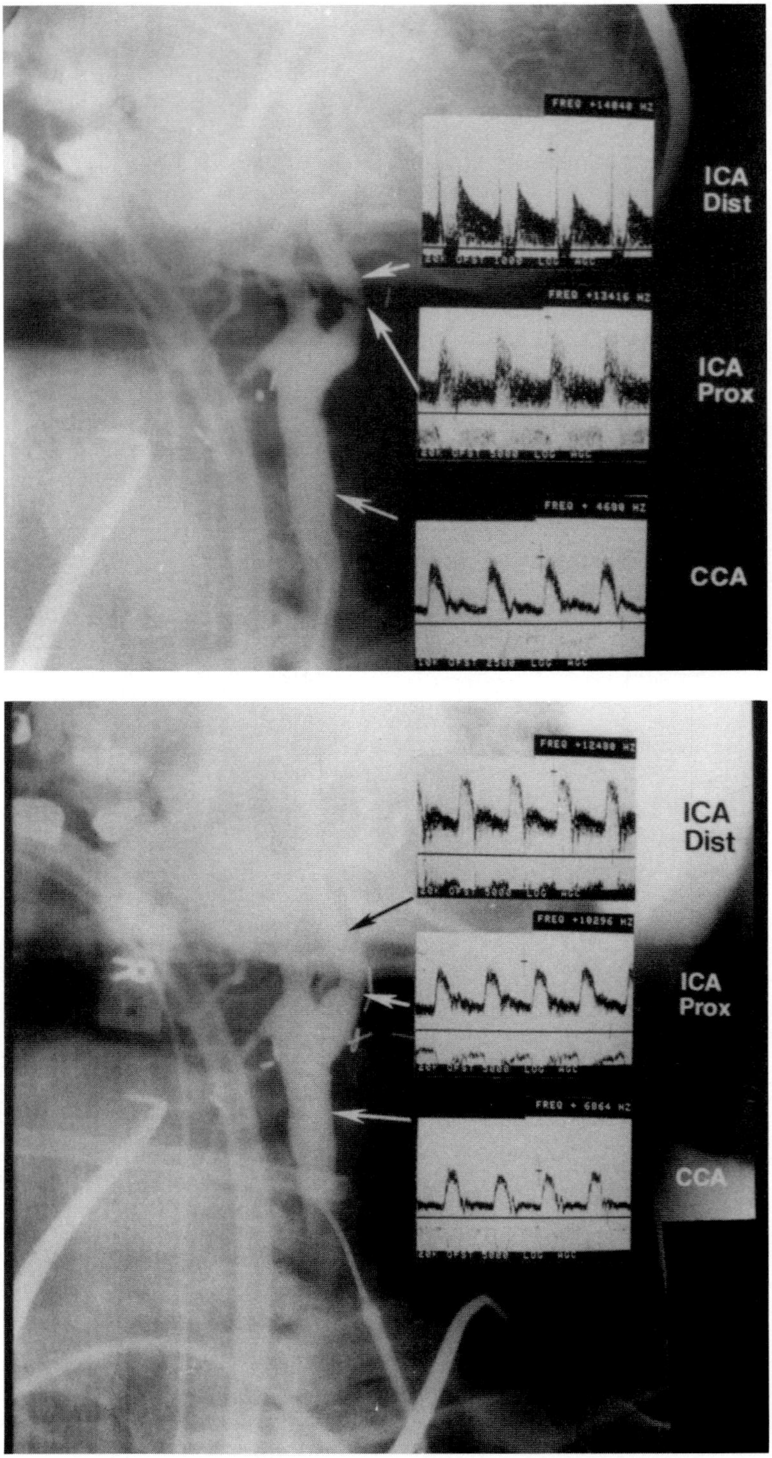

Figure 25-2. *A.* Intraoperative carotid arteriogram and accompanying pulsed Doppler spectral analysis recordings following carotid endarterectomy. The arteriogram demonstrates a focal high-grade stenosis in the internal carotid artery consistent with an intimal flap. The common carotid (CCA) waveform is normal, but the proximal internal carotid (ICA Prox) and distal internal carotid (ICA Dist) show increases in peak systolic frequency and marked spectral broadening. *B.* Intraoperative carotid arteriogram and pulsed Doppler recordings following repair of the lesion shown in *A.* The arteriogram shows a good technical result. Doppler spectral analysis shows a reduction in spectral broadening and peak systolic frequency. (*From Zierler et al.*[7] *Reproduced by permission.)*

nificantly lower ischemic neurologic morbidity and a decreased incidence of reoperation for recurrent stenosis.[8]

If the decision is made to correct an abnormality found by arteriography, the arteriotomy usually is reopened and the shunt replaced if one was originally used. External carotid artery defects, however, often can be repaired without occlusion of the internal carotid by clamping the origin of the external carotid and making a new arteriotomy distal to the clamp. The arteriographic appearance of the artery usually will dictate how the defect is repaired. This may require tacking an intimal flap, extending the endarterectomy, performing patch angioplasty, or removing platelet-fibrin aggregates. The arteriogram also may show internal carotid artery spasm, which has been identified in up to 10 percent of intraoperative arteriograms.[9] This usually involves the segment of internal carotid artery distal to the reconstruction. Although carotid spasm is most likely a transient event, severe cases may be associated with perioperative internal carotid artery occlusion.

In 1967, Blaisdell and associates reported a 25 percent prevalence of unacceptable technical results in a series of intraoperative arteriograms obtained during 100 carotid endarterectomies.[3] This proportion of technical defects is too high by current standards, and a number of more recent studies based on intraoperative arteriography have indicated that defects occur in 5 to 10 percent of carotid endarterectomies.[1,2,7,10,11] These defects are found with about equal frequency in the internal and external carotid arteries but are rare in the common carotid artery.

The argument in favor of not performing routine intraoperative arteriography is based on the risk of the procedure. These risks are associated mainly with the injection of the contrast material and include subintimal injection, embolization, and allergic reaction. Roon and Hoogerwerf reported no complications in 535 cases.[8] While complications are extremely rare in experienced hands, their occurrence has discouraged some surgeons from performing intraoperative arteriography routinely.[2,12] This has led to a selective approach in which intraoperative arteriography is performed only when the endarterectomy has been difficult or a technical defect is suspected.[2] Limiting the contrast load may be accomplished by digital techniques, and a portable digital processor has been used for intraoperative assessment after carotid endarterectomy.[8,13] However, this equipment is not readily available in most operating rooms. The key factor for successful and low-risk use of intraoperative arteriography is proper education of the radiology technician, surgical team, and anesthesiologist.

B-Mode Ultrasound

Anatomic imaging of the carotid artery after endarterectomy also can be accomplished with B-mode ultrasound. This technique has been used in the operating room for numerous surgical procedures, including those on the liver, pancreas, biliary tree, and vascular system.[14–16] When used to image the carotid artery after endarterectomy, the risks of arteriography theoretically can be avoided.

B-mode imaging requires additional equipment in the operating room. A compact, small-parts scanner and a hand-held probe that can be gas-sterilized or covered with a sterile plastic sheath are typically used.[17] High-frequency imaging systems with 7.5 or 10 MHz probes are satisfactory because there is no tissue between the vessel and the scanhead. Acoustic coupling is achieved by filling the operative incision with warm saline solution, and transverse and sagittal images can be obtained and recorded for later review.

There are few well established objective criteria for determining the significance of a defect seen on a B-mode image, and interpretation depends primarily on the experience of the examiner. After the presence of a defect has been established, its size, location, and type will help determine whether surgical revision is necessary. Coelho and associates showed that B-mode ultrasound was highly accurate in the detection of intimal flaps, stenoses, and thrombi.[18]

Dilley and Bernstein studied 158 patients with B-mode imaging and arteriography after carotid endarterectomy.[19] Twelve patients had internal carotid artery abnormalities and 57 had defects in the external carotid (Fig. 25-3). All the internal carotid defects and 14 of the external carotid defects were repaired. Flanigan and coworkers used B-mode scanning to examine 48 carotid arteries after endarterectomy and noted defects in 13.[17] Only two of these defects, however, were felt to require revision, and none of the 13 patients suffered any perioperative neurologic morbidity. Lane and Appelberg conducted a similar study in which B-mode scanning revealed defects in nine of 60 arteries (15 percent), although only three of the defects required correction.[20] It should be noted that this technique identifies more defects than intraoperative arteriography, but the number of defects actually repaired is similar to the proportion of unacceptable technical results found by arteriography.

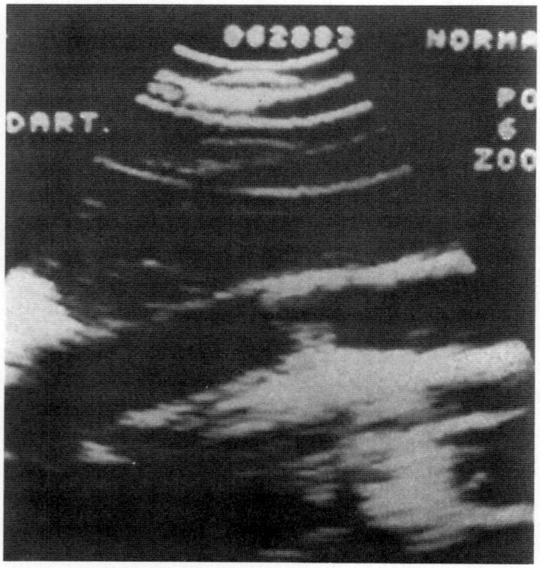

Figure 25-3. This longitudinal real-time B-mode image shows an intimal flap at the upper end of the endarterectomy site. (*From Dilley and Bernstein,*[19] *by permission of Mosby-Year Book, Inc.*)

The arguments against routine use of intraoperative B-mode scanning to assess carotid reconstructions are the high equipment costs, the need for the surgeon to learn and interpret a new technique, and the inability to evaluate any arterial segment beyond the confines of the neck incision. Another major limitation of B-mode scanning is that it does not differentiate reliably between fresh thrombus and flowing blood,[21] so an acutely thrombosed artery may appear patent on the B-mode image. This error is avoided if flow detection methods are employed as an adjunct to the B-mode image.[7,15] The major advantages to this technique are its high accuracy in experienced hands and the ability to avoid the risks of intraoperative arteriography.

Vascular Endoscopy

Endoscopic techniques have been used during biliary tract operations[22] and urologic procedures,[23] as well as vascular reconstruction.[24–27] This method of direct inspection of the lumen of the vessel rather than an image of it also has been used to assess arterialized vein grafts in infrainguinal reconstructions. Towne and Bernhard used a rigid choledochoscope and arthroscope to evaluate the technical results of 42 carotid endarterectomies prior to completing closure of the arteriotomy.[26] Atheromatous shreds felt to have embolic potential were found in two internal carotid arteries, and elevated distal intimal flaps were found in 17 external carotid arteries. The examination was reportedly associated with no operative morbidity and required only a few minutes to perform.

Newer and more sophisticated endoscopic equipment has been developed, including a video-assisted flexible device that has the capability for instrumentation and intervention through the endoscope. Mehigan and Olcott reported a series of 21 carotid endarterectomies that had been assessed with flexible endoscopes.[27] Four of 21 internal carotid artery end-points were shown to have strandlike debris which was removed through the endoscope. All 21 external carotid end-points were felt to be poor, and 18 were improved with the video-assisted instrumentation. For surgeons who are experienced, endoscopy does provide an alternative to intraoperative arteriography for assessment of carotid reconstructions. The major disadvantage is that this technique allows only a visual inspection of the luminal surface, and it is performed before the arteriotomy is completely closed and flow has been re-established. Therefore, endoscopy is not a technique that can assess a carotid reconstruction under conditions of physiologic pressure and flow.

FLOW DETECTION

The intraoperative assessment techniques discussed above provide no information on the hemodynamic flow pattern or rate of blood flow in the endarterectomized vessel. There are obvious potential benefits of techniques that test the adequacy of blood flow in the carotid system, as the goal of operation is to restore or preserve cerebral blood flow in addition to removing potentially embolic material.

Electromagnetic Flowmeter

This device has been widely used in research and for assessing the results of peripheral arterial reconstruction[28] and carotid endarterectomy.[10,29,30] Hobson and coworkers measured internal carotid artery blood flow with an electromagnetic flow probe before and after 25 carotid endarterectomies performed under regional anesthesia.[10] The mean flow rate was 126 ± 17 cc/min before endarterectomy and 159 ± 15 cc/min after endarterectomy, but this was not a statistically significant increase. Although improvement in flow rates did occur after operation, particularly in patients with severe carotid stenoses, accurate diagnostic criteria for intraoperative assessment could not be established.

Archie and Feldtman reported 143 carotid endarterectomies in which blood flow measurements were used to assess the results.[30] If postendarterectomy internal carotid artery blood flow was less than 100 cc/min or less than 70 percent of preendarterectomy flow (when the stenosis present was less than 70 percent diameter-reducing), a flow-limiting technical defect was said to be present. Six patients had abnormal internal carotid artery blood flow criteria, and after immediate revision all had normal flow measurements. They did not attempt any repair of external carotid artery defects, even if the flow was less than 25 cc/min.

The major limitation of this technique is that it probably cannot be applied to all patients. There are patients whose preoperative internal carotid artery flow is normal, even though they are candidates for endarterectomy. This may be due in part to the fact that a 50 percent diameter reduction (75 percent cross-sectional area reduction) is needed before flow rates will drop.[31] Many lesions with embolic manifestations may not cause any drop in preoperative flow rates, especially those with stenoses of less than 50 percent diameter reduction. As a single technique, blood flow measurement is probably not suitable for routine assessment after carotid endarterectomy.

Continuous-Wave Doppler

Intraoperative assessment methods that utilize a continuous-wave Doppler instrument are the supraorbital Doppler examination and the audible interpretation of Doppler signals from the endarterectomy site.[32–34] The supraorbital Doppler examination is capable only of detecting lesions that ultimately result in reduced pressure and flow in the carotid arterial system, and many technical defects such as platelet-fibrin aggregates, adventitial webs, or residual atherosclerosis may not result in major hemodynamic alterations. In addition, false-positive tests can occur in patients with ophthalmic artery occlusive disease.[32] Therefore, this technique has limited value in the intraoperative assessment of carotid endarterectomy.

A gas-sterilized Doppler probe can be brought into the operative field and coupled acoustically to the outer surface of any vessel with a small amount of blood or sterile saline. The normal quality of the Doppler signal in each carotid bifurcation vessel is recognizable, and the harsh, high-frequency flow patterns associated with stenoses also are easy to learn. Keitzer and coworkers used this technique to assess 93 peripheral vascular reconstructions and compared the results to 49 operations performed without the use of this instrument.[34] Reoperation was necessary in 31 percent of the patients in the latter group, but only 9 percent of the patients in the former group. Both the reoperation and mortality rates were significantly lower for those patients who had the benefit of intraoperative Doppler assessment.

Barnes and Garrett used audible interpretation of continuous-wave Doppler signals to assess the technical outcome of 42 carotid endarterectomies.[32] All of the internal carotid signals were considered normal, but obstructive signals were noted in three external carotid arteries. In these three cases, the external carotid defect was repaired and satisfactory audible signals were then confirmed by repeat Doppler examination. An 8.5-MHz probe was used by Seifert and Blackshear to assess 229 carotid endarterectomies.[35] Ten internal carotid and 20 external carotid arteries were felt to have either absent signals indicating occlusion, high-frequency signals indicating stenosis, or monophasic poststenotic signals. Seven internal and 19 external carotid defects were managed by immediate repair. The authors concluded that the use of continuous-wave Doppler for intraoperative assessment of carotid endarterectomy has a high positive predictive value for detecting defects; it is also safe, inexpensive, and avoids the problems associated with intraoperative arteriography.

The audible interpretation of continuous-wave Doppler signals is very subjective, and major frequency shifts must occur in order for a stenotic lesion or technical defect to be apparent. Abnormal or equivocal results may be further evaluated by intraoperative arteriography. The main advantages of the direct continuous-wave Doppler technique are that it is simple, does not prolong the operation, and only relatively inexpensive equipment is required.

Pulsed Doppler Ultrasound and Spectral Analysis

The use of a pulsed Doppler instrument with signal processing by spectral analysis can provide more objective and quantifiable data than that obtained with the audibly interpreted continuous-wave Doppler instrument. While a continuous-wave Doppler examines flow patterns across an entire vessel,[36] pulsed Doppler systems detect blood flow at a discrete site referred to as the "sample volume." This sample volume may be positioned in the center of the arterial stream, thereby avoiding the velocity gradients adjacent to the vessel wall, and providing a signal better suited to spectral analysis than that from a continuous-wave device.

Signal processing is performed by a spectrum analyzer that displays the entire range of frequencies and amplitudes in the Doppler signal. As discussed in Chap. 11, the severity of various carotid stenoses has been correlated with the spectral characteristics of this center stream flow signal.[36,37] Spectral broadening, or a widening of the frequency band, occurs when a lesion disrupts the normal laminar flow pattern. Increased peak systolic frequencies with spectral broadening reflect the increased flow velocity and turbulence associated with high-grade stenoses (Fig. 25-2*A* and *B*).

A direction-sensitive 20-MHz pulsed Doppler has been developed especially for intraoperative use.[7,36,38] The probe consists of a small ultrasonic transducer mounted on the end of a 16-gauge needle, and the sample volume is approximately 0.2 cubic millimeters in size. To assess the reconstruction after the arteriotomy is closed and flow reestablished, the transducer is placed directly on the outer surface of the artery, and the sample volume is positioned in the center of the flow stream. The spectrum analyzer then processes and displays the signal for visual interpretation (Fig. 25-2*A* and *B*). Zierler and associates used this technique to assess the immediate technical result of 50 carotid endarterectomies.[7] Using intraoperative arteriography as the standard, pre- and postendarterectomy spectra from the internal carotid artery showed improved flow patterns in most cases. Flow disturbances consistent with technical errors were noted in seven internal carotid arteries, and arteriography confirmed a significant technical problem in two of these seven cases before immediate repair was carried out. No other technical errors were encountered in this group, nor was there any neurologic morbidity or mortality.

Intraoperative assessment with pulsed Doppler and spectral analysis is a sensitive method for detecting technical errors. This particular clinical situation requires a screening test that has a low false-negative rate. When the false-negative rate is low, few, if any, technical errors will be missed, and those patients with false-positive screening tests can be identified by arteriographic confirmation. Bandyk and coworkers examined the technical adequacy of 250 carotid endarterectomy sites in 235 patients with this technique.[39] There were 68 arteries in which a residual flow disturbance was identified, and this group of patients had an increased risk of developing recurrent carotid stenosis when compared to patients with normal flow patterns. Operative arteriography in these 68 patients revealed only 10 correctable abnormalities. This method of assessment allows selective use of intraoperative arteriography to minimize injection- and contrast-related complications. As with any new technique, there is an associated learning curve, and the proper acquisition and interpretation of pulsed Doppler data requires considerable experience.

Duplex Ultrasonography and Color Doppler Imaging

As discussed previously, both B-mode ultrasound and pulsed Doppler with spectral analysis are of value in assessing the carotid bifurcation immediately after endarterectomy, and their combined use (duplex ultrasonography) is well established in the detection of carotid stenosis (Chap. 11). The main advantage of intraoperative duplex scanning is that the two modalities are available in a single instrument. The pulsed Doppler can be used to assess the hemodynamics of the internal carotid artery, and the results can be compared to the preoperative study (Figs. 25-4*A* and *B*). B-mode imaging is also helpful in identifying flaps and overt luminal narrowing (Fig. 25-4*C*). Since many duplex units are now equipped with color Doppler imaging systems, this modality also can be used to assess the overall flow characteristics of the carotid vessels (Fig. 25-4*D*).

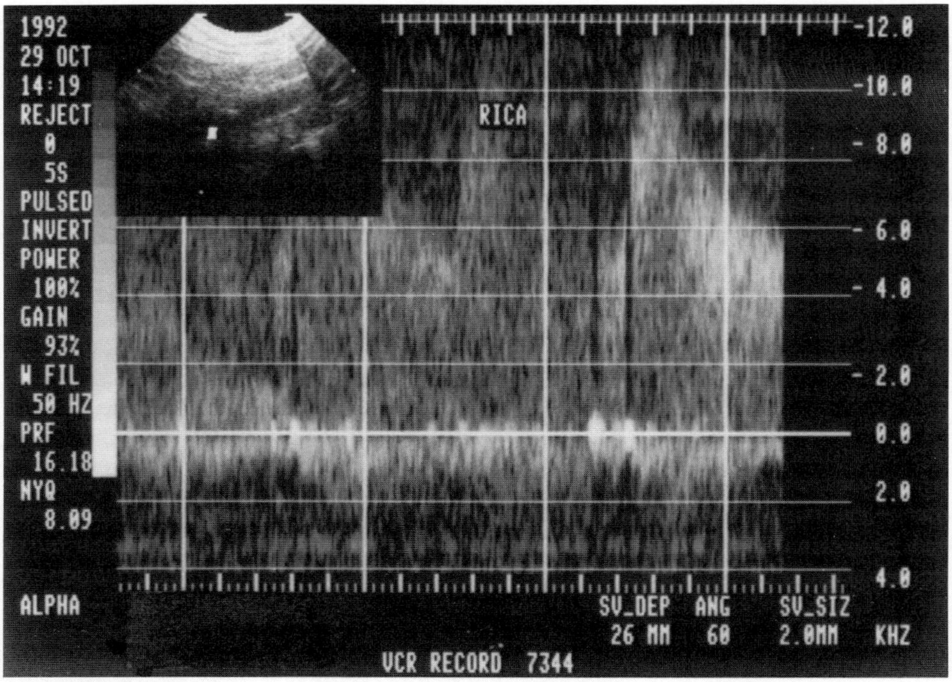

A

Figure 25-4. *A.* Internal carotid stenosis. Preoperative duplex ultrasound evaluation shows a peak systolic frequency of greater than 12 kHz and an end-diastolic frequency of 6 kHz. These findings are consistent with a high-grade (≥80 percent diameter reduction) internal carotid stenosis which was confirmed by angiography. *B.* Following carotid endarterectomy of the vessel represented in panel *A,* intraoperative duplex examination was performed. The spectral analysis recording shown here documents a fall in peak systolic frequency to 4 kHz and end-diastolic frequency to 1.8 kHz. Mild-to-moderate spectral broadening persists, which, in our experience, is common following carotid endarterectomy. *C.* B-mode image component of the intraoperative duplex examination shown in panel *B.* The internal carotid artery is imaged and shows no evidence of stenosis, thrombus, or flap. The dilated portion (*arrow*) is the region repaired by a vein patch angioplasty. *D.* Black and white representation of a color Doppler image from the same case illustrated in *A–C.* There is no residual stenosis or technical defect. Some disturbed flow is present at the point where the vein patch ends (*arrow*).

Reilly and colleagues used this technique to assess both anatomic and hemodynamic parameters intraoperatively after endarterectomy.[40] They compared the presence of wall defects and intraoperative spectral characteristics with the subsequent development of recurrent carotid stenosis. Spectral characteristics did not predict recurrent stenosis, but defect size greater than 40 percent of the lumen diameter was correlated with more severe degrees of stenosis.

Duplex scanning with color-flow Doppler imaging also has been used to assure technical adequacy after carotid endarterectomy. Bandyk reported his experience with this technique in 95 patients and found that 8 percent of the studies were abnormal.[41] A wedge-shaped scanhead wrapped in a sterile sheath

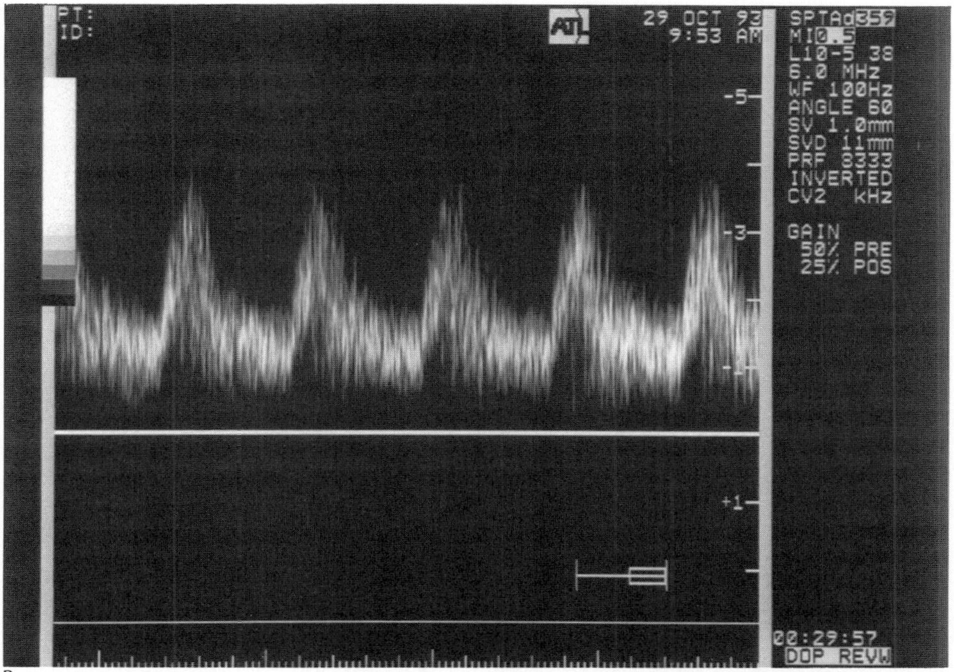

B

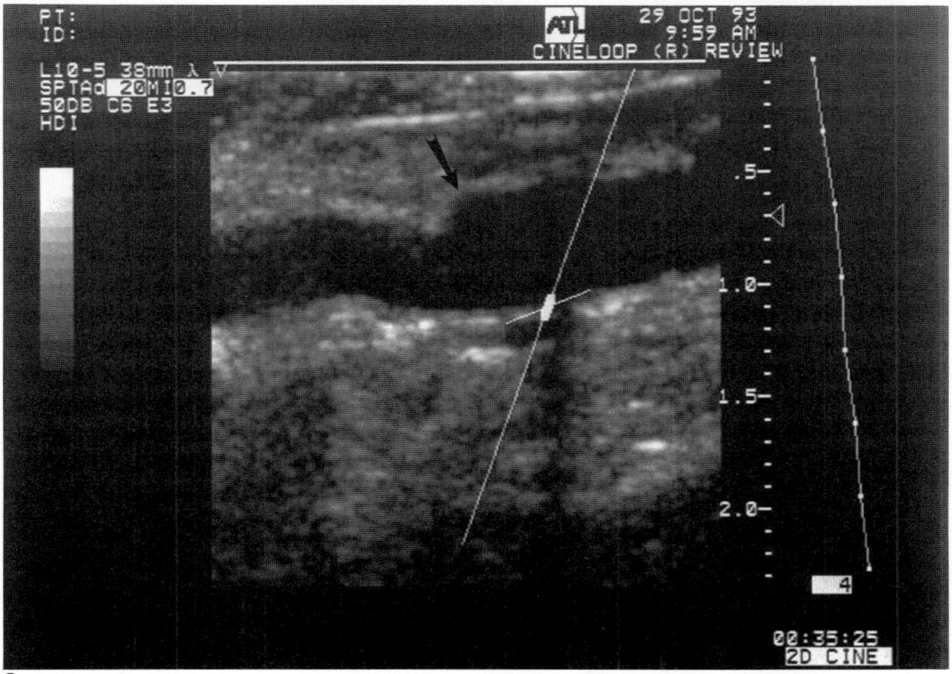

C

Figure 25-4. (*Continued*)

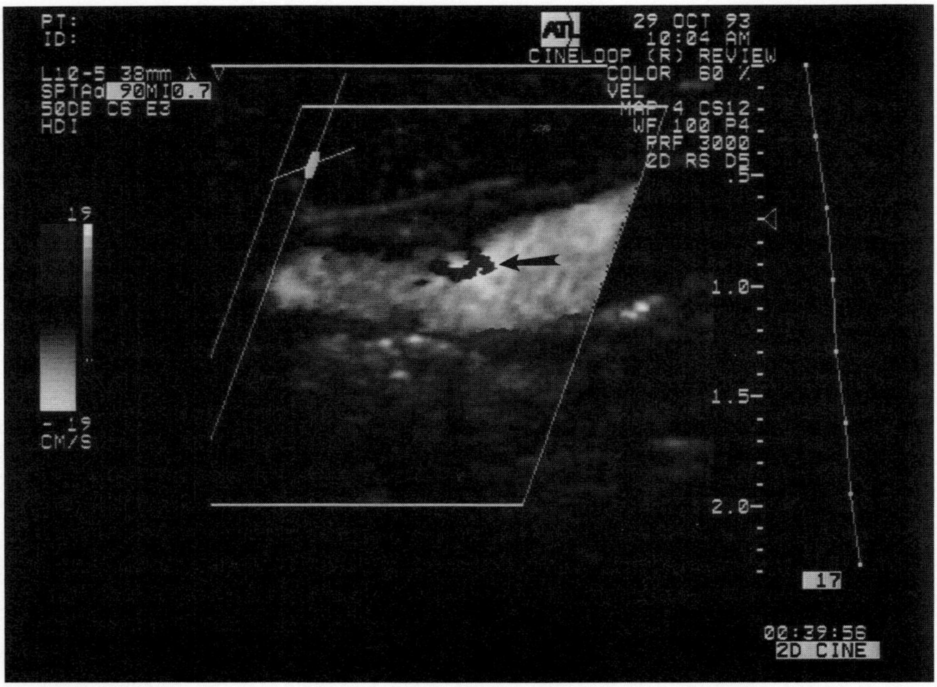

D

Figure 25-4. (*Continued*)

worked best, and both longitudinal and transverse images were obtained. The technique relies on the color-flow image to look for nonhomogeneous areas of flow during each pulse cycle. Using color Doppler information alone, frequency shifts indicating possible defects can be recognized. However, Bandyk concluded that when an abnormality is found either by spectral analysis or color-flow imaging, additional assessment by the surgeon is necessary to decide which defects require immediate revision.

Using a combination of spectral analysis, color-flow imaging, and high resolution B-mode imaging, Bandyk recommended the following: (1) mild or moderate flow disturbances associated with normal B-mode images require no further evaluation; (2) moderate flow disturbances with abnormal B-mode images should be further investigated with arteriography; (3) severe flow disturbances with normal B-mode images should be evaluated with arteriography; and (4) severe flow disturbances with abnormal B-mode images require immediate surgical revision without further delay.[41]

Duplex ultrasonography and color-flow Doppler imaging in the assessment of carotid endarterectomy do have some disadvantages. First, they require expensive equipment and a trained nurse or technologist to operate the machine. In addition, they may add significantly to the overall operating time. Despite these considerations, duplex ultrasonography is probably the best single intraoperative testing modality, since it combines two methods of evaluation in a single examination. Although the equipment is expensive, most hospitals where carotid endarterectomy is performed already have vascular laboratories with ultrasonic duplex scanners readily adaptable to the operating room environment.

The long-term outcome of patients having intraoperative assessment during carotid endarterectomy was studied by Bandyk.[41] In 90 patients (60 duplex scanning alone and 30 color-flow Doppler imaging) there were 21 abnormalities: one in the common carotid artery; six in the internal carotid artery; and 14 in the external carotid artery. Twelve defects were revised and one patient whose defect was not revised suffered a postoperative internal carotid occlusion and stroke. The ultrasound studies did not predict perioperative stroke risk in the carotid territory, suggesting other mechanisms of stroke morbidity. Over long-term follow-up, patients with abnormal studies and those who had no study done were at increased risk for recurrent carotid stenosis and ipsilateral stroke.

CONCLUSIONS

Carotid endarterectomy can be justified only if morbidity and mortality rates remain low. Perioperative neurologic deficits should not exceed 4 percent, and death rates should be less than 1 percent.[42] When trying to achieve such a low incidence of perioperative complications, the identification of even one defect may have a significant effect on overall perioperative complication rates.

Anatomic imaging and physiologic blood flow measurement techniques for intraoperative assessment of carotid endarterectomy are complementary, since each adds important information to assure technical adequacy. Operative arteriography gives an anatomic picture but no functional information about blood flow. There are risks involved with its use, but it can be safely applied in a routine or selective fashion.

An attractive alternative to intraoperative arteriography is the use of noninvasive techniques. Ideally, such tests should provide both hemodynamic and imaging information. Many of the noninvasive tests described above provide hemodynamic or imaging information that can help the operating surgeon. Duplex ultrasonography provides both spectral analysis of flow patterns (hemodynamic assessment) and imaging information, and is the single best noninvasive test for intraoperative use. Not all defects must be repaired, since minor abnormalities rarely result in neurologic deficits. However, any technical error that is a potential cause for internal carotid artery thrombosis or embolism should be identified if this can be done with minimal harm to the patient. Equivocal duplex studies should prompt intraoperative arteriography, while clearly abnormal postendarterectomy duplex results indicate the need for immediate repair. Color Doppler imaging, which is incorporated in many duplex scanners, may add another dimension to the intraoperative assessment of carotid endarterectomy.

As long as assessment techniques are safe and result in the correction of technical defects that might otherwise lead to neurologic morbidity or mortality, their use is justified. Intraoperative assessment of technical adequacy is especially important for documentation on a teaching service and also should serve as a constant reminder of the need for meticulous surgical technique when performing carotid endarterectomy.

REFERENCES

1. Rosental JJ, Gaspar MM, Movius HJ: Intraoperative arteriography in carotid thromboendarterectomy. *Arch Surg* 106:806, 1973.
2. Anderson CA, Collins GJ, Rich NM: Routine operative arteriography during carotid endarterectomy: A reassessment. *Surgery* 83:67, 1978.

3. Blaisdell FM, Lim R, Hall AD: Technical result of carotid endarterectomy-arteriographic assessment. *Am J Surg* 114:239, 1967.
4. Courbier R, Jausseran JM, Reggi M: Detecting complications of direct arterial surgery—the role of intraoperative arteriography. *Arch Surg* 112:1115, 1977.
5. Plecha FR, Pories WJ: Intraoperative angiography in the immediate assessment of arterial reconstruction. *Arch Surg* 105:902, 1972.
6. Fischer HW, Cornell SH: The toxicity of the sodium and methylglucamine salts of diatrizoate, iothalamate, and metrizoate—an experimental study of the circulatory effects following intracarotid injection. *Radiology* 85:1013, 1965.
7. Zierler RE, Bandyk DF, Thiele BL: Intraoperative assessment of carotid endarterectomy. *J Vasc Surg* 1:73, 1984.
8. Roon AJ, Hoogerwerf D: Intraoperative arteriography and carotid surgery. *J Vasc Surg* 16:239, 1992.
9. Lye CR, Marrow IM, Downs AR: Carotid artery spasm—a cause of postendarterectomy thrombosis? *Arch Surg* 117:1531, 1982.
10. Hobson RW, Rich NM, Wright CB, Fedde CW: Operative assessment of carotid endarterectomy—internal carotid artery back pressure, carotid arterial blood flow, and carotid arteriography. *Am Surg* 41:603, 1975.
11. Larson SR, Movius HJ, Bell OD, et al: Intraoperative arteriography in cerebrovascular surgery, in Bergan JJ, Yao JT (eds): *Cerebrovascular Insufficiency*. New York, Grune & Stratton, pp 353–365, 1983.
12. Collins GJ, Rich NM, Anderson CA, McDonald PT: Stroke associated with carotid endarterectomy. *Am J Surg* 135:221, 1978.
13. Meguno K, Tsukada A, Matsumura A, et al: Portable digital subtraction angiography in the operating room and intensive care unit. *Neurolog Med Chir* 31:768, 1991.
14. Sigel B, Coelho JCU, Machi J, et al: The application of real-time ultrasound imaging during surgical procedures. *Surg Gynecol Obstet* 157:33, 1983.
15. Lane RJ: Intraoperative B-mode scanning. *J Clin Ultrasound* 8:427, 1980.
16. Sigel B, Coelho JCU, Flanigan DP, et al: Ultrasonic imaging during vascular surgery. *Arch Surg* 117:764, 1982.
17. Flanigan DP, Sigel B, Schuler JJ: Intraoperative ultrasonic carotid artery imaging, in Bergan JJ, Yao JST (eds): *Cerebrovascular Insufficiency*. New York, Grune & Stratton, pp 343–352, 1983.
18. Coelho JCU, Sigel B, Flanigan DP, et al: An experimental evaluation of arteriography and imaging ultrasonography in detecting arterial defects at operation. *J Surg Res* 32:130, 1982.
19. Dilley RB, Bernstein EF: A comparison of B-mode real-time imaging and arteriography in the intraoperative assessment of carotid endarterectomy. *J Vasc Surg* 4:457, 1986.
20. Lane RJ, Appleberg M: Real-time intraoperative angiosonography after carotid endarterectomy. *Surgery* 92:5, 1982.
21. Anderson JC, Baltaxe HA, Wolf GL: Inability to show clot—one limitation of ultrasonography of the abdominal aorta. *Radiology* 132:693, 1979.
22. Shore JM, Berci G, Morgenstern L: The value of biliary endoscopy. *Surg Gynecol Obstet* 140:601, 1975.
23. Vatz A, Berci G, Shore JM: Operative nephroscopy. *J Urol* 107:355, 1972.
24. Vollmar JF, Storz LW: Vascular endoscopy—possibilities and limitations of its clinical application. *Surg Clin North Am* 54:111, 1974.
25. Towne JB, Bernhard VM: Vascular endoscopy—an adjunct to carotid surgery. *Stroke* 8:569, 1977.
26. Towne JB, Bernhard VM: Vascular endoscopy—useful tool or interesting toy? *Surgery* 82:415, 1977.
27. Mehigan JT, Olcott C: Video angioscopy as an alternative to intraoperative arteriography. *Am J Surg* 152:139, 1986.
28. Dean RH, Yao JST, Stanton PE, Bergan JJ: Prognostic indicators in femoropopliteal reconstruction. *Arch Surg* 110:1287, 1975.
29. Owens ML, Wilson SE: Prevention of neurologic complications after carotid endarterectomy. *Arch Surg* 117:551, 1982.
30. Archie JP Jr, Feldtman RW: Intraoperative assessment of carotid endarterectomy by electro-

magnetic blood flow measurements. *Surg Gynecol Obstet* 158:457, 1984.
31. May AG, Van de Berg L, DeWeese JA, Rob CG: Critical arterial stenosis. *Surgery* 54:250, 1963.
32. Barnes RW, Garrett WV: Intraoperative assessment of arterial reconstruction by Doppler ultrasound. *Surg Gynecol Obstet* 146:896, 1978.
33. Mozersky DJ, Sumner DS, Barnes RW, Strandness DE Jr: Intraoperative use of a sterile ultrasonic flow probe. *Surg Gynecol Obstet* 136:279, 1973.
34. Keitzer WF, Lichti EL, Brossart FA, DeWeese MS: Use of the Doppler ultrasonic flowmeter during arterial vascular surgery. *Arch Surg* 105:308, 1972.
35. Seifert KB, Blackshear WM Jr: Continuous-wave Doppler in the intraoperative assessment of carotid endarterectomy. *J Vasc Surg* 2:817, 1985.
36. Zierler RE, Roederer GO, Strandness DE Jr: The use of frequency spectral analysis in carotid artery surgery, in Bergan JJ, Yao JST (eds): *Cerebrovascular Insufficiency*. New York, Grune & Stratton, pp 137–161, 1983.
37. Fell G, Phillips DJ, Chikos PM, et al: Ultrasonic duplex scanning for disease of the carotid artery. *Circulation* 64:896, 1978.
38. Zierler RE, Bandyk DF, Berni GA, Thiele BL: Intraoperative pulsed Doppler assessment of carotid endarterectomy. *Ultrasound Med Biol* 9:65, 1983.
39. Bandyk DF, Kaebnick HW, Adams MB, Towne JB: Turbulence occurring after carotid bifurcation endarterectomy: A harbinger of residual and recurrent carotid stenosis. *J Vasc Surg* 7:261, 1988.
40. Reilly LM, Okuhn SP, Rapp JH, et al: Recurrent carotid stenosis: A consequence of local or systemic factors? The influence of unrepaired technical defects. *J Vasc Surg* 11:448, 1990.
41. Bandyk DF: Intraoperative monitoring and completion studies. San Diego Symposium on Vascular Diagnosis, Feb. 1992.
42. Thompson JE, Talkington CM: Carotid endarterectomy. *Ann Surg* 184:1, 1976.

26

Complications of Carotid Endarterectomy

William J. Quiñones-Baldrich

Carotid endarterectomy has been shown to be effective in the treatment of symptomatic extracranial arterial occlusive disease. The benefits of operation, however, may be negated by a high complication rate—specifically, perioperative stroke and death. As a group, patients operated upon for symptomatic carotid stenosis will benefit from a reduction in the future risk of stroke if the perioperative complication rate is maintained below 5 percent.[1] A higher complication rate can render the procedure ineffective. Perioperative complications and long-term results of carotid endarterectomy depend on patient selection, technical expertise, and perioperative management. This chapter will focus on recognition, prevention, and management of complications associated with carotid endarterectomy.

MYOCARDIAL INFARCTION

The most significant cause of perioperative death after carotid endarterectomy is myocardial infarction (MI) secondary to severe coronary artery disease. Clearly, prevention of this complication depends on proper patient selection and careful preoperative preparation. Patients operated upon electively should have an adequate cardiac evaluation. This may consist initially of clinical assessment and electrocardiography, with more extensive evaluation reserved for selected patients considered to be at high risk for significant coronary artery disease. Using this approach, Yeager[2] noted an incidence of fatal perioperative MI of 0.4 percent and nonfatal MI of 3.6 percent in 249 consecutive carotid endarterectomies. It is the responsibility of the surgeon, however, to screen these patients clinically so that those deserving a more aggressive evaluation with radionuclide studies or coronary arteriography can be identified prior to surgery. This group includes patients with prior MI, angina, a history of congestive heart failure, or ischemia noted on the resting electrocardiogram.

Adequate control of hypertension prior to surgery is of paramount importance, not only in reducing the incidence of post-carotid endarterectomy hypertension, but also the risk of MI. The practice of artificially elevating the systemic blood pressure during carotid clamping to increase collateral cerebral blood flow instead of using a temporary shunt increases the incidence of myocardial ischemia and the risk of MI. Similarly, poor control of hypertension following carotid surgery increases the risk of both stroke and MI. Thus, blood pressure should be maintained at physiologic levels (systolic blood pressure no greater than 160 mmHg) throughout the perioperative period.

The choice of anesthetic technique also may influence the risk of coronary events around the time of surgery (Chap. 22). Local anesthesia with cervical block may be preferable in patients requiring urgent carotid endarterectomy who have marginal cardiac function secondary to uncorrectable coronary artery disease. Although general anesthesia is safe for most patients, carotid endarterectomy may be carried out safely under local anesthesia in patients who would not tolerate a general anesthetic.[3]

STROKE AND TRANSIENT ISCHEMIC ATTACK

Risk of Perioperative Neurologic Symptoms

A neurologic event in the perioperative period after carotid endarterectomy, either stroke or transient ischemic attack (TIA), may be secondary to embolic phenomena or carotid thrombosis with subsequent ischemia. Stroke may also be due to intracranial bleeding from conversion of a bland ischemic infarct into a hemorrhagic infarct. The incidence of stroke in the perioperative period correlates directly with the indication for the procedure, with the status of the contralateral carotid artery having little influence on overall outcome.[4–6] Whereas asymptomatic patients operated upon for severe carotid stenosis have a risk of perioperative stroke usually less than 2 percent, the corresponding risk for patients operated upon for TIAs is between 3 and 5 percent. Patients operated upon electively after a stroke with neurologic recovery may have an incidence of perioperative stroke as high as 7.5 percent. This latter group is at an increased risk for perioperative stroke secondary to poor perfusion of peri-infarct collaterals during carotid clamping. Most surgeons would recommend routine use of a temporary shunt during carotid clamping for patients in whom the indication for operation is a prior stroke.

The timing of carotid endarterectomy following a completed stroke will also influence the risk of perioperative stroke. Although patients undergoing carotid endarterectomy more than six weeks after an acute cerebral infarction may be operated upon with a risk similar to that of patients with a history of stroke in the remote past, patients having surgery within six weeks of an acute cerebral infarction are at higher risk for perioperative stroke.[7] There is also a significant incidence of early recurrent stroke (up to 21 percent) when operation is routinely delayed for six weeks after an acute stroke; however, patients suffering a stroke ipsilateral to an appropriate carotid lesion can be safely operated upon in the early interval when a head computed tomography (CT) scan is negative.[8] The role of CT in the timing of carotid endarterectomy is also discussed in Chap. 13. In patients with a completed stroke, we recommend that intervention be delayed until a plateau is reached in neurologic recovery, and then proceeding with surgery. This may be a few days in some patients or a few weeks in others. A negative head CT scan in this clinical situation is reassuring. The exception would be patients with either crescendo TIAs or stroke in evolution, in whom proceeding to surgery without delay is recommended. This latter group is clearly at increased risk for perioperative stroke, but these patients will benefit significantly from surgery compared with the natural history of stroke-in-evolution.[9]

The risk of perioperative stroke associated with carotid endarterectomy must take into account the small but real incidence of stroke secondary to preoperative angiography. In a study prospectively evaluating 382 patients with symptomatic carotid artery disease undergoing cerebral angiography, reversible stroke occurred in three patients (0.8 percent) and permanent stroke in five (1.3 percent).[10] Significant risk factors for postangiographic stroke were stroke before angiography and the presence of greater than 50 percent symptomatic internal carotid artery stenosis. This significant risk of stroke secondary to angiography can be decreased by selective use of preoperative angiography. The ability of duplex scanning to identify and characterize significant carotid lesions has allowed use of this modality as the only preoperative study in many patients who are candidates for carotid endarterectomy (Chap. 21).[11–13] However, this practice assumes that the results of the laboratory performing the duplex scans have been validated by correlations with angiography. Even when high-quality duplex scanning is available, preoperative angiography must be used selectively in patients with unusual or atypical symptoms, a history of radiation therapy, and in those with recurrent carotid disease. This approach may reduce the overall incidence of stroke related to preoperative angiography in patients who are candidates for surgery.

Prevention of Perioperative Neurologic Events

Prevention of perioperative neurologic events is one of the most important issues in surgery for extracranial arterial occlusive disease. Many factors will influence the occurrence of this devastating complication. Perioperative management of both hypotension and hypertension is of paramount importance. Both have been associated with an increased risk of stroke in patients undergoing elective carotid endarterectomy. The mechanism of post-carotid endarterectomy hypertension has not been completely elucidated. Both increased cerebral renin and cerebral norepinephrine have been postulated as important mechanisms.[14,15] In a retrospective review, Skydell and associates noted that diabetes mellitus, isoflurane anesthesia, peripheral arterial occlusive disease, and the presence of either TIAs or high-grade ipsilateral carotid stenosis were associated with a higher incidence of post-carotid endarterectomy hypertension.[16] In these patients, monitoring blood pressure during and after intervention is essential. We strongly recommend the routine use of a radial artery line for continuous blood pressure monitoring in all patients undergoing carotid endarterectomy. Hypotension is less frequent, but should be managed with equal aggressiveness.

One of the most debated issues surrounding carotid endarterectomy has been the use of intraoperative shunting during carotid clamping (Chap. 24). It should be emphasized that the most common cause of an intraoperative or perioperative neurologic event related to carotid endarterectomy is embolism or thrombosis, not decreased ipsilateral hemispheric perfusion.[17] When carotid endarterectomy is performed under local anesthesia with continuous neurologic assessment of the awake patient, only about 8 percent of patients require the use of a temporary shunt.[18] Thus, although routine shunting has its merits in that the surgeon becomes facile with the technique, in reality more than 85 percent of the patients do not require shunting. Furthermore, shunting has been associated with complication rates as high as 0.5 percent, including shunt thrombosis and intimal dissection.[19,20] Care must be taken during shunt insertion so that no air or particulate matter is allowed in the shunt. It is our practice to insert the distal (internal carotid) end of the shunt first, allowing backbleeding to fill the cul-de-sac in the common carotid artery prior to retrograde insertion into that vessel. We prefer the use of extraluminal shunts, so that a clamp may be placed on the shunt during proximal insertion. This clamp is released while the shunt tubing is under direct vision, proceeding with immediate reclamping if any particulate matter or air is seen.

Patients with a history of stroke as an indication for surgery should be routinely shunted. The peri-infarct zone usually is supplied by high resistance collaterals dependent on a high perfusion pressure, and these patients may be at risk for extending the infarcted area during carotid clamping. An exception to this practice may be made when patients are continuously monitored with electroencephalography or brain mapping during surgery. In spite of such monitoring, we prefer to use a shunt routinely in patients operated upon for stroke. If high dissection of the internal carotid is required and the shunt is an impediment to a complete endarterectomy, continuous electroencephalographic monitoring is reassuring in this group of patients when no changes are noted. Otherwise, perfusion should be assured to protect the ipsilateral hemisphere during carotid clamping.

Perhaps the most important consideration in the prevention of a perioperative neurologic event following carotid endarterectomy is assurance of an adequate technical result. Both perioperative carotid thrombosis and embolic sources must be eliminated to minimize the risk of perioperative stroke. Whenever possible, the endarterectomy should be complete, without the need for tacking sutures at the distal end-point. The need for such sutures usually implies an incomplete endarterectomy, which can be avoided by further dissection and complete removal of plaque. The endarterectomy site should be thoroughly irrigated with heparinized saline, removing all loose debris. It is our practice to use antiplatelet agents around the time of surgery, including aspirin and dextran. This may prevent the development of significant platelet aggregation on the endarterectomized site occasionally seen as a filling defect on completion arteriography.

Some type of intraoperative assessment of the technical result should be undertaken in all patients undergoing carotid endarterectomy (Chap. 25). Completion arteriography is routinely used in our hands, with correction of all significant defects identified (Fig. 26-1). Significant defects in the internal carotid artery will be seen in as many as 10 percent of cases. This correlates well with findings based on ultrasound techniques.[21] The presence of these defects has been correlated with both early and late results, and immediate correction has been shown to decrease perioperative and late

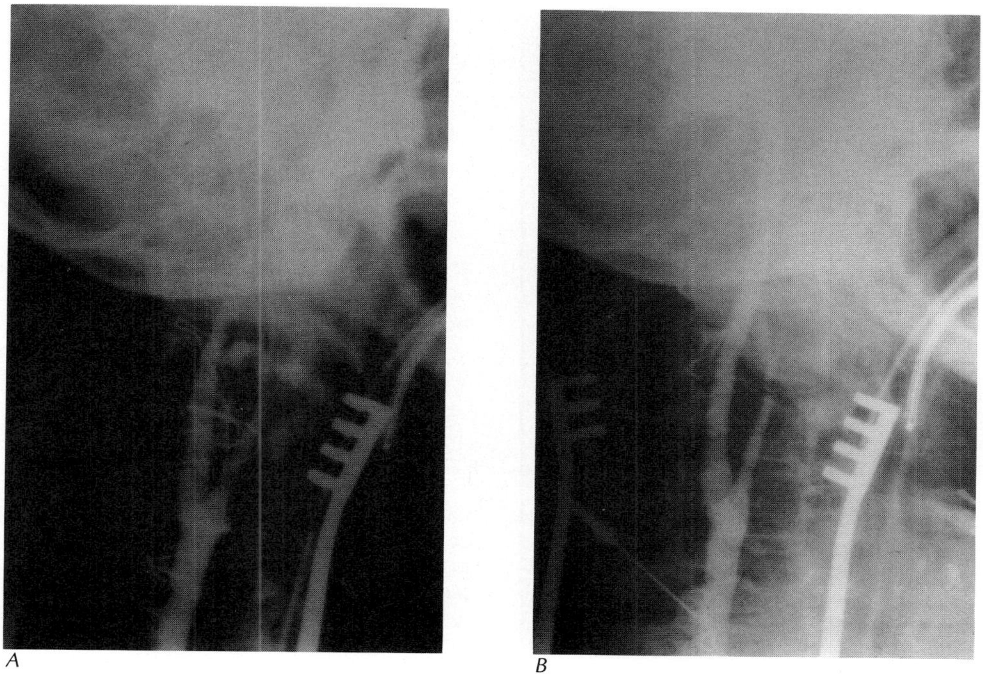

A B

Figure 26-1. *A.* Intraoperative completion arteriogram after carotid endarterectomy for a preocclusive stenosis. Note distal spasm of the internal carotid artery. *B.* Intraoperative arteriogram of the same patient after reopening the endarterectomy site and dilatation of the internal carotid artery.

complications such as recurrent stenosis and stroke.[22] Whereas not all these defects require correction, those that appear to compromise the lumen or to represent significant flaps should be corrected. Performance of a technically successful endarterectomy, as demonstrated by either arteriography or other types of assessment such as duplex scanning, is clearly the responsibility of the operating surgeon. It is curious that many vascular surgeons are willing to perform arteriography after a lower extremity bypass but are reluctant to assess their technical result after carotid endarterectomy.

Recently, occlusion of the external carotid artery has been identified as a cause of perioperative and even late strokes following carotid endarterectomy (Fig. 26-2).[23,24] Thrombosis at the origin of the external carotid artery will lead to an area of thrombus that may shed material into the internal carotid circulation and produce a neurologic event. Thus, it is of extreme importance that endarterectomy of the external carotid be performed with the same care as that of the internal carotid artery. Technical defects in the external carotid identified on arteriography or duplex scanning may be corrected without reclamping the internal carotid artery. The use of a curved vascular clamp allows selective occlusion at the origin of the external carotid artery. This permits direct repair through a longitudinal arteriotomy with patch angioplasty or removal of any residual plaque or intimal flap in the external carotid.

There has been considerable debate over

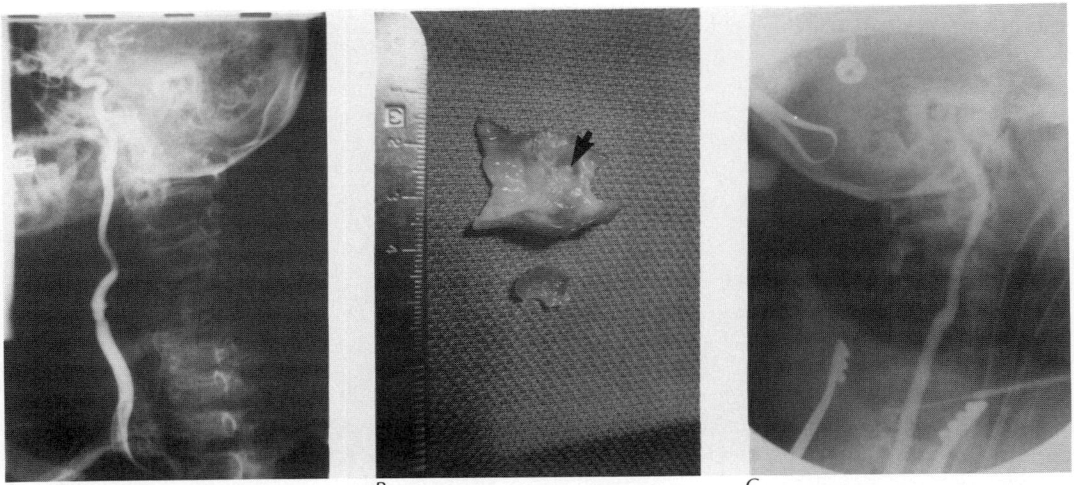

Figure 26-2. *A.* Arteriogram of a patient with right hemispheric transient ischemic attacks presenting two years after a right carotid endarterectomy. Note occlusion of the external carotid artery with relatively benign appearing bulb irregularity. *B.* Specimen after exploration of the carotid artery because of recurring symptoms with right hemispheric stroke one month after the original arteriogram. The carotid bulb was resected, and the occluded origin of the external carotid artery was found to be covered by a soft thrombus that has been removed (*arrow*). *C.* Intraoperative completion arteriogram after replacement of the carotid bulb with a 6-mm PTFE graft. Patient is alive and asymptomatic on follow-up 55 months later.

whether or not patching of the arteriotomy at the time of endarterectomy reduces the incidence of early and late complications. Regardless of the method used to close the arteriotomy, the goals are to avoid narrowing with primary closure or significant enlargement of the bulb with patch closure. Both of these can predispose to early and late neurologic events by thrombus formation. Certainly, patching with either prosthetic or autogenous material is indicated for small arteries, particularly in women, and during repair of a recurrent stenosis (Chap. 27), especially when secondary to intimal hyperplasia (Chap. 28).

Use of antithrombotic regimens around the time of carotid endarterectomy is recommended. Heparin should be used routinely during carotid clamping. Most patients operated upon at our institution are placed on aspirin prior to operation and maintained on this regimen postoperatively. An exception may be patients who cannot tolerate aspirin because of gastrointestinal complications. In most patients, particularly in the latter group, use of dextran intraoperatively may be of benefit. An occasional patient will show a strong tendency to form platelet aggregates on the endarterectomy site. The exact mechanism of this is unclear; however, it may be prevented by an aggressive antiplatelet regimen. Heparin may be selectively used postoperatively, although its benefit remains to be proved. A potential hazard of such regimens in patients with a prior history of stroke, particularly the use of postoperative heparin, is an increased incidence of intracranial bleeding.[25]

A rare but important mechanism of perioperative stroke is intracranial bleeding. This devastating complication can occur—especially in patients with uncontrolled hypertension or recent cerebral infarction. If the patient is on heparin when intracranial bleeding is detected, this should be discontinued immediately. Blood pressure should be adequately controlled. Use of calcium channel blockers or other agents to control cerebral vasospasm may be of benefit. Intracranial bleeding should be suspected in any patient complaining of significant headache following carotid endarterectomy, especially when accompanied by seizures. This problem is discussed further with the hyperperfusion syndrome. Risk factors for postendarterectomy intracranial bleeding include severe carotid stenosis, postoperative systemic hypertension, and administration of anticoagulant or antiplatelet medication. The mortality rate from intracranial hemorrhage following carotid endarterectomy is extremely high, with some series reporting 100 percent mortality.[25]

The effect of intracranial carotid disease on the incidence of stroke remains unclear. In a series of 91 carotid endarterectomies performed in 79 patients, no significant difference in complication rate was seen among patients with or without concomitant carotid siphon stenosis. Thus, the contribution of carotid siphon stenosis to perioperative stroke risk appears to be low. Most patients with significant tandem carotid bifurcation and siphon lesions will be relieved of their symptoms by repair of the bifurcation lesion.[26]

Management of Perioperative Neurologic Deficits

Management of a patient with a perioperative neurologic deficit following carotid endarterectomy should include assessing the patency of the operated artery and a detailed neurologic evaluation. When intraoperative arteriography has documented an adequate technical result, demonstration of patent vessels by duplex scanning after a neurologic episode occurs suggests an embolic event. If an intracranial bleed is excluded by CT scan, anticoagulation is indicated. Conversely, if an adequate technical result has not been documented intraoperatively, assessment of patency alone is insufficient without further evaluation. Proceeding with either immediate reoperation or arteriography is the best alternative. In most situations, exploration of the carotid bifurcation by reoperation is the most expedient method of assessment within the first few hours after the original operation. The severity of the neurologic deficit also may dictate the best alternative. Whereas patients with a minor transient neurologic deficit may be worked up with duplex scanning, arteriography, or both to determine the need for intervention, patients with a significant hemispheric deficit require immediate intervention.

The most important step in diagnostic evaluation is the exclusion of intracranial hemorrhage, a process that may be aggravated by reoperation and anticoagulation. In patients with loss of consciousness, proceeding with an expeditious CT scan to exclude this possibility, especially in those at high risk for intracranial hemorrhage, is essential. Once intracranial hemorrhage has been excluded, exploration of the operative site is most prudent in patients with a significant neurologic deficit following operation. An algorithm for management of perioperative neurologic deficits based on immediate duplex examination is presented in Fig. 26-3.

Occasionally, a patient will do well for the first 24 to 48 h after carotid endarterectomy and then experience a TIA. This type of event is usually secondary to a small embolus. Documentation of patency and adequacy of the endarterectomy site by duplex scanning may be all that is necessary in this situation—perhaps with an increase in the antithrombotic regimen if intracranial bleeding has been excluded. If carotid thrombosis is evident, reoperation is indicated in the patient with a persistent neurologic deficit or recurrent symptoms. In the stable patient with complete recovery after the initial postoperative event, considerable judgment is required before pro-

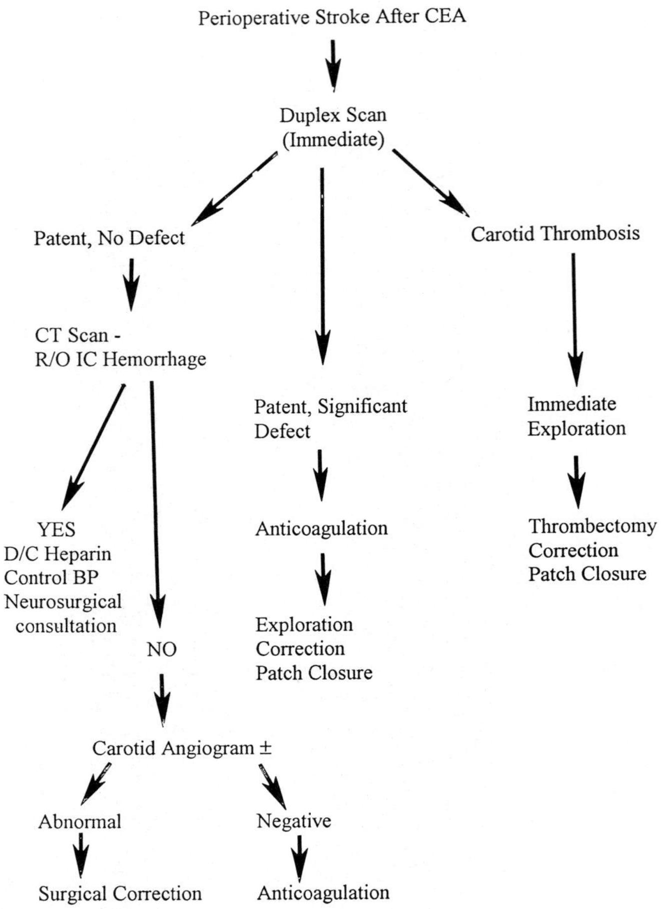

Figure 26-3. Algorithm for management of patients with minor to moderate neurologic deficits developing within the first few hours after carotid endarterectomy (CEA). Patients with severe deficits immediately after carotid endarterectomy are probably best managed by immediate exploration (see text).

ceeding with carotid thrombectomy, since this is a relatively high-risk procedure. When exploration is not undertaken and intracranial bleeding has been excluded, long-term anticoagulation may reduce the incidence of subsequent symptoms.

In summary, management of the patient with a neurologic deficit following carotid endarterectomy should be individualized. Stroke is second to MI as a cause of death following carotid endarterectomy. In general, management is guided by the availability of various diagnostic tools. When arteriography or duplex scanning may delay necessary intervention, immediate exploration remains the best alternative. Upon exposure of the artery, if pulses are present in the internal carotid, an arteriogram may be performed, avoiding carotid clamping in what may be an evolving stroke. If no defects are identified, the diagnosis of an embolic event is assured and the patient may be appropriately treated with anticoagulation once intracranial hemorrhage has been excluded. When carotid thrombosis is the initial finding, local thrombectomy and immediate insertion of an indwelling shunt should be undertaken. Whatever technical defect is identified should be corrected and the carotid closed, preferably with a patch. If no technical defects are identified, the antithrombotic regimen should be increased and the carotid artery closed, preferably with an autogenous patch.

CRANIAL AND PERIPHERAL NERVE INJURY

Figure 26-4 shows the relationships of the various cranial and peripheral nerves within the operative site typically exposed during carotid endarterectomy. Knowledge of the anatomy of this area is essential to avoid damage to these nerves. The incidence of cranial and cervical nerve injury following carotid endarterectomy was studied prospectively in 43 carotid endarterectomies. A 25 percent incidence of temporary vocal cord palsy, 5 percent incidence of hypoglossal nerve damage, and a 60 to 69 percent incidence of either greater auricular or transverse cervical nerve injury was documented.[27] Much lower incidences have been reported in other studies.

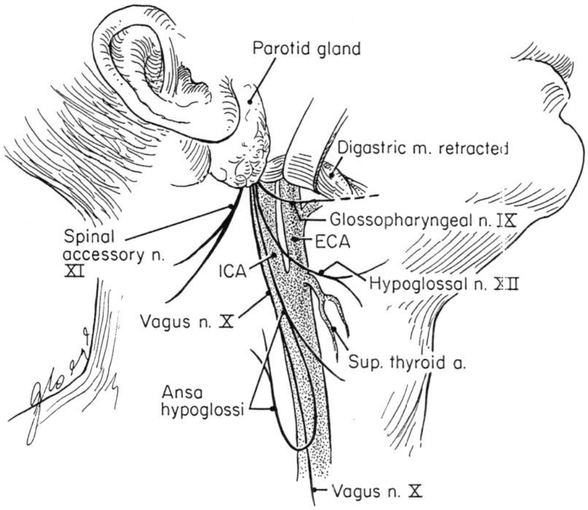

Figure 26-4. Typical exposure during carotid endarterectomy showing the relationships of cranial nerves and other important structures.

Clearly, the occurrence of nerve injury during carotid endarterectomy will depend on how carefully the patient is evaluated postoperatively to document this complication. When the routine postoperative examination is supplemented with detailed evaluation by a speech pathologist, the incidence of vocal cord palsy may be as high as 27 percent.[28]

Return of function is common, although this may not be due to complete recovery when the recurrent laryngeal nerve is involved. Rather, there is compensation with apposition of the contralateral vocal cord to allow return of normal speech, even with continued presence of a unilateral vocal cord palsy.[29] Thus, return of voice alone is an unreliable guide to resolution of a vocal cord palsy. This underscores the importance of preoperative screening with examination of the larynx before proceeding with a contralateral operation in patients undergoing bilateral staged carotid endarterectomies. Such an approach will help to avoid the devastating complication of bilateral vocal cord palsy and respiratory compromise. Damage to the vagus nerve, and thus to the recurrent laryngeal nerve, can be avoided by dissection of the common and internal carotid arteries using the periadventitial plane and separating this nerve from the arterial structures to avoid crushing the nerve in a vascular clamp. Refraining from grasping these nerves with forceps during dissection is also of utmost importance. An occasional patient may have a nonrecurrent laryngeal nerve, which can be identified anterior to the carotid and which may be confused with the ansa hypoglossi (Chap. 2).

The superior laryngeal nerve may be injured during control of the external carotid artery. This will produce tiredness of the voice and an inability to reach high pitches. Injury to this nerve is avoided by careful dissection around the origin of the external carotid artery, avoiding adjacent tissues during passage of a right-angle clamp for control.

Management of patients with persistent hoarseness after carotid endarterectomy should be conservative. Most patients will recover a normal voice within six months of surgery. After that, if hoarseness persists, Teflon injection of the ipsilateral cord to allow better apposition can be carried out safely and will benefit the occasional patient who does not recover from this deficit.

The incidence of hypoglossal nerve injury is approximately 5 percent.[30] This nerve may be injured during dissection of the middle to high portions of the internal carotid artery. Most commonly, it is injured when the nerve is inadvertently included under the retractor in the superior aspect of the operative field. Hypoglossal nerve injury is manifested by paralysis of the ipsilateral tongue musculature, with deviation of the tongue to the ipsilateral side. Although usually transient, this degree of dysfunction may make mastication difficult, as well as producing speech and deglutition difficulties. When mobilization of this nerve is required during high dissections of the internal carotid artery, care should be taken to ligate the small arterial and venous branches that tether the nerve laterally. This allows the nerve to move away from the internal carotid artery and facilitates high exposure. As cephalad dissection proceeds, the hypoglossal nerve becomes closely related to the vagus nerve where the ansa hypoglossi originates (Fig. 26-4). If separation of the vagus and hypoglossal nerves is necessary, care must be taken to do so along their anatomic plane, and no nerve fibers should be divided. Division of the digastric muscle, a maneuver necessary for high exposure of the carotid artery, is associated with an increased incidence of hypoglossal and glossopharyngeal nerve injury.[31] Thus, care must be taken to identify these structures prior to division of the digastric muscle.

High dissection of the internal carotid artery is associated with an increased incidence of glossopharyngeal nerve injury. In most patients, this leads to difficulty swallowing. Although most commonly a transient deficit, glossopharyngeal nerve injury is associated with a prolonged hospital stay and delayed recovery. This complication is best avoided by knowledge of the anatomy, identification of the nerve, and protection during dissection.

Damage to the spinal accessory nerve also is associated with high exposure of the internal carotid artery. Injury to this nerve may lead to difficulty in turning the head to the contralateral side. During high dissections of the carotid artery, it is important that cautery be avoided in control of any minor bleeding as this is one of the more common mechanisms for injury to the spinal accessory nerve. Knowledge of the anatomic relationships of these cranial nerves is essential for safe exposure of the high internal carotid artery (Fig. 26-4).

Division of the *ansa hypoglossi* is required for adequate exposure of the carotid bifurcation in most patients, but this is usually of no clinical consequence. An exception may be in patients undergoing a contralateral carotid endarterectomy in whom bilateral division of the *ansa hypoglossi* can produce difficulty with mastication. An occasional patient who has had prior head and neck surgery for malignancy may require carotid endarterectomy. Some of these patients have esophageal speech or have learned other means of speech following laryngectomy. It is of utmost importance in these patients to avoid division of the *ansa hypoglossi*. This will assure their ability to continue to use their learned speech modality following carotid endarterectomy. Otherwise, a period of intense retraining may be necessary.

Damage to the mandibular branch of the facial nerve usually is secondary to a retraction injury along the anterior portion of the wound. This is seen most commonly with transverse cervical incisions. During retraction of the wound, care should be taken not to place any retractor against the midportion of the mandible. Damage to the mandibular branch of the facial nerve leads to a drooping of the ipsilateral corner of the mouth most evident when the patient is asked to smile. In the most severe cases, the patient may be unable to keep food and saliva from spilling. Although recovery is common, permanent deficits can occur.

Injury or division of peripheral cervical nerves is common during carotid endarterectomy. Most patients will have an area of numbness anterior to the wound. Although of no clinical consequence, this is an annoying complication of which patients frequently complain following surgery. In most instances, it is not avoidable. When large branches of the cervical nerves are identified, an attempt should be made to preserve them. Otherwise, the patient should be reassured that this problem will improve with time, decreasing the area of numbness to a small oval anterior to the incision.

The greater auricular nerve is found in the upper third of the cervical incision. Although occasionally it must be divided to expose the high internal carotid artery, in most instances it can be preserved by mobilization along its subcutaneous course, allowing retraction to the highest portion of the incision. Care must be taken not to include this nerve in the approximation of the platysma during closure. Division of the greater auricular nerve produces an area of numbness over the lower portion of the earlobe. Although this has no significant clinical consequences, it is an annoying symptom that may be avoided in most patients by mobilization of the nerve rather than division. Patients should be warned preoperatively of these potentially annoying deficits.

BLEEDING

The major factors that increase the incidence of wound hematomas following carotid endarterectomy are use of such antithrombotic regimens as antiplatelet agents or heparin and postoperative hypertension.[32] Most patients undergoing carotid endarterectomy are on aspirin preoperatively, and the potential benefits of such therapy cannot be ignored. Careful attention to hemostasis at the completion of the procedure must be emphasized. Use of a drain for the first 24 h after surgery usually does not prevent the development of a hematoma. However, a drain may decrease the amount of fluid in the incision and improve patient comfort.

Most significant hematomas that occur following carotid artery surgery are related to bleeding from the suture line. Thus, the surgeon must make sure that the arteriotomy closure is hemostatic, with or without a patch. We have seen several patients bleed from puncture sites in the common carotid artery after intraoperative arteriography; therefore, we recommend routine placement of a polypropylene stitch at the site of needle puncture. It is important to avoid vigorous coughing during extubation, if the procedure was performed under general anesthesia. Keeping the patient in a semi-Fowler position in the immediate postoperative period aids in reduction of overall edema of the operative site and may assist in reducing the incidence of venous bleeding.

Reversal of intraoperative heparinization with protamine sulfate has both benefits and potential complications. A severe protamine reaction can be lethal and is seen more often in patients with diabetes mellitus owing to prior exposure from insulin preparations. Otherwise, judicious use of protamine may benefit patients in whom continued oozing is encountered toward completion of the procedure. It is the author's practice to limit heparin reversal to these patients.

Management of post-carotid endarterectomy wound hematomas should be individualized. Small hematomas that cause no significant discomfort, no compromise of the airway, and are otherwise asymptomatic may be managed conservatively with the expectation that they will resolve in four to six weeks. Patients with considerable discomfort, difficulty swallowing, or respiratory compromise should be immediately explored. Exploration may be carried out under local anesthesia. Often, no specific bleeding site is encountered, and evacuation of the hematoma, assurance of overall hemostasis, and reclosure of the wound are all that is necessary. Clearly, if a bleeding point is identified, it should be properly secured. Placement of a drain after evacuation of a wound hematoma is commonly advised, although not universally practiced. Temporary use of hemostatic agents is helpful, although leaving such agents in the wound is unlikely to be of benefit and potentially increases the risk of infection.

INFECTION

Infection following carotid endarterectomy is extremely rare. Prophylactic use of antibiotics did not show any benefit in a prospective randomized study, and routine use is not recommended.[33] However, if prosthetic material is used for arteriotomy closure, prophylactic antibiotics are advocated, given the serious nature of an infection in this setting. This highlights one of the disadvantages of a prosthetic patch. In the absence of prosthetic material, infection after carotid endarterectomy should be handled according to the clinical condition. If erythema without abscess formation is present, appropriate antibiotic therapy should resolve the process. On the other hand, if a subcutaneous fluid collection is documented by ultrasound, prompt drainage and debridement with appropriate systemic antibiotics is necessary. Covering the carotid artery with either healthy surrounding tissue or, in extreme cases, a flap is an essential part of management.

When infection is suspected in the presence of a prosthetic patch, an initial trial of aggressive antibiotic therapy may be appropriate. Persistence of symptoms, or other evidence of continued infection, is probably best handled by operative debridement, drainage, and replacement of the prosthetic patch with autogenous tissue. Very little experience with this complication is reported in the literature; thus, the general principles for management of infections in vascular surgery should be followed.

False aneurysm complicating carotid endarterectomy has been associated with chronic infection. The overall incidence of false aneurysm after carotid surgery may be as high as 0.3 percent.[34] No significant difference in the incidence of this complication appears to exist between primary arteriotomy closure and patch closure. Successful repair of the pseudoaneurysm with a saphenous vein patch has been reported.[35] Ligation of the artery may be necessary in patients who fail to respond to autogenous patch closure or replacement with a vein graft; however, this form of management is associated with a morbidity and mortality of about 50 percent.[34] Liberal use of antibiotics in these cases is strongly recommended.

The risk of infection following carotid endarterectomy is definitely increased when concomitant head and neck procedures are carried out. This is most commonly seen in patients requiring carotid surgery in the presence of gastrointestinal or respiratory stomas. In these instances, prophylactic antibiotics should be routine and prosthetic materials should be avoided.

COMPLICATIONS OF CLOSURE

Closure of the arteriotomy following carotid endarterectomy may be carried out primarily or with a patch of autogenous or synthetic material. Complications have been described for all three alternatives, including pseudoaneurysm, rupture, stenosis, and dilatation.

In a comparison of saphenous vein patch, polytetrafluoroethylene (PTFE) patch, and primary arteriotomy closure after carotid endarterectomy, neurologic complications were slightly more frequent in the primary closure group, although the differences were not statistically significant.[36] Stenoses of 30 to 50 percent diameter reduction occurred in 17 percent of the primarily closed arteries and none of the patched arteries. On the other hand, dilatation of the common or internal carotid artery to more than twice the normal diameter was absent in the primary closure group but present in 17 percent of the saphenous vein patch closures and 9 percent of the PTFE patch closures. Thus, abnormalities may be associated with any of these three closure techniques. Certainly, primary closure of the arteriotomy requires careful and meticulous technique to avoid narrowing. It is the author's practice to patch patients with small arteries (especially women) and patients operated upon for recurrent stenosis following carotid endarterectomy. Primary closure may be performed safely and effectively, provided narrowing of the artery is avoided by small bites with fine (7–0) monofilament suture.

Rupture of the vein patch used for carotid arteriotomy closure has been reported. Infection does not seem to play a significant role in this complication.[37] The most common finding at reoperation is necrosis of the mid portion of the patch, with spontaneous rupture. In a study of patch closure, it was suggested that veins harvested from the ankle have a much higher incidence of rupture than saphenous veins harvested from the thigh. In fact, rupture of an ankle vein patch has been treated successfully with a repeat patch using saphenous vein obtained from the groin.[38] Thus, when autogenous tissue is used, it is best to harvest the vein from the groin in preference to the ankle.

Pseudoaneurysm formation can be a complication of any carotid arteriotomy closure, and repair is indicated to prevent rupture or embolization. Infection may play a significant role in up to 14 percent of patients, especially when prosthetic material has been used.[35] In the absence of infection, treatment should consist of closure with either an autogenous or prosthetic patch. An occasional patient will require resection and placement of an interposition saphenous vein graft. In the presence of infection, recurrence after prosthetic patch closure has been reported, and autogenous tissue must be used for any reconstructive procedure.

The long-term results with each type of carotid artery closure in terms of recurrent carotid stenosis remain uncertain. There are reported series suggesting that the incidence of recurrent stenosis is reduced by patch closure,[39,40] although excellent results with low rates of recurrent stenosis also have been achieved using primary closure.[41] With respect to this controversy it is important to remember that narrowing of the carotid artery must be avoided and an assessment of the technical result carried out, regardless of the method of closure.

RECURRENT STENOSIS

The incidence of recurrent stenosis following carotid endarterectomy has been estimated to be between 5 and 25 percent, depending on the method of postoperative assessment.[42,43] In patients routinely followed with duplex scanning, significant recurrent stenosis of greater than 50 percent diameter reduction has been identified in 12 to 18 percent of patients.[44] These lesions, when they occur within the first two years, usually are associated with intimal hyperplasia. Their natural history tends to be benign, with the possible exception of the most severe stenoses. Recurrent lesions developing more than two years following the initial operation may be associated with atherosclerotic changes, and their natural history is more likely to resemble that of the original lesion.[45] In a study of 120 patients who underwent 143 carotid endarterectomies, the incidence of symptomatic recurrence was low, with only two of 14 recurrent stenoses being associated with symptoms. The incidence of ipsilateral symptoms was similar for those arteries that did not develop recurrent stenoses; thus, by life-table analysis, there was no increased risk of TIA, stroke, or death in patients with recurrent stenosis.[44]

The incidence of recurrent stenosis appears to be higher in patients who continue to smoke following carotid endarterectomy, in women, and in patients with hypertension or hypercholesterolemia.[46,47] The latter two risk factors have not been universally accepted, although some studies show a significant correlation.[48] Aspirin has not been shown conclusively to reduce the incidence of recurrent stenosis, although it is routinely recommended in the overall management of patients with both coronary and carotid artery disease.[49]

Turbulent flow through the endarterectomized segment can be identified by duplex scanning, either intraoperatively or in the immediate postoperative period. This finding suggests either technical defects or residual disease, and is a risk factor for recurrent stenosis. The technical adequacy of 250 endarterectomy sites in 235 patients was assessed at operation by pulsed Doppler spectral analysis and arteriography. The incidence of residual lesions, recurrent stenoses, and variations in clinical outcome were documented in these patients. Residual flow disturbances at the endarterectomy site correlated with both perioperative thrombosis and stroke.[50] The incidence of occlusion and recurrent stenosis was increased in arteries with residual flow disturbances identified at operation. Thus, completeness of the endarterectomy and adequacy of the technical result represent the most important factors under the surgeon's control to prevent recurrent carotid stenosis. If primary closure is elected, one must document that the artery is not narrowed. Otherwise, patch closure should be performed.

Management of recurrent carotid stenosis depends on the timing of the recurrence, the degree of narrowing, and the presence or absence of symptoms. Asymptomatic patients with less than approximately 80 percent stenosis should be managed conservatively, especially for recurrent lesions within the first six months following endarterectomy. Some of these lesions have actually been shown to regress on later evaluations.[51] Symptomatic patients with significant recurrent lesions should be managed operatively. Similarly, asymptomatic patients who have shown progression to a greater than 80 percent stenosis should be considered for operation. Management of stenoses that recur more than two years following carotid endarterectomy should be similar to that for primary lesions of the carotid bifurcation.

Recurrent carotid stenoses secondary to intimal hyperplasia are best managed by longitudinal transection of the lesion and patch closure. Repeat endarterectomy of these lesions usually is not possible and carries the risk of injury to the remaining arterial wall. Lesions with a significant atherosclerotic component are best managed by repeat endarterectomy and patch closure. Results of operations for recurrent carotid stenosis suggest that effective control of symptoms can be achieved. However, perioperative risks are generally higher than for primary operations, and a higher incidence of cranial nerve injury has been reported.[52] More detailed discussions of recurrent carotid stenosis and reoperative carotid surgery are presented in Chaps. 27 and 28.

HYPERPERFUSION SYNDROME

Some patients complain of severe ipsilateral headache following carotid endarterectomy. This may result from the mild-to-moderate brain edema that can follow removal of a highly stenotic lesion at the carotid bifurcation. These patients are at significant risk for intracranial hemorrhage and should be observed in the hospital. The syndrome may progress to focal seizures requiring anticonvulsant medication. Anticoagulation must be avoided to minimize the risk of intracranial hemorrhage. Although hypertension has not been correlated with the incidence of hyperperfusion syndrome, adequate control of blood pressure is important for minimizing the risk of other complications. Methods to reduce brain swelling appear reasonable, although they are of unproven value. In the absence of intracranial hemorrhage, the syndrome is usually self-limited and resolves spontaneously.

The pathophysiology of hyperperfusion syndrome is not well understood, but it is believed to be secondary to a loss of autoregulation of cerebral perfusion. Elevated flow velocities in the ipsilateral cerebral vasculature, with abnormally low peripheral vascular resistance, have been documented by transcranial Doppler in patients with hyperperfusion syndrome following carotid endarterectomy.[53] Electroencephalographic evaluation of patients with this syndrome who have experienced seizures reveals periodic lateralizing epileptiform discharges on the side of the brain ipsilateral to the endarterectomy.[54] Autopsy findings in patients with this syndrome have shown hypercellularity and edema of the arterial and arteriolar walls, with extravasation of erythrocytes and exudation of fibrin.[55] This suggests a lack of autoregulation with hyperperfusion similar to the condition found in severely hypertensive patients that results in hypertensive encephalopathy. This forms the basis for recommending rapid control of blood pressure when this syndrome is recognized.

HYPERTENSION

The influence of uncontrolled hypertension on the complications of carotid endarterectomy is well documented. Hypertensive patients are at increased risk for stroke, wound hematoma, MI, and intracranial hemorrhage. Thus, perioperative control of blood pressure is extremely important, and arterial line monitoring is highly recommended. Postoperative hypertension occurs more frequently in patients with poor preoperative blood pressure control, when peripheral arterial occlusive disease is present, after removal of a highly stenotic carotid lesion, and in patients with diabetes mellitus. One of the postulated mechanisms for post-carotid endarterectomy hypertension suggests that reperfusion of chronically ischemic brain tissue results in release of renin and norepinephrine.[14,15] Some investigators have suggested that preservation of the intercarotid neural bundle supplying the carotid baroreceptors may influence the incidence of post-carotid endarterectomy hypertension.[56] They advocated placement of catheters to block the carotid sinus nerves in order to minimize extremes of blood pressure. However, the true value of this type of intervention is unclear.

The adequacy of the cerebral collateral circulation during carotid clamping also has been mentioned as a factor that may be associated with post-carotid endarterectomy hypertension. Others have found no significant difference between patients who are shunted and those who are not.[16] Thus, the relationship between postoperative blood pressure changes and intraoperative brain ischemia is not known.

We routinely use an arterial line for blood pressure monitoring in patients undergoing carotid endarterectomy. Systolic blood pressure is maintained between 100 mmHg and 140 mmHg. Treatment with sodium nitroprusside or nitroglycerin is started if systolic blood pressure rises above 160 mmHg. Patients are restarted on oral antihypertensive medications postoperatively as soon as they can tolerate oral intake.

PAROTID INJURY

Injury to the parotid gland is an extremely rare complication following carotid endarterectomy. It may be manifested by a swelling in the upper portion of the wound, with eventual drainage of clear fluid through the incision. The drainage typically is increased by oral intake and may persist as a fistula. This complication is avoided by curving the upper portion of the incision well behind the ear, thus avoiding the tail of the parotid gland. Glandular tissue characteristic of the parotid may be recognized when the dissection inadvertently is carried forward in the upper portion of the incision. This glandular tissue may be the source of significant bleeding. Careful repair of a parotid injury with monofilament sutures may prevent postoperative complications. The author has repaired two such injuries by this method without sequelae. The presence of a parotid injury can be confirmed in the postoperative period by sialography. A parotid fistula may be seen as extravasation of contrast through the wound.

Management of a parotid fistula should be individualized and is based on experience with this complication after other types of surgery or trauma. When drainage is limited, conservative management consists of no oral intake, with intravenous or enteral nutritional support, to allow spontaneous closure. With traumatic parotid fistula, conservative management has been successful in over 90 percent of cases for minor injuries without major duct involvement.[57] Otherwise, various techniques have been described, including resection and vein graft repair.[58]

CONCLUSIONS

Complications of carotid endarterectomy are mostly preventable by careful attention to detail in the preoperative preparation of the patient, knowledge of the anatomy and potential pitfalls during dissection, and proper perioperative management of patients with generalized atherosclerosis. Carotid endarterectomy is mostly a prophylactic operation. Thus, it is incumbent on surgeons performing this procedure to keep complications to a minimum. In preoperative discussions with patients, it is important for surgeons to present their own experience, not just numbers quoted from the literature. Surgeons performing carotid endarterectomy should routinely evaluate their results to be sure that they are consistent with those attained in centers of excellence. Only then will patients benefit from carotid endarterectomy.

REFERENCES

1. North American Symptomatic Carotid Endarterectomy Trial (NASCET) Steering Committee: North American Symptomatic Carotid Endarterectomy Trial: Methods, patient characteristics, and progress. *Stroke* 22:611–720, 1991.
2. Yeager RA, Moneta GL, McConnell DB, et al: Analysis of risk factors for myocardial infarction following carotid endarterectomy. *Arch Surg* 124(10):1142–1145, 1989.
3. Zuccarello M, Yeh HS, Tew JM: Morbidity and mortality of carotid endarterectomy under local anesthesia: A retrospective study. *Neurosurgery* 23(4):445–450, 1988.
4. Quiñones-Baldrich WJ, Moore WS: Asymptomatic carotid stenosis: Rationale for management. *Arch Neurol* 42:378–382, 1985.
5. Moore DJ, Modi JR, Finch WT, Sumner DS: Influence of the contralateral carotid artery on neurologic complications following carotid endarterectomy. *J Vasc Surg* 1(3):409–414, 1984.
6. McKittrick JE, MacLean WB, Lim RA: Carotid endarterectomy in patients with contralateral carotid occlusion: Is the risk increased? *Ann Vasc Surg* 3(4):324–327, 1989.
7. Giordano JM, Trout HH III, Kozloff L, DePalma RG: Timing of carotid artery endarterectomy after stroke. *J Vasc Surg* 2(2):250–255, 1985.
8. Dosick SM, Whalen RC, Gale SS, Brown OW: Carotid endarterectomy in the stroke patient: Computerized axial tomography to determine timing. *J Vasc Surg* 2(1):214–219, 1985.
9. Mentzer RM, Finkelmeier BA, Crosby IK, et al: Emergency carotid endarterectomy for fluctuating neurologic deficits. *Surgery* 89:60, 1981.

10. Hankey GJ, Warlow CP, Molynex AJ: Complications of cerebral angiography for patients with mild carotid territory ischaemia being considered for carotid endarterectomy. *J Neurol Neurosurg Psychiat (England)* 53(7):542–548, 1990.
11. Wagner WH, Treiman RL, Crossman DV, et al: The diminishing role of diagnostic arteriography in carotid artery disease: Duplex scanning as definitive preoperative study. *Ann Vasc Surg* 5(2):105–110, 1991.
12. Goodson SF, Flanigan DP, Bishara RA, et al: Can carotid duplex scanning supplant arteriography in patients with focal carotid territory symptoms? *J Vasc Surg* 5(4):551–557, 1987.
13. Flanigan DP, Schuler JJ, Vogel M, et al: The role of carotid duplex scanning in surgical decision making. *J Vasc Surg* 2(1):15–25, 1985.
14. Smith BL: Hypertension following carotid endarterectomy: The role of cerebral renin production. *J Vasc Surg* 1(5):623–627, 1984.
15. Ahn SS, Marcus DR, Moore WS: Post-carotid endarterectomy hypertension: Association with elevated cranial norepinephrine. *J Vasc Surg* 9 (2):351–360, 1989.
16. Skydell JL, Machleder HI, Baker JD, et al: Incidence and mechanism of post-carotid endarterectomy hypertension. *Arch Surg* 122(10):1153–1155, 1987.
17. Rosenthal D, Zeichner WD, Lamis PA, Stanton PE Jr: Neurologic deficit after carotid endarterectomy: Pathogenesis and management. *Surgery* 94(5):776–780, 1983.
18. Hafner CD: Minimizing the risks of carotid endarterectomy. *J Vasc Surg* 1(3):392–397, 1984.
19. Loftus CM, Dyste GN, Reinarz SJ, Hingtgen WL: Distal cervical carotid dissection after carotid endarterectomy: A complication of indwelling shunt? *Neurosurgery* 19(3):441–445, 1986.
20. Sundt TM Jr, Ebersold MJ, Sharbrough FW, et al: The risk-benefit ratio of intraoperative shunting during carotid endarterectomy. Relevancy to operative and postoperative results and complications. *Ann Surg* 203(2):196–204, 1986.
21. Zierler RE, Bandyk DF, Thiele BL: Intraoperative assessment of carotid endarterectomy. *J Vasc Surg* 1(1):73–83, 1984.
22. Courbier R, Jausseran JM, Reggi M, et al: Routine intraoperative carotid angiography: Its impact on operative morbidity and carotid restenosis. *J Vasc Surg* 3(2):343–350, 1986.
23. Countee RW, Vijayanathan T, Wu SZ: External carotid occlusion as a cause of recurrent ischemia after carotid endarterectomy. *Neurosurgery* 11(4):518–521, 1982.
24. Moore WS, Martello JY, Quiñones-Baldrich WJ, Ahn SS: Etiologic importance of the intimal flap of the external carotid artery in the development of postcarotid endarterectomy stroke. *Stroke* 21(10):1497–1502, 1990.
25. Hafner DH, Smith RB III, King OW, et al: Massive intracerebral hemorrhage following carotid endarterectomy. *Arch Surg* 122(3):305–307, 1987.
26. Schuler JJ, Flanigan DP, Lim LT, et al: The effect of carotid siphon stenosis on stroke rate, death, and relief of symptoms following elective carotid endarterectomy. *Surgery* 92(6): 1058–1067, 1982.
27. Dehn TC, Taylor GW: Cranial and cervical nerve damage associated with carotid endarterectomy. *Br J Surg* 70(6):365–368, 1983.
28. Evans WE, Mendelowitz DS, Liapis C, et al: Motor speech deficit following carotid endarterectomy. *Ann Surg* 196(4):461–464, 1982.
29. Sannella NA, Tober RL, Cipro RP, et al: Vocal cord paralysis following carotid endarterectomy: The paradox of return of function. *Ann Vasc Surg* 4(1):42–45, 1990.
30. Maniglia AJ, Han DP: Cranial nerve injuries following carotid endarterectomy: An analysis of 336 procedures. *Head Neck* 13(2):121–124, 1991.
31. Rosenbloom M, Friedman SG, Lamparello PJ, et al: Glossopharyngeal nerve injury complicating carotid endarterectomy. *J Vasc Surg* 5(3):469–471, 1987.
32. Welling RE, Ramadas HS, Gansmuller KJ: Cervical wound hematoma after carotid endarterectomy. *Ann Vasc Surg* 3(3):229–231, 1989.
33. Pitt HA, Postier RG, MacGowan WL, et al: Prophylactic antibiotics in vascular surgery—topical, systemic or both? *Ann Surg* 192:356–364, 1980.
34. Branch CL Jr, Davis CH Jr: False aneurysm

complicating carotid endarterectomy. *Neurosurgery* 19(3):421–425, 1986.

35. Graver LM, Mulcare RJ: Pseudoaneurysm after carotid endarterectomy. *J Cardiovasc Surg* 27(3):294–297, 1986.
36. Lord RS, Raj TB, Stary DL, et al: Comparison of saphenous vein patch, polytetrafluoroethylene patch, and direct arteriotomy closure after carotid endarterectomy. Part I. Perioperative results. *J Vasc Surg* 9(4):521–529, 1989.
37. Riles TS, Lamparello PJ, Giangola G, Imparato AM: Rupture of the vein patch: A rare complication of carotid endarterectomy. *Surgery* 107 (1):10–12, 1990.
38. O'Hara PJ, Hertzer NR, Krajewski LP, Beven EG: Saphenous vein patch rupture after carotid endarterectomy. *J Vasc Surg* 15(3):504–509, 1992.
39. Ouriel K, Green RM: Clinical and technical factors influencing recurrent carotid stenosis and occlusion after endarterectomy. *J Vasc Surg* 5(5):702–706, 1987.
40. Hertzer NR, Beven EG, O'Hara PJ, Krajewski LP: A prospective study of vein patch angioplasty during carotid endarterectomy. Three-year results for 801 patients and 917 operations. *Ann Surg* 206(5):628–635, 1987.
41. Atnip RG, Wengrovitz M, Gifford RR, et al: A rational approach to recurrent carotid stenosis. *J Vasc Surg* 11(4):511–516, 1990.
42. Das MB, Hertzer NR, Ratliff NB, et al: Recurrent carotid stenosis. A five-year series of 65 reoperations. *Ann Surg* 202(1):28–35, 1985.
43. Bertin VJ, Plecha FR, Rogers GJ, et al: Recurrent stenosis by duplex scan following carotid endarterectomy. *Arch Surg* 124(7):866–869, 1989.
44. Cook JM, Thompson BW, Barnes RW: Is routine duplex examination after carotid endarterectomy justified? *J Vasc Surg* 12(3):334–340, 1990.
45. Washburn WK, Mackey WC, Belkin M, O'Donnell TF Jr: Late stroke after carotid endarterectomy: The role of recurrent stenosis. *J Vasc Surg* 15(6):1032–1036, 1992.
46. Reilly LM, Okuhn SP, Rapp JH, et al: Recurrent carotid stenosis: A consequence of local or systemic factors? The influence of unrepaired technical defects. *J Vasc Surg* 11(3):448–459, 1990.
47. Clagett GP, Rich NM, McDonald PT, et al: Etiologic factors for recurrent carotid artery stenosis. *Surgery* 93(2):313–318, 1983.
48. Rapp JH, Qvarfordt P, Krupski WC, et al: Hypercholesterolemia and early restenosis after carotid endarterectomy. *Surgery* 101(3):277–282, 1987.
49. Archie JP Jr: Prevention of early restenosis and thrombosis-occlusion after carotid endarterectomy by saphenous vein patch angioplasty. *Stroke* 17(5):901–905, 1986.
50. Bandyk DF, Kaebnick HW, Adams MB, Towne JB: Turbulence occurring after carotid bifurcation endarterectomy: A harbinger of residual and recurrent carotid stenosis. *J Vasc Surg* 7(2):261–274, 1988.
51. Healy DA, Zierler RE, Nicholls SC, et al: Long-term follow-up and clinical outcome of carotid restenosis. *J Vasc Surg* 10(6):662–668, 1989.
52. Piepgras DG, Sundt TM Jr, Marsh WR, et al: Recurrent carotid stenosis. Results and complications of 57 operations. *Ann Surg* 203 (2):205–213, 1986.
53. Powers AD, Smith RR: Hyperperfusion syndrome after carotid endarterectomy: A transcranial Doppler evaluation. *Neurosurgery* 26 (1):56–59, 1990.
54. Reigel MM, Hollier LH, Sundt TM Jr, et al: Cerebral hyperperfusion syndrome: A cause of neurologic dysfunction after carotid endarterectomy. *J Vasc Surg* 5(4):628–634, 1987.
55. Bernstein M, Fleming JF, Deck JH: Cerebral hyperperfusion after carotid endarterectomy: A cause of cerebral hemorrhage. *Neurosurgery* 15(1):50–56, 1984.
56. Cafferata HT, Merchant RF Jr, DePalma RG: Avoidance of postcarotid endarterectomy hypertension. *Ann Surg* 196(4):465–472, 1982.
57. Parekh D, Glezerson G, Stewart M, et al: Posttraumatic parotid fistulae and sialoceles. A prospective study of conservative management in 51 cases. *Ann Surg* 209(1):105–111, 1989.
58. Ananthakrishnan N: Vein graft repair of a chronic parotid duct fistula. *J Oral Maxillofac Surg* 41(4):266–267, 1983.

27

Clinical Outcome and Recurrent Stenosis after Carotid Endarterectomy

Mark Wengrovitz
Dean A. Healy

Despite all the information available regarding the natural history of carotid bifurcation atherosclerosis, the role of carotid endarterectomy remains controversial. The efficacy of this procedure depends on the inherent associated perioperative risks, the reduction in neurologic events it achieves, and the long-term durability of the repair. These issues will be addressed here by reviewing the natural history of extracranial carotid disease by clinical subsets and the reported results of medical and surgical therapy. In a second section, the pathogenesis, incidence, clinical impact, and therapy of recurrent carotid stenosis will be considered.

CLINICAL OUTCOME

Asymptomatic Carotid Stenosis

It is now generally accepted that the mere presence of a stenotic lesion affecting the carotid artery is not sufficient cause for performing a carotid endarterectomy. However, it is also becoming clear that some patients with asymptomatic carotid stenosis have a significant chance of developing cerebral ischemic symptoms if followed over time. Roederer and coworkers followed 167 asymptomatic patients with serial duplex scans.[1] All patients had cervical bruits but were included regardless of the degree of carotid disease present. The overall rate for development of neurologic symptoms was 4 percent per year for this group, but almost all patients (89 percent) who developed symptoms either had, or showed progression to, a severe stenosis (greater than 80 percent diameter reduction) at the appropriate carotid bifurcation. In this same series, progression to a greater than 80 percent diameter-reducing lesion was associated with a 46 percent chance of developing cerebral ischemic symptoms or going on to internal carotid artery occlusion. Patients with lesions that remained less than 80 percent diameter-reducing had only a 1.5 percent chance of developing symptoms. Others have reported similar rates of stroke (approximately 20 percent over five years) in patients with asymptomatic disease and carotid lesions of greater than 50 percent diameter reduction.[2,3]

Bock and associates also followed a group of patients with carotid artery disease by noninvasive testing.[4] The group of patients with stenoses greater than 80 percent did indeed have a much higher rate of stroke and transient ischemic events, but many of these events were in the distribution of the contralateral internal carotid artery. These findings confirm the accepted idea that many patients with known severe internal carotid stenoses do not have a benign course, and that their clinical outcome can be unpredictable.

Numerous authors have reported their results of carotid endarterectomy for asymptomatic stenosis. Mattos and colleagues described a series of 544 carotid endarterectomies on 478 patients with follow-up in 83 percent of patients over a mean period of 44 months.[5] Of those patients still alive five and ten years after endarterectomy done for asymptomatic carotid stenosis, stroke-free rates were 96 percent and 92 percent, respectively. This translates to a stroke rate of less than 1 percent per year. Among these patients, 50 percent of all deaths were related to cardiac disease, and stroke-free rates were significantly greater than stroke-free survival rates, indicating that most deaths were not related to cerebrovascular accidents.

Similar results have been reported by Bernstein and coworkers, who followed 456 patients for a mean of 45 months.[6] The surgically treated asymptomatic patients had a 3.2 percent incidence of stroke during follow-up and a 1.6 percent incidence of transient ischemic events over a period up to 11 years postoperatively. In addition, series by Moore,[7] and Hertzer[8] report a similar incidence of postoperative cerebral ischemic events during long-term follow-up. Patients who undergo carotid endarterectomy for asymptomatic carotid stenoses have a long-term risk of stroke of approximately 1 percent per year and therefore can expect a three- to fourfold reduction in stroke rate.

A Veterans Affairs cooperative study determined the fate of asymptomatic patients with internal carotid stenoses greater than 50 percent diameter reduction who were randomized to either surgery followed by aspirin or aspirin therapy alone.[9] Although there appeared to be a large reduction in stroke rate in the surgical group during long-term follow-up, the difference did not achieve statistical significance (*p*

< .06). However, this study did not stratify patients with more severe carotid stenoses, in whom the natural history is thought to be associated with a substantially higher stroke risk.

Moneta and associates studied the effect of carotid endarterectomy in the management of high-grade (80 to 99 percent) asymptomatic internal carotid stenosis.[10] Endarterectomy was performed in 56 patients, while 73 patients were followed nonoperatively for at least 24 months. Although this was not a randomized study, life table analysis revealed a higher rate of stroke, transient cerebral ischemia, and carotid occlusion in the nonoperated group. Statistical significance was not achieved for stroke alone, but it can be argued that transient cerebral ischemia is a marker for impending stroke and that these results are still meaningful. This suggests that preservation of neurologic status can be improved by carotid endarterectomy in the asymptomatic patient with high-grade carotid stenosis. Table 27-1 summarizes these studies in asymptomatic patients.

Most surgeons favor the operative management of carotid disease in asymptomatic patients only if the stenoses are greater than 80 percent diameter reduction, as these lesions are most likely to give rise to symptoms or progress to internal carotid artery occlusion. In this group of patients, carotid endarterectomy can be performed with acceptable perioperative morbidity and mortality rates to achieve a reduction in the symptom and stroke rate over long-term follow-up. This also improves upon the results gained with the sole use of antiplatelet agents.[9] However, this practice has not been universally accepted by all vascular surgeons and neurologists, and it continues to undergo randomized prospective study (Chap. 17).

Transient Cerebral Ischemia

Patients who experience transient cerebral ischemic events (ipsilateral hemispheric symptoms or amaurosis fugax) have an increased risk of stroke. Whisnant and colleagues reported 118 patients who were followed with nonoperative therapy after experiencing a transient ischemic event.[11] Over the five-year study period, stroke rates in this group of patients were as high as 45 percent, representing a 16- to 20-fold higher risk of stroke as compared to the general age-matched population. Most neurologic deficits occurred in the first year, and the risk of permanent ischemic damage then lessened each year thereafter. Other series[12,13] have reported similar results for untreated transient cerebral ischemia due to carotid stenosis, with stroke rates of approximately 10 percent in the first year and 5 percent each year thereafter.

The aforementioned Mattos study[5] revealed that perioperative stroke rates were low (1.3 percent) for their group of patients operated

Table 27-1 Clinical Outcome after Endarterectomy for Asymptomatic Carotid Stenosis

Study (yr, ref)	# Arteries	Mean follow-up (months)	Survival (%)	Stroke rate (%/year)
Mattos, 1992[5]	146	44	92.4 (10 yr)	1.0
Bernstein, 1981[6]	87	43	70 (7 yr)	1.5
Moore, 1979[7]	78	15 yr total	83 (42 mo)	0.3
Hertzer, 1985[8]	126	14 yr total	44 (10 yr)	1.0
VA Coop, 1993[9]	211	48	66 (8 yr)	1.25
Moneta, 1987[10]	56	24	85 (2 yr)	2.0

on for transient cerebral ischemic events. Of those patients followed, the five-year post-endarterectomy stroke rate was 7 percent, and this increased to 13 percent at 10 years. This compares favorably with medically managed patients, who have a five-year stroke rate that may approach 45 percent, as reported above.[11] Similar beneficial results following carotid endarterectomy for transient cerebral ischemia have been reported by others,[6,8,14] even though the postoperative rate for ischemic stroke is somewhat higher than in asymptomatic patients. On the average, 15 percent of patients (1.5 percent/year) undergoing carotid endarterectomy for this indication will experience transient cerebral ischemia, and 20 percent of patients (2 percent/year) will experience stroke over a ten-year postoperative period.

It is well established that transient cerebral ischemia is a valid indication for carotid endarterectomy, but this may hold true only if the patient has a high-grade carotid stenosis. In the North American Symptomatic Carotid Endarterectomy Trial (NASCET), in which one arm was prematurely halted in 1991,[15] a significant benefit was observed in the group of patients whose carotid lesions were greater than 70 percent diameter-reducing. Patients who had lesser degrees of stenosis may have had transient cerebral ischemia from some other cause, and the outcome of surgery in this group of patients is still being investigated (Chap. 16). No long-term studies have stratified patients according to the specific indication for surgery as well as degree of stenosis to see whether the results are different for each group. Thus, the presence of transient cerebral ischemia as the indication for carotid endarterectomy may not be the only factor that affects long-term outcome in this group of patients. Table 27-2 summarizes the studies that include endarterectomy for symptomatic patients.

Completed Stroke

This group of patients has the highest risk of suffering a subsequent stroke, regardless of the treatment modality implemented. Such patients may be candidates for carotid endarterectomy if a bifurcation lesion is the likely cause of stroke and if neurologic impairment is mild. The patient with hemodynamic instability or severe neurologic disability after a cerebrovascular accident is usually not considered a candidate for surgery. Patients who suffer a stroke and survive, and who are then followed without intervention, continue to be at major risk for recurrent stroke over the

Table 27-2 Clinical Outcome after Endarterectomy for Symptomatic Cerebral Ischemia

Study (yr,ref)	# Arteries	Follow-up (total)	Survival (%)	Stroke rate (%/year)
Transient Ischemic Attacks				
Mattos, 1992[5]	231	14 yr	52.9	1.3
Bernstein, 1981[6]	228	10 yr	50	1.5
Hertzer, 1985[8]	123	14 yr	49	0.6
Takolander, 1983[14]	142	5 yr	90	1.3
NASCET, 1991[15] (incl nondisabling stroke)	328	18 mos	95	0.8
Completed Stroke				
Mattos, 1992[5]	126	14 yr	52.9	2.7
Hertzer, 1985[8]	80	14 yr	30	0.6
Takolander, 1983[14]	60	5 yr	75	2.0

course of their lives. Natural history studies have estimated a recurrent stroke rate of 5 to 20 percent per year.[16–19]

Higher perioperative stroke rates occur in this group of patients, with a range of 4 to 7 percent.[5,8,14] After operation, follow-up studies show that this group of patients also has the highest long-term stroke rate. Mattos reported that 20 and 27 percent of patients followed five and ten years after operative therapy, respectively, suffered recurrent strokes.[5] Both Takolander and Hertzer[8,14] have reported similar results over the long term. It has become accepted that these patients have the highest stroke risk both before and after surgery, but the likelihood of stroke without surgery is so high that endarterectomy should be considered in properly selected patients. Table 27-2 also lists studies in which carotid endarterectomy was performed for completed stroke.

Acute Stroke

In the past, carotid endarterectomy was commonly performed for acute stroke. In 1964 Wylie reported that the risk of converting a stable acute stroke into an unstable hemorrhagic stroke was higher if carotid endarterectomy was performed.[20] This indication for carotid endarterectomy was further studied, and it is now known that there is an interval after an acute stroke during which carotid endarterectomy should not be performed. Giordano showed that if endarterectomy is performed less than five weeks after the acute neurologic event, the mortality and morbidity of the surgery is higher than if surgery is delayed for at least five weeks.[21] This series included 22 patients operated on for stroke at a later stage (5 to 20 weeks) and 27 patients operated on for stroke at an earlier stage (less than 5 weeks). The early group had an increased incidence of new neurologic morbidity that approached 20 percent, while the later group had no new neurologic morbidity in the perioperative period.

This was further investigated by Dosick and coworkers, who found that perioperative morbidity was much less in the early period following stroke as long as computed tomography (CT) showed no cerebral infarction,[22] and the diagnosis of stroke was made on clinical grounds alone. This has been substantiated by others as well.[23] Therefore, as discussed in Chap. 13, patients presenting with a persistent new neurologic deficit may be candidates for surgery in this early post-stroke period if their CT scans are negative. Sannella reported interesting findings regarding 13 patients with severe bilateral carotid disease who presented with acute hemispheric stroke symptoms and a positive CT scan.[24] Contralateral carotid endarterectomy was performed in these patients an average of seven days after presentation. No patient was made worse by this intervention, but no benefit was shown. Thus, it is not clear at this time whether contralateral carotid reconstruction in the early post-stroke period is of any long-term benefit.

For the most part, carotid endarterectomy in the immediate (within 5 weeks) post-stroke period is contraindicated. This is especially true if the patient is hemodynamically unstable, has a dense neurologic deficit, or if the level of consciousness is altered. However, if a patient has a mild deficit, is lucid, and is otherwise stable, early carotid endarterectomy can be considered if the CT scan is negative for cerebral infarction.

Stroke-in-Evolution

Stroke-in-evolution identifies another group of patients previously believed not to benefit from carotid endarterectomy. These patients present with a neurologic deficit but have a changing examination indicating neurologic instability. The natural history of stroke-in-evolution without intervention is known to be poor, with very high morbidity and mortality rates. Goldstone and Moore reported on a group of patients with this presentation who had an unstable condition noted angiographically[25] consisting of a free-floating thrombus with a patent distal internal carotid artery. These patients were operated on despite their neurologic status and had uniformally good outcomes.

In a review of the literature, Mentzer and coworkers reported on the results of carotid endarterectomy in patients with stroke-in-evolution.[26] They found a 55 percent rate of neurologic improvement, a 25 percent rate of neurologic stabilization, a 10 percent worsening of neurologic status, and a 10 percent operative mortality. Although the perioperative morbidity is high, the natural history of this problem is so uniformally poor that the improvement and stabilization rate of 80 percent was considered favorable.

Nonhemispheric Symptoms

Carotid endarterectomy is sometimes performed in patients with carotid stenoses who have symptoms not classically in the middle cerebral artery distribution. When vertebrobasilar events occur in patients with both vertebral and carotid occlusive disease, the carotid bifurcation is usually treated first. When the circle of Willis is intact, posterior circulation transient ischemia may be relieved by improving anterior circulation flow. However, according to Mattos and colleagues, such patients with nonhemispheric symptoms have a higher operative morbidity rate, with a 4.9 percent perioperative stroke rate, and a five-year stroke-free rate of 92 percent.[5] Results of carotid endarterectomy in this group of patients lie between the asymptomatic group and the completed stroke group with respect to long-term stroke-free survival.

Tandem Lesions

This term refers to the situation in which two (or more) significant stenoses occur in series in the carotid circulation. It may represent simultaneously existing common and internal carotid lesions, but usually refers to coexisting lesions of the carotid siphon and internal carotid artery. Consequently, tandem carotid lesions are most often identified during arteriography. It appears that the potential harm of a carotid bifurcation lesion is significant and outweighs the presence of a siphon lesion.[27]

Moore reported good results when performing carotid endarterectomy in the presence of a siphon lesion.[28] Schuler and associates[29] reported a series of 44 carotid endarterectomies in 35 patients, all of whom had a tandem siphon lesion. Although follow-up was limited to a mean of 15.9 months, there was no statistically significant increased risk of stroke or death following endarterectomy when compared to a simultaneous surgical group with carotid stenosis only. All symptomatic patients also had complete relief of symptoms after operation, indicating that the cause was most likely the bifurcation lesion.

Contralateral Internal Carotid Occlusion

One might expect an increase in neurologic complications during carotid endarterectomy in patients with contralateral internal carotid occlusion. Perler and associates reviewed their experience with 36 patients in this clinical situation and compared the outcome with a group of patients who had a patent contralateral vessel.[30] The perioperative stroke rate was the same in both groups, and stroke and death rates were no different after an average follow-up of 23 months. Sillesen and coworkers also reported a series of similar patients and arrived at similar conclusions.[31]

Conclusions

As discussed above, when performed by experienced surgeons, carotid endarterectomy is a durable operation. The long-term results in most cases give patients an improvement in their quality of life and a statistically significant reduction in stroke rate. Patient selection criteria remain controversial in the absence of proper prospective trials. Although carotid endarterectomy seems to benefit symptomatic patients with high-grade lesions (>70 percent diameter reduction), the benefit rendered to symptomatic patients with lesser lesions is not known at this time. Endarterectomy for asymptomatic individuals is usually reserved for high-grade lesions, but data proving benefit are not yet available.

Carotid endarterectomy is an important therapeutic tool in treating patients with extracranial cerebrovascular disease, and as long as perioperative stroke and death rates remain acceptably low, the long-term outlook is certainly good. The objective of prevention of ipsilateral disabling stroke will be met in the great majority of patients.

RECURRENT STENOSIS

Recurrent stenosis after carotid endarterectomy is a well-described clinical entity. Many series have reported this phenomenon,[32–35] and it is usually considered significant if the lumen diameter of the endarterectomized vessel is reduced by 50 percent or more. Two proposed pathophysiologic mechanisms might give rise to these stenotic lesions, each one causing a distinct arterial wall process resulting in a narrowed internal carotid artery. Recurrent lesions are also classified by the interval after endarterectomy at which they appear. Early recurrent stenoses, defined as those occurring within two years of endarterectomy, tend to resemble myointimal proliferative lesions, whereas those occurring later tend to resemble atheromatous plaques.[36–38]

A great deal has been learned about this clinical entity in recent years as routine noninvasive follow-up has become commonplace. In retrospect, the incidence of this condition was probably underestimated in early series. Modern series have emphasized the need for serial follow-up on all patients and the use of life-table data analysis.

Incidence of Recurrent Carotid Stenosis

The initial studies that defined the incidence of recurrent stenosis after endarterectomy were based primarily on patients who presented with recurrent neurologic symptoms and underwent arteriography (Table 27-3). This incidence was about 1 to 4 percent of the postendarterectomy population, but it failed to include the much larger group of patients who did not have symptoms.[32,36,39] Therefore, the true incidence was felt to be higher, and the availability of noninvasive testing and surveillance programs provided larger postendarterectomy groups for study.

If noninvasive testing is used to make the diagnosis, and asymptomatic patients are also included, the incidence of these lesions is increased markedly from earlier series, as shown in Table 27-4. This incidence in contemporary series has been reported to range from 9 to 32 percent of endarterectomized vessels.[33,34,40–44] This wide disparity is in part due to the different criteria and methods used for establishing the diagnosis and probably does not reflect a change in technical factors or patient selection for operation.

Table 27-3 Incidence of Recurrent Carotid Stenosis Based on Recurrent Neurologic Symptoms

Study (yr,ref)	# Arteries	Incidence (%)	2–24 Months (%)	>24 Months (%)
Hertzer, 1979[32]	1250	1.3	56	44
Stoney, 1976[36]	1654	1.5	35	65
Cossman, 1978[39]	361	3.6	100	—

SOURCE: Reprinted from Zierler RE, Chap. 48, in *Vascular Surgery Principles and Practice,* 1987, Wilson, Veith, Hobson, Williams (eds), p 609 by permission of McGraw-Hill.

Table 27-4 Incidence of Recurrent Carotid Stenosis Using Noninvasive Testing Methods

Study (yr,ref)	# Arteries	Method[a]	Overall restenosis incidence (%)	Symptomatic restenosis incidence (%)
Degroote, 1987[33b]	310	OPG-G Doppler B-mode	32	1.6
Healy, 1989[34b]	301	Duplex	31	3.7
Zierler, 1982[40]	89	Duplex	19	4.5
Baker, 1983[41]	133	SOD, OPG-K Doppler	10[c]	3[d]
Cantelmo, 1981[42]	199	OPG-K, CPA UA	12	4.5
Kremen, 1979[43]	173	OPG-K	10	1.7
Turnipseed, 1980[44]	80	UA	9	2.5

[a]SOD: Supraorbital Doppler; OPG-K: Kartchner oculoplethysmography; CPA: Carotid phonoangiography; UA: Ultrasonic arteriography; Doppler: Direct Doppler exam; OPG-G: Gee oculoplethysmography.
[b]Life-table analysis.
[c]Excludes patients with abnormal initial study.
[d]Includes patients operated on for symptomatic recurrence.
SOURCE: Reprinted from Healy DA, Zierler RE, Chap. 56, in *Vascular Surgery Principles and Practice,* 1993, Wilson, Veith, Hobson, Williams, eds, by permission of McGraw-Hill.

Etiology and Pathology

Numerous factors have been implicated in the development of recurrent lesions, none of which has been universally accepted. At least theoretically, recurrent stenoses could occur as a result of operative technical factors, local processes in the arterial wall, or such systemic factors as gender, hypertension, diabetes, and cigarette smoking.

Technical factors that possibly could contribute to the development of these lesions include vascular clamp injury, incomplete endarterectomy, intimal flaps, and suturing faults. However, the incidence of significant technical defects may be too low for these factors to be responsible for most recurrent lesions. When intraoperative methods are used to detect significant technical errors, their incidence is surprisingly low, ranging from 5 to 10 percent in a number of clinical series. Thus, such defects could not be responsible for the reported incidence of recurrent stenoses, which may approach 30 percent.[45–47] Nevertheless, suture tacking of a distal intimal flap has been associated with recurrent lesions.[48,49] A detailed analysis of unrepaired technical defects followed with postoperative duplex scanning revealed that larger defects created by endarterectomy correlated with recurrent carotid stenoses, and the operated segment usually fared worse than the unoperated segment of the artery.[50] The number of defects, use of a shunt, or reopening of the arteriotomy did not correlate with development of restenosis.

Female gender has been described as a predisposing factor in the development of recurrent carotid lesions.[34,51–54] Certainly a significant correlation exists between female gender and recurrent stenosis, but a cause and effect relationship has not been established. Most likely this finding is related to the smaller diameter of the internal carotid artery in females, and the artery may become even smaller after primary closure and therefore more susceptible to recurrent disease. However, this observation may also be related to increases in platelet number, or a difference in platelet aggregation between the sexes.[55,56]

Other systemic factors have been correlated or associated with recurrent stenosis, but little evidence of a cause and effect relationship for any of these exists. Cigarette smoking, hyperlipidemia, hypertension, and diabetes have been the most frequently mentioned systemic factors associated with this condition, but no studies have investigated risk factor management or its effect on preventing the development of restenosis.[35,51,54,57,58] Table 27-5 presents the etiologic factors thought to play a role in the development of recurrent carotid stenosis.

Two types of lesions have been recognized as causing recurrent carotid stenosis: myointimal hyperplasia in the early postoperative period and recurrent atherosclerosis in the later period.[35,59,60] The early lesions typically appear in the first two years and may be an uncontrolled proliferative reaction to the endarterectomy procedure. The gross appearance of these lesions is smooth, rubbery, and pale in color with a glistening surface. There are usually no ulcerations, which may in part be responsible for the infrequent occurrence of symptoms. Histologically, the lesions contain large amounts of smooth muscle cells and fibroblasts in a relatively homogeneous, acellular matrix. This is different from the atheromatous lesion, which has hemosiderin and fibrin deposition, foam cells, neovascularization, and is more prone to ulceration.

Table 27-5 Etiologic Factors Implicated in the Development of Recurrent Carotid Stenosis

Technical factors:	Vascular clamp injury
	Incomplete endarterectomy
	Intimal flap and suture tacking
	Suturing faults
Female gender:	Small arterial diameter
	Platelet function differences
Cigarette smoking	
Hyperlipidemia	
Hypertension	
Diabetes mellitus	

There is some evidence, however, that all recurrent stenoses begin as proliferative lesions and eventually become atheromatous.[42] Clagett and coworkers noted increasing amounts of collagen, calcium, foam cells, and neovascularization in recurrent carotid lesions examined at longer and longer intervals after initial endarterectomy.[61] The role of active thrombus was not completely defined, but the authors felt that mural thrombus might play a role in the development of these lesions. Thrombus was identified in virtually all recurrent lesions, regardless of age.

Tissue culture studies have yielded information that may be relevant to the pathophysiology of recurrent carotid lesions. Anastomotic stenoses involving prosthetic bypass grafts in the lower extremity appear to be related to mitogenic factors for vascular smooth muscle.[62] Cells removed from these lesions produce substances that stimulate bovine aortic smooth muscle cells in vitro. Nearby native endothelial cells also appear to produce mitogenic substances. This overabundance of the healing process may be primarily involved in the development of intimal proliferative lesions of the carotid artery as well.

Diagnosis

Although no uniform diagnostic criteria exist for recurrent stenosis after carotid endarterectomy, most series define it as the presence of a lesion that occupies more than 50 percent of the diameter of the arterial lumen.[34,54,63] The diagnosis of significant recurrent stenosis can be made by a variety of methods. The most common is probably the incidental finding of a lesion when routine postoperative follow-up studies are being done or the patient is being evaluated for contralateral carotid disease.

Asymptomatic patients do not have historical or physical findings likely to alert a clinician that this condition exists. The presence of a cervical bruit over the carotid bifurcation is a common postoperative finding, but it is not generally considered to be a reliable sign of recurrent stenotic lesions.[64] Cervical bruits after endarterectomy are more likely related to scarring and remodeling of the arterial wall in the area of the endarterectomy which result in localized turbulence. The presence of a new postoperative cervical bruit warrants noninvasive testing to see whether a recurrent stenosis is present.

The diagnostic tests that can confirm the presence of recurrent carotid lesions include arteriography,[36] duplex scanning,[34] ultrasonic arteriography,[44] and oculoplethysmography.[43] Figure 27-1 shows the typical arteriographic appearance of early recurrent carotid stenosis. Each method used has its own diagnostic accuracy reflecting both the sensitivity of the test and the skill of the examiner. The accuracy of duplex scanning in detecting carotid arterial disease is well known and well accepted (Chap. 11). Roederer and colleagues investigated the clinical utility of duplex scanning to diagnose recurrent carotid stenotic lesions.[63] They found that duplex scanning had an accuracy of 94 percent in detecting lesions of greater than 50 percent diameter reduction or internal carotid artery occlusion when compared to conventional angiography. Thus, du-

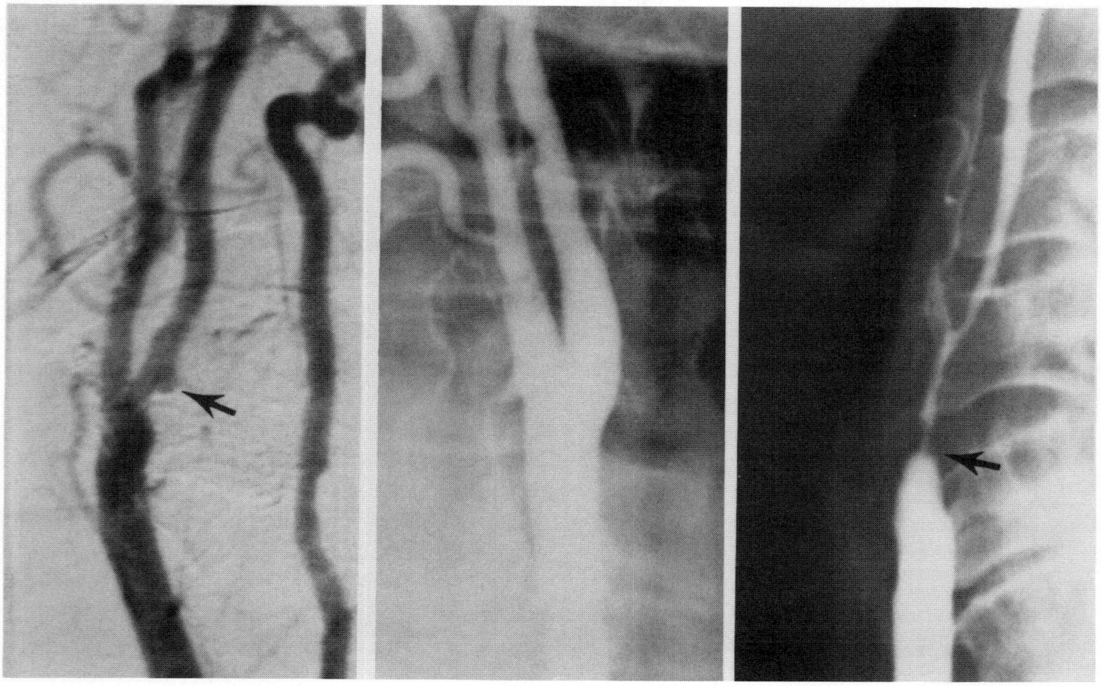

A *B* *C*

Figure 27-1. Sequence of arteriograms illustrating a patient with recurrent carotid stenosis. *A.* Preoperative carotid arteriogram showing ulcerated plaque (arrow) in a patient with amaurosis fugax. *B.* Intraoperative arteriogram after carotid endarterectomy showing widely patent internal carotid artery. *C.* Arteriogram 8 months postoperatively showing extensive asymptomatic early recurrent carotid stenosis beginning in common carotid artery (arrow) and extending into external and internal carotid arteries.

plex ultrasonography has about the same accuracy for detecting recurrent stenosis as it has in the detection of primary atherosclerotic lesions of the carotid bifurcation.[59] We believe that this is the diagnostic test of choice if recurrent lesions are suspected.

Natural History

Patients with recurrent stenosis have been followed over time with serial noninvasive tests, and it has become possible to describe the natural history of this disorder. One large study indicated that some high-grade stenoses noted in the early postoperative period became less severe over time.[34] This observation is consistent with the remodeling process of the postoperative arterial wall.

Clinically, it may become apparent that a patient has a recurrent carotid stenosis. About 10 to 20 percent of patients with recurrent stenosis will manifest ipsilateral hemispheric ischemic symptoms.[33–35,40,52,53] However, comparing postendarterectomy patients with and without recurrent stenosis, there is no statistically significant indication that recurrent disease is associated with a higher incidence of symptoms.[34] In fact, the opposite may even be true. In a study by Bernstein and coworkers, 49 of 566 endarterectomized carotid arteries developed recurrent stenosis.[65] The presence of a recurrent lesion was associated with a significantly longer life expectancy and a lower incidence of stroke, although the latter did not achieve statistical significance. By combining these end-points, patients with recurrent lesions were significantly less likely to have late symptoms, early death, or stroke than were patients with normal postoperative studies. This apparently beneficial or protective effect of restenosis is intriguing, but has not been substantiated in other series. It has been speculated that the myointimal covering of the lesion might actually protect the arterial wall from subsequent atheromatous degeneration with ulceration, embolization, and the development of symptoms. Thus, the natural history of this condition usually is benign, and most patients can look forward to a long-term favorable outcome without further surgery.

Prevention of Recurrent Stenosis

Prevention of recurrent carotid stenosis might be the most effective method of management. Pharmacologic manipulation has been studied in limited series. In a double-blind randomized study, Pratesi and coworkers reported that excessive platelet accumulation on the endarterectomized surface might be an early sign of recurrent stenosis.[66] Antiplatelet therapy with indobufen begun preoperatively resulted in a beneficial effect in the early postoperative period; however, late results were not reported, and this was not a large series. Harker and associates reported 175 patients who were randomized to receive aspirin plus dipyridamole or placebo for one year after carotid endarterectomy.[67] By duplex follow-up there was no significant reduction in the development of stenosis in the treated group (16 percent) versus the placebo group (14 percent). By using intention-to-treat analysis, they showed that the arteries treated with antiplatelet therapy actually had an observed risk increase of 110 percent. At the present time, there is no accepted rationale for postoperative pharmacologic therapy to prevent recurrent stenosis.

A different approach for the prevention of recurrent stenosis entails the use of patch angioplasty for arteriotomy closure at the time of the primary endarterectomy. There is evidence in some series that patch closure can decrease the incidence of postoperative stenosis. Archie reported 200 endarterectomies in which half were closed with a patch angioplasty.[68] He showed that 10 percent of primary closures and none of the patched arteries developed stenosis after one year of follow-up. No long-term data were presented in this series, but others have shown a similar beneficial effect with patching.[69] Long-term results were reported in a retrospective series of 1000 cases, including 750 arteries that were patched with autogenous vein or prosthetic material.[70] There were no statistically significant differences between the group with primary closure and the group having a patch closure, regardless of the material used. With a mean follow-up of 38 months, there was also no difference in the late ipsilateral stroke rate between patients with and without restenosis.

Hans and coworkers reported a series of 78 patients who underwent 83 carotid endarterectomies with autogenous vein patch angioplasty between 1980 and 1985.[71] By intermediate follow-up at a mean of 21 months, eight of 69 arteries had stenosed or occluded, and by 55 months three additional patients had developed recurrent stenoses. This indicated that the use of patch angioplasty did not significantly alter the frequency with which this condition developed.

Clagett and colleagues also reported a series of 152 endarterectomized arteries randomized to patch closure, primary closure, or obligatory patch closure if the internal carotid artery diameter was less than 5 mm, the arteriotomy extended beyond 3 cm from the internal carotid artery origin, or the artery was excessively kinked or tortuous.[72] Only one patient in the series was female, so the effect of patch closure and gender on the development of stenosis was not investigated. However, patch closure in this series was associated with a 13 percent incidence of early recurrent stenosis, as compared to 1.7 percent for those with primary closure. In addition, operative time was significantly increased in the patch closure group. Most stenoses were moderate, asymptomatic, and did not require reoperation. Thus, they concluded that patch closure in selected patients with anatomic or systemic risk factors for recurrent disease is more appropriate than routine patching.

Based on these studies, preventing stenosis of the carotid artery after endarterectomy does not appear possible at this time. There is no effective pharmacologic regimen to prevent recurrent stenosis, and the commonly used antiplatelet agents may actually increase its incidence. In addition, patch angioplasty, regardless of the material used, does not appear convincingly to decrease the incidence of recurrent carotid stenosis. Meticulous surgical technique and a selective approach to patch closure seem most justified.

Management

Most vascular surgeons will treat asymptomatic recurrent carotid lesions nonoperatively with careful clinical follow-up and serial noninvasive testing. Reoperation usually has been advocated for "preocclusive lesions" or those with symptomatic disease.[34] Ipsilateral neurologic symptoms have been reported in up to 20 percent of patients, and therefore at least 80 percent of patients will remain asymptomatic. As long as they remain so or do not progress to a critical stenosis, they can be managed in a nonoperative fashion. Long-term follow-up studies have shown that early recurrent lesions may even regress over time.[34] Thus, a conservative approach to the asymptomatic recurrent lesion seems prudent.

If a patient develops symptoms after carotid endarterectomy, further diagnostic evaluation is indicated. Other embolic sources must be considered, particularly those related to the heart. It has been estimated that up to 20 percent of patients with cardiac and cerebrovascular disease have a potential cardiac source for emboli.[73] Arteriography should always be performed before reoperative carotid surgery, as the nature and extent of each lesion must be known.

Because two types of recurrent carotid lesions have been identified, the surgical management of this condition must be tailored to the individual lesion. Even with preoperative arteriography, the exact technique needed to repair or remove the lesion may not be known until the artery is opened in the operating room. The early fibrointimal lesions are characteristically smooth and rubbery, and an endarterectomy plane cannot be developed. The primary goal of operation is to enlarge the lumen rather than remove an embolic source. This can be accomplished by incising through the primary arteriotomy closure and then performing a patch angioplasty, preferably with autogenous saphenous vein. In contrast, the recurrent atheromatous lesion is more likely to resemble the primary lesion, and an endarterectomy usually can be performed. It is still recommended that the arteriotomy then be closed with a patch.[74] Carotid artery excision and replacement with an interposition graft of autogenous vein has also been reported with good results.[75] The technical aspects of reoperative carotid surgery are discussed further in Chap. 28.

Reoperative carotid surgery is generally more technically demanding than the primary operation. In early series, operative complications such as stroke, transient ischemic events, and cranial nerve injury were reported to have an increased incidence in this group of patients.[76,77] Nitzberg and coworkers reviewed their series of 27 patients with recurrent carotid stenosis who underwent reoperation.[78] They showed that reoperation for symptomatic or preocclusive lesions (> 75 percent diameter reduction) allowed patients to retain the stroke-free rates afforded by primary carotid endarterectomy. Their perioperative stroke rate was 3.4 percent, and they reported no surgical mortality. These findings have been confirmed by others.[79] Thus, reoperative carotid surgery by experienced surgeons can be performed with a morbidity and mortality similar to the primary operation and with a long-term stroke-free outcome.

Conclusions

Recurrent carotid artery stenosis occurs in up to 30 percent of patients after primary endarterectomy, depending on the criteria and testing methods used to make the diagnosis. This incidence has increased in recent years owing to more widespread noninvasive follow-up of asymptomatic patients. Numerous risk factors have been associated with the development of recurrent lesions, including technical defects, female gender, cigarette smoking, hyperlipidemia, hypertension, and diabetes mellitus. However, none of the factors has consistently been found in all series, and there has not been a study reported in which risk factor modification reduced the incidence of recurrent stenosis.

The pathologic process in these lesions has been characterized according to the time of occurrence: early lesions (< 2 years) are usually fibrointimal and proliferative; later lesions are atheromatous. Whether or not these lesions represent a continuum of the same disease process is unknown. It has been reported that fibrointimal lesions may convey some protection against symptoms, but this is presently unproven.

Patients with recurrent stenoses can expect a relatively benign course. Symptoms such as transient cerebral ischemia or stroke are rare and can be expected in about 10 percent of patients. The asymptomatic patient found to have a recurrent lesion can be managed nonoperatively with careful clinical follow-up and serial noninvasive examinations. The patient with ipsilateral cerebral ischemic symptoms or a "preocclusive lesion" may be a candidate for reoperation.

Endarterectomy usually cannot be performed on an artery with a fibroproliferative lesion and these cases are best treated by patch angioplasty, preferably with autogenous saphenous vein. Lesions occurring later may indeed be amenable to endarterectomy, but the artery should also be closed with a patch. Reoperative carotid surgery has been reported to have a much higher incidence of complications including stroke, death, and cranial nerve injury, but more recent studies have shown that a low perioperative morbidity and mortality can be obtained with excellent long-term stroke prevention.

At present, there is no effective method to prevent recurrent carotid disease from developing after endarterectomy. Antiplatelet agents have not been shown to change the incidence of this process, nor does mandatory closure of the primary endarterectomy with a patch angioplasty. It can be recommended that selective patch closure be performed in patients felt to be at higher risk for developing recurrent stenosis. If a recurrent lesion is found, it should be followed clinically and noninvasively, but the great majority of these patients can expect long-term stroke-free survival without intervention.

REFERENCES

1. Roederer GO, Langlois YE, Jager KA, et al: The natural history of carotid arterial disease in asymptomatic patients with cervical bruits. *Stroke* 15:605, 1984.
2. Moore DJ, et al: Non-invasive assessment of stroke risk in asymptomatic and nonhemispheric patients with suspective carotid disease: Five year follow-up of 294 unoperated and 81 operated patients. *Ann Surg* 202:491, 1985.
3. Chambers BR, Norris JW: Outcome in patients with asymptomatic neck bruits. *N Engl J Med* 315:860, 1986.
4. Bock RW, Gray-Weale AC, Mock PA, et al: The natural history of asymptomatic carotid artery disease. *J Vasc Surg* 17:160, 1993.
5. Mattos MA, Hodgson KJ, Londrey GL, et al: Carotid endarterectomy: Operative risks, recurrent stenosis, and long term stroke rates in a modern series. *J Cardiovasc Surg* 33:387, 1992.
6. Bernstein EF, et al: Influence of preoperative factors on late neurologic events after carotid endarterectomy, in *International Vascular Symposium, Programs and Abstracts*. New York, Macmillan, p 460, 1981.
7. Moore WS, Boren C, Malone JM, et al: Asymptomatic carotid stenosis: Immediate and long term results after prophylactic endarterectomy. *Am J Surg* 138:228, 1979.
8. Hertzer NR, Arison R: Cumulative stroke and survival ten years after carotid endarterectomy. *J Vasc Surg* 2:661, 1985.
9. Hobson RW, Weiss DG, Fields WS, et al: Efficacy of carotid endarterectomy for asymptomatic carotid stenosis. *N Engl J Med* 328:221, 1993.
10. Moneta GL, Taylor DC, Nicholls SC, et al: Operative versus nonoperative management of asymptomatic high-grade internal carotid artery stenosis: Improved results with endarterectomy. *Stroke* 18:1005, 1987.
11. Whisnant JP, Matsumoto M, Elveback LR: The effects of anticoagulant therapy on the prognosis of patients with transient cerebral ischemic attacks in a community, Rochester, Minnesota 1965–69. *Mayo Clinic Proc* 48:844, 1973.
12. Hass WK, Jonas S: Caution—falling rock zone: An analysis of the medical and surgical management of threatened stroke. *Proc Inst Med* 33:80, 1980.
13. Loeb C, Priano A, Albana C: Clinical features and long term follow-up of patients with reversible ischemic attacks. *Acta Neurol Scand* 57:471, 1978.
14. Takolander RJ, Bergentz SE, Ericsson BF: Carotid artery surgery in patients with minor stroke. *Br J Surg* 70:13, 1983.
15. NASCET Collaborators: Beneficial effect of carotid endarterectomy in symptomatic patients with high-grade stenoses. *N Engl J Med* 325:445, 1991.
16. Sacco RL, Wolf PA, Kannel WB, McNamara PM: Survival and recurrence following stroke: The Framingham study. *Stroke* 13:290, 1982.
17. Robinson RE, et al: Natural history of cerebral thrombosis. 9-19 year follow-up. *J Chronic Dis* 21:221, 1968.
18. Schmidt EV, Smirnov VE, Ryabova VS: Results of the seven-year prospective study of stroke patients. *Stroke* 19:942, 1988.
19. Swedish Cooperative Study: High dose acetylsalicylic acid after cerebrarl infarction. *Stroke* 18:325, 1987.

20. Wylie EJ, Hein MF, Adams JE: Intracranial hemorrhage following surgical revascularization for treatment of acute strokes. *J Neurosurg* 21:212, 1964.
21. Giordano JM, et al: Timing carotid arterial endarterectomy after stroke. *J Vasc Surg* 2:250, 1985.
22. Dosick SM, et al: Carotid endarterectomy in the stroke patient: Computerized axial tomography to determine timing. *J Vasc Surg* 2:214, 1985.
23. Whittmeore AD, Ruby ST, Couch NP, et al: Early carotid endarterectomy in patients with small fixed neurologic deficits. *J Vasc Surg* 1:795, 1984.
24. Sanella NA: Bilateral severe carotid stenosis or occlusion and computed tomographic scan positive hemispheric stroke with neurologic deficit: Immediate contralateral carotid endarterectomy. *Ann Vasc Surg* 6:252, 1992.
25. Goldstone J, Moore WS: Emergency carotid artery surgery in neurologically unstable patients. *Arch Surg* 111:1284, 1976.
26. Mentzer RM, et al: Emergency carotid endarterectomy for fluctuating neurologic deficits. *Surgery* 89:60, 1981.
27. Schuler JJ, et al: The effect of carotid siphon stenosis on stroke rate, death, and relief of symptoms following elective carotid endarterectomy. *Surgery* 92:1058, 1982.
28. Moore WS: Does tandem lesion mean tandem risk in patients with carotid artery disease? *J Vasc Surg* 7:454, 1988.
29. Schuler JJ, Flanigan DP, Lim LT, et al: The effect of carotid siphon stenosis on stroke rate, death, and relief of symptoms following elective carotid endarterectomy. *Surgery* 92:1058, 1982.
30. Perler BA, Burdick JF, Williams GA: Does contralateral internal carotid artery occlusion increase the risk of carotid endarterectomy? *J Vasc Surg* 16:347, 1992.
31. Sillesen H, Schroeder T, Rasmussen L, Burchardt Hansen HJ: Carotid endarterectomy in patients with occlusion of the contralateral carotid artery. Perioperative risk and late results. *Eur J Vasc Surg* 1:85, 1987.
32. Hertzer NR, Martinez BD, Beven EG: Recurrent stenosis after carotid endarterectomy. *Surg Gynecol Obstet* 149:360, 1979.
33. DeGroote RD, Lynch JG, Jamil Z, Hobson RW III: Carotid restenosis: Long term noninvasive follow-up after carotid endarterectomy. *Stroke* 18:1031, 1987.
34. Healy DA, Zierler RE, Nichols SC, et al: Long-term follow-up and clinical outcome of carotid restenosis. *J Vasc Surg* 10:662, 1989.
35. Atnip RG, Wengrovitz M, Gifford RRM, et al: A rational approach to recurrent carotid stenosis. *J Vasc Surg* 11:511, 1990.
36. Stoney RJ, String ST: Recurrent carotid stenosis. *Surgery* 80:705, 1976.
37. Hunter GC, Palmaz JC, Hayashi HH, et al: The etiology of symptoms in patients with recurrent carotid stenosis. *Arch Surg* 122:;311, 1987.
38. Das MB, Hertzer NR, Ratliff NB, et al: Recurrent carotid stenosis. A five year series of 65 reoperations. *Ann Surg* 202:28, 1985.
39. Cossman D, Callow AD, Stein A, Matsumoto G: Early restenosis after carotid endarterectomy. *Arch Surg* 113:275, 1978.
40. Zierler RE, Bandyk DF, Thiele BL, Strandness DE Jr: Carotid artery restenosis following endarterectomy. *Arch Surg* 117:1408, 1982.
41. Baker WH, Hayes AC, Mahler DM, Littooy FN: Durability of carotid endarterectomy. *Surgery* 94:112, 1983.
42. Cantelmo NL, Cutler BS, Wheeler HB, et al: Non-invasive detection of carotid stenosis following endarterectomy. *Arch Surg* 116:1005, 1981.
43. Kremen JE, Gee W, Kaupp HA, McDonald KM: Restenosis or occlusion after carotid endarterectomy—A survey with ocular pneumoplethysmography. *Arch Surg* 114:608, 1979.
44. Turnipseed WD, Berkhoff HA, Crummy A: Postoperative occlusion after carotid endarterectomy. *Arch Surg* 115:573, 1980.
45. Zierler RE, Bandyk DF, Thiele BL: Intraoperative assessment of carotid endarterectomy. *J Vasc Surg* 1:73, 1984.
46. Keitzer WF, Lichti EL, Brossart FA, DeWeese MS: Use of the Doppler ultrasonic flowmeter during arterial vascular surgery. *Arch Surg* 105:308, 1972.
47. Barnes RW, Garrett WV: Intraoperative as-

sessment of arterial reconstruction by Doppler ultrasound. *Surg Gynecol Obstet* 146:896, 1978.

48. Salvian A, Baker JD, Machleder HI, et al: Cause and noninvasive detection of restenosis after carotid endarterectomy. *Am J Surg* 146: 29, 1983.
49. Ackroyd N, Lane R, Appleberg M: Intraoperative ultrasound during carotid artery surgery. *Austr N Z J Surg* 55:321, 1985.
50. Reilly LM, Okuhn SP, Rapp JH, et al: Recurrent carotid stenosis: A consequence of local or systemic factors? The influence of unrepaired technical defects. *J Vasc Surg* 11:448, 1990.
51. Claggett GP, Rich NM, McDonald PT, et al: Etiologic factors for recurrent carotid artery stenosis. *Surgery* 93:313, 1983.
52. Nicholls SC, Phillips DJ, Bergelin RO, et al: Carotid endarterectomy: relationship of outcome to early restenosis. *J Vasc Surg* 2:374, 1985.
53. Zbornikova V, Elfstrom J, Lassvik C, et al: Restenosis and occlusion after carotid surgery assessed by duplex scanning and digital subtraction angiography. *Stroke* 17:1137, 1986.
54. Maki HS, Kruger RA, Kuehner ME: The problem of recurrent stenosis following carotid endarterectomy. *Wis Med J* 90:583, 1991.
55. Johnson M, Ramwell PW: Androgen mediated sex differences in platelet aggregation. *Physiologist* 17:256, 1974.
56. Johnson M, Ramey E, Ramwell PW: Sex and age differences in human platelet aggregation. *Nature* 253:355, 1975.
57. Salenius JP, Haapanen A, Harju E, et al: Late carotid restenosis: Aetiologic factors for recurrent carotid stenosis during long-term follow-up. *Eur J Vasc Surg* 3:271, 1989.
58. Rapp JH, Qvarfordt P, Krupski WC, et al: Hypercholesterolemia and early restenosis after carotid endarterectomy. *Surgery* 101:277, 1987.
59. Bandyk DF, Moldenhauer P, Lipchik E, et al: Accuracy of duplex scanning in the detection of stenosis after carotid endarterectomy. *J Vasc Surg* 8:696, 1988.
60. French BN, Rewcastle NB: Recurrent stenosis at site of carotid endarterectomy. *Stroke* 8:597, 1977.
61. Clagett GP, Bobinowitz M, Yonkey JR, et al: Morphogenesis and clinicopathologic characteristics of recurrent carotid disease. *J Vasc Surg* 3:10, 1986.
62. Birinyi LK, Warner SJC, Salomon RN, et al: Observations on human smooth muscle cell cultures from hyperplastic lesions of prosthetic bypass grafts: Production of a platelet-derived growth factor-like mitogen and expression of a gene for PDGF-receptor: A preliminary study. *J Vasc Surg* 10:157, 1989.
63. Roederer GO, Langlois Y, Chan ATW, et al: Postendarterectomy carotid ultrasonic duplex scanning—concordance with contrast angiography. *Ultrasound Med Biol* 9:73, 1983.
64. McBride K, Callow AD: Recurrent stenosis after carotid endarterectomy—A limited survey, in Bernhard VM, Towne JB (eds): *Complications in Vascular Surgery*. New York, Grune & Stratton, pp 259–273, 1980.
65. Bernstein EF, Torem S, Dilley RB: Does carotid restenosis predict an increased risk of late symptoms, stroke, or death? *Ann Surg* 212:629, 1990.
66. Pratesi C, Pulli R, Milanesi G, et al: Indobufen versus placebo in the prevention of restenosis after carotid endarterectomy: A double-blind pilot study. *J Int Med Res* 19:202, 1991.
67. Harker LA, Bernstein EF, Dilley RB, et al: Failure of aspirin plus dipyridamole to prevent restenosis after carotid endarterectomy. *Ann Int Med* 116:731, 1992.
68. Archie JP Jr: Prevention of early restenosis and thrombosis-occlusion after carotid endarterectomy by saphenous vein patch angioplasty. *Stroke* 17:901, 1986.
69. Hertzer NR, Beven EG, O'Hara PJ, Krajewski LP: A prospective study of vein patch angioplasty during carotid endarterectomy. Three-year results for 801 patients and 917 operations. *Ann Surg* 206:628, 1987.
70. Rosenthal D, Archie JP Jr, Garcia-Rinaldi R, et al: Carotid patch angioplasty: Immediate and long-term results. *J Vasc Surg* 12:326, 1990.
71. Hans SS, Girishkumar H, Hans B: Venous patch grafts and carotid endarterectomy: A critical appraisal. *Arch Surg* 122:1134, 1987.
72. Clagett GP, Patterson CB, Fisher DF Jr: Vein patch versus primary closure for carotid endarterectomy. A randomized prospective study in

a selected group of patients. *J Vasc Surg* 9:213, 1989.

73. Bogousslavsky J, Hachinski VC, Boughner DR, et al: Cardiac and arterial lesions in carotid transient ischemic attacks. *Arch Neurol* 43:223, 1986.
74. Callow AD, Nitzberg R, Prendiville E, Mackey WC: Surgical treatment of cerebral ischemia secondary to recurrent carotid stenosis, in Ernst CB, Stanley JC (eds): *Current Therapy in Vascular Surgery,* 2d ed. Philadelphia, BC Decker pp 111–112, 1991.
75. Treiman GS, Jenkins JM, Edwards WH, et al: The evolving surgical management of recurrent carotid stenosis. *J Vasc Surg* 16:354, 1992.
76. Piepgras DG, Sundt TM, Marsh WR, et al: Recurrent carotid stenosis: Results and complications of 57 operations. *Ann Surg* 203:205, 1986.
77. Shumway SJ, Edwards WH, Jenkins JM, et al: Recurrent carotid stenosis: Incidence and management. *Am Surg* 53:61, 1987.
78. Nitzberg RS, Mackey WC, Prendiville E, et al: Long-term follow-up of patients operated on for recurrent carotid stenosis. *J Vasc Surg* 13:121, 1991.
79. Kazmers A, Zierler RE, Huang TW, et al: Reoperative carotid surgery. *Am J Surg* 156:346, 1988.

28

Reoperative Carotid Surgery

Christopher DeMaioribus
Andris Kazmers

Though the first reports of successful carotid endarterectomies were published in 1953[1] and 1954,[2] symptomatic recurrent carotid stenosis was not described until 1967.[3] In 1976, Stoney and String drew attention to this problem by reporting reoperation for symptomatic recurrent stenosis in 1.6 percent of 1654 primary carotid endarterectomies.[4] Using the occurrence of neurologic symptoms or the appearance of a new bruit to prompt a clinical evaluation, others documented a similar proportion of recurrent stenoses requiring reoperation, ranging from 1.2 to 3.5 percent.[5,6]

The advent of widespread noninvasive testing for extracranial carotid artery disease allowed detection of asymptomatic recurrent stenoses. As expected, the incidence of asymptomatic recurrent stenosis was much higher than that of symptomatic recurrent disease.[5,6] Using a variety of techniques (ocular plethysmography, periorbital Doppler, carotid phonoangiography, ultrasonic angiography, B-mode imaging, and duplex scanning) various authors reported recurrent stenosis or occlusion rates of 2.5 to 25 percent during follow-up periods extending to 16 years.[7–12] In this same group of studies, the incidence of neurologic symptoms referable to the side of the primary endarterectomy was 1.7 to 13.3 percent.[7–10,12] The wide variation in the incidence of recurrent stenosis can be attributed in part to a lack of serial follow-up testing,[7–11] combining carotid stenoses with occlusions,[9,11–12] and the inclusion of nonhemodynamically significant stenoses.[9] Similarly, when reporting the incidence of neurologic symptoms, several studies included symptomatic patients without hemodynamically significant recurrent stenoses[10,12] or with carotid occlusions.[7–9,12]

More precise information regarding the incidence of recurrent carotid stenosis has been gained from reports based on serial noninvasive follow-up examinations. In these studies, the overall incidence of stenosis varies from 7.5 to 36 percent.[13–22] However, recurrent stenoses were found to be dynamic lesions, and often were noted to regress.[13–16,19–23] Zierler and coworkers reported that 20 percent of hemodynamically significant recurrences (≥50 percent diameter reduction) became less than 50 percent in diameter reduction during follow-up.[13] When this type of lesion regression was included, the incidence of persistent hemodynamically significant recurrent stenosis was in the range of 7 to 19 percent.[13–16,19–22,24] In addition, these reports demonstrated that the majority of these lesions reached their maximum severity in the first two years after primary carotid endarterectomy, with little progression thereafter.[13–16,20–22]

It has been pointed out that the use of crude incidence rates—since they are independent of the duration and frequency of follow-up—tends to underestimate the actual incidence of recurrent carotid stenosis.[21] Using life-table methods, Ackroyd[17] and Healy[21] and their associates reported the incidence of significant recurrent stenosis to be 15 percent at five years and 21 percent at seven years (including regressions), respectively. Similarly, DeGroote and coworkers[18] showed cumulative significant recurrent stenosis rates of 8, 17, 19, and 32 percent at 1, 3, 5, and 7 years, respectively.

Despite the relatively high incidence of recurrent carotid stenosis, the rate of reoperation in the reported series is low, ranging from 1.3 to 2.9 percent of primary carotid endarterectomies.[7,9,14–16,18,20–22]

INDICATIONS FOR REOPERATION

As discussed in Chap. 27, recurrent carotid stenosis appears to have a clinical course different from that of primary carotid atherosclerosis. This different natural history serves as a basis for decisions about routine follow-up of patients after carotid endarterectomy, the monitoring of recurrent stenoses when detected, and surgical management.

After carotid endarterectomy, all patients should be followed with duplex scanning. This allows serial evaluations of the endarterectomy site as well as documenting the progression of contralateral disease. However, Mattos and colleagues found frequent duplex examinations in the first postoperative year not to be cost-effective, and in their series this approach did not alter management or clinical outcome.[20] Thus, after an early postoperative examination to detect technical failures, the optimal timing for subsequent duplex scans to detect recurrent carotid stenosis has not been determined. In this era of cost-containment, it is worth noting that in 1988 the estimated savings from limiting follow-up to two scans in the first postoperative year would have been approximately $50 million.[20]

Early recurrent stenoses commonly are defined as those lesions which appear during the first two years after carotid endarterectomy and are generally attributed to myointimal hyperplasia. Stenoses occurring later in the postoperative period are more likely to be associated with recurrent atherosclerosis, although, as noted in Chap. 27, elements of both these processes may be found in a single lesion.

When an early recurrent stenosis is detected

in an asymptomatic patient, continued conservative management is indicated. Most reports suggest that early lesions, even if hemodynamically significant, are not an indication for further diagnostic evaluation or surgical therapy.[13,15–17,21,22,24–35] This approach may be recommended for several reasons. In most patients, recurrent carotid stenosis is well-tolerated, not directly related to recurrent symptoms or stroke,[16] and may even have a protective effect.[21,22] Since the natural history of recurrent lesions appears to differ from that of primary carotid stenoses, prophylactic reoperation to prevent neurologic events is not indicated. Furthermore, there is no convincing evidence that these lesions are especially likely to progress to complete occlusion.[5,16,21] Finally, in many cases of early recurrent stenosis there is significant regression within the first year as myointimal hyperplasia remodels.[13,15,16,20–22]

Since asymptomatic critical recurrent stenoses (>90 percent diameter reduction) are rare, there are not enough data to predict confidently the natural history of these lesions. However, because of the perceived risk of subsequent thrombosis, many authors consider the finding of a critical lesion on follow-up duplex scanning to be an indication for a full evaluation, including arteriography and possible surgical intervention.[9,11,15,22,28,31,35] Such an approach certainly should be considered if a high-grade recurrent stenosis shows progression on serial noninvasive studies. Others contend that the need for further therapy depends on the condition of the remaining cerebral arteries and the patient's operative risk.[13,22] In these circumstances, a transcranial Doppler examination (Chap. 12) may be helpful to assess the adequacy of the cerebral collateral circulation.[22] The arteriographic appearance of a high-grade recurrent carotid stenosis is shown in Fig. 28-1.

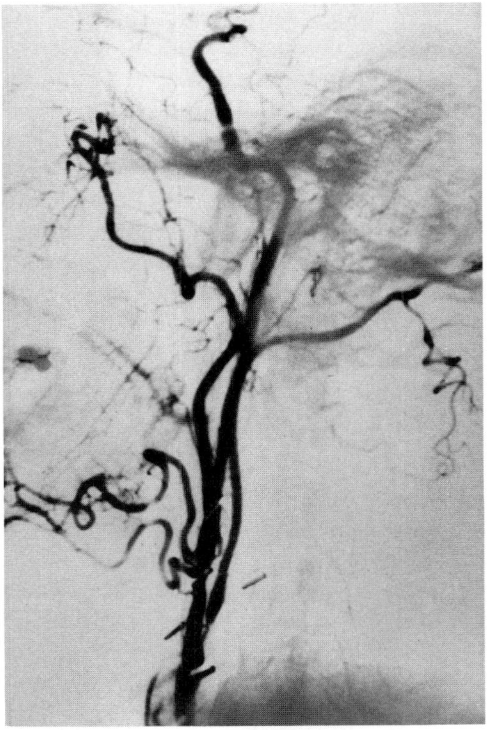

Figure 28-1. Arteriogram of a severe early recurrent carotid stenosis. This patient developed ipsilateral hemispheric symptoms eight months after the primary endarterectomy. A relatively smooth and tapered narrowing is seen in the proximal internal carotid artery.

If ipsilateral or contralateral focal neurologic symptoms occur in the presence of a recurrent carotid stenosis, a full diagnostic evaluation is warranted. Alternative sources of cerebral emboli should be considered, particularly if symptoms occur in the absence of a hemodynamically significant ipsilateral lesion. Symptomatic recurrent carotid stenosis generally is regarded as an indication for reoperation.[9,11,13,15,21,22,24,28,31,34,35] Patients with vertebrobasilar symptoms and recurrent carotid stenosis should be considered for surgery if correction of the stenosis can be expected to compensate for inadequate collateral circulation.

In summary, all patients with symptomatic

recurrent carotid stenoses and selected patients with asymptomatic critical recurrent stenoses should undergo arteriography and reoperation. However, in the latter group of patients, there are at present no objective data on which to base this decision. Those with asymptomatic recurrent stenoses of less than approximately 90 percent diameter reduction, even if hemodynamically significant, should be managed conservatively and followed with serial duplex scanning.

SURGICAL TECHNIQUE

Whenever possible, the operative note from the previous procedure should be reviewed before undertaking reoperative carotid surgery. This can be very useful to help define the local structures and the extent of the earlier dissection. Procedures for recurrent carotid stenosis are best performed under general anesthesia, with hemodynamic monitoring appropriate to the patient's medical condition. Shunts may be used routinely, or standard criteria applied for selective shunting (Chap. 24).

As with all reoperative vascular surgery, great care must be taken during the dissection to avoid injury to the vessels and surrounding structures. The vagus nerve may be in an unusual position or adherent to the carotid artery; similarly, the hypoglossal nerve and marginal mandibular branch of the facial nerve may be encased in scar tissue and more vulnerable to injury. If possible, exposure of the common, internal, and external carotid arteries should extend outside the previous operative field for proximal and distal control. Extension of the previous skin incision and the use of loupe magnification may facilitate the dissection. Antibiotic prophylaxis should be considered in all patients, particularly if use of prosthetic material is anticipated. Postoperative care is identical to that for primary carotid endarterectomy.

Operative techniques for managing recurrent carotid stenosis include patch angioplasty alone, repeat endarterectomy with or without patch angioplasty, and carotid resection with placement of an interposition graft. The specific approach chosen depends on the surgeon's preference, the clinical situation, and the underlying disease. In many cases, the final decision must be made intraoperatively. Regardless of the method used, the technical result should be assessed with intraoperative duplex scanning or arteriography at the completion of the operation (Fig. 28-2).

Patch Angioplasty

This procedure is most often chosen when recurrent carotid stenosis is due to myointimal hyperplasia and there are no focal symptoms referable to the lesion. Myointimal hyperplasia is a direct extension of the media, and the development of a proper endarterectomy plane may be very difficult, although in some cases myointimectomy can be performed.[28] Patch angioplasty without endarterectomy can be used because the smooth surface of the myointimal lesion is unlikely to ulcerate or to act as a source for cerebral emboli. When the goal is to increase flow, as in a patient with vertebrobasilar symptoms associated with recurrent carotid stenosis, patch angioplasty is the procedure of choice. The preferred patch material is autogenous vein; prosthetic material can be used when suitable vein is unavailable.

Repeat Endarterectomy

Lesions composed primarily of degenerated atherosclerotic plaque or adherent thrombus may lend themselves to repeat endarterectomy. Recurrent stenoses occurring more than two years after the primary carotid endarterectomy are more likely to show these features. In contrast to the situation described above for smooth myointimal lesions, removal of an irregular atherosclerotic plaque

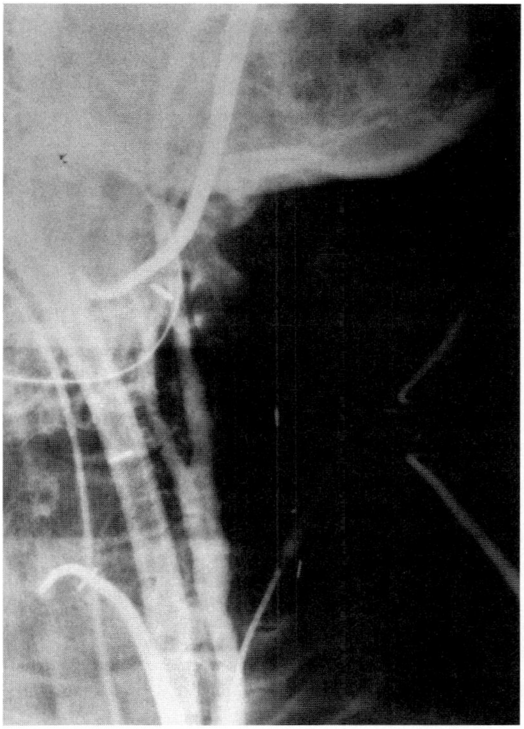

Figure 28-2. Intraoperative arteriogram from the reoperation on the lesion shown in Fig. 28-1. The early recurrent stenosis has been managed by vein patch angioplasty without repeat endarterectomy. A widely patent lumen has been restored.

and any overlying thrombus is desirable. An endarterectomy plane usually can be readily established.[15,25,28,30,36] Patch angioplasty for arteriotomy closure is strongly recommended in conjunction with repeat endarterectomy.[6,25,28,30,36] Again, autogenous vein should be used for patching whenever possible.

Carotid Resection

Resection of the diseased carotid segment and reconstruction by interposition graft placement is a third surgical option. This procedure should be considered whenever recurrent atherosclerosis with extensive calcification and scarring renders repeat carotid endarterectomy difficult. It also may be necessary for treating the uncommon but technically challenging secondary and tertiary recurrent stenoses.[36] When recurrent carotid stenosis is associated with dense periarterial fibrosis, carotid resection may be the only feasible approach.

Treiman and associates reported a large series, comparing carotid resection and autogenous vein graft interposition with repeat carotid endarterectomy.[34] Three theoretical advantages were cited for carotid resection: (1) removing the diseased area of the carotid bifurcation may minimize the effects of hemodynamic factors on recurrent carotid stenosis; (2) the intima of a vein graft may be less thrombogenic than an endarterectomy site; and (3) some patients may have an abnormal response to vessel injury and therefore may develop secondary or tertiary stenoses due to myointimal hyperplasia. The results of the comparison showed no significant difference in perioperative morbidity or mortality between the two treatment groups, but there was a higher rate of secondary recurrent stenosis for repeat endarterectomy attributed in part to longer follow-up. It was concluded that carotid resection and interposition grafting was a safe and effective alternative to repeat endarterectomy in patients undergoing operation for recurrent carotid stenosis.

RESULTS OF REOPERATION

The perioperative results for reoperative carotid surgery are shown in Table 28-1.[25–28,30,34–37] It is evident that operative morbidity and mortality are low; the mean incidence of perioperative death (0.8 percent), stroke (3.7 percent), and transient ischemic attack (2.7 percent) compare favorably with those of primary carotid endarterectomy. Piepgras and cowork-

Table 28-1 Perioperative Results of Reoperative Carotid Surgery

Study	Patients	Procedures	Death (%)	Stroke (%)	TIA (%)	CN (%)
Clagett (1983)[37]	27	29	0	1/29 (3.4)	2/29 (6.9)	1/29 (3.4)
Das (1985)[25]	61	65	2/65 (3.1)	1/65 (1.5)	1/65 (1.5)	7/65 (10.7)
Piepgras (1985)[36]	51	57	0	6/57 (10.5)	2/57 (3.5)	Not stated
Bartlett (1987)[28]	99	116	2/116 (1.7)	5/116 (4.3)	0	23/116 (19.8)
Kazmers (1988)[30]	14	14	0	0	0	2/14 (14.3)
Nitzberg (1991)[35]	27	29	0	1/29 (3.4)	2/29 (6.8)	5/29 (17.2)
Treiman (1992)[34]	162	162	1/162 (0.6)	4/162 (2.5)	0	4/162 (2.5)
Overall			(0.8)	(3.7)	(2.7)	(11.3)

NOTE: TIA = Transient ischemic attack; CN = Cranial nerve injury.

ers related perioperative stroke risk to the underlying disease process.[36] In their series, four of six perioperative strokes occurred when soft atherosclerotic plaque or thrombus was present, but no strokes occurred with operations for myointimal hyperplasia. In addition, several of the strokes listed in Table 28-1 followed reoperative carotid surgery combined with coronary artery bypass[28] or an additional arterial reconstructive procedure.[35] The inci-

Table 28-2 Late Results of Reoperative Carotid Surgery

Study	Patients	Primary reoperations	Mean follow-up (range)	Ipsilateral events: Stroke (%)	Ipsilateral events: TIA (%)	Secondary recurrent carotid stenosis (%)	Secondary reoperations
Clagett (1983)[37]	27	29	2.1 yrs (0.3–9)	0	0	0	0
Das (1985)[25]	61	65	22 mo. (1–137)	1/59 (1.7)	1/59 (1.7)	Not stated	0
Bartlett (1987)[28]	94	103	Not stated	Not stated	Not stated	6/103[a] (5.8)	6[a]
Kazmers (1988)[30]	14	14	27.4 mo. (4–87)	0	0	1/12 (8.3)	0
Nitzberg (1991)[35]	26	28	47.2 mo. (1–127)	1/28 (3.6)	1/28 (3.6)	1/28 (3.6)	1
Treiman (1992)[34]							
Resection	57	57	35 mo. (3–99)	1/54 (1.9)	1/54 (1.9)	8/54[b] (14.8)	0
Repeat CEA	105	105	64 mo. (2–149)	4/103 (3.9)	21/103 (20)	23/103[c] (22.3)	20

[a]One of these patients developed tertiary restenosis and required a second reoperation
[b]Includes five >50 percent interposition graft stenoses and three occlusions
[c]Noninvasive follow-up available on 54/103 patients
NOTE: TIA = Transient ischemic attack.

dence of cranial nerve injuries was relatively high (mean 11.3 percent), as would be expected; however, the majority of these were transient palsies.

The late results of reoperative carotid surgery have been reported by several groups and are summarized in Table 28-2.[25,28,30,34,35,37] The incidence of late ipsilateral stroke in these series varies from 0 to 3.9 percent. Nitzberg and associates compared the late stroke rate in patients undergoing reoperation to that in patients who did not develop recurrent carotid stenosis and found no significant difference.[35] Using life-table analysis to compare patients undergoing either carotid resection or repeat endarterectomy, Treiman and coworkers found low stroke rates in both groups (0.0064/year and 0.011/year, respectively).[34] The incidence of late ipsilateral transient ischemic attacks is also low in most series, between 0 and 3.6 percent.[25,30,35,37] Only one study reported a relatively high rate of late transient ischemic attacks (20 percent), which paralleled the high incidence of secondary recurrent stenoses.[34]

The true incidence of secondary recurrent carotid stenosis is not known. In the studies that report late results of reoperative carotid surgery, the absolute numbers of patients who develop secondary recurrences are low. In addition, although clinical follow-up is available on nearly all patients after the first reoperation, noninvasive follow-up is less complete.[34,35] Except for one series that reported a secondary recurrence rate of 22.3 percent,[34] the incidence ranges between 0 and 8.3 percent.[28,30,35,37] It seems reasonable to suspect that the incidence of secondary recurrent carotid stenosis parallels that of primary recurrent stenosis. The incidence of tertiary recurrent stenosis appears to be extremely low. The diagnostic and therapeutic approach to secondary and tertiary recurrent carotid stenosis is identical to that discussed above for primary recurrent stenosis.

CONCLUSIONS

Reoperative carotid surgery can be performed with excellent perioperative morbidity and mortality rates, and it can be anticipated that the long-term clinical outcome will be comparable to that after primary carotid endarterectomy. Patients with hemispheric symptoms ipsilateral to a recurrent carotid stenosis represent the predominant population in which carotid reoperation is indicated, although patients with nonhemispheric symptoms associated with significant recurrent carotid stenosis also may be considered for surgery. Nonoperative management is indicated for nearly all asymptomatic recurrent stenoses.

REFERENCES

1. Strully KJ, Hurwith ES, Blankenberg HW: Thrombo-endarterectomy for thrombosis of the internal carotid artery in the neck. *J Neurosurg* 10:474, 1953.
2. Eastcott HHG, Pickering GW, Rob CG: Reconstruction of internal carotid artery in a patient with intermittent attacks of hemiplegia. *Lancet* 2:994, 1954.
3. Edwards WS, Wilson TAS, Bennett A: The long-term effectiveness of carotid endarterectomy in the prevention of strokes. *Ann Surg* 168:765–70, 1968.
4. Stoney RJ, String ST: Recurrent carotid stenosis. *Surgery* 80:705–710, 1976.
5. Cossman D, Callow AD, Stein A, Matsumoto G: Early restenosis after carotid endarterectomy. *Arch Surg* 113:275–278, 1978.
6. Hertzer NR, Martinez BD, Benjamin SP, Beven EG: Recurrent stenosis after carotid endarterectomy. *Surg Gynecol Obstet* 149:722–725, 1979.
7. Kremen JE, Gee W, Kaupp HA, McDonald KM: Restenosis or occlusion after carotid endarterectomy. *Arch Surg* 114:608–610, 1979.
8. Turnipseed WD, Berkoff HA, Crummy A: Postoperative occlusion after carotid endarterectomy. *Arch Surg* 115:573–574, 1980.
9. Cantelmo NL, Cutler BS, Wheeler HB, et al: Noninvasive detection of carotid stenosis fol-

lowing endarterectomy. *Arch Surg* 116:1005–1008, 1981.

10. Colgan P, Kingston V, Shanik G: Stenosis following carotid endarterectomy. *Arch Surg* 119: 1033–1035, 1984.
11. Keagy BA, Edrington RD, Poole MA, Johnson G: Incidence of recurrent or residual stenosis after carotid endarterectomy. *Am J Surg* 149: 722–725, 1985.
12. Zbornikova V, Elfstrom , Lassvik C, et al: Restenosis and occlusion after carotid surgery assessed by duplex scanning and digital subtraction angiography. *Stroke* 17:1137–1142, 1986.
13. Zierler RE, Bandyk DF, Thiele BL, Strandness DE: Carotid artery stenosis following endarterectomy. *Arch Surg* 117:1408–1415, 1982.
14. Baker WH, Hayes AC, Mahler D, Littooy FN: Durability of carotid endarterectomy. *Surgery* 94:112–115, 1983.
15. Thomas M, Otis SM, Rush M, et al: Recurrent carotid stenosis following endarterectomy. *Ann Surg* 200:74–79, 1984.
16. Nicholls SC, Phillips DJ, Bergelin RO, et al: Carotid endarterectomy. Relationship of outcome to early restenosis. *J Vasc Surg* 2:375–381, 1985.
17. Ackroyd N, Lane R, Appleberg M: Carotid endarterectomy. Long-term follow-up with specific reference to recurrent stenosis, contralateral progression, mortality, and recurrent neurologic episodes. *J Cardiovasc Surg* 27: 418–425, 1986.
18. DeGroote RD, Lynch TG, Jamil Z, Hobson RW: Carotid restenosis: Long-term noninvasive followup after carotid endarterectomy. *Stroke* 18:1031–1036, 1987.
19. Sanders EACM, Hoeneveld H, Eikelboom BC, et al: Residual lesions and early recurrent stenosis after carotid endarterectomy: A serial follow-up study with duplex scanning and intravenous digital subtraction angiography. *J Vasc Surg* 5:731–737, 1987.
20. Mattos MA, Shanma AR, Rossi N, et al: Is duplex follow-up cost-effective in the first year after carotid endarterectomy? *Am J Surg* 156:91–95, 1988.
21. Healy DA, Zierler RE, Nicholls SC, et al: Long-term follow-up and clinical outcome of carotid restenosis. *J Vasc Surg* 10:662–669, 1989.
22. Bernstein EF, Torem S, Dilley RB: Does carotid restenosis predict an increased risk of late symptoms, stroke, or death? *Ann Surg* 212: 629–636, 1990.
23. Reilly LM, Okuhn SP, Rapp JH, et al: Recurrent carotid stenosis: A consequence of local or systemic factors? The influence of unrepaired technical defects. *J Vasc Surg* 11:448–460, 1990.
24. Ricotta JJ, O'Brien MS, DeWeese JA: Natural history of recurrent and residual stenosis after carotid endarterectomy: Implications for post-operative surveillance and surgical management. *Surgery* 112:656–663, 1992.
25. Das MH, Hertzer NR, Ratliff NB, et al: Recurrent carotid stenosis: A five-year series of 65 reoperations. *Ann Surg* 202:28-35, 1985.
26. Clagett GP, Robinowitz M, Youkey JR, et al: Morphogenesis and clinicopathologic characteristics of recurrent carotid disease. *J Vasc Surg* 3:10–23, 1986.
27. Imparato AM, Weinstein GS: Clinicopathologic correlation in postendarterectomy recurrent stenosis. A case report and bibliographic review. *J Vasc Surg* 3:657–662, 1986.
28. Bartlett FF, Rapp JH, Goldstone J, et al: Recurrent carotid stenosis: Operative strategy and late results. *J Vasc Surg* 5:452–456, 1987.
29. Callow AD: Recurrent stenosis after carotid endarterectomy. *Arch Surg* 117:1082–1085, 1982.
30. Kazmers A, Zierler RE, Huang TW, et al: Reoperative carotid surgery. *Am J Surg* 156:346–352, 1988.
31. Curley S, Edwards WS, Jacob TP: Recurrent carotid stenosis after autologous tissue patching. *J Vasc Surg* 6:350–354, 1987.
32. Courbier R, Jausseran J-M, Reggi M, et al: Routine intraoperative carotid angiography: Its impact on operative morbidity and carotid restenosis. *J Vasc Surg* 3:343–350, 1986.
33. Edwards WS: Discussion of Reilly LM, Okuhn SP, Rapp JH, et al: Recurrent carotid stenosis: A consequence of local or systemic factors? The influence of unrepaired technical defects. *J Vasc Surg* 11:448–460, 1990.
34. Treiman GS, Jenkins JM, Edwards WH, et al:

The evolving surgical management of recurrent carotid stenosis. *J Vasc Surg* 16:354–363, 1992.

35. Nitzberg RS, Mackey WC, Prindeville E, et al: Long-term follow-up of patients operated on for recurrent carotid stenosis. *J Vasc Surg* 13: 121–127, 1991.
36. Piepgras DG, Marsh WR, Mussman LA, et al: Recurrent carotid stenosis. Results and complications of 57 reoperations. *Ann Surg* 203: 205–213, 1986.
37. Clagett GP, Rich NM, McDonald PT, et al: Risk factors for recurrent carotid artery stenosis. *Surgery* 93:313–318, 1983.

29

Approaches to Innominate and Common Carotid Disease

Henry Veldenz
Andris Kazmers

Although the surgical management of cerebrovascular disease most commonly involves carotid bifurcation endarterectomy, arterial lesions that may adversely affect the cerebral circulation also can arise in the more proximal vessels. As a result, surgical treatment of innominate and proximal common carotid artery disease occasionally may be necessary.[1-4] The disease processes affecting the aortic arch and its major branches include atherosclerosis, giant cell arteritis, and aortic dissection. Atherosclerotic lesions of the aortic arch branches may cause hemodynamically significant stenoses or may serve as sources of emboli, much like carotid bifurcation disease (Fig. 29-1). Aneurysmal dilatation also is possible. This review will be directed primarily toward surgical management of atherosclerotic occlusive disease of the aortic arch branches proximal to the common carotid bifurcation.

PATIENT EVALUATION AND INDICATIONS FOR SURGERY

Innominate and proximal common carotid artery disease may become apparent during the work-up of patients with cerebrovascular symptoms (Fig. 29-2). Focal symptoms such as transient ischemic attacks, amaurosis fu-

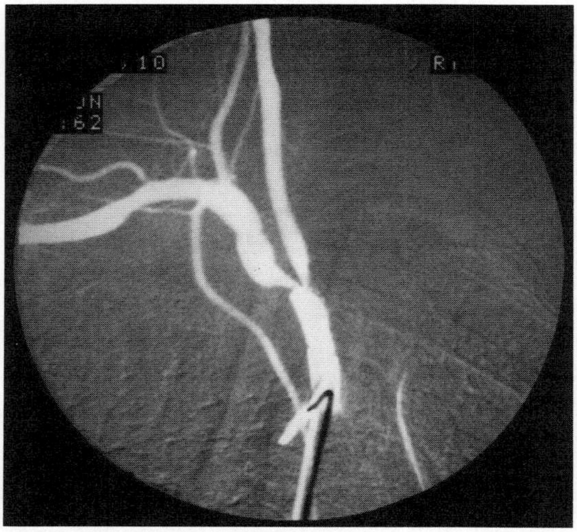

Figure 29-1. Selective innominate artery injection revealing a stenosis at the bifurcation of the innominate into the right subclavian and right common carotid arteries. The appearance of the lesion is similar to that of a carotid bifurcation plaque.

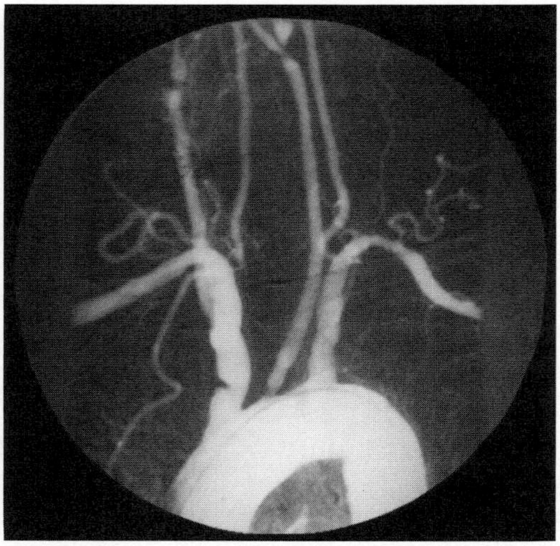

Figure 29-2. Aortic arch injection revealing innominate, proximal left common carotid, and bilateral carotid bifurcation disease.

gax, or cerebral infarction may result from atherosclerotic disease proximal to the carotid bifurcation.[5] Symptoms of vertebrobasilar insufficiency also may result from occlusive disease of the innominate, common carotid, or subclavian arteries.[5–7] Patients can present with upper extremity ischemia from either arterial occlusion or embolism associated with innominate or proximal subclavian disease.[7] In addition, subclavian artery stenosis may promote retrograde flow in the ipsilateral vertebral artery and the "subclavian steal" syndrome (Chap. 7). A combination of the presenting symptoms just mentioned can occur with aortic arch disease.

The indications for surgical correction of innominate and proximal common carotid artery lesions are somewhat controversial. Unfortunately, there have been no randomized clinical trials to define the best approach to aortic arch occlusive disease. If work-up reveals an innominate or proximal carotid stenosis associated with focal neurologic symptoms, then operative treatment of these proximal lesions may be indicated, provided there are no significant lesions present in the ipsilateral carotid bifurcation.[1,5–6,8–12] When disease is present at both sites, decisions about surgical treatment are more difficult, but correction of the arterial disease at both anatomic levels may be required (Fig. 29-2). A history of prior stroke in the distribution of an innominate or proximal common carotid lesion in the absence of ipsilateral carotid bifurcation disease may justify a proximal revascularization. Symptoms of global cerebral hypoperfusion also may warrant direct proximal revascularization if cerebral blood flow cannot be increased by extrathoracic surgical approaches.

The management of high-grade stenotic lesions of the aortic arch branches in patients without cerebrovascular or upper extremity symptoms is even more controversial than that for symptomatic patients. Unlike symptomatic or asymptomatic carotid bifurcation stenoses, about which there are substantial data from retrospective and prospective studies, few reports have examined the natural history of asymptomatic disease of the aortic arch branches. Some have recommended repair of severe asymptomatic aortic arch branch stenoses in patients who appear to be at low operative risk.[6] Repair of asymptomatic innominate or proximal carotid stenoses of greater than 75 percent diameter reduction has been recommended when such lesions occur proximal to symptomatic carotid bifurcation disease requiring endarterectomy.[5,6,8,13] In two series, 20 percent of aortic arch branch operations were performed in conjunction with surgical treatment of carotid bifurcation stenoses.[8,12] However, the true benefit of treating these asymptomatic proximal lesions remains to be determined.

Work-up of patients with possible occlusive disease of the aortic arch branches requires aortic arch angiography as well as selective angiography with visualization of the origins and entire extent of the innominate, carotid, vertebral, and subclavian arteries. Definitive cardiac evaluation, including coronary angiography, should be considered for patients who will require a median sternotomy, since it may be easier to carry out a coronary artery bypass procedure at the time of aortic arch reconstruction than it would be in staged procedures. This consideration is important because a reoperative median sternotomy is both technically more difficult and associated with increased risk of great vessel and cardiac injury. In addition, reoperative median sternotomy may carry an increased risk of infection, which would be disastrous for a patient with an arch reconstruction involving prosthetic graft material.

ANATOMY AND EXPOSURE

To achieve a better understanding of the surgical approaches to innominate and proximal common carotid artery occlusive disease, the anatomy of the great vessels and mediastinum will be briefly reviewed (Fig. 29-3). Since the surgical options involve transthoracic, transsternal, and extraanatomic approaches, the anatomic relationships of the aortic arch branches and adjacent structures are important considerations in obtaining adequate exposure.

As shown in Fig. 29-3, the innominate artery originates from the aortic arch deep to the left brachiocephalic vein, and divides into the right subclavian and right common carotid arteries behind the medial head of the right clavicle.[14] In rare cases, the right common carotid artery arises directly from the aorta. The origin of the left common carotid artery is at the level of the aortic arch in 70 percent of patients, usually in close proximity to the origin of the innominate. In about 27 percent, the left common carotid artery originates from the innominate artery, forming a "bovine arch." The first branch of the common carotid artery is at or just proximal to its bifurcation.[15] In the

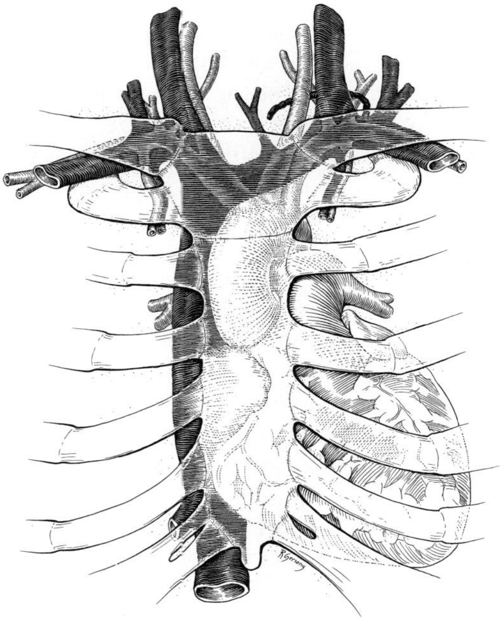

Figure 29-3. Mediastinal structures of importance for cerebral and upper extremity revascularization.

mediastinum, the aortic arch runs diagonally through the chest, thus placing the origins of the innominate and left common carotid arteries in a relatively anterior position compared with the origin of the left subclavian artery, which is more posterior.[14]

The right vagus nerve is closely related to the right common carotid and innominate arteries. This nerve usually runs along the posterior or lateral aspect of the right common carotid artery down to the common carotid origin, where it lies anteriorly and crosses the origin of the right subclavian artery. At this point, the right recurrent laryngeal nerve turns posteriorly beneath the subclavian artery and ascends out of the chest in the tracheoesophageal groove. The right vagus nerve then courses into the chest deep to the right brachiocephalic vein.

A median sternotomy is used for elective exposure of the innominate artery. For median sternotomy, the patient should be placed supine with arms at the sides. The head is turned to the right for exposure of the left common carotid, and vice versa. An incision is made over the midline of the sternum from the sternal notch to a point past the xiphoid process. The retrosternal space is opened by bluntly dissecting the mediastinal tissues before using a sternal saw to divide the sternum. The underlying mediastinal fat and thymic tissue remnants are dissected from the left brachiocephalic vein, and this vein is mobilized by dissection and ligation of its minor tributaries. Division of the left brachiocephalic vein may cause venous hypertension in the left arm and face, but such division may be necessary for access to the more distal aortic arch, including the proximal left subclavian artery. Once the brachiocephalic vein is dissected and mobilized, it may be retracted superiorly or inferiorly as needed. Exposure of the innominate artery to its bifurcation can then be obtained, with identification and preservation of the right vagus and recurrent laryngeal nerves. The pericardium usually is entered to achieve adequate exposure of the ascending aorta.

Concomitant exposure of the left or right common carotid artery bifurcation requires extension of the midline sternotomy incision into the neck along the anterior border of the ipsilateral sternocleidomastoid muscle. A second, noncontinuous neck incision allows exposure of the contralateral carotid artery bifurcation, if needed.

ENDARTERECTOMY

In some cases the treatment of localized atherosclerotic lesions in the aortic arch branches can be done effectively by endarterectomy. For innominate artery endarterectomy, exposure of the innominate artery is obtained as described above. The proximal innominate artery is clamped, with the jaws of the clamp extending onto the aortic arch but without compromising cardiac output. Care must be taken not to occlude the left common carotid artery at its origin (Fig. 29-4). The distal innominate artery is controlled at its bifurcation or by clamping the right subclavian and common carotid arteries. A longitudinal arteriotomy is made on the anterior aspect of the innominate artery, and an endarterectomy plane is developed—with care not to make the arterial wall adjacent to the arteriotomy excessively thin. Definition of the distal end-point may require extension of the arteriotomy onto the right common carotid artery. Tacking sutures may be required in the innominate, right subclavian, or right common carotid arteries, depending on the extent of the disease. Proximally, the atherosclerotic plaque typically is contiguous with involvement of the aortic arch and must be divided sharply without raising a flap in the aorta which could initiate an aortic arch dissection. After completion of the endarterectomy the artery may be closed primarily or with a patch. Innominate endarterec-

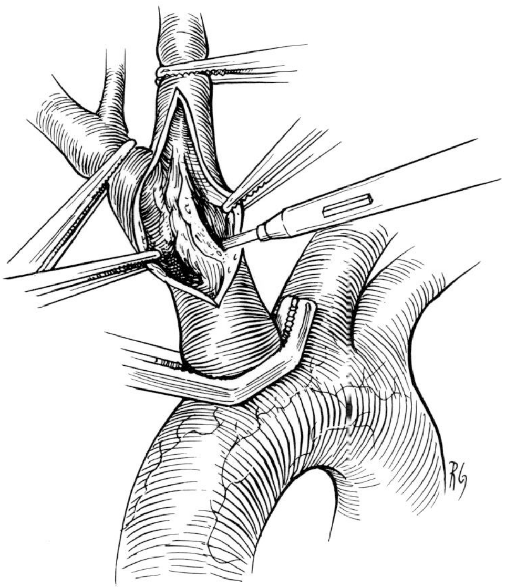

Figure 29-4. Innominate artery endarterectomy. Note the proximity of the vascular clamp to the origin of the left common carotid artery.

tomy is recommended only for relatively localized lesions involving the more distal innominate artery (Figs. 29-1 and 29-4).

DIRECT INTRATHORACIC BYPASS

Ordinarily, bypass grafts are preferred for management of more extensive atherosclerotic lesions involving the aortic arch branches. Unlike endarterectomy, bypass may be useful for treating multiple or diffuse sites of involvement, whether atherosclerotic or inflammatory. In most cases, disease of the proximal left and right common carotid arteries is best treated with a bypass graft or carotid reimplantation. Common carotid endarterectomy can be combined with innominate endarterectomy in some circumstances, although multiple bypasses may be preferable.[16]

Bypass of innominate and carotid artery lesions has been well described.[1–4,10–13,16] For innominate bypass, the ascending aorta is used as the inflow source (Fig. 29-5). A side-biting clamp is applied to the ascending aorta so as not to interfere with aortic valve function, cardiac output, or the placement of any planned coronary artery vein grafts. It is crucial to choose a side-biting clamp big enough not to slip off the aorta. A small bifurcated graft may be used, as shown in Fig. 29-5. If only a single graft limb is needed, one limb of a bifurcated graft can be transected so that its hood is fashioned from the larger graft segment. An end-to-end configuration typically is used for a distal anastomosis at the innominate artery bifurcation (Fig. 29-5). If necessary, the distal anastomosis also can serve as a patch onto the right common carotid or right subclavian artery.

Aorto-carotid bypass may be used in conjunction with bypasses to other brachiocephalic arteries or with concomitant carotid endarterectomy. An extraanatomic bypass or

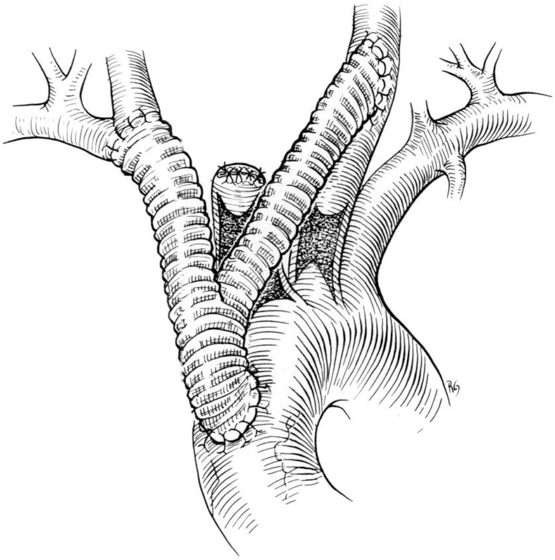

Figure 29-5. Use of a bifurcated prosthetic graft for a complex aortic arch revascularization. The ascending aorta is used as the inflow source, and the graft limbs are anastomosed to the distal innominate and left common carotid arteries.

carotid reimplantation should be considered when only a single aorto-carotid bypass is needed; however, a single graft can be used to bypass a lesion in the innominate artery. When multiple lesions are being bypassed, one possible configuration is a single "parent" graft to a target vessel, with side limbs placed as indicated (Fig. 29-6). Some of the side limb anastomoses usually can be performed by an extrathoracic approach. This technique requires less space in the anterior medastinum than a bifurcated graft originating from the aortic arch, and it may be useful for avoiding compression of the graft or adjacent structures under the sternum.[8,11,13,16] Usually prosthetic graft material is chosen for bypass of innominate and proximal carotid artery lesions. Autogenous vein is typically too small and may be prone to reduced long-term patency when used in this location.

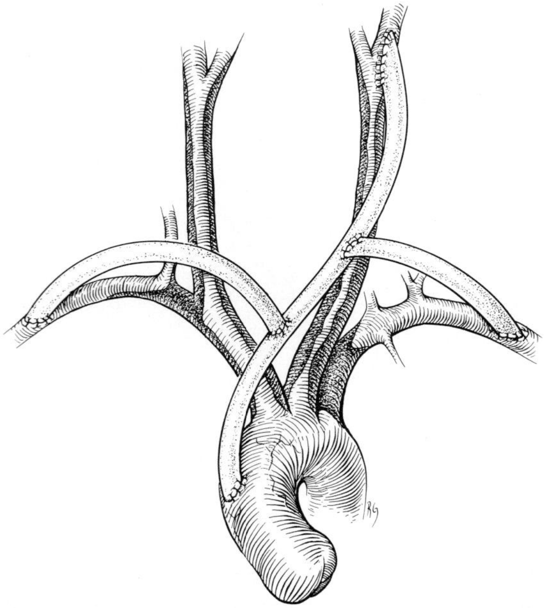

Figure 29-6. Multiple side-grafts taken off a single "parent" graft from the ascending aorta to the left carotid bifurcation.

Direct bypass from the aorta to the carotid or innominate arteries has produced good results in many centers. Reul and coworkers reported no postoperative neurologic deficits in the innominate distribution in a series of patients undergoing bypass grafting for innominate artery disease.[1] These authors had a 9 percent occlusion rate after endarterectomy, while the 30-day graft occlusion rate was 7 percent. All patients with graft occlusion were salvaged by secondary reconstructions. Crawford and colleagues found that 88 percent of their patients with intrathoracic bypasses were asymptomatic at 30 days; at a mean of seven years, just over 75 percent were asymptomatic.[8] Other series report less than 5 percent early and approximately 20 percent late (5 years or more) neurologic morbidity.[7,9,11,13,17] Graft patency also ranges from 90 to 96 percent at five years. Perioperative mortality rates have been higher for direct aortic arch repairs using bypass or endarterectomy than for extraanatomic bypass, but the long-term results also have been somewhat more favorable for the direct procedures in most reports.

EXTRAANATOMIC BYPASS

Extraanatomic approaches to innominate and proximal carotid reconstruction have merit when either anatomic or systemic factors make an intrathoracic approach more difficult or hazardous. Reasons to select an extraanatomic bypass include prior median sternotomy and poor cardiac or pulmonary status. The extrathoracic procedures have had good results when properly applied, and the long-term results often overlap with those reported for direct aortic arch reconstruction.[5,6,18,19]

For a proximal common carotid stenosis or occlusion with a patent ipsilateral subclavian artery, a subclavian-carotid bypass provides excellent inflow to the carotid circulation (Fig. 29-7). Many surgeons prefer this type of bypass for the treatment of isolated proximal ca-

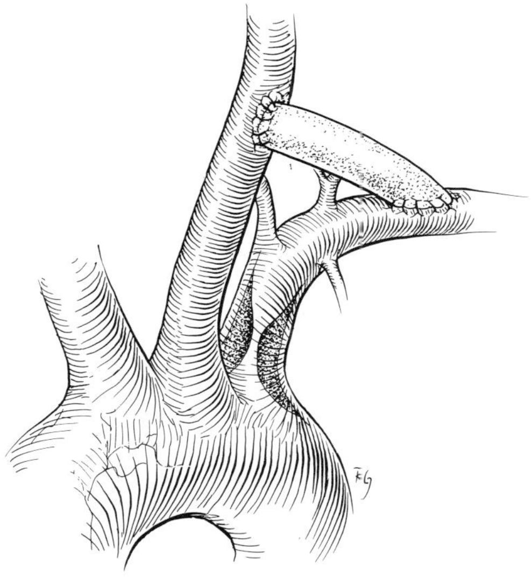

Figure 29-7. Carotid-subclavian bypass graft. This technique can be used to treat proximal subclavian lesions associated with upper extremity ischemia or subclavian-steal syndrome. The same procedure also is useful for treating proximal common carotid lesions when the ipsilateral subclavian artery is widely patent (subclavian–carotid bypass).

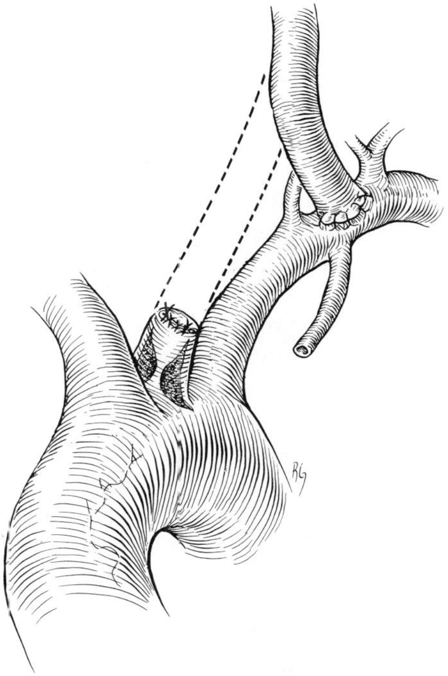

Figure 29-8. Common carotid artery transposition. This technique occasionally is useful for proximal common carotid lesions when the ipsilateral subclavian artery is not significantly diseased.

rotid lesions. Common carotid revascularization also can be accomplished by transposition of the proximal common carotid to the adjacent subclavian artery (Fig. 29-8). The supraclavicular approach can be used to treat proximal right subclavian disease if the innominate and right common carotid arteries are free of occlusive lesions. The subclavian artery lateral to the thyrocervical trunk is one potential outflow site for a carotid-subclavian bypass. In this procedure, the graft can be passed either behind or in front of the internal jugular vein. When the subclavian artery is used as an inflow source, the anastomosis to the common carotid artery can be either end-to-end or end-to-side; if a concomitant carotid bifurcation endarterectomy has been performed, the subclavian-carotid bypass graft may be used as a patch over the carotid arteriotomy. The contralateral carotid or subclavian arteries also may serve as inflow sources for carotid bypasses.

Patency of carotid–subclavian (or subclavian–carotid) bypasses ranges from 89 to 100 percent at 30 days, with an average neurologic morbidity rate of 4 percent.[5] Long-term patency ranges from 86 to 100 percent for prosthetic grafts and 58 to 100 percent for vein grafts. The lower reported patency rates for venous conduits in this position warrant preferential use of prosthetic grafts in those patients without a contraindication. Some authors report that subclavian-carotid transposition is a better procedure than bypass, with 100 percent short-term patency, 97 percent long-term patency, and less than 1 per-

mortality from neurologic causes.[5,18] Transposition procedures often require ligation and division of such subclavian artery branches as the internal mammary artery, and this may be of clinical significance in patients who require coronary artery bypass. Consequently, a transposition would not be suitable for patients who have had their ipsilateral internal mammary artery used in a coronary artery bypass procedure.

Another surgical approach to proximal carotid or innominate lesions is a carotid–carotid bypass graft.[6] This can be useful for a carotid stenosis or occlusion limited to the mediastinal portion of the artery. It is carried out through two standard cervical carotid exposures utilizing a retropharyngeal tunnel for the bypass. A subcutaneous tunnel can be used, but is longer and less appealing cosmetically. Because of the short length of carotid–carotid bypass grafts, the results generally are good.[6]

Innominate or unilateral subclavian artery disease also can be bypassed with an axillary–axillary graft.[18] This requires two infraclavicular incisions with subcutaneous tunneling of the graft over the upper portion of the sternum (Fig. 29-9). The most proximal or first portion of the axillary artery is the desired site for each anastomosis. As with the other extraanatomic bypasses, this procedure has a reported morbidity and mortality rate of less than 5 percent. The reported patency of axillary–axillary bypass grafts has been variable and occasionally poor, but excellent patency rates and clinical results also have been reported, approaching 100 percent in some series. This technique has the advantage of allowing cerebral or upper extremity revascularization without dissection or clamping of either the carotid arteries or intrathoracic structures. If a subsequent median sternotomy is necessary, it usually is possible to mobilize and retract an axillary–axillary bypass, and division of the graft should not be required.

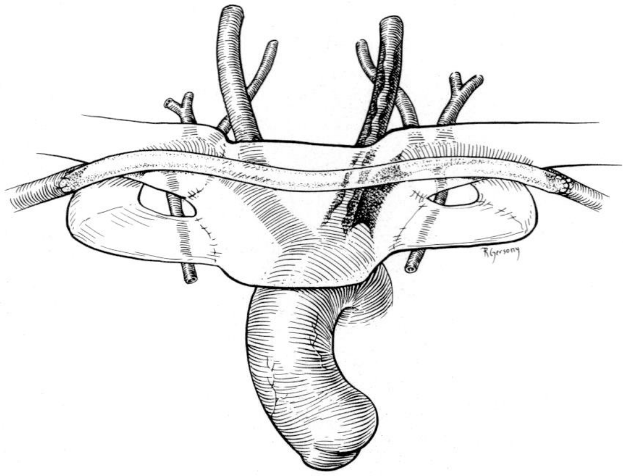

Figure 29-9. Axillary–axillary bypass graft. Arterial exposure is achieved with bilateral infraclavicular incisions, and the graft is tunneled subcutaneously over the upper portion of the sternum.

CONCLUSIONS

Many options are available for the treatment of innominate and common carotid occlusive disease. One recent trend has been to utilize direct intrathoracic bypass for diffuse, multiple, or complex patterns of disease (Fig. 29-10). This practice can be attributed to the generally superior long-term patency rates and acceptable complication rates that many centers have achieved. Endarterectomy remains useful for more localized disease. Many effective extraanatomic bypass techniques are also available for managing patients with aortic arch branch disease. Unlike carotid bifurcation endarterectomy, the indications for these procedures cannot be based on the results of large clinical trials or detailed natural history studies.

Operative complications consist primarily of neurologic events and injury to adjacent structures. Perioperative neurologic complications have been infrequent with all techniques for revascularization of the aortic arch branches.[5,6,8,10,11,13,16] Potential nerve injuries

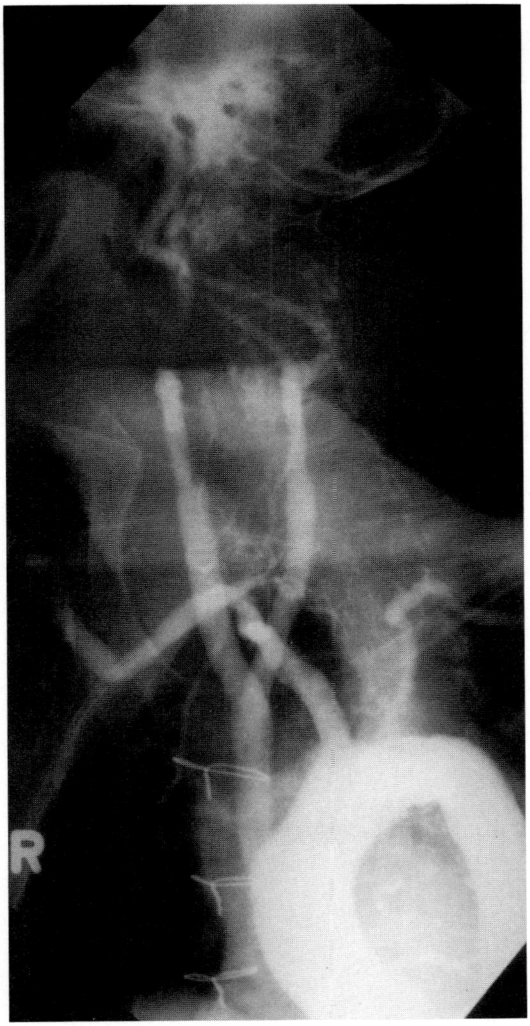

Figure 29-10. Postoperative arteriogram after an aorto-carotid bypass graft. The graft originates from the ascending aorta and gives off separate limbs to the right and left common carotid arteries.

include damage to the vagus, recurrent laryngeal, and phrenic nerves, or the brachial plexus. The thoracic duct may be damaged during procedures involving the left carotid or subclavian arteries and should be repaired or ligated if an injury is recognized intraoperatively. Most of these procedures require general anesthesia. Temporary carotid shunting is rarely needed during aortic arch branch reconstructions, particularly if the sequence of revascularization is planned appropriately.[16]

Many surgeons believe that aortic arch branch lesions will behave like carotid bifurcation lesions, but this represents a clinical impression, not a scientific conclusion. Although extraanatomic bypasses have a lower perioperative risk of stroke and death, they appear to be somewhat less durable. It is certainly reasonable to perform a direct intrathoracic reconstruction when alternative approaches are not feasible or would not correct the anatomic problem. Some reports suggest that direct innominate artery reconstructions are preferable to the extraanatomic alternatives, but both approaches can achieve therapeutic success. While the proper role of direct intrathoracic procedures will continue to be debated, such reconstructions are certainly appropriate, and in many cases necessary, to effectively treat patients with cerebrovascular and upper extremity ischemia.

REFERENCES

1. Reul GH, Jacobs MJH, Gregoric ID, Cooley DA: Innominate artery bypass: A ten year follow-up, in Yao JST, Pearce WH (eds): *Long-term Results in Vascular Surgery*. Norwalk: Appleton & Lange, chap 2, pp 97–107.
2. Oudet J, Roge R, Delahaye G, Cormier JM: Greffe vasculaire en y pour aneurysme traumatique du tronc brachio-céphalique. *Presse Méd* 61:449–451, 1953.
3. Davis JB, Grove WJ, Julian OC: Thrombotic occlusion of the branches of the aortic arch. Martorell's syndrome: Report of a case treated surgically. *Ann Surg* 144:124–126, 1956.
4. DeBakey ME, Crawford ES: Resection and homograft replacement of innominate and carotid arteries with use of shunt to maintain circulation. *Surg Gynecol Obstet* 105:129–135, 1957.

5. Colburn MD, Moore WS: Late results of vascular reconstruction of the proximal carotid and subclavian arteries, in Yao JST, Pearce WH (eds): *Long-term Results in Vascular Surgery.* Norwalk, Appleton & Lange, chap 7, pp 81–96, 1993.
6. Berguer R: Reconstruction of the supraaortic trunks and vertebrobasilar system, in Moore WS (ed): *Vascular Surgery: A Comprehensive Review,* 3d ed. Philadelphia, WB Saunders, chap 27, pp 473–486, 1992.
7. Cormier F, Ward A, Cormier JM, Laurian C: Long-term results of aortoinnominate and aortocarotid polytetrafluoroethylene bypass grafting for atherosclerotic lesions. *J Vasc Surg* 10: 135–142, 1989.
8. Crawford ES, Stowe CL, Powers RW: Occlusion of the innominate, common carotid, and subclavian arteries: Long-term results of surgical treatment. *Surgery* 94:781–791, 1983.
9. Farina C, Sterpetti AV, Schultz RD, et al: Extrathoracic and transthoracic management of vascular disease of the aortic arch branches: A 16 year experience. *Ann Thorac Surg* 47:580–585, 1989.
10. Courbier R, Jausseran JM, Poyen V: Current status of vascular grafting in supraaortic trunks: Personal experience. *Int Surg* 73:210–212, 1988.
11. Evans WE, Williams TE, Hayes JP: Aortobrachiocephalic reconstruction. *Am J Surg* 156(8): 100–102, 1988.
12. Vogt DP, Hertzer NR, O'Hara PJ, Bevern EG: Brachiocephalic arterial reconstruction. *Ann Surg* 196(5):541–552, 1982.
13. Zelenock GB, Cronenwett JL, Graham LM, et al: Brachiocephalic arterial occlusions and stenoses: Manifestations and management of complex lesions. *Arch Surg* 120:370–376, 1985.
14. Wind GG, Valentine RJ: Thoracic aorta, in *Anatomic Exposures in Vascular Surgery.* Baltimore, Williams & Wilkins, chap 3, pp 73–104, 1991.
15. Wind GG, Valentine RJ: Carotid arteries, in *Anatomic Exposures in Vascular Surgery.* Baltimore, Williams & Wilkins, chap 1, pp 23–48, 1991.
16. Reul GJ, Jacobs MJH, Gregoric ID, et al: Innominate artery occlusive disease: Surgical approach and longterm results. *J Vasc Surg* 14(3):405–412, 1991.
17. DeSobregrau RC, Collado ML, Docampo MM, et al: Surgery of the innominate artery. *J Cardiovasc Surg* 27:31–37, 1986.
18. Schanzer H, Chung-Loy H, Kotok M, et al: Evaluation of axillo-axillary artery bypass for the treatment of subclavian or innominate artery occlusive disease. *J Cardiovasc Surg* 28: 258–261, 1987.
19. Sandmann W, Kniemeyer HW, Jaeschock R, et al: The role of subclavian-carotid transposition in surgery for supra-aortic occlusive disease. *J Vasc Surg* 5(1):53–58, 1987.

30

Surgical Procedures for Vertebral Artery Disease

Stephen C. Nicholls

Elective ligation of the proximal vertebral artery was first reported in 1864 by Smyth.[1] This procedure was performed for arterial erosion and hemorrhage following a prior ligation of the subclavian and common carotid arteries for a subclavian aneurysm. The first direct vertebral reconstruction was carried out in 1957 by Cate and Scott, who performed an endarterectomy of the left subclavian and vertebral arteries.[2] However, this case was not reported until 1959, and in 1958 Crawford and DeBakey performed and reported a vertebral endarterectomy.[3] A successful series of vertebral artery reconstructions was not reported until 1972 by Edwards and Wright.[4]

Numerous operations have been devised to correct the problem of vertebrobasilar insufficiency, including carotid endarterectomy as the initial procedure (Chap. 19).[5–7] Direct approaches to the diseased vertebral artery involve endarterectomy with or without patch angioplasty, transposition or reimplantation, and bypass grafting. Since most atherosclerotic lesions of the vertebral artery are located at its origin from the subclavian, most of these procedures are on the proximal or V1 segment (Fig. 30-1). Extrinsic lesions usually are managed by decompression or correction of tortuosity and kinks. Decompression may involve either osteotomies at single or multiple levels from C6 to C1, or relief of compression by the longus colli or anterior scalene muscles. A variety of intracranial bypass procedures also has been performed to treat occlusions or stenoses in the fourth portion of the vertebral artery (Table 30-1).

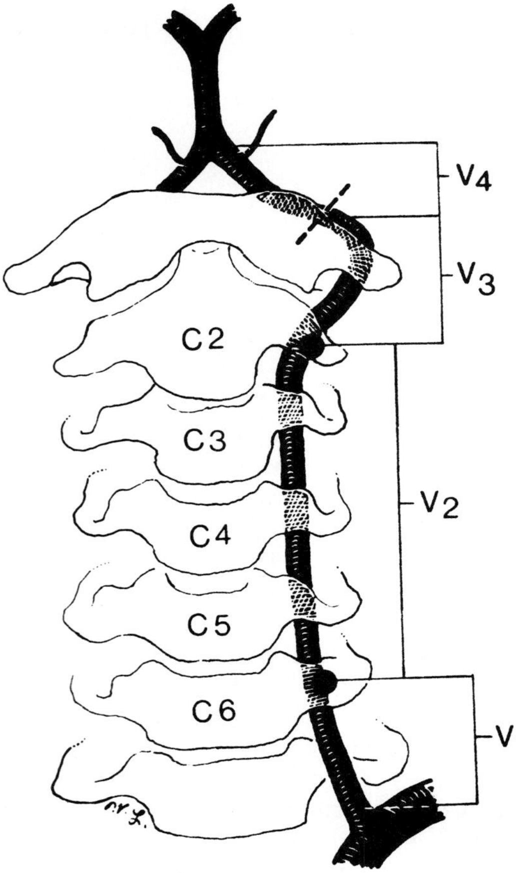

Figure 30-1. The four anatomic segments of the vertebral artery. [*From Berguer R: Surgical management of the vertebral artery, in Moore WS (ed): Surgery for Cerebrovascular Disease (Chapter 60). Reproduced by permission of Churchill Livingstone, Inc., New York, 1986.*]

SURGICAL APPROACHES

Supraclavicular

This approach is required when the subclavian artery is to be used as a source of inflow or for direct access to the proximal vertebral artery (Fig. 30-2*A* and *B*). The incision is made approximately 2 cm above and parallel to the clavicle, extending from its medial head laterally. The platysma muscle is divided, and the anterior or external jugular veins are ligated and divided. The sternocleidomastoid muscle is then divided, and the prescalene fat pad is entered. Better exposure is obtained by excising this latter structure with its associ-

Table 30-1 Surgical Procedures for Correction of Vertebral Artery Lesions

Cervical: Intrinsic Lesions
1. Subclavian/vertebral endarterectomy with or without patch angioplasty
2. Transposition of the vertebral artery to the:
Subclavian artery
Thyrocervical trunk
Common carotid artery
3. Carotid or subclavian to vertebral bypass
Proximal bypass to the distal first or proximal second segment at the C5–C6 level
Distal bypass to the third segment at the C1–C2 level
Cervical: Extrinsic Lesions
1. Decompression
2. Correction of tortuosity and kinks
3. Unroofing of the bony canal—spondylolisthesis, spurs, herniation
4. Sympathectomy
Intracranial Procedures
1. Occipital to PICA anastomosis
2. Superficial temporal to superior cerebellar anastomosis
3. Intracranial vertebral endarterectomy
4. External carotid to posterior cerebral bypass

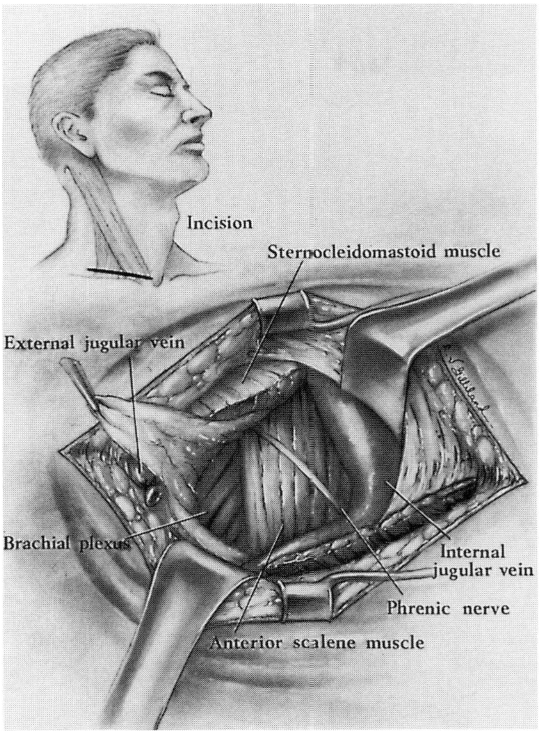

A

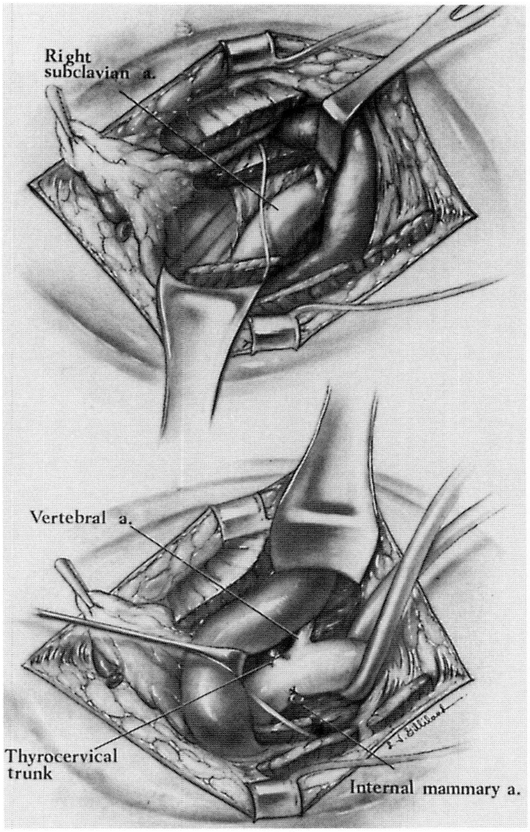

B

Figure 30-2. *A.* Supraclavicular approach to the right vertebral artery. *B.* Exposure can be improved by ligation and division of selected arterial branches. [*From Wylie EJ, Ehrenfeld WK (eds): Extracranial Occlusive Cerebrovascular Disease: Diagnosis and Management. Reproduced by permission of WB Saunders Company, Philadelphia, 1970.*]

ated lymph nodes. The transverse cervical vessels running through the prescalene fat pad also are divided. The phrenic nerve is identified on the anterior aspect of the anterior scalene muscle and is mobilized, isolated with a Silastic loop, and gently retracted. This allows the muscle to be divided without damage to the phrenic nerve. After division of the anterior scalene muscle, the subclavian artery is readily exposed, and the thyrocervical trunk, internal mammary, and vertebral arteries can be isolated. The subclavian artery is typically thin-walled and friable.

During the supraclavicular approach on the left side, care must be taken to avoid damage to the thoracic duct, which arches laterally at the level of C7 and passes in front of the left vertebral artery, phrenic nerve, and anterior scalene muscle before joining the left internal jugular or subclavian vein. On the right side, the recurrent laryngeal nerve may be injured as it winds around the subclavian artery just medial to the origin of the vertebral. The origins of the vertebral arteries are located posteromedially on the subclavian arteries. On the left, the vertebral origin tends to be deeper and more posterior than on the right. Care also must be taken to avoid a Horner's syndrome resulting from damage to the sympathetic trunk, which is located anterior to the proximal vertebral artery. Dissection of the vertebral artery is carried up to the longus colli muscle, which may compress the vessel. If necessary, the tendon of this muscle can be divided to avoid angulation. The transverse process of C6 is at this level.

The proximal portion of the vertebral artery also may be approached through a median sternotomy or, on the left, by a lateral thoracotomy (Fig. 30-3).

Low Anterior Neck Incision

This approach is required for exposure of the second portion of the vertebral artery. The in-

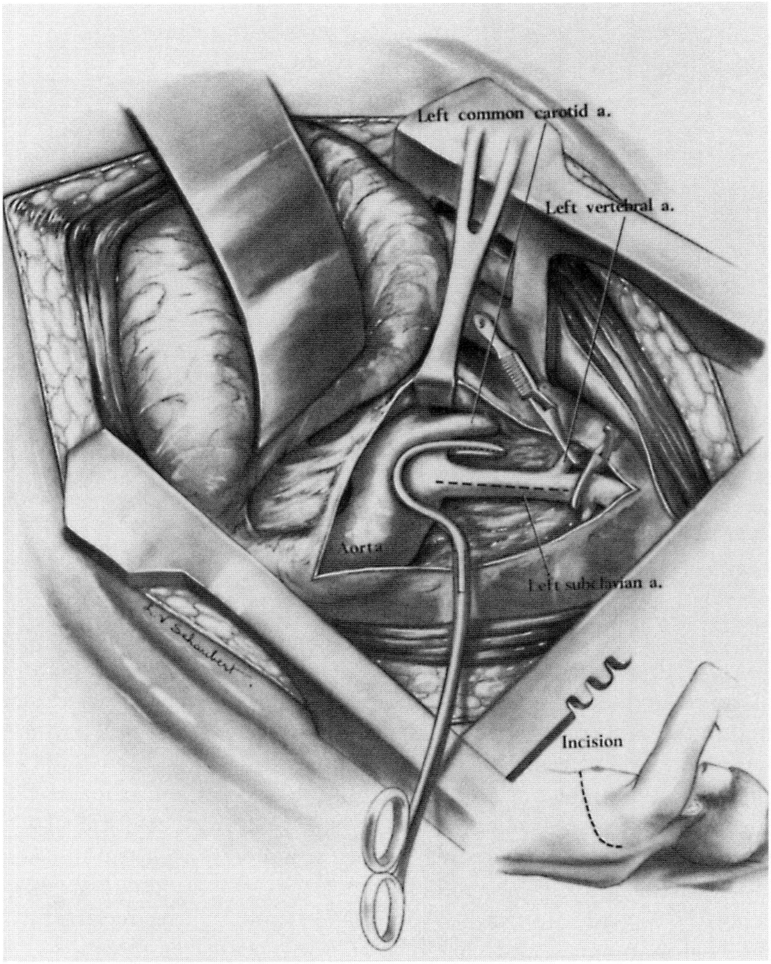

Figure 30-3. Incision site and exposure of the left subclavian and left vertebral arteries through a left thoracotomy. [*From Wylie EJ, Ehrenfeld WK (eds): Extracranial Occlusive Cerebrovascular Disease: Diagnosis and Management. Reproduced by permission of WB Saunders Company, Philadelphia, 1970.*]

cision is made along the anterior border of the sternocleidomastoid from the medial head of the clavicle to approximately half-way up the muscle. Dissection is continued along the anterior border of the sternocleidomastoid, which is retracted laterally. The internal jugular vein and vagus nerve are identified and mobilized along their lateral margins. On the left side, the thoracic duct is identified and best managed by careful ligation and division. As with the supraclavicular approach, the sympathetic trunk must be carefully preserved, and dissection is continued distally to the longus colli muscle.

Exposure of the V2 segment is accomplished by medial retraction of the common carotid artery, internal jugular vein, and vagus nerve to uncover the prevertebral fascia. The anterior spinal ligament is then incised. Mobilization of the longus colli and longus capitis muscles exposes the transverse processes, which may be partly removed with a rongeur to gain access to the vertebral artery in the bony canal. Careful dissection is required to separate the vertebral artery from the accompanying veins.

Exposure of the Distal Vertebral

The incision for this exposure is placed over the upper two-thirds of the anterior border of the sternocleidomastoid muscle, and the parotid gland is mobilized and retracted superiorly. The great auricular nerve may be identified and preserved near the upper end of the incision. A plane is then developed between the sternocleidomastoid muscle and internal jugular vein, where the spinal accessory nerve is identified near its entrance to the muscle. This nerve is retracted gently with a Silastic loop. The posterior belly of the digastric muscle is then identified and retracted upward. The transverse process of C1 may be palpated under the digastric and marks the upper limit of this exposure.

The internal jugular vein is retracted laterally and the common facial vein divided. The levator scapulae muscle is then identified by retracting the sternocleidomastoid and spinal accessory nerve laterally and removing the fat pad which overlies it. The ventral ramus of nerve C2 emerges from under the belly of the levator scapulae which inserts on the C1 transverse process. The levator scapulae may be divided by inserting an instrument over the nerve and under the muscle at the level of the C2 transverse process (Fig. 30-4*A*). The exposure of the vertebral artery can be improved by excising the proximal stump of the levator scapulae muscle up to its insertion on C1. The exposure gained enables the ventral ramus of nerve C2 to be seen running transversely in the intertransverse space adjacent to the vertebral artery. This nerve is then mobilized and exposure of the artery achieved by cutting the ventral ramus of C2 over the artery (Fig. 30-4*B*). This does not result in a clinical deficit because of the interconnections between the first three cervical nerves. Once exposed, the vertebral artery is surrounded by thin-walled veins from which it must be separated (Fig. 30-4*C*). To facilitate this, 3.5 power magnification is recommended.

VERTEBRAL ARTERY PROCEDURES

The surgical procedures for correction of vertebral artery lesions are listed in Table 30-1. Some of the technical details of these procedures are summarized below.

Endarterectomy

As discussed in Chap. 19, atherosclerotic plaques most commonly involve the origin of the vertebral artery. An endarterectomy of such a lesion may be performed by either of two approaches.[8] The standard approach involves a longitudinal arteriotomy across the origin of the vertebral artery extending onto the subclavian. This permits the plaque to be followed distally and the end-point established under direct vision, as described for carotid

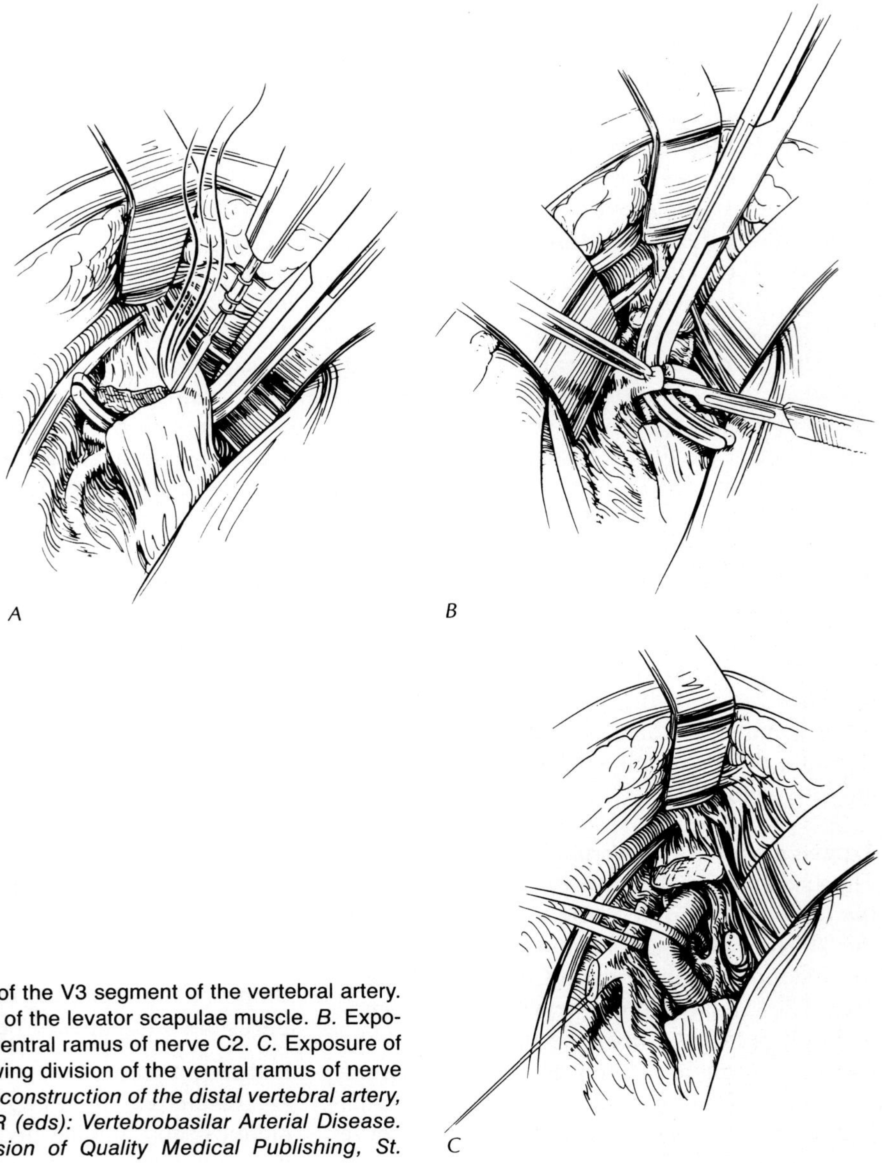

Figure 30-4. Exposure of the V3 segment of the vertebral artery. *A.* Exposure and division of the levator scapulae muscle. *B.* Exposure and division of the ventral ramus of nerve C2. *C.* Exposure of the vertebral artery following division of the ventral ramus of nerve C2. [*From Berguer R: Reconstruction of the distal vertebral artery, in Berguer R, Caplan LR (eds): Vertebrobasilar Arterial Disease. Reproduced by permission of Quality Medical Publishing, St. Louis, 1992.*]

endarterectomy (Chap. 23). The end-point should be secured with tacking sutures if necessary. The arteriotomy usually is closed with a vein patch to avoid narrowing at the endarterectomy site.

For a stenotic lesion limited to the orifice of the vertebral artery, a trans-subclavian endarterectomy may be performed through a longitudinal incision curving slightly toward the origin of the vertebral artery (Fig. 30-5). The plaque is everted from the orifice of the vertebral into the lumen of the subclavian artery. The main disadvantage of this technique is that the distal end-point is not directly visual-

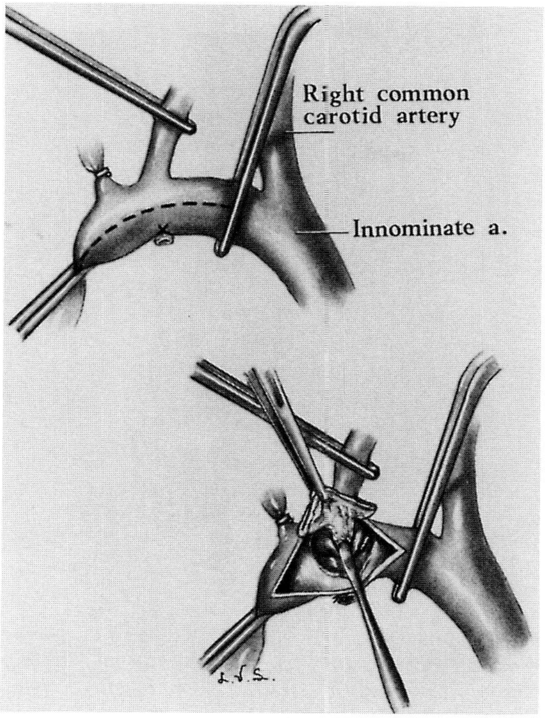

Figure 30-5. Trans-subclavian endarterectomy of the vertebral artery orifice. [*From Wylie EJ, Ehrenfeld WK (eds): Extracranial Occlusive Cerebrovascular Disease: Diagnosis and Management. Reproduced by permission of WB Saunders, Philadelphia, 1970.*]

ized, and a residual intimal flap may result in an arterial dissection. In addition, the endpoint in the subclavian artery may need to be taken into areas which would not otherwise require treatment.

Subclavian-Vertebral Angioplasty

This procedure is designed to correct the kinking associated with redundancy in the first portion of the vertebral artery.[9] The arteriotomy is extended from the subclavian artery up onto the vertebral. It usually is advisable to excise the origin of the thyrocervical trunk along with an ellipse of the subclavian arterial wall extending up into the vertebral segment of the arteriotomy. The normal intima of the vertebral is then plicated to the intima of the subclavian artery across the stenotic ostium, thus excluding any ostial plaque and eliminating the kink. The arterial defect is closed with a vein patch.

Reimplantation of the Vertebral Artery

Transposition to the Subclavian Artery If there is sufficient length of the V1 segment, the vertebral artery may be divided above the plaque and reimplanted into another site on the subclavian artery. This is possible when the first portion of the vertebral artery is redundant. The advantages of this approach are that it eliminates the need for manipulation of the carotid artery and requires only one anastomosis. When this technique is used, the vertebral artery must be dissected up to the longus colli muscle to obtain as much length as possible. The divided end of the vertebral artery is spatulated, and a site on the superior and anterior aspect of the subclavian artery that is free of disease is chosen for the anastomosis. The subclavian arteriotomy may be performed with a punch or by direct excision of a piece of the artery.

If the thyrocervical trunk is free of disease and of adequate size, it may offer a suitable reimplantation site. The branches of the thyrocervical trunk must be ligated and divided to mobilize the vessel. Spatulating the ends of the thyrocervical trunk and vertebral artery facilitates the anastomosis.

Transposition to the Common Carotid Artery This technique probably is the one most commonly used for proximal vertebral artery reconstruction. It requires only one anastomosis and eliminates the need for vein harvesting. The common carotid artery is a large vessel and is usually relatively free of disease. Exposure for this approach is also simple, involving only division of the omohyoid muscle and possibly ligation of the thoracic duct. When the vertebral artery enters the bony canal at C7, transposition may be difficult owing to inadequate length, and alternative reconstruction techniques must be considered.

A potential disadvantage of this approach is that clamping of the common carotid artery may be hazardous. However, problems are most likely to occur when the contralateral internal carotid artery is occluded. Thus, the status of the contralateral carotid system must be known, and information on the intracerebral crossover circulation also is desirable. Monitoring of the ipsilateral middle cerebral artery by transcranial Doppler during the procedure is helpful. Despite earlier concerns, experience has shown that flows in the common carotid artery are more than adequate to accommodate the increased run-off to the ipsilateral vertebral circulation following vertebral artery reimplantation.

After adequate mobilization of the proximal segment, the vertebral artery is divided above the stenosis. Care should be taken to avoid disturbing the fibers of the sympathetic trunk. The common carotid artery may be rotated between clamps to facilitate performance of the anastomosis (Fig. 30-6). Careful flushing maneuvers must be used after the anastomosis is completed to eliminate air and debris before releasing the clamps and allowing flow to the intracerebral circulation.

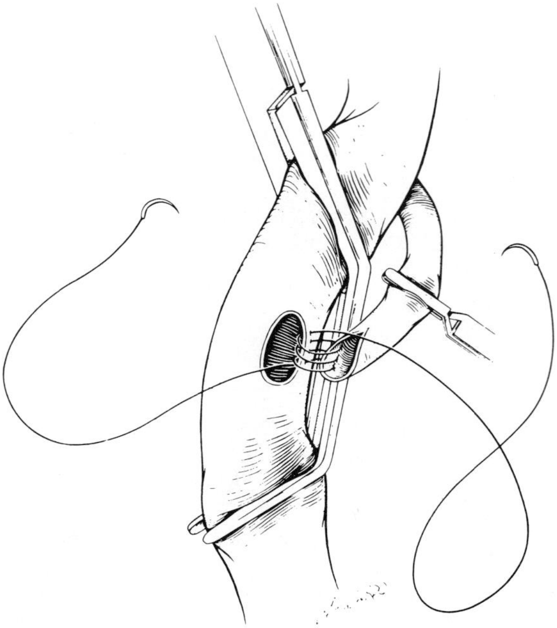

Figure 30-6. Vertebral-common carotid artery anastomosis. [*From Lee RE: Reconstruction of the proximal vertebral artery, in Berguer R, Caplan LR (eds): Vertebrobasilar Arterial Disease. Reproduced by permission of Quality Medical Publishing Inc., St. Louis, 1992.*]

Carotid or Subclavian to Vertebral Bypass

Proximal Bypass In some cases there may be an inadequate length of vertebral artery to perform a transposition or reimplantation procedure. This may occur if the plaque extends for a significant distance up the vertebral artery of if there is complete occlusion of the proximal segment. In these situations bypass may be the best option. Care must be taken to make the distal anastomosis well beyond the site of disease. Dissection of the vertebral artery in the bony canal is difficult, owing to the plexus of veins surrounding it. It may be necessary to unroof one or more of the transverse processes (usually C5 and C6) and then perform the distal anastomosis of the saphenous vein graft to the transected end of the vertebral artery. As with transposition procedures, the common carotid artery generally is preferred over the subclavian as the inflow source due to the better quality of the common carotid and the greater ease in obtaining exposure and control.

Reconstruction of the Distal Vertebral Artery Options for reconstruction of the distal vertebral artery include vein bypass from the common carotid artery to the third segment at the C1–C2 level (Fig. 30-7). An alternative approach is to anastomose the distal external carotid artery to the distal vertebral artery (Fig. 30-8). Occasionally the occipital artery, a branch of the external carotid, may be used for this purpose. These latter techniques require a normal carotid bifurcation, and the external carotid must not be serving as a ma-

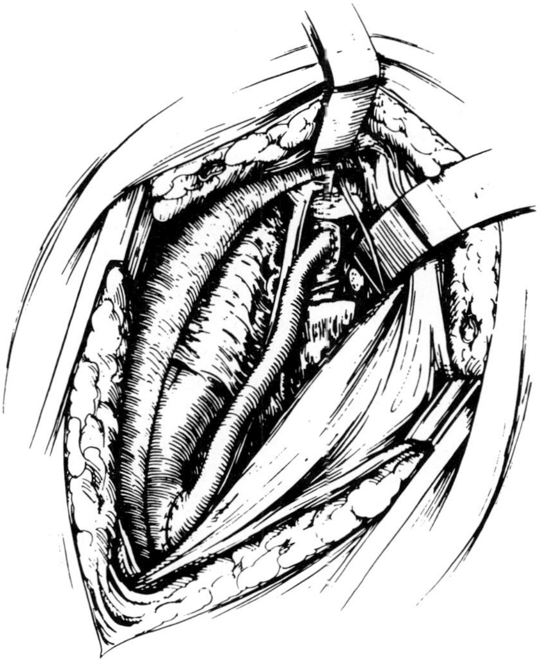

Figure 30-7. Common carotid artery to V3 segment bypass at C1–C2 level. [*From Berguer R: Reconstruction of the distal vertebral artery, in Berguer R, Caplan LR (eds): Vertebrobasilar Arterial Disease. Reproduced by permission of Quality Medical Publishing Inc., St. Louis, 1992.*]

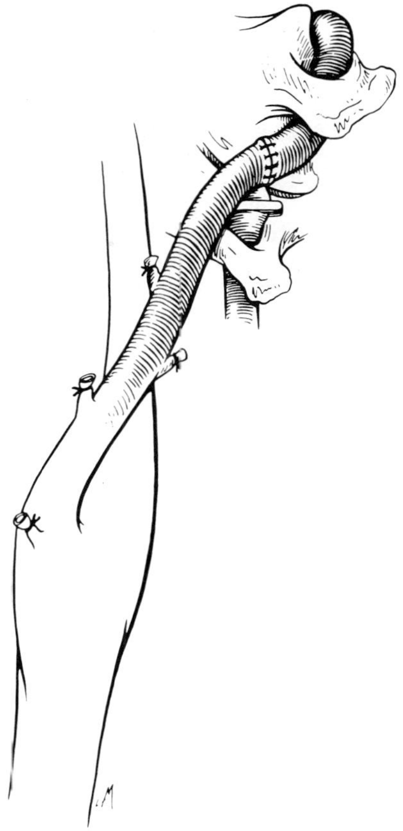

Figure 30-8. Distal external carotid artery to distal vertebral artery transposition. [*From Berguer R: Reconstruction of the distal vertebral artery, in Berguer R, Caplan LR (eds): Vertebrobasilar Arterial Disease. Reproduced by permission of Quality Medical Publishing Inc., St. Louis, 1992.*]

jor collateral to the intracranial circulation through the orbit, as occurs in some cases of internal carotid occlusion. Another option is transposition of the distal vertebral artery to the side of the internal carotid artery (Fig. 30-9).

The advantage of vertebral reconstruction at the C1–C2 level is that most pathologic conditions affect the artery proximal to this site. The C1–C2 interval is the widest between the transverse processes, and it is at this level that the distal vertebral artery reconstitutes by collaterals when its proximal segments are occluded. There is also a range of rotational mobility at this level, resulting in some redundancy (called the "safety loop" by the French), and this allows exposure of a reasonable length of the artery. Rarely, the abnormality is at the level of C1, in which case the reconstruction must be made where the artery runs over the posterior arch of the atlas.

Exposure of the vertebral artery for these procedures is achieved as previously described, through a neck incision along the anterior border of the sternocleidomastoid muscle.

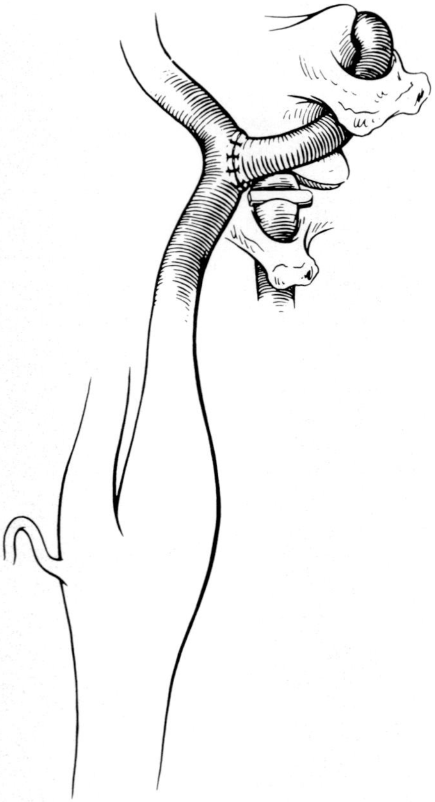

Figure 30-9. Transposition of the distal vertebral artery to the internal carotid artery. [*From Berguer R: Reconstruction of the distal vertebral artery, in Berguer R, Caplan LR (eds): Vertebrobasilar Arterial Disease. Reproduced by permission of Quality Medical Publishing Inc., St. Louis, 1992.*]

RESULTS

Proximal Reconstruction

Reports based on large series of vertebral artery operations are still relatively rare. Branchereau and Magnan reported the immediate and long-term results of 191 vertebral reconstructions.[10] Among 179 patients undergoing surgery, 170 presented with symptoms of vertebrobasilar insufficiency. These were associated with hemispheric symptoms in 29 patients. Five patients had hemispheric symptoms only, and four patients were asymptomatic. Procedures involved the proximal segment of the vertebral artery in 148 cases and the distal segment in 43 cases. There were eight deaths (4 percent). Of these, only one occurred in the group of 118 patients undergoing isolated vertebral artery reconstruction, while seven occurred in a group of 72 patients undergoing combined vertebral and carotid surgery ($p<.01$). During a mean follow-up period of 34.6 months, 118 patients were asymptomatic and 15 were improved, for a success rate of 80 percent. Overall survival at seven years was 89 percent, and patency at seven years was 90 percent. Results were better for proximal reconstructions compared to distal repairs (94 vs. 77 percent). The authors of this report concluded that in patients with vertebrobasilar symptoms, arteriographic findings compatible with a hemodynamic etiology, and no general contraindications to surgery, vertebral artery reconstruction resulted in symptom resolution in more than 80 percent of cases. Patients with associated hemispheric symptoms and carotid lesions constituted a high-risk population for vertebral artery reconstruction.

The results from the same center were reviewed two years later, at which time 240 vertebral artery procedures had been performed, including 110 isolated proximal reconstructions with no concomitant carotid arterial reconstruction.[11] All but one of the patients presented with symptoms of vertebrobasilar insufficiency characterized by a combination of balance and visual disturbances in 35 patients (32 percent). The mortality rate at 30 days was 1 percent of patients and 0.9 percent of procedures performed. Patency for all reconstructions, including operative failures, was 93 percent at five years and 87 percent at 10 years, based on follow-up information on 97 patients. The main conclusion from this analysis was that proximal vertebral artery reconstruction is a safe procedure which provides better than 95 percent immediate patency and a mortality rate below 1 percent.

Long-term failure of the reconstructions was rare, with a patency rate of over 80 percent at 10 years. Life expectancy was over 80 percent at 10 years, justifying operation for relief of symptoms to improve quality of life.

In the series summarized above, the choice of procedure was determined by the status of the vertebral, subclavian, and carotid arteries as documented by angiography. When both vertebral arteries were diseased, the dominant vertebral was reconstructed, except when it ended in a posterior inferior cerebellar artery (PICA). The presence of intrinsic and extrinsic lesions affecting the second segment of the vertebral artery had to be carefully determined, since a distal vertebral artery bypass was indicated in these cases. Underestimating the severity of more distal vertebral lesions resulted in failures in two cases. When the vertebral lesions were bilateral and equivalent, the right vertebral artery, which is easier to approach than the left, was the one reconstructed. In these cases, a left-sided reconstruction was reserved for patients who were not relieved of symptoms by the initial procedure. With a normal subclavian artery, transposition of the vertebral artery to the thyrocervical trunk was a simple procedure with good results. Transposition of the vertebral artery to the ascending portion of the subclavian was performed when the vertebral was elongated and without distal obstructive lesions. It was felt that, in most cases, carotid transposition was more feasible, and vein bypass grafts from the carotid artery were performed in two circumstances: (1) if there was insufficient vertebral artery length; and (2) the atheromatous lesion in the vertebral artery was unusually long.

Edwards and Mulherin reported on 498 proximal subclavian and vertebral artery procedures in 411 patients.[12] There were 317 operations performed for vertebral artery lesions involving direct anastomosis of the vertebral to the common carotid artery. Of these, 215 (68 percent) were rendered asymptomatic, 83 (26 percent) had improvement of their symptoms, and 19 (6 percent) were not improved. There was an exceedingly low incidence of complications, which included three cases of hemorrhage, one lymph fistula, one neurologic deficit, and only one death.

Imparato reported the results of 120 operations: 108 subclavian-vertebral angioplasties with vertebral plication and patching; five carotid-vertebral bypasses with reversed saphenous vein; five reimplantations of the vertebral artery into the common carotid; and two procedures for unroofing of the bony canal.[9] The early postoperative mortality was three patients or 2.5 percent (one from myocardial infarction, one due to pulmonary embolus, and one associated with cerebral infarction). There was one asymptomatic occlusion of a bypass graft to the mid-vertebral artery. During a follow-up period of two months to 19 years, overall survival was 88 percent at five years, 69 percent at 10 years, and 69 percent at 15 years. One case of permanent Horner's syndrome was noted, but transient Horner's syndrome occurred in 40 percent and transient elevation of the ipsilateral hemidiaphragm in 30 percent of cases. No vocal cord paralyses were reported.

Diaz and Ausman reported vertebral to carotid transpositions at the first or second portion of the vertebral artery in 118 patients.[13] Of these, 107 (91 percent) became asymptomatic and there was one death (0.8 percent). One patient developed a brain stem infarct, and nine had recurrent symptoms of vertebrobasilar insufficiency (7.6 percent). Postoperative angiography revealed occlusion at the anastomosis in four of 107 patients. Long-term survival and late stroke rates were not given.

Distal Reconstruction

Kieffer and coworkers reported the results of 222 patients having 241 distal vertebral reconstructions between 1978 and 1989.[14] Most of these patients (93 percent) had a unilateral vertebral operation. A bypass graft was performed in 160 cases (66 percent), usually with saphenous vein. Transposition of the transected distal vertebral artery to the internal carotid artery was performed in 73 cases (31 percent). Transposition of an endarterectomized previously occluded internal carotid to the distal vertebral artery was performed in five cases (2 percent). Reconstruction was accomplished by simple freeing of the V3 segment in three cases (1 percent). Reconstruction was carried out at the C1–C2 level in 27 cases (11 percent) and above C1 in 14 cases (6 percent). Simultaneous internal carotid artery reconstruction was performed in 64 cases (27 percent). There were four postoperative deaths (1.8 percent). All neurologic complications except one vertebrobasilar stroke occurred in the 64 cases of combined carotid and vertebral reconstruction ($p<.05$ percent).

In the series of Kieffer and coworkers accessory nerve injuries occurred in 21 cases (9 percent), but all regressed within three months.[14] Horner's syndrome occurred in 10 cases (4 percent). Early postoperative occlusions were noted in 18 (7.5 percent) of the 241 reconstructions, and in all cases the occlusion was extensive (up to and including the V4 segment). The five-year cumulative survival rate was 93 percent. There was complete cure of vertebrobasilar insufficiency in 118 patients (53 percent), and significant improvement was obtained in 73 patients (33 percent). The five-year cumulative patency rate for the distal vertebral reconstructions was 85 percent.

Kieffer and coworkers concluded that the early postoperative morbidity and mortality were largely dependent on concomitant surgical treatment of associated carotid artery disease.[14] The early combined death and stroke rate was 2.5 percent overall, but only 0.6 percent for the isolated vertebral artery reconstructions. The early postoperative occlusion rate of 7.5 percent was attributed to improper indications leading to competitive flow situations or technical problems including extremely small distal vertebral arteries or the occurrence of distal spasm or dissection. Based on this experience, it was recommended that operation be avoided in all small (less than 2 mm) vertebral arteries.

Berguer recently reviewed an experience with 233 vertebral artery reconstructions performed since 1975, most having been done during the last 10 years.[15] These included 176 proximal and 57 distal procedures. All patients undergoing distal vertebral artery reconstructions presented with symptoms of vertebrobasilar insufficiency. The anatomic indication for distal vertebral reconstruction was severe stenosis of the intraspinal vertebral artery segment that was either fixed (plaque, thrombus) or transient (external compression). Common carotid to distal vertebral artery vein bypass grafting was the surgical technique used in 41 cases. Other methods used were transposition of the external carotid to the distal vertebral artery (10 cases), internal carotid to distal vertebral bypass (one case), transposition of the occipital to the distal vertebral artery (two cases), transposition of the distal vertebral artery to the internal carotid (two cases), and carotid to contralateral distal vertebral artery retroesophageal bypass (one case).

There were three deaths in Berguer's series, for an operative mortality rate of 1.3 percent.[15] There were five early occlusions (8.5 percent) after distal vertebral artery reconstructions. Two of these occurred in patients who died; the other three occlusions were attributed to competitive flow between the bypass graft and collaterals from the occipital artery. One patient had recurrence of symptoms two years after a successful bypass graft and was found to have intimal hyperplasia. This vein graft was replaced and remained patent for seven years. Dysesthesia or anesthesia in the territory of the great auricular nerve was present in approximately 30 percent of patients. No other peripheral nerve deficits were described. Clinical cure or substantial improvement was reported in 58 percent of the patients, and an additional 20 percent had improvement to the point of being able to carry on with daily activities and work. Thus, 78 percent of the patients were considered as cured or improved after 10 years. The early occlusion rate of 8.5 percent in this series was very similar to the 7.5 percent rate reported by Kieffer and coworkers.[14]

CONCLUSIONS

The natural history of patients with vertebrobasilar insufficiency has not been clearly established. Accurate diagnosis of vertebrobasilar insufficiency is essential, and the symptoms must be ascribed not only to the vertebrobasilar territory but also to specific vascular lesions within that territory. Other causes of vertebrobasilar insufficiency must be excluded. Available data suggest that the stroke risk for untreated patients with symptomatic vertebrobasilar ischemia is 35 percent within four years from the onset of symptoms and that stroke risk is decreased to 15 percent in symptomatic patients treated with anticoagulants.[16] However, no angiographic documentation of the relationship between symptoms of vertebrobasilar insufficiency and significant vertebral artery lesions is available. The frequency of vertebrobasilar ischemic symptoms and infarction is increased in patients with unilateral vertebral artery occlusion associated with contralateral vertebral stenosis and in patients with severe basilar artery stenosis or occlusion.

Surgical morbidity for patients with significant vertebral or basilar artery lesions is approximately 8 percent, and surgical mortality is in the range of 1 to 5 percent. Combined carotid and vertebral artery operations appear to have significantly higher surgical complication rates. A multiplicity of surgical approaches has been used to treat patients with vertebrobasilar insufficiency and concomitant vertebral artery lesions demonstrated by angiography. However, no attempt has been made to carry out a controlled, randomized clinical trial on the treatment of vertebral artery disease. Such a study would be necessary to demonstrate conclusively that surgical management is most appropriate for these patients. In the absence of a definitive clinical trial, the reported experience suggests that operative treatment offers significant benefits over either the expected natural history or medical management alone.

REFERENCES

1. Smyth AW: A case of successful ligation of the innominate artery. *N Orleans J Med* 22:464–469, 1869.
2. Cate WR, Scott HW: Cerebral ischemia of central origin: Relief by subclavian vertebral artery thromboendarterectomy. *Surgery* 45:19–30, 1959.
3. Crawford ES, DeBakey MS, Fields WS: Roentgenographic diagnosis and surgical treatment of basilar insufficiency. *JAMA* 168:509–514, 1958.
4. Edwards WH, Wright R: A new surgical technique for relief for subclavian stenosis. *Hosp Pract* 7:78–87, 1972.
5. Humphries AW, Young JR, Beven EG, et al: Relief of vertebrobasilar symptoms by carotid endarterectomy. *Surgery* 57:48–52, 1965.
6. Ford JJ Jr, Baker WH, Ehrenhaft JL: Carotid endarterectomy for nonhemispheric transient ischemic attacks. *Arch Surg* 110:1314–1317, 1975.
7. McNamara JO, Heyman A, Silver D, Mandell ME: The value of carotid endarterectomy in treating transient ischemia of the posterior circulation. *Neurology* 27:682–684, 1977.
8. Thevenet A, Ruotolo C: Surgical repair of vertebral artery stenosis. *J Cardiovasc Surg* 25: 101–110, 1984.
9. Imparato AM: Vertebral artery surgery reconstruction: A nineteen-year experience. *J Vasc Surg* 2:626–634, 1985.
10. Branchereau A, Magnan PE: Results of verte-

bral artery reconstruction. *J Cardiovasc Surg* 31:320–326, 1990.

11. Branchereau A, Rosset LD, Magnan DE, et al: Proximal reconstructions, in Berguer R, Caplan LR (eds): *Vertebrobasilar Arterial Disease*. St. Louis, Quality Medical Publishing, chap 24, 1992.
12. Edwards WH, Mulherin JL: The surgical reconstruction of the proximal subclavian and vertebral artery. *J Vasc Surg* 2:634–639, 1985.
13. Diaz FG, Ausman JI: Cerebral revascularization of the vertebrobasilar circulation, in Berguer R, Caplan LR (eds): *Vertebrobasilar Arterial Disease*. St. Louis, Quality Medical Publishing, chap 26, 1992.
14. Kieffer E, Koskas F, Rancurel G, et al: Reconstruction of the distal cervical vertebral artery, in Berguer R, Caplan LR (eds): *Vertebrobasilar Arterial Disease*. St. Louis, Quality Medical Publishing, chap 25, 1992.
15. Berguer R: Long-term results of reconstruction of the vertebral artery, in *Long-Term Results in Vascular Surgery*. Appleton and Lange, 1993.
16. Whisnant TP, Cartlidge NEF, Elvebach LR: Carotid and vertebrobasilar transient ischemic attacks. Effects of anticoagulations, hypertension and cardiac disorders on survival and stroke occurrence. A population study. *Ann Neurol* 3:107–115, 1978.

31

Vascular Injury in the Neck: Evaluation and Management

Kaj H. Johansen

Trauma to the large arteries and veins of the neck constitutes a significant medical, surgical, and public health concern. Except for immediately lethal trauma to the heart or central nervous system, no injuries are associated with as high a likelihood of early death as those of the cervicothoracic great vessels. Even in injuries that are not immediately apparent, a predisposition toward crippling or even lethal late complications is an ever-present threat. This chapter will discuss "state of the art" techniques in evaluation and management of extracranial cerebrovascular and cervicothoracic vascular trauma.

EPIDEMIOLOGY

Vascular injuries in the neck represent about 1 percent of all blood vessel trauma.[1] A large majority of patients suffering extracranial cervical vascular trauma have *penetrating* neck injuries. Carotid artery injury is discovered during evaluation in up to 13 percent of patients with such trauma,[2] an incidence that has led to the common practice of routine neck exploration for subplatysmal penetrating cervical injury.

The consequences of penetrating cervical carotid artery trauma are well documented. Hospital mortality associated with penetrating trauma to these arteries ranges from 6 to 22 percent in several series reported over the past 15 years.[2–4] Up to 50 percent of patients with penetrating trauma to the extracranial carotid or aortic arch vessels may die at the trauma scene.[5] The vast majority of patients who survive penetrating trauma to the neck vessels ultimately appear to do well, although follow-up frequently is incomplete.

Much less is known about the prevalence of *blunt* trauma to the extracranial carotid and vertebral arteries. This is probably because a substantial number of such patients may have intimal flaps, pseudoaneurysms of varying sizes, arterial dissections, or even vessel occlusions without manifesting any symptoms. Less than 5 percent of carotid injuries collected in cumulative reviews result from blunt trauma.[6] Occasionally, a devastating neurologic injury in a severely injured patient is found at postmortem examination to have resulted from carotid artery disruption and occlusion; patients with blunt craniocerebral, maxillofacial, or cervical spine trauma may be at special risk for silent carotid artery injury.[7]

Injury to the vertebral artery is relatively uncommon. In the report by Reid and Weigelt, only 43 such injuries were recorded at Parkland Hospital in Dallas during an 11-year period.[8] As in the case of blunt trauma to the carotid and other brachiocephalic vessels, unilateral vertebral artery injury is often silent because excellent collateral circulation through the contralateral vertebral artery and other vessels supplying the circle of Willis makes unilateral vertebral artery blood flow redundant in more than 95 percent of the population.[8,9] The proximity of the vertebral artery and vein seems to result in an unusual predilection for vertebral arteriovenous fistula following penetrating neck trauma.[10] Concurrent penetrating carotid and vertebral artery injuries are rare but are associated with a 50 percent mortality.[11]

Iatrogenic trauma—unintended arterial damage during diagnostic or therapeutic maneuvers—is an increasingly frequent cause of injury to the arteries of the neck. Arteriography may result in dissection of atherosclerotic plaques or may cause embolization in the presence of intrinsic carotid disease. For example, the risk of disabling permanent stroke associated with carotid arteriography is 1 percent.[12] Insertion of catheters into the neck or subclavian region for hemodynamic monitoring or administration of fluids, parenteral nutrition, or chemotherapy may result in damage to nearby vessels. Tonsillectomy and other intraoral operations are carried out relatively close to the internal carotid artery, which occasionally is damaged in the course of such procedures. Chiropractic manipulation of the neck also has resulted in damage to the extracranial cervical arteries,[13] sometimes with catastrophic results involving dissection followed by thrombosis. External beam irradiation to treat head and neck tumors can clearly result in an accelerated cervical carotid occlusive process.[14] These latter disorders are discussed in more detail in Chap. 5.

MECHANISMS OF INJURY

The means by which penetrating trauma damages the extracranial carotid and brachiocephalic vessels is relatively straightforward: the same weapon or missile that causes the penetrating trauma damages the artery in the course of its path through the neck. Vascular injury also may result from secondary missiles, such as fragments of bullets or bone. Wound contamination may occur when trauma penetrates clothing or the oral cavity. Penetrating arterial injuries of the neck generally involve the common carotid artery or internal jugular vein.

As for arteries elsewhere in the body, penetrating trauma to the neck can result in laceration of arteries with massive bleeding. Occasionally, complete transection of vessels results only in minimal hemorrhage, owing to arterial constriction and vessel thrombosis. Hematoma formation following penetrating trauma may compress or even occlude arteries, and arterial flow may be reduced or blocked completely if an atherosclerotic plaque is elevated by needles or catheters inserted for diagnostic or therapeutic purposes.

Blunt trauma to the arteries of the neck and upper trunk may result in stenoses, dissections, embolization, or vessel occlusions. The vast majority of such injuries are at or above the common carotid artery bifurcation. Rotational stress combined with lateral excursion of the head may be particularly likely to damage the contralateral internal carotid artery as it is stretched over the lateral processes of the cervical vertebrae.[15] Although the two outer layers of the arterial wall are relatively elastic, the intima is not, and axial stretch of an artery may lead to intimal fracture followed by partial thrombosis, embolization, or even complete occlusion. In a series of blunt carotid artery injuries, 7 percent resulted from shoulder safety belt trauma.[7]

A specific form of "blunt" vessel trauma may result from cavitation effects along the paths of missiles fired from high muzzle-velocity firearms. Even though the bullet does not directly impact the artery, disruption of the vessel wall with intimal fracture, pseudoaneurysm formation, or thrombosis may occur. Although military-style weapons are becoming more common in civilian strife, such cavitation injuries secondary to the high kinetic energy missiles fired from them remain relatively rare.

CLINICAL PRESENTATION AND DIAGNOSIS

As previously mentioned, the clinical presentation following trauma to the large arteries of the neck ranges from vessel disruption and immediate exsanguination at the trauma scene to a totally asymptomatic patient whose silent arterial occlusion or pseudoaneurysm may become evident only weeks, months, or even years later. Patients who present with "hard" signs of cervical vascular trauma—rapidly expanding hematoma, arterial bleeding from a wound, obvious signs of distal ischemia—should be subjected to few diagnostic delays on the way to the operating room. As in all trauma patients, large-bore venous access lines should be inserted and volume resuscitation initiated while immediately life-threatening injuries of the head, chest, and abdomen are simultaneously evaluated and managed.[16]

Patients with few, subtle, or evanescent signs of vascular trauma—pulse deficits, nonexpanding hematoma, concurrent peripheral nerve injury—present more of a diagnostic challenge. A substantial proportion of such patients will have only trivial or otherwise clinically insignificant vascular injuries, and many will have no vascular injury at all. How to make the diagnosis of the occasional occult cervical arterial injury most accurately and efficiently remains in dispute.

Two general approaches have been validated over the past 15 years for the diagnostic evaluation of penetrating trauma to the neck and upper trunk. They are based on classifying the injury according to three anatomic regions or Zones, as illustrated in Fig. 31-1: injuries below the cricoid cartilage (Zone I); injuries between the cricoid cartilage and the angle of the mandible (Zone II); and injuries above the level of the angle of the mandible (Zone III).[17]

Zone I penetrating injuries primarily threaten the great vessels of the upper mediastinum; injuries to the trachea and upper thoracic esophagus are possible but uncommon. Potential injuries in this region include trauma to the brachiocephalic artery and vein, the proximal (V1) segment of the vertebral artery,

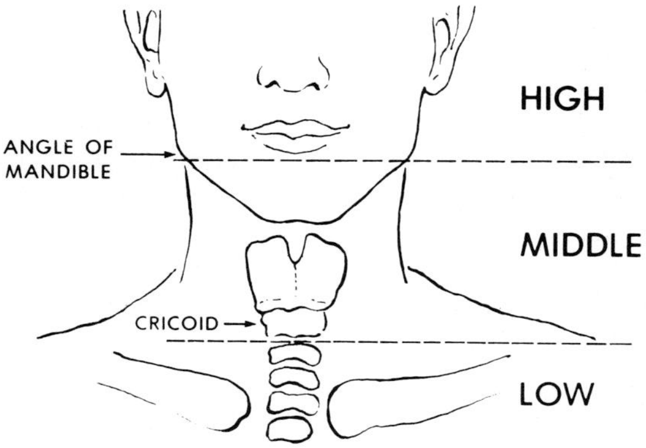

Figure 31-1. The three anatomic zones of the neck for classification of penetrating cervical trauma. Low: Zone I; Middle: Zone II; High: Zone III. *(From Roon and Christensen.*[17] *Reproduced by permission.)*

the brachial plexus, and the pleural cavities and their contents. Zone II injuries threaten the common carotid artery and its primary branches, the V2 segment of the vertebral artery, the internal jugular vein, the cervical esophagus, and the larynx. Zone III injuries are generally presumed to involve structures of the upper neck at the skull base or above; vascular injuries at this level involve the high extracranial internal carotid artery and the V3 segment of the vertebral artery.

From a diagnostic perspective, clinically stable Zone I injuries warrant emergency arteriography and a thoracic surgery consultation. Zone II injuries penetrating the platysma should undergo either "routine" ("mandatory") neck exploration, or a battery of invasive nonoperative examinations with selective operation based on the results of these tests. Zone III injuries require arteriography and a neurosurgery consultation.

For penetrating Zone II cervical injuries, the yield of positive findings on "routine" neck exploration approximates 50 percent.[2] Because of this relatively low yield and the expense associated with routine operative exploration, alternative diagnostic approaches—usually involving triple endoscopy, barium swallow, and contrast arteriography—have been proposed. The debate over whether mandatory operative exploration or selective operation based on the results of nonoperative diagnostic tests should be used for penetrating Zone II injuries revolves primarily around the absolute necessity to diagnose occult esophageal and airway injuries, and is beyond the scope of this discussion. Either approach provides excellent (although not perfect) results in the detection of cervical arterial injuries. In addition, the hospital charges are not significantly different, and the mortality rates are virtually identical for the two approaches. Selective exploration raises the yield of positive findings by about 16 percent over that of routine exploration.[2] The arteriogram of a patient with a penetrating Zone II injury is shown in Figs. 31-2 and 31-3. One potential advantage of using arteriography as a screening test, even when mandatory neck exploration is practiced, is that it may reveal occult vertebral artery injuries that often cannot be diagnosed by operative exploration alone.[18]

As previously indicated, blunt injuries to the arteries of the neck and upper thorax are more poorly understood than penetrating trauma, primarily because neither the incidence of these injuries nor their mechanisms have been well established. The clinical presentation of patients with blunt trauma to the arteries of the neck and upper chest may be subtle, often with nonspecific or waxing and waning neurologic symptoms. Less commonly, transient ischemic attack or stroke is the presenting event.

Because the mechanism of injury is obscure, it is not clear which blunt trauma patients are at high risk and should undergo screening evaluations for occult arterial injuries. Patients that appear to be at increased risk include those with closed head or cervical spine injuries, clavicular or first rib fractures, or massive maxillofacial trauma. Contrast ar-

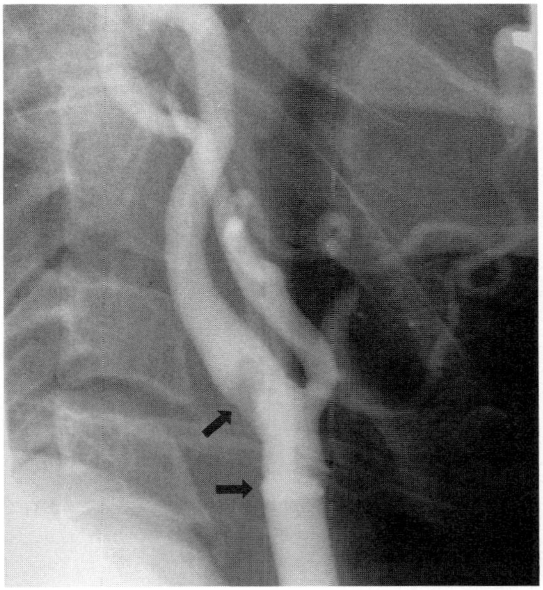

Figure 31-2. Right carotid arteriogram of a 48-year-old woman with a self-inflicted stab wound to Zone II of the neck. She presented with a right hemispheric stroke and a right cortical infarct on CT scan. Lateral view shows defects in the distal common and proximal internal carotid arteries (*arrows*).

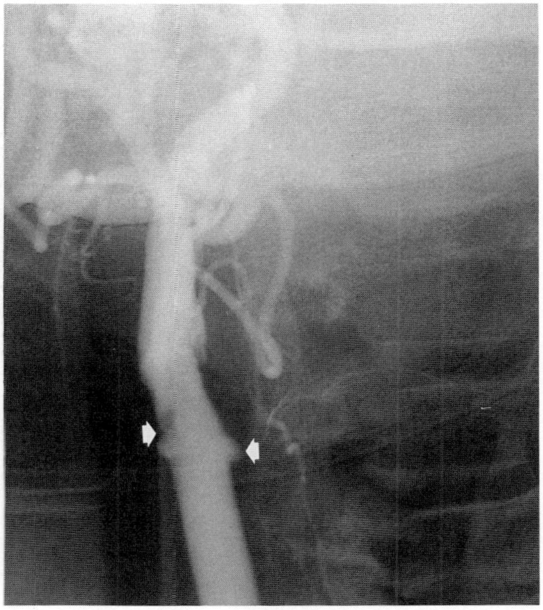

Figure 31-3. Oblique view from the right carotid arteriogram of the same patient shown in Fig. 31-2. A small pseudoaneurysm is seen in the distal common carotid artery (*arrows*). At operation, an intimal flap and thrombus were removed from the proximal internal carotid artery, and a laceration in the common carotid was debrided and repaired with a vein patch.

teriography is recommended in trauma victims presenting with symptoms that might be associated with blunt trauma to the carotid or vertebral arteries. Duplex scanning, a diagnostic modality that has been extensively validated for chronic arterial disease, may be valuable.[19] The appearance of an intimal flap on a B-mode image obtained during carotid duplex scanning is illustrated in Fig. 31-4.

OPERATIVE MANAGEMENT

Emergency management of carotid or brachiocephalic arterial trauma may be mandated by several of the symptoms or signs previously noted—massive arterial bleeding from an open wound, a rapidly expanding cervical hematoma, or shock in association with trauma to the root of the neck. In such circumstances the patient must be brought urgently to the operating room and occasionally must undergo simultaneous resuscitation and operative exploration. Large-bore intravenous lines must be inserted; however, when penetrating trauma might involve the brachiocephalic veins or the superior vena cava, insertion of lines into the greater saphenous vein at the ankle or the common femoral vein is prudent. Because bleeding from the carotid or brachiocephalic vessels can be torrential, these patients should be typed and cross-matched for large amounts of banked blood, and the availability of cell-saving devices should be assured.[16]

Airway control by endotracheal intubation may be extremely difficult in these patients. Bleeding from intraoral or pharyngeal wounds

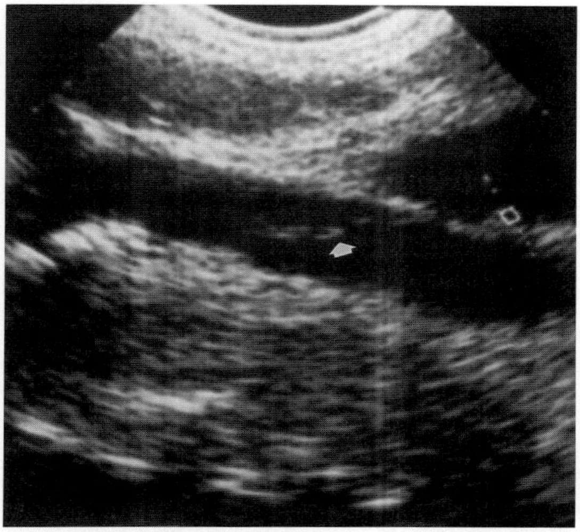

Figure 31-4. B-mode image from a carotid duplex scan of an elderly man with left brain transient ischemic attacks following shoulder safety harness trauma in an automobile accident. An intimal flap is visualized in the common carotid artery (*arrow*).

may obscure the anesthesiologist's view of the airway, or a rapidly expanding neck hematoma may cause tracheal deviation and complicate endotracheal intubation. In this situation the impulse to gain airway control by cricothyroidotomy must be weighed against the potentially catastrophic consequences of suddenly decompressing a tamponaded neck hematoma. Oxygenation by mask or percutaneous cricothyroidotomy may be reasonable alternatives in this unusual setting.

As for vascular trauma elsewhere in the body, adequate exposure and proximal control of the injured cervical arteries are of critical importance. The patient should be prepared and draped from the mandible to the umbilicus so that, if necessary, median sternotomy or left thoracotomy can be performed. Preparation and draping of one lower extremity permits harvesting of saphenous vein for use as an autogenous patch or bypass graft.

Carotid artery injuries in Zone II should be approached through an oblique neck incision along the anterior border of the sternocleidomastoid muscle. Injuries at the root of the neck may require arterial control in the upper mediastinum, and extension of the neck incision to the suprasternal notch and continuation as a median sternotomy offers excellent proximal control of all the arteries on the right side of the upper torso (Fig. 31-5).

Because of the obliquity of the transverse aortic arch, access to the proximal left common carotid artery, and especially the proximal left subclavian artery, cannot be achieved dependably through the neck incision and median sternotomy approach described above. In fact, if control cannot be obtained through a left neck incision, these latter two vessels are best controlled through a left second or third intercostal space thoracotomy combined with a left supraclavicular incision (Fig. 31-5). If wider access to the proximal left common carotid and subclavian arteries is required, a partial median sternotomy joining the medial ends of the supraclavicular and left upper thoracotomy incisions produces an "open-book" or "trapdoor" thoracotomy, which provides excellent exposure for proximal arterial control (Fig. 31-5). If injuries to the middle or distal segments of the left subclavian artery are not accessible through a supraclavicular incision, more adequate exposure can be gained following resection of the medial third or half of the clavicle. This technique generally has minimal negative functional or cosmetic impact. Subsequent to clavicular resection for exposure of the left subclavian artery, care must be taken to avoid damage to the thoracic duct, phrenic nerve, and brachial plexus.

With important exceptions, obtaining distal arterial control is more straightforward for most cervical vascular injuries. However, penetrating or blunt trauma to the internal carotid artery above the angle of the mandible (Zone III) creates special problems for the surgeon because the artery is nearly inaccessible in its last several centimeters before entering

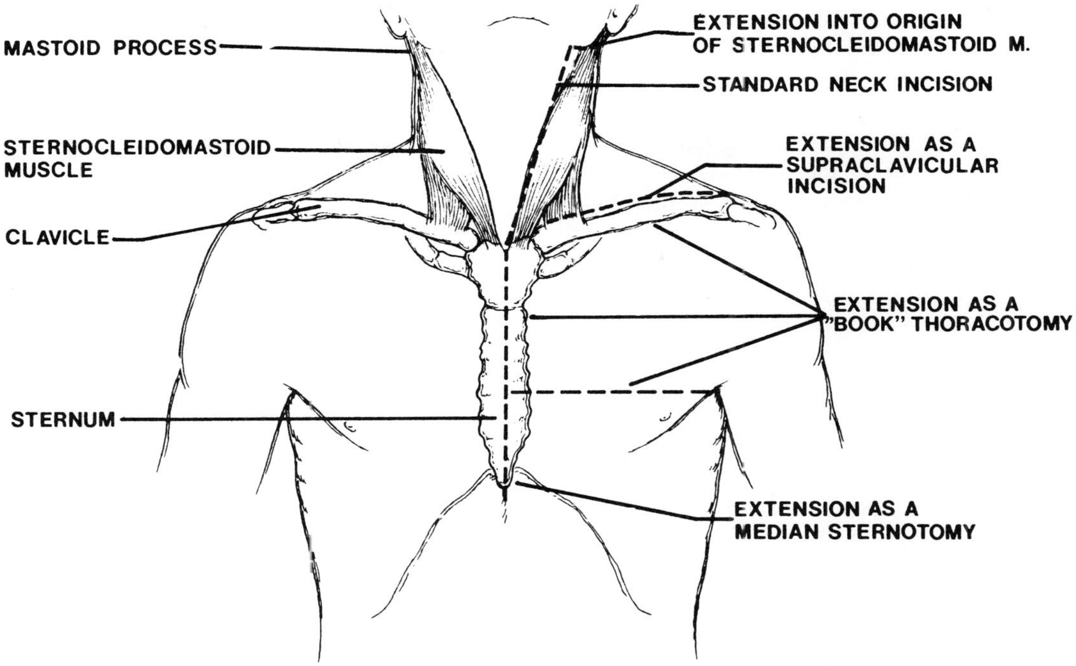

Figure 31-5. Operative incisions for exposure of Zone I and Zone II penetrating neck injuries. A standard oblique neck incision continued as a median sternotomy suffices for injuries to the right of midline. The obliquity of the transverse aortic arch requires left thoracotomy or even "open-book" or "trapdoor" thoracotomy for left-sided exposure of injured great vessels. (*From Asensio et al.*[2] *Reproduced by permission.)*

the base of the skull. The standard diagonal neck incision should be carried upward and slightly posteriorly so that the distal internal carotid artery can be approached from behind the upper sternocleidomastoid muscle. Alternatively, the origin of the sternocleidomastoid can be separated from the mastoid process to provide reasonable exposure of the distal internal carotid, especially with simultaneous division of the digastric muscle. Other maneuvers to facilitate this distal exposure include: anterior dislocation of the temporomandibular joint with the retromandibular space kept open by the placement of arch bars or a mandibulator wielded by a surgical assistant[20]; vertical osteotomy of the mandible[21]; and partial resection of the temporal bone.[22]

The performance of an extracranial-intracranial arterial bypass procedure using superficial temporal artery or a reversed vein graft to the middle cerebral artery, as described by Gewertz and coworkers, may be useful in the presence of a carotid injury at the skull base when it is apparent that the ipsilateral cerebral hemisphere has inadequate collateral blood supply to tolerate carotid artery ligation.[23] However, this technique is rarely practical in the acute trauma setting.

Access to the injured vertebral artery is difficult, and the exposure becomes increasingly complicated with more distal injuries.[8] The vertebral artery can be identified low in the neck by dissection lateral and posterior to the sternocleidomastoid muscle; the anterior scalene muscle must be retracted or divided, and care must be taken to avoid damage to the phrenic nerve. At the level of the sixth cervical vertebra, the vertebral artery deviates dorsally into the interosseous canal formed by the transverse foramina of the cervical vertebrae. Access within this bony canal is extremely difficult and may require osteotomy.[24] Above the second cervical vertebra the vertebral arteries exit from the bony canal and may be approached through a posterolateral incision.[25] The relative inaccessibility of the vertebral artery and its general functional redundancy[8,9] make arteriographic catheterization and embolization a useful therapeutic alternative when vascular control of the vertebral artery is required. This may be the preferred treatment for persistent bleeding or an arteriovenous fistula involving the vertebral artery (Fig. 31-6). Proximal ligation of the vertebral artery should be avoided if there is a possibility that a trans-catheter approach may be needed.[10]

The use of temporary shunts during elective carotid surgery for atherosclerotic disease is widespread, although recent data suggest that the vast majority of such patients have adequate collateral blood supply to tolerate temporary carotid clamping.[26] Whether these data can be extended to the generally young, nonatherosclerotic trauma patient population is unclear. In the setting of common carotid artery trauma, ipsilateral cerebral hemisphere perfusion is maintained not only by the usual posterior and contralateral collateral sources, but also by reversed flow in the ipsilateral external carotid artery. Accordingly, temporary arterial shunts are not used for common carotid artery injuries in our trauma center. However, injuries to the internal carotid artery may not be tolerated as well, and we measure the distal carotid "stump" pressure and insert a shunt for stump pressures less than 50 mmHg. Other methods for monitoring cerebral perfusion—EEG, transcranial Doppler, and "awake" anesthesia—should be considered as supplementary techniques for assuring adequate cerebral perfusion during carotid clamping but may be less applicable in the emergency setting.

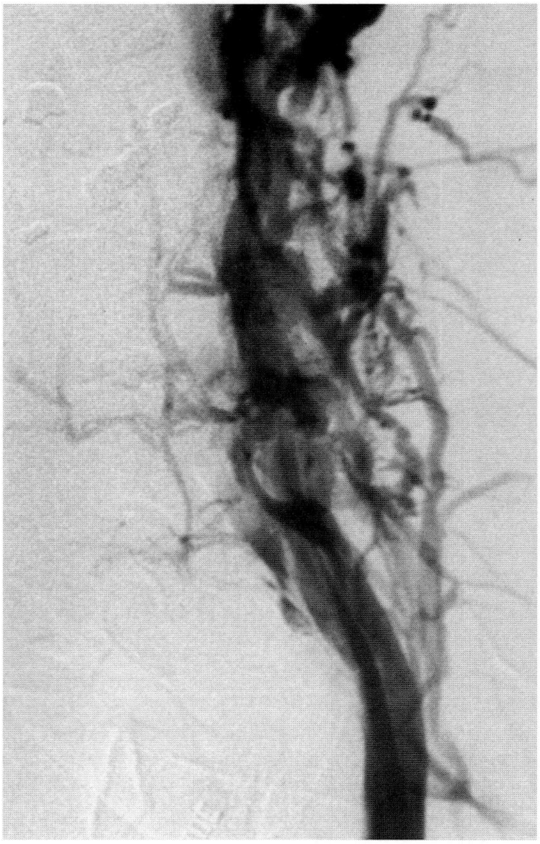

Figure 31-6. Intraarterial digital subtraction arteriogram showing a vertebral arteriovenous fistula (selective left vertebral injection). The patient is a 36-year-old man who suffered a stab wound to the left neck. A high-flow vertebral artery to vein fistula is present at the level of C_5 with filling of the vertebral artery and adjacent paravertebral veins. This was successfully treated by trans-catheter balloon embolization.

Although the indications and techniques for balloon catheter thrombectomy are well established, nowhere are the potential risks of balloon catheter thrombectomy more evident than in the carotid artery system. For example, it is crucial not to pass the balloon catheter above the level of the base of the skull, since the risk of a traumatic carotid artery–cavernous sinus fistula is very high following injudicious inflation of the balloon in the supraclinoid segment of the internal carotid artery. Management of a carotid–cavernous fistula requires skilled radiologic and neurosurgical involvement.[27]

OPERATIVE TECHNIQUES

The specific technical approach to management of an injured carotid or brachiocephalic artery depends primarily on the urgency of repair, the location of vascular damage, and the presence of associated injuries and shock. For injuries of the extracranial carotid arteries, the presence, duration, and severity of any neurologic deficit are additional factors that influence management.

The operative techniques for repair of vascular injuries in the neck are based on the same general principles that apply to vascular procedures elsewhere in the body. Proximal and distal arterial control should be obtained; disrupted or damaged arterial wall should be debrided; and a dependable, hemostatic reconstitution of arterial flow should be assured. With certain limited arterial injuries, resection of the damaged segment and end-to-end anastomosis can be accomplished. However, the arterial anastomosis must not be under any tension, so insertion of an interposition graft is often a more satisfactory approach. Greater saphenous vein is the preferred graft material, although polytetrafluoroethylene grafts may be of equivalent utility in all but the most grossly contaminated wounds.[28,29] A simple arteriorrhaphy or lateral repair may suffice for puncture wounds, but care must be taken to ensure that the arterial lumen is not narrowed. When this type of repair could create a focal stenosis, patch angioplasty with vein, polytetrafluoroethylene, or woven Dacron should be considered.

Venous injury in the neck is most appropriately treated by ligation unless a laceration can be managed by simple lateral venorrhaphy. Bilateral internal jugular vein ligation should be avoided, if at all possible, to avoid the risks of cerebral edema.

Debate continues over the merits of arterial reconstruction versus ligation for damaged cervicothoracic arteries. For the innominate and subclavian arteries, simple ligation will almost always be tolerated if clinical circumstances warrant. The collateral blood supply to the upper extremities is so well-developed that only in unusual circumstances, such as massive crush injury to the fore-quarter or iatrogenic interruption of upper extremity blood supply, is upper extremity viability threatened.[30] Similarly, ligation of the vertebral artery is rarely associated with neurologic sequelae, and operative or even trans-catheter occlusion of the vertebral artery is almost always tolerated.[8,9,29]

Early experience with neurologic deterioration or even death following revascularization for acute traumatic or thrombotic carotid occlusion led to the recommendation of simple proximal arterial ligation for carotid artery trauma.[31,32] However, subsequent clinical experience supports a much larger role for carotid artery reconstruction following injuries to the neck. This has resulted not only from the generally favorable neurologic outcomes following such reconstructions in patients whose preoperative neurologic status was normal, but also from the observation that carotid artery ligation could be associated with postoperative stroke, presumably due to embolization from thrombus distal to the ligature.

CLINICAL OUTCOME

Cohen and coworkers were the first to suggest that the outcome following carotid artery reconstruction for trauma was related to the preoperative neurologic status.[33] While Bradley[32] cautioned that carotid revascularization in the presence of a preoperative neurologic deficit led to deterioration or death in up to one-third of patients, the careful literature review of 233 cases by Liekweg and Greenfield[34] suggested that an improved neurologic outcome is more likely following repair (85 percent) than ligation (50 percent). This study also revealed that extension of cerebral infarction or conversion to a hemorrhagic stroke following revascularization is uncommon. The outcome in patients presenting with carotid injury and coma was poor no matter which operative approach was utilized. A multicenter study reported by Richardson and colleagues arrived at similar conclusions[35]: patients with carotid artery trauma who are neurologically intact preoperatively usually remain so following carotid artery reconstruction; those with recent-onset, mild, or waxing and waning neurologic deficits are generally improved following successful carotid reconstruction; and patients who are comatose preoperatively fare poorly with either ligation or direct repair.

As previously noted, untreated cervical arterial injuries are frequently lethal. Bladergroen and associates showed that, while mortality rates are acceptably low for patients arriving alive at the hospital with major penetrating trauma to the vessels of the neck and upper torso, fully 50 percent of such patients had already died at the trauma scene or during transport to the hospital.[5] Asensio and coworkers reviewed 11 series totaling 1584 carotid artery injuries and found an average mortality rate of 17 percent.[2] In a review of 100 cases of blunt carotid trauma, the mortality rate was 12 percent and the morbidity rate was 46 percent.[7]

Few data are available regarding the long-term outcome of patients who have suffered carotid or vertebral artery trauma. As for arterial injury at other sites, the natural history of arterial reconstruction for cervical arterial trauma remains obscure. While late complications such as thrombosis and pseudoaneurysm formation seem to occur at a relatively low rate, the incomplete long-term follow-up inherent to all populations of trauma victims prevents drawing firm conclusions. Two different populations of patients undergoing elective carotid artery surgery offer some insights on this problem. As discussed in Chap. 27, an elderly atherosclerotic population undergoing successful carotid endarterectomy has a risk of up to 20 percent for developing recurrent carotid stenosis, usually as a consequence of an uncontrolled neointimal hyperplastic response.[36] At the opposite end of the age spectrum are infants who have survived extracorporeal membrane oxygenator support, a technology that generally requires sacrifice of the right common carotid artery. These infants demonstrate a low but disturbing incidence of neurologic dysfunction, which can be reduced substantially by elective carotid artery reconstruction.[37]

SUMMARY

Trauma to the extracranial cerebrovascular vessels has a significant associated mortality risk, although most patients who arrive at the hospital alive and neurologically intact will survive and function normally. Trauma victims with neurologic dysfunction in the setting of carotid artery trauma fare much less well, and those who are comatose do very poorly no matter how they are managed. Penetrating trauma to the neck primarily involves the common carotid artery, while blunt trauma more frequently damages the internal carotid artery. Whether penetrating neck trauma should be routinely or selectively explored remains unclear, and either approach can be accurate, safe, and cost-effective.

While the specific indications for operative management of the damaged carotid artery have changed over time, the current consensus appears to support a liberal operative intervention policy. Most patients should undergo arterial reconstruction when technically feasible, with carotid ligation reserved for the occasional patient with a devastating neurologic injury in whom torrential bleeding must be controlled. Vertebral artery trauma is both less common and of less concern from a clinical perspective, since the majority of such injuries can be successfully ligated or even embolized by angiographic techniques.

REFERENCES

1. Rich N, Spencer FC: Carotid and vertebral artery injuries, in Rich N, Spencer FC (eds): *Vascular Trauma*. Philadelphia, WB Saunders, chap 11, pp 260–286, 1978.
2. Asensio JA, Valenziano CP, Falcone RE, Grosh JD: Management of penetrating neck injuries. *Surg Clin North Am* 71:267, 1991.
3. Richardson JD, Simpson C, Miller FB: Management of carotid artery trauma. *Surgery* 104:673, 1988.
4. Demetriades D, Skalkides J, Sofianos C, et al: Carotid artery injuries: Experience with 124 cases. *J Trauma* 29:91, 1989.
5. Bladergroen M, Brockman R, Luna G, et al: A twelve-year survey of cervicothoracic vascular trauma. *Am J Surg* 157:483, 1989.
6. Flanigan JP, Baraniewski HM, Schuler JJ, Meyer JP: Neck injuries, in Flanigan JP (ed): *Civilian Vascular Trauma*. Philadelphia, Lea & Febiger, chap 13, 1992.
7. Li MS, Smith BM, Espinosa J, et al: Non-penetrating trauma to the carotid artery: Seven cases and a literature review. *J Trauma* 36:265, 1994.
8. Reid JS, Weigelt JA: Forty-three cases of vertebral artery trauma. *J Trauma* 28:1007, 1988.
9. Thomas GI, Anderson KN, Hain RF, et al: The significance of anomalous vertebral-basilar artery communications on operations on the heart and great vessels: An illustrative case with review of the literature. *Surgery* 46:747, 1959.
10. Golueke P, Sclafani S, Phillips T, et al: Vertebral artery injury—diagnosis and management. *J Trauma* 27:856, 1987.
11. Landreneau RJ, Weigelt JA, Megison SM, et al: Combined carotid–vertebral arterial trauma. *Arch Surg* 127:301, 1992.
12. Hankey GJ, Warlow CP, Sellar RJ: Cerebral angiographic risk in mild cerebrovascular disease. *Stroke* 21:209, 1990.
13. Raskind R, North CM: Cerebral artery injuries following chiropractic cervical spine manipulations. *Angiology* 41:445, 1990.
14. McCready RA, Hyde GL, Bivins B, et al: Radiation-induced arterial injuries. *Surgery* 93: 306, 1982.
15. Martin RF, Eldrup-Jorgensen J, Clark D: Blunt trauma to the carotid arteries. *J Vasc Surg* 14:789, 1991.
16. Committee on Trauma, American College of Surgeons: *Advanced Trauma Life Support Instructors Manual*. Chicago, American College of Surgeons, 1992.
17. Roon AJ, Christensen N: Evaluation and treatment of penetrating cervical injuries. *J Trauma* 19:391, 1979.
18. Meier DE, Brink B, Fry WJ: Vertebral arterial trauma: Acute recognition and treatment. *Arch Surg* 116:236, 1981.
19. Meissner M, Paun M, Johansen K: Duplex scanning for arterial trauma. *Am J Surg* 161: 552, 1991.
20. Fisher DF, Claggett JP, Parker JI, et al: Mandibular subluxation for high carotid exposure. *J Vasc Surg* 1:727, 1984.
21. Schwartz JA, Turner D, Sheldon GF, et al: Penetrating trauma of the internal carotid artery at the base of the skull. *J Cardiovasc Surg* 28:542, 1987.
22. Lambert PR, Johns ME, Winn HR: Infralabyrinthine approach to skull-base lesions. *Otolaryngol Head Neck Surg* 93:250, 1985.
23. Gewertz BL, Samson DS, Ditmore QM: Management of penetrating injuries of the internal carotid artery at the base of the skull utilizing extracranial-intracranial bypass. *J Trauma* 20: 365, 1980.
24. Brink BE: Approach to the second segment of the vertebral arteries, in Berguer R, Bauer RB (eds): *Vertebrobasilar Arterial Occlusive Disease*. New York, Raven Press, 1984.

25. Berguer R: Distal vertebral artery bypass: Technique, the 'occipital connection,' and potential uses. *J Vasc Surg* 2:621, 1985.
26. Anthony T, Johansen K: Optimal outcome for "high-risk" carotid endarterectomy. *Am J Surg* 167:469, 1994.
27. Brosnahan D, McFadzean RM, Teasdale E: Neuro-ophthalmic features of carotid-cavernous fistulas and their treatment by endoarterial balloon embolization. *J Neurol Neurosurg Psychiatry* 55:553, 1992.
28. Brown MF, Graham JM, Feliciano DV, et al: Carotid artery injuries. *Am J Surg* 144:748, 1982.
29. Rao PM, Ivatury RR, Sharma P, et al: Cervical vascular injuries: A trauma center experience. *Surgery* 114:527, 1993.
30. Geiss D, Williams WG, Lindsay WK, Rowe RD: Upper extremity gangrene: A complication of subclavian artery division. *Ann Thorac Surg* 30:487, 1978.
31. Wylie EJ, Hein MF, Adams JE: Intracranial hemorrhage following surgical revascularization for treatment of acute stroke. *J Neurosurg* 21:212, 1964.
32. Bradley EL III: Management of penetrating carotid injuries: An alternative approach. *J Trauma* 13:248, 1973.
33. Cohen A, Brief D, Mathewson C: Carotid artery injuries. *Am J Surg* 120:210, 1970.
34. Liekweg WG, Greenfield LJ: Management of penetrating carotid arterial injury. *Ann Surg* 188:587, 1978.
35. Richardson R, Obeid FN, Richardson JD, et al: Cerebrovascular injury: Neurologic consequences. *J Trauma* 42:901, 1991.
36. Das MB, Hertzer NR, Ratliff NB, et al: Recurrent carotid stenosis: A five-year series of 65 operations. *Ann Surg* 202:28, 1985.
37. Crombleholme TM, Adzick NS, de Lorimier AA, et al: Carotid artery reconstruction following extracorporeal membrane oxygenation. *Am J Dis Child* 144:872, 1990.

32

Tumors of the Carotid Body

R. Eugene Zierler

PATHOLOGY
CLINICAL PRESENTATION
DIAGNOSTIC EVALUATION
THERAPEUTIC CONSIDERATIONS
SURGICAL TECHNIQUE
CLINICAL OUTCOME AND PROGNOSIS
CONCLUSIONS

The carotid bodies, oval-shaped nodules of chemoreceptor tissue measuring approximately 3 to 6 mm across, are located on the posteromedial aspect of the distal common carotid artery. Although tumors of the carotid body are uncommon, neoplasia is the only major pathologic process that involves these structures. The carotid body develops in the adventitia of the vessel, and its blood supply is derived predominantly from the external carotid artery.[1] Embryologically, the carotid bodies appear to originate from neural crest cells that migrate in close association with the autonomic ganglion cells. Similar clusters of chemoreceptor cells are also found in the aortic bodies, the jugular body, and the ganglion nodosum of the vagus nerve (Fig. 32-1).

It is important to distinguish between the carotid body and the carotid sinus. While these structures are closely related anatomically, the carotid sinus is strictly a pressure receptor which responds to increases in blood pressure by slowing the heart rate. The carotid bodies respond to chemical changes in the blood, specifically those resulting from hypoxia. Thus, a fall in O_2 tension, a rise in CO_2 tension, or a decrease in pH, produce an in-

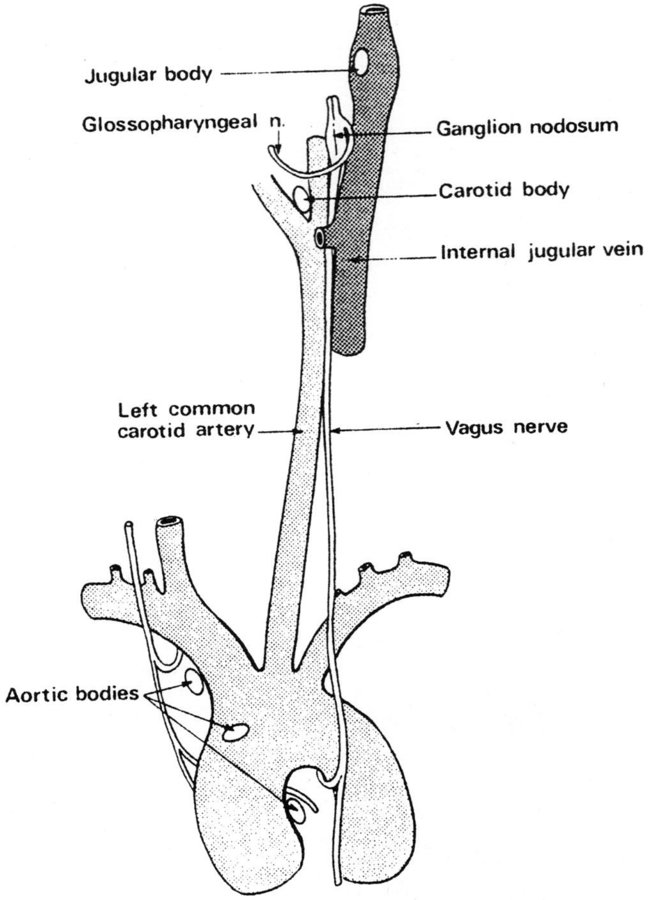

Figure 32-1. Locations of chemoreceptor tissue. (*From Krupski et al.*[24] *Reproduced by permission.*)

crease in cardiac rate and the depth and rate of respiration.

Their infrequent occurrence and varying biologic behavior have given rise to a variety of terms for tumors of the carotid body. The lesions have been called glomus tumors, paragangliomas, nonchromaffin paragangliomas, and chemodectomas. Based on their cells of origin and the observation that the carotid body is the most common site for extraadrenal paraganglionic tumors, "paraganglioma" appears to be a correct name for these lesions. "Nonchromaffin" is also appropriate, since the cells of these tumors do not react with dichromate salts. The term "chemodectoma" reflects the fact that the tumors originate from chemoreceptor tissue.[2]

PATHOLOGY

The pathologic processes involving the carotid body include both hypertrophy and neoplasia. Physiologic hypertrophy of the carotid body is associated with chronic hypoxia and has been observed in individuals living at high altitudes, patients with cyanotic heart disease, and patients with chronic obstructive lung disease.[3–7] While carotid body tumors have been reported in patients who have been subject to chronic hypoxic stimulation, most of these lesions have no identifiable predisposing factors.

Carotid body tumors occasionally are familial, with autosomal dominant genetic transmission.[8,9] Familial carotid body tumors are more frequently bilateral than are the nonfamilial type, with bilateral involvement in about 35 percent of familial tumors and in 5 percent of nonfamilial cases. There does not appear to be any significant difference in gender distribution or mean age at diagnosis for familial and nonfamilial tumors. However, familial carotid body tumors are more likely to be associated with other paraganglionic tumors, including pheochromocytomas.[10–12] Thus, some carotid body tumors may be considered as part of a combined syndrome of multiple paragangliomas.

Carotid body tumors appear grossly as round encapsulated masses of firm tan-gray tissue. As the carotid body enlarges, it extends superiorly above the common carotid bifurcation and fills the space between the internal and external carotid arteries, producing a characteristic widening of the bifurcation (Figs. 32-2 and 32-3). These lesions typically do not penetrate the arterial media. Occasionally, carotid body tumors infiltrate the surrounding structures, but invasive characteristics usually are found only in recurrent lesions.[13]

Microscopically, carotid body tumors contain clusters of cells called *Zelballen* (cell balls) surrounded by an abundant capillary network that renders the lesion extremely vascular (Fig. 32-4). Two cell types are present: a

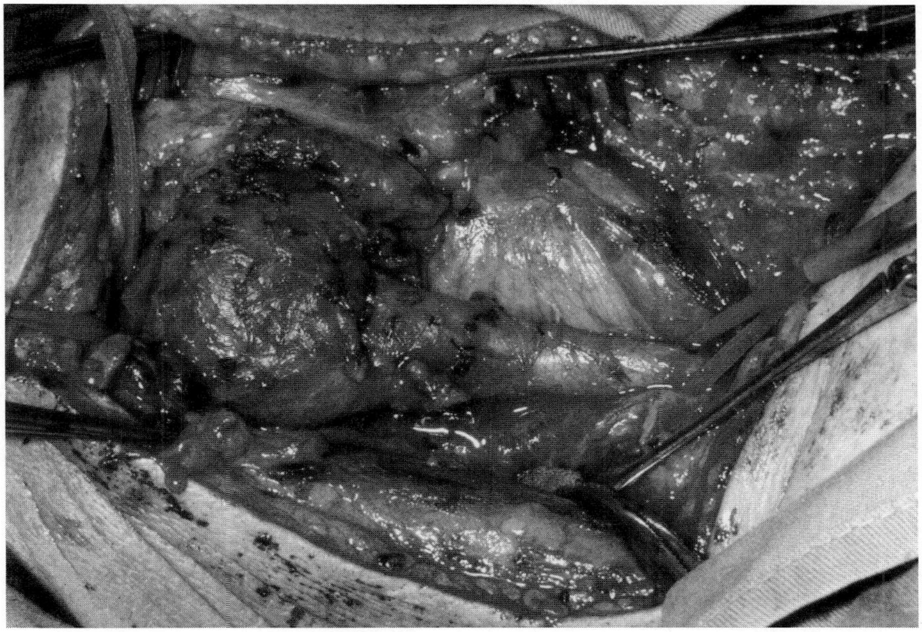

Figure 32-2. Operative photograph of a carotid body tumor after exposure but before resection. The common carotid artery is to the right, the internal carotid artery lies below and to the left, and the external carotid is largely covered by the tumor. All three arteries are controlled with umbilical tapes. The tumor mass occupies the space between the internal and external carotid arteries.

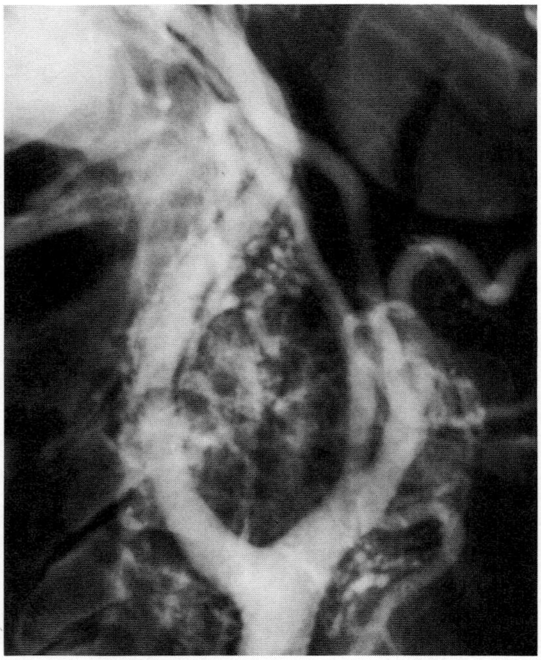

A

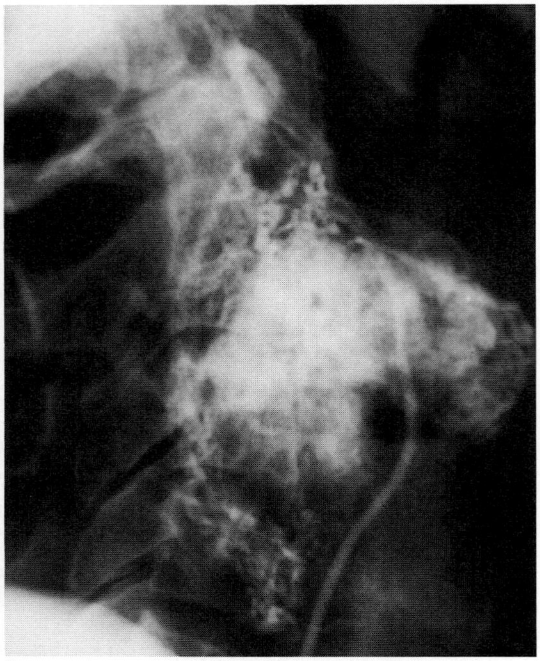

B

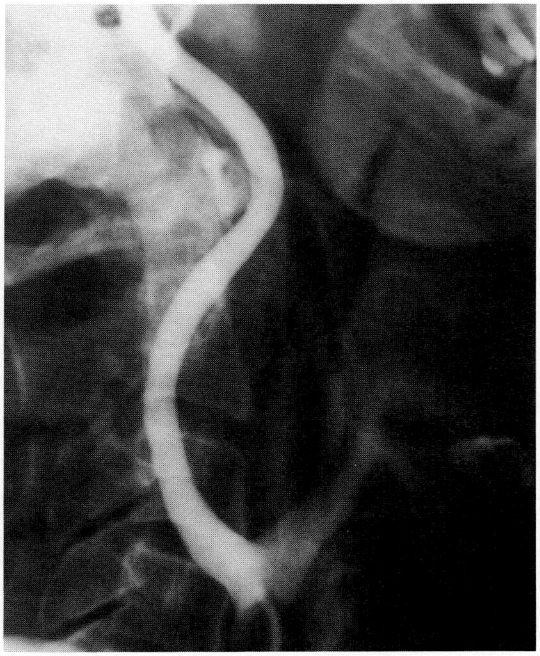

C

Figure 32-3. Carotid arteriogram in a patient with a carotid body tumor. *A.* Common carotid injection showing the internal and external carotid arteries splayed apart by the tumor mass. *B.* External carotid injection with tumor blush, indicating the extreme vascularity of the lesion. *C.* Selective injection of the internal carotid artery, showing that the blood supply to the tumor originates from the external carotid.

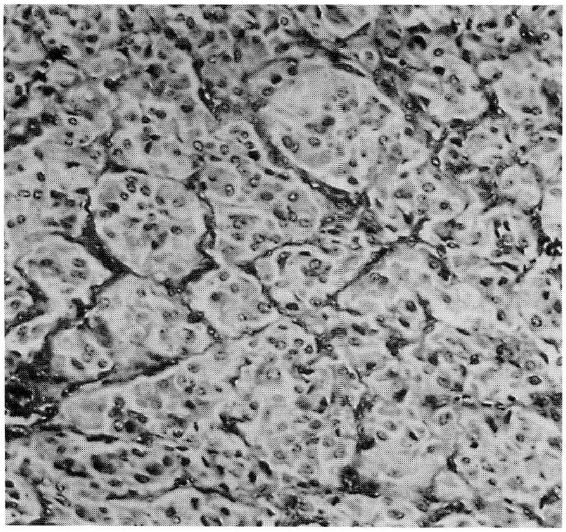

Figure 32-4. Photomicrograph of a carotid body tumor. Reticulin stain demonstrates the typical Zelballen (cell balls) which create a glandular pattern. (Magnification × 140.)

sustenacular or supporting cell and an epithelioid or chief cell. Neurosecretory granules, a distinctive feature of cells derived from the neural crest, are found in the chief cells. Although cytochemical techniques have shown that chief cells contain epinephrine, norepinephrine, and serotonin, functioning carotid body tumors that produce hypertension are exceedingly rare.[14–16] In contrast, retroperitoneal paragangliomas often secrete catecholamines and are associated with hypertension.[17]

There has been considerable controversy over the malignant potential of carotid body tumors, and the reported prevalence of malignancy ranges from 2 to 30 percent.[18–20] This variation can be attributed in part to differences in the extent of patient follow-up and the lack of any accepted histologic criteria for malignancy. In particular, the presence of nuclear pleomorphism or mitotic activity in the cells of a carotid body tumor does not correlate with metastatic behavior, and metastases may not become apparent for many years after the initial diagnosis.[14,19,21] Since the malignant potential of carotid body tumors cannot be predicted from their histologic features, this determination can be made only by the presence of lymph node or distant metastatic spread.

The large majority of carotid body tumors grow slowly and exhibit benign characteristics. While some patients may survive for protracted periods without surgical treatment, these tumors can cause significant disability and death, even in the absence of malignancy. It is important to distinguish between true malignant behavior and the occurrence of multiple tumors, especially in familial cases. Although local tumor invasion does not satisfy the strict criteria for malignancy, the ultimate effect on the patient can be just as serious. Deaths due to asphyxia and intracranial extension of carotid body tumors have been reported.[18,22,23] Local recurrence following surgical resection also has been described, even after prolonged disease-free intervals.[18,22] In general, the size of a carotid body tumor and the severity of symptoms at the time of diagnosis appear to be the best predictors of future biologic behavior.[24]

CLINICAL PRESENTATION

Because carotid body tumors are extremely rare, it is impossible to define a true incidence. They appear to occur with equal frequency in both sexes. Although these tumors have been reported in patients ranging in age from the teens to the eighth decade, the typical age at the time of initial diagnosis is in the fifth decade. Bilateral carotid body tumors and multiple paragangliomas are most likely to represent familial cases. Marked hypertension or elevated serum catecholamine levels suggest the presence of additional paragangliomas, particularly pheochromocytomas.

The most common clinical presentation of a carotid body tumor is with a painless mass in the location of the common carotid bifurcation adjacent to the angle of the mandible. When present, symptoms are generally nonspecific, and may include neck or ear pain, local tenderness, dysphagia, hoarseness, or tinnitus. A history of slow enlargement is typical, and many years may elapse between initial recognition of the mass and surgical treatment.[19,24] Cranial nerve dysfunction is rare with unoperated carotid body tumors, but involvement of the vagus, hypoglossal, and cervical sympathetic nerves has been reported.[25,26]

The most important finding on physical examination is a firm, rubbery lateral cervical mass. Because of its attachment to the carotid bifurcation, a carotid body tumor tends to be more mobile in the horizontal than the vertical direction. It also may appear to be pulsatile, owing to its close relationship to the carotid artery. A bruit in the area of the mass most likely represents underlying arterial occlusive disease. Since carotid body tumors are relatively uncommon, other causes of neck masses must always be considered. The differential diagnosis includes branchial cleft cysts, lymphomas, thyroid lesions, metastatic tumors, and carotid artery aneurysms.

DIAGNOSTIC EVALUATION

The clinical presentation of a slowly enlarging mass in the neck at the level of the carotid bifurcation should raise the suspicion of a carotid body tumor and lead to a prompt diagnostic evaluation. Because of the extreme vascularity of these tumors and their close relationship to the carotid vessels, percutaneous needle aspiration or incisional biopsy is strongly contraindicated. These procedures have resulted in such complications as massive hemorrhage, pseudoaneurysm formation, and carotid thrombosis.[22,25,27] Routine screening for elevated serum catecholamines is unwarranted, since most carotid body tumors are nonfunctional. However, in the presence of severe hypertension or other symptoms suggestive of a functioning paraganglionic tumor, appropriate studies should be obtained.

Noninvasive evaluation by duplex scanning with color-flow imaging (Chap. 11) is useful for documenting the presence of a highly vascular mass in the area of the carotid bifurcation.[28–30] The characteristic ultrasound feature of a carotid body tumor is a soft tissue mass that separates the internal and external carotid arteries and widens the carotid bifurcation. The vascularity of these tumors is readily demonstrated by color-flow imaging, a finding that helps differentiate them from such relatively nonvascular masses as lymph node metastases, salivary gland tumors, and branchial cleft cysts.[30] Duplex scanning also can provide information on the dimensions of the tumor and can indicate whether there is any concurrent arterial occlusive disease. However, it is difficult to identify the specific origin of the blood supply to carotid body tumors by duplex scanning, and arteriography is required to provide additional anatomic detail. Although the clinical role of the indirect noninvasive tests for carotid artery disease is limited (Chap. 10), the oculopneumoplethysmograph may be useful for evaluating the cerebral collateral circulation and the ability of a patient to tolerate carotid artery occlusion.[31]

Computed tomography (CT) can be useful for the general evaluation of neck masses. Rapid bolus infusion of intravenous contrast may help to identify carotid body tumors, although they can be difficult to distinguish from carotid artery aneurysms by this technique.[32] While the reported experience with magnetic resonance imaging (MRI) of carotid body tumors is limited, this approach may be superior to CT scanning for demonstrating the relationship of the tumor to adjacent structures.[33,34] The highly vascular nature of carotid body tumors produces a characteristic appearance on

MRI that readily differentiates them from the other soft tissue lesions involving the neck and skull base.[33]

Conventional contrast arteriography with selective arterial injections is the definitive diagnostic test for carotid body tumors.[22,24–26,35] The typical arteriographic findings include an early tumor blush at the carotid bifurcation, with splaying of the proximal internal and external carotid arteries (Fig. 32-3). Arteriography also can delineate the blood supply to the tumor and coexisting atherosclerotic lesions or extrinsic compression of the carotid artery. This information is essential for planning surgical treatment. The blood supply of carotid body tumors characteristically originates from the external carotid artery (Fig. 32-3); however, contributions also can arise from the internal carotid, vertebral, and thyrocervical arteries.[35,36]

THERAPEUTIC CONSIDERATIONS

Because their malignant potential is unpredictable and local extension can occur even in the absence of true malignancy, all carotid body tumors should be considered for surgical resection. The natural history of these tumors is one of progressive enlargement, with eventual erosion of the skull base and involvement of the surrounding structures, including pharynx, muscles, and cranial nerves. Although radiotherapy generally has been considered inadequate as primary treatment of carotid body tumors, some satisfactory results have been reported for local control of residual or recurrent disease.[37,38] However, the use of radiotherapy prior to surgery makes operative treatment more difficult. Chemotherapy does not appear to be of any value.

Carotid body tumors have been classified according to their size and local extent into three groups.[19] Group I tumors are small and readily separated from the surrounding structures. Group II lesions are more adherent to the adjacent vessels, and sacrifice of the external carotid may be necessary during resection. Group III tumors are large and densely adherent to the carotid vessels. Removal of Group III tumors usually requires reconstruction of the internal carotid artery with an autogenous vein graft. Unfortunately, most carotid body tumors are in Groups II and III at the time of clinical presentation.[24] The results of partial resection are poor, but postoperative radiotherapy may be beneficial in cases where total resection is technically impossible.[26,37,38] Selective arteriographic embolization of carotid body tumors has been reported to decrease subsequent operative blood loss and technical difficulties.[39–41] While this is clearly a useful preoperative measure, cerebral embolization is a potential complication.

SURGICAL TECHNIQUE

The first surgical resection of a carotid body tumor was performed in 1880; however, the procedure included carotid ligation, and the patient developed hemiplegia and died three days after the operation.[42] Tumor resection with survival was described in 1886.[42] In 1947, a mortality rate of 33 percent and a stroke rate of 50 percent were reported in patients requiring carotid ligation during tumor excision.[43] Based on the dismal results of resection with carotid ligation, aggressive surgical treatment of carotid body tumors could not be advocated until techniques for reconstructing the carotid vessels were available.[44] Continued improvements in vascular surgical techniques, cerebral protection during carotid surgery, and critical care now make resection the treatment of choice for carotid body tumors.

The anatomic and technical aspects of surgery for carotid body tumors are similar to those for carotid endarterectomy (Chaps. 2 and 23). Tumor resection usually is associated with considerably more blood loss than carotid endarterectomy, so at least four units of blood should be available. Use of an autotransfusion system can reduce the requirements for banked blood. Resection of extremely large tumors may require exposure of the carotid artery at the base of the skull or carotid ligation. In these cases, evaluation of the cerebral collateral circulation may be useful in predicting which patients are likely to tolerate carotid occlusion.[31] Preoperative planning with an oral surgeon or otolaryngologist allows expeditious subluxation of the temporomandibular joint to facilitate distal carotid exposure. One or both legs should be prepared for harvesting of saphenous vein. If the suitability of the saphenous vein is uncertain, vein mapping by duplex scanning should be performed preoperatively. In the rare patient with a functioning tumor, alpha- and beta-adrenergic blockade is required.

General endotracheal anesthesia is used routinely, and in cases where the need for temporomandibular subluxation is anticipated, nasotracheal intubation is preferred. Patient positioning is identical to that for a carotid endarterectomy, with a roll between the scapulae, the neck extended, and the head turned away from the side of the tumor. An incision along the anterior border of the sternomastoid muscle and curving behind the ear gives optimal exposure of the carotid vessels. After proximal control of the common carotid artery is achieved, the internal and external carotid arteries distal to the tumor are mobilized. Control of the external carotid may be particularly difficult, since the blood supply to the tumor characteristically originates from this vessel. Preoperative tumor embolization decreases blood loss during this stage of the operation. In some cases, early ligation and division of the external carotid artery also reduces blood loss and facilitates further dissection of the tumor (Fig. 32-5).[24] If the distal internal carotid is inaccessible, arterial reconstruction is impossible, and tumor resection requires sacrifice of the internal carotid artery. Whether this extreme measure is warranted will depend on the extent of the tumor elsewhere in the neck and the assessment of the cerebral collateral circulation.

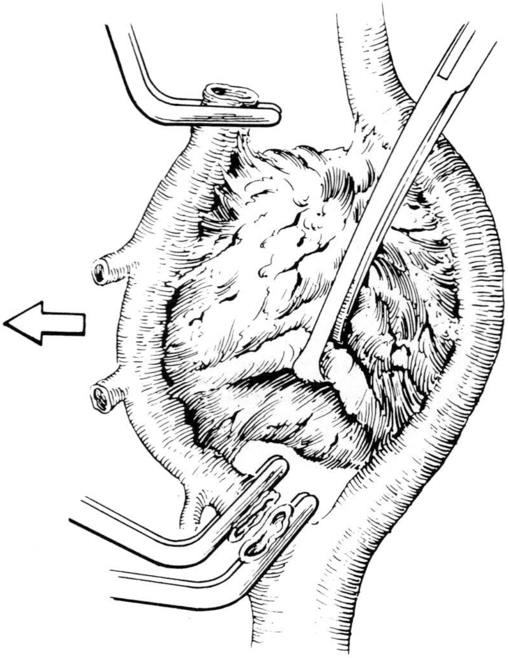

Figure 32-5. Operative technique of carotid body tumor resection. The blood supply to the tumor is controlled by dividing the external carotid artery, and this vessel is then removed with the tumor. (*From Krupski et al.*[24] *Reproduced by permission.*)

Prior to separating the tumor from the vessels, the carotid bifurcation and tumor mass are mobilized circumferentially to assess the local extent of disease. During this dissection, the hypoglossal and vagus nerves must be identified and protected. The tumor is resected by developing a relatively avascular plane between the tumor and the common carotid artery and proceeding distally up the internal carotid. Although this plane is traditionally described as "subadventitial," it actually involves the most superficial adventitial layers.[45] Group I tumors are easily removed with this technique. With Group II and III lesions, the internal carotid is partly or totally surrounded by the tumor, and a longitudinal incision through the tumor is required to develop the proper dissection plane. If this plane cannot be continued along the internal carotid, invasion of the arterial wall must be suspected, and carotid resection is necessary.

In this situation, a segment of greater saphenous vein is harvested from the thigh and prepared for use as a reversed interposition graft. The need for temporary shunting is assessed in the same manner as for carotid endarterectomy. An internal carotid stump pressure of 50 mmHg or more is generally considered adequate for proceeding without a shunt. When the stump pressure is low, a straight shunt is placed through the lumen of the vein graft. After systemic heparinization, vascular clamps are applied, and the tumor is removed along with the adherent portions of the internal, external, and common carotid arteries. If shunting is necessary, the shunt tubing is inserted into the transected ends of the internal and common carotid arteries, taking care to remove all air prior to allowing antegrade flow. The shunt tubing can be held in place with vessel loops or shunt clamps. The distal internal carotid artery and appropriate end of the vein graft are spatulated, and an end-to-end anastomosis is carried out using 6-0 or 7-0 monofilament suture. The anastomosis between the common carotid artery and the vein graft is done in a similar fashion with 5-0 or 6-0 suture. Prior to completion of the proximal anastomosis, the shunt is rapidly removed and the graft flushed to eliminate all air and debris.

Reconstruction of the external carotid artery following tumor removal is not necessary, and the external carotid stump is oversewn. If heparin has been given for vascular grafting, it should be reversed at the conclusion of the procedure to avoid postoperative hematoma formation. Drains are generally not needed, but may be beneficial if there is residual dead space after resection of large tumors.

CLINICAL OUTCOME AND PROGNOSIS

Cranial nerve injuries are more common after resection of carotid body tumors than following carotid endarterectomy. This is probably related to the more extensive dissection required for tumor removal. The most frequently involved nerves are the hypoglossal and vagus, but damage to the accessory, facial, and cervical sysmpathetic nerves also has been reported.[24,25,39,46] The overall rate of cranial nerve dysfunction after surgery for carotid body tumors is in the range of 40 percent, and the risk for such complications is significantly higher for larger tumors.[46] In contrast, the stroke and death rates following resection of carotid body tumors since the advent of vascular reconstruction have been extremely low and are similar to those associated with carotid endarterectomy.

Complete surgical removal of carotid body tumors, when technically possible, is generally curative. However, since the natural history and malignant potential of these tumors is quite variable, periodic clinical observation is indicated to detect multicentric or recurrent disease. Examination of the patient's relatives is advisable in suspected familial cases. Metastases may appear many years after primary treatment, and patients can survive for prolonged periods with evidence of metastatic disease.[20] Patients with interposition vein grafts can be followed with duplex scanning to identify any problems with the arterial reconstruction.

CONCLUSIONS

While an individual vascular surgeon can expect to encounter only a small number of carotid body tumors, these lesions are readily identified if the diagnosis is suspected. Noninvasive tests are valuable for screening, but arteriography is still required for definitive diagnosis and planning of operative therapy. Biopsy is hazardous and unnecessary when the characteristic features are present.

In most patients, surgical removal prevents both progressive local enlargement and development of metastatic lesions. Resection usually can be done without sacrifice of the common or internal carotid; however, when necessary, standard vascular surgical techniques are used to reconstruct the internal carotid artery. Since the perioperative complication rate is acceptably low and the prognosis following surgical treatment is favorable, resection should be offered to all but the most elderly and debilitated patients with carotid body tumors.

REFERENCES

1. Boyd JH: The development of the human carotid body. *Contrib Embryo* 26:1–31, 1937.
2. Mulligan RM: Chemodectoma in the dog. *Am J Pathol* 26:680–681, 1950.
3. Heath D, Edwards C, Harris P: Postmortem size and structure of the human carotid body. *Thorax* 25:129–140, 1970.
4. Edwards C, Heath D, Harris P: The carotid body in emphysema and left ventricular hypertrophy. *J Pathol* 104:1–13, 1971.
5. Hirsh JM, Killien FC, Troupin RH: Bilateral carotid body tumors and cyanotic heart disease. *Am J Radiol* 134:1073–1075, 1980.
6. Saldana MJ, Salem LE, Travezan R: High altitude hypoxia and chemodectomas. *Hum Pathol* 4:251–263, 1973.
7. Nissenblatt MJ: Cyanotic heart disease: Low altitude risk for carotid body tumor? *Johns Hopkins Med J* 142:18–21, 1978.
8. Parry DM, Li FP, Strong LC, et al: Carotid body tumors in humans: Genetics and epidemiology. *J Natl Cancer Inst* 68:573–578, 1982.
9. Grufferman S, Gillman AB, Pasternak R, et al: Familial carotid body tumors: Case report and epidemiologic review. *Cancer* 46:2116–2122, 1980.
10. Pritchett JW: Familial concurrence of carotid body tumor and pheochromocytoma. *Cancer* 49:2578–2579, 1982.
11. Jensen JC, Choyke PL, Rosenfeld M, et al: A report of familial carotid body tumors and multiple extra-adrenal pheochromocytomas. *J Urol* 145:1040–1042, 1991.
12. Sobol SM, Dailey JC: Familial multiple cervical paragangliomas: A report of a kindred and review of the literature. *Otolaryngol Head Neck Surg* 102:382–390, 1990.
13. Merino MJ, Livolsi VA: Malignant carotid body tumors: Report of two cases and review of the literature. *Cancer* 47:1403–1414, 1981.
14. Grimley PM, Glenner GG: Histology and ultrastructure of carotid body paragangliomas; comparison with the normal gland. *Cancer* 20:1473–1488, 1967.
15. Fries JC, Chamberlin JA: Extra-adrenal pheochromocytoma: Literature review and report of a cervical pheochromocytoma. *Surgery* 63:268–279, 1968.
16. Levit SA, Sheps SG, Espinosa RE, et al: Catecholamine secreting paraganglioma of glomus-jugular rgion. *N Engl J Med* 281:805–811, 1969.
17. Brantigan CO, Katase RY: Clinical and pathologic features of paragangliomas of the organ of Zuckerkandl. *Surgery* 65:898–902, 1969.
18. Martin CE, Rosenfeld L, McSwainB: Carotid body tumors: A 16 year follow-up of seven malignant cases. *South Med J* 66:1236–1243, 1973.
19. Shamblin WR, ReMine WH, Sheps SG, et al: Carotid body tumor (chemodectoma): clinicopathologic analysis of ninety cases. *Am J Surg* 122:732–739, 1971.
20. Gaylis H, Mieny CJ: Incidence of malignancy in carotid body tumors. *Br J Surg* 64:885–889, 1977.
21. Staats EF, Brown RL, Smith RR: Carotid body tumors, benign and malignant. *Laryngoscope* 76:907–916, 1966.
22. Dent TL, Thompson NW, Fry WJ: Carotid body tumors. *Surgery* 80:365–372, 1976.
23. Monro RS: Natural history of carotid body tumors and their diagnosis and treatment. *Br J Surg* 37:445–453, 1950.
24. Krupski WC, Effeney DJ, Ehrenfeld WK, et al: Cervical chemodectoma: Technical consider-

ations and management options. *Am J Surg* 144:215–220, 1982.
25. Padberg FT Jr, Cady B, Persson AV: Carotid body tumor. *Am J Surg* 145:526–528, 1983.
26. Farr HW: Carotid body tumors—a 40 year study. *CA* 30:260–265, 1980.
27. Engzell U, Franzen S, Zajicek J: Aspiration biopsy of tumors of the neck. II Cytologic findings in 13 cases of carotid body tumor. *Acta Cytol* 15:25–30, 1971.
28. Worsey MJ, Laborde AL, Bower T, et al: An evaluation of color duplex scanning in the primary diagnosis and management of carotid body tumors. *Ann Vasc Surg* 6:90–94, 1992.
29. Steinke W, Hennerici M, Aulich A: Doppler color-flow imaging of carotid body tumors. *Stroke* 20:1574–1577, 1989.
30. Gritzmann N, Herold C, Haller J, et al: Duplex sonography for tumors of the carotid body. *Cardiovasc Intervent Radiol* 10:280–284, 1987.
31. Gee W, Mehigan JT, Wylie EJ: Measurement of collateral cerebral hemispheric blood pressure by ocular pneumoplethysmography. *Am J Surg* 130:121–127, 1975.
32. Shugar MA, Mafee MF: Diagnosis of carotid body tumors by dynamic computerized tomography. *Head Neck Surg* 4:518–521, 1982.
33. Olsen WL, Dillon WP, Kelly WM, et al: MR imaging of paragangliomas. *Am J Roentgenol* 148:201–204, 1987.
34. Vogl T, Bruning R, Schedel H, et al: Paragangliomas of the jugular bulb and carotid body: MR imaging with short sequences and Gd-DTPA enhancement. *Am Roentgenol* 153:583–587, 1989.
35. Rosen IB, Palmer JA, Goldberg M, et al: Vascular problems associated with carotid body tumors. *Am J Surg* 142:459–463, 1981.
36. Chambers RG, Mahoney WD: Carotid body tumors. *Am J Surg* 116:548–554, 1968.
37. Schild SE, Foote RL, Buskirk S, et al: Results of radiotherapy for chemodecetomas. *Mayo Clin Proc* 67:537–540, 1992.
38. Valdagni R, Amichetti M: Radiation therapy of carotid body tumors. *Am J Clin Oncol* 13:45–48, 1990.
39. LaMuraglia GM, Fabian RL, Brewster DC, et al: The current surgical management of carotid body paragangliomas. *J Vasc Surg* 15:1038–1044, 1992.
40. Robison JG, Shagets FW, Beckett WC Jr, et al: A multidisciplinary approach to reducing morbidity and operative blood loss during resection of carotid body tumor. *Surg Gynecol Obstet* 168:166–170, 1989.
41. Smith RF, Shetty PC, Reddy DJ: Surgical treatment of carotid paragangliomas presenting unusual technical difficulties. The value of preoperative embolization. *J Vasc Surg* 7:631–637, 1988.
42. Gratiot JM: Carotid body tumors: Collective review. *Surg Gynecol Obstet* 77:177–186, 1943.
43. Lahey FH, Warren KM: Tumors of the carotid body. *Surg Gynecol Obstet* 85:281–288, 1947.
44. Eastcott HHG, Pickering GW, Rob CG: Reconstruction of internal carotid artery in a patient with intermittent attacks of hemiplegia. *Lancet* 2:994–996, 1954.
45. Gordon-Taylor G: On carotid body tumors. *Br J Surg* 28:163, 1940.
46. Hallett JW, Nora JD, Hollier LH, et al: Trends in neurovascular complications of surgical management for carotid body and cervical paragangliomas: A fifty year experience with 153 tumors. *J Vasc Surg* 7:284–291, 1988.

Index

The letter *t* following a page number indicates that a table is being referenced; a page number in *italic* indicates that a figure is being referenced.

ISBN 0-07-072792-9

90000>

9 780070 727922